# Medical Back Office Procedure

Blesi | Wise | Kelley-Arney | Brasin | Favreau

CENGAGE Learning

Australia • Brazil • Japan • Korea • Mexico • Singapore • Spain • United Kingdom • United States

CENGAGE Learning

**Medical Back Office Procedure**

Senior Project Development Manager:
Linda deStefano

Market Development Manager:
Heather Kramer

Senior Production/Manufacturing Manager:
Donna M. Brown

Production Editorial Manager:
Kim Fry

Sr. Rights Acquisition Account Manager:
Todd Osborne

Printed in the United States of America



For product information and technology assistance, contact us at
**Cengage Learning Customer & Sales Support, 1-800-354-9706**
For permission to use material from this text or product,
submit all requests online at **cengage.com/permissions**
Further permissions questions can be emailed to
**permissionrequest@cengage.com**

This book contains select works from existing Cengage Learning resources and was produced by Cengage Learning Custom Solutions for collegiate use. As such, those adopting and/or contributing to this work are responsible for editorial content accuracy, continuity and completeness.



ISBN-13: 978-1-285-91983-6

ISBN-10: 1-285-91983-1

**Cengage Learning**
5191 Natorp Boulevard
Mason, Ohio 45040
USA

Cengage Learning is a leading provider of customized learning solutions with office locations around the globe, including Singapore, the United Kingdom, Australia, Mexico, Brazil, and Japan. Locate your local office at: **international.cengage.com/region.**

Cengage Learning products are represented in Canada by Nelson Education, Ltd.

For your lifelong learning solutions, visit **www.cengage.com/custom.**

Visit our corporate website at **www.cengage.com.**

# Brief Contents


| | | |
|---|---|---|
| Chapter 1 | *Infection Control and Medical Asepsis* | 1 |
| Chapter 1 Workbook | *Infection Control and Medical Asepsis* | 39 |
| Chapter 2 | *The Medical History and Patient Screening* | 41 |
| Chapter 2 Workbook | *The Medical History and Patient Screening* | 57 |
| Chapter 3 | *Body Measurements and Vital Signs* | 58 |
| Chapter 3 Workbook | *Vital Signs and Measurements* | 97 |
| Chapter 4 | *Preparing for Examinations* | 98 |
| Chapter 4 Workbook | *Preparing for Examinations* | 115 |
| Chapter 5 | *The Physical Exam, Specialty Exams, and Procedures* | 118 |
| Chapter 5 Workbook | *The Physical Exam, Specialty Exams, and Procedures* | 159 |
| Module 5 | *Working in the Patient Electronic Medical Record* | 161 |
| Module 7 | *Recording Therapeutic Injections and Immunizations* | 177 |
| Chapter 6 | *OB/GYN Examinations* | 185 |
| Chapter 6 Workbook | *OB/GYN Examinations* | 203 |
| Chapter 7 | *Pediatric Examinations* | 204 |
| Chapter 7 Workbook | *Pediatric Examinations* | 233 |
| Chapter 8 | *Preparing for Surgery* | 234 |
| Chapter 8 Workbook | *Preparing for Surgery* | 255 |

| | | |
|---|---|---|
| Chapter 9 | ***Assisting with Minor Surgery*** | 256 |
| Chapter 9 Workbook | ***Assisting with Minor Surgery*** | 271 |
| Chapter 10 | ***Emergencies in the Medical Office*** | 272 |
| Chapter 10 Workbook | ***Emergencies in the Medical Office*** | 295 |
| Chapter 11 | ***First Aid for Accidents and Injuries*** | 298 |
| Chapter 11 Workbook | ***First Aid for Accidents and Injuries*** | 321 |
| Appendix A | ***Measurements and Abbreviations*** | A-1 |
| Glossary | | G-1 |

Chapter 1

# Infection Control and Medical Asepsis

## OBJECTIVES

In this chapter, you will learn the following:

### KB KNOWLEDGE BASE

1. Spell and define, using the glossary in the back of the text, all the Words to Know in this chapter.
2. Locate and interpret from the communicable disease chart the means of transmission, incubation time, symptoms, and treatment for a given disease.
3. Describe the infection control cycle and chain of infection links, giving an example of how to break each link.
4. Name five common infectious agents and give an example of each.
5. Explain what direct and indirect contact is.
6. List the five steps in the infectious disease process and give an explanation of each.
7. List the growth requirements of microorganisms and methods of controlling their growth.
8. Explain how used needles, lancets, capillary tubes, glass slides, and other sharp instruments are to be handled.
9. Describe the recommended universal and standard precautions to be taken when you are exposed to human tissue, blood, and body fluids and explain why it is important to follow these precautions.
10. Explain the process for disposal of biohazardous material.
11. List the habits a medical assistant should practice to reduce and prevent disease transmission, including patient education suggestions.
12. Describe the body's defense mechanisms against disease.
13. Define medical asepsis.
14. Explain the importance of proper hand washing and the purpose of wearing gloves and other personal protective equipment (PPE).
15. Explain the preventive measures for health care professionals to protect against the hepatitis B virus.
16. Explain the difference between sanitization, disinfection, and sterilization and the purpose of each.
17. Explain the function of the autoclave and the steps and safety precautions to follow when using the autoclave.
18. Explain the purpose of using sterilization and biological indicators for autoclaving.

### S SKILLS

1. Demonstrate the proper procedure for completing an incident exposure report form.
2. Demonstrate proper hand washing.
3. Demonstrate proper removal of non-sterile gloves.
4. Demonstrate application and removal of appropriate personal protective equipment (PPE) when working in potentially infectious situations.
5. Demonstrate sanitization procedures.
6. Demonstrate disinfection procedures.
7. Demonstrate the proper procedure for preparing and wrapping instruments to be autoclaved.
8. Demonstrate the proper procedure for sterilization of instruments by use of an autoclave.

## WORDS TO KNOW

aerobe
airborne
anaerobes
asepsis
autoclave
bacteria
biohazardous
bloodborne
Clinical Laboratory Improvement Amendments (CLIA)
coma
communicable
disinfection
droplet infection
exudative
fecal
flora
fomite
fungi
hygiene
incineration
incubation
invasive
malaise
microorganism
morphology
nits
obligate
Occupational Safety and Health Administration (OSHA)
parasites
pathogens
personal protective equipment (PPE)
petechial
pH
protozoa
pruritic
pustular
rickettsiae
resuscitation
sanitization
seizures
serrations
shelf life
spores
Standard Precautions
sterilization
susceptible
vector
vigilant
virulence
viruses
vulnerable

## THE INFECTION CYCLE AND DISEASE TRANSMISSION

Infection control is an ongoing aspect of health care for both the patient and the health care provider that is of the utmost importance. As a medical assistant, always be mindful of the necessity of **asepsis** (a state of being free from all pathogenic **microorganisms**) when performing clinical procedures. Although maintaining a completely sterile environment throughout an entire medical facility might not be realistic, the facility must be clean and safe for all who enter.

Table 36–1 lists **communicable** diseases and their means of transmission, **incubation** time, symptoms, and treatment. Becoming familiar with this information will help you serve patients better. Incubation time refers to the time between the initial exposure to the disease-causing microbes and the appearance of the first symptoms or signs of the disease. If a person is **susceptible** to a disease, that person is receptive, or **vulnerable**, to catching it. Generally, the susceptible person is weakened because of a preexisting illness or condition, is overall run down and worn out, or has poor **hygiene** and health habits.

Microorganisms that are the cause of disease are called **pathogens**. They have certain requirements for growth and multiplication. If steps are taken to interrupt and prevent their growth, disease transmission can be reduced. A microorganism's power to produce a disease is know as **virulence**.

It is important to note that not all microorganisms are pathogenic. Some microorganisms are helpful and necessary to normal **flora** in humans and animals because they provide a balance in the body and destroy pathogens. Normal flora is the cohabitation of microorganisms (nonpathogenic and pathogenic in balance) that live in or within an organism to provide a natural immunity against certain infections. Infection occurs when this balance is disturbed.

In the effort to prevent disease transmission, it is helpful to have an idea of what you are trying to prevent. All living organisms have requirements to sustain life and facilitate growth and development. These requirements are:

- *Oxygen*. Microorganisms that need oxygen to grow are called **aerobes**, and those that grow best in the absence of oxygen are called **anaerobes**.
- *pH*. The body has a 6.0 average **pH**, which is an acidic level high enough to protect the body from microorganism invasion. If the pH level is higher, it indicates that microbial growth is present. As bacteria grow and multiply, the pH level becomes higher in alkalinity. A low pH reading, one less than 6, can be the result of ketosis or of not eating for a long period. An environment that is too acidic will not support microbial growth.
- *Temperature (98.6°F)*. Microorganisms grow best at the average body temperature (37°C or 98.6°F ). The human body has not only a desirable temperature for microbial growth but also darkness and moisture, other growth requirements.
- *Nutrients*.
- *Water*.
- *A host to inhabit*.

### Stages of the Infection Cycle

Study the infection cycle (also known as the "chain of infection") in Figure 36–1 and follow the cycle to see how easily diseases can be transferred from one person to another unless the cycle is broken. Taking care of yourself is extremely important in the scope of disease

## TABLE 36–1 Communicable Diseases

| Disease | Means of Transmission | Incubation | Symptoms | Treatment |
|---|---|---|---|---|
| AIDS (acquired immunodeficiency syndrome)* | Direct contact: sexual, anal, or vaginal intercourse; sharing IV drug needles; infected mother to child (childbirth); blood to blood (from cuts, scrapes, punctures of skin). Indirect contact: blood transfusions | Onset of AIDS following infection with human immunodeficiency virus (HIV) from 6 months to 10+ years | Early—loss of appetite, weight loss, fever, night sweats, skin rashes, diarrhea, fatigue, poor resistance to infections, swollen lymph nodes. Later—cough, fever, shortness of breath, dyspnea, purple blotches on the skin | Research and new developments continue in the search for a cure and a vaccine. The current most commonly used treatments are antiretroviral drugs. (Visit the CDC website for the most up-to-date treatment regimes.) |
| Chickenpox* (deaths only reportable) (varicella zoster virus) | Direct or indirect contact, droplet, or **airborne** secretion of infected person | 2–3 weeks, usually 13–17 days | Crops of **pruritic** vesicular eruptions on the skin, slight fever and headache, **malaise** | Bed rest, topical anti-pruritics |
| Common cold (upper respiratory infection—URI) | Direct or indirect contact with infected person | 12–72 hours (some viruses 2–7 days), usually 24 hours | Slight sore throat, watery eyes, runny nose, sneezing, chills, malaise, low-grade fever | Rest, decongestant, mild analgesics, increased fluid intake |
| Conjunctivitis (pink eye) | Direct or indirect contact with discharge from eyes or upper respiratory tract of infected person | Viral: 24 hours to days; bacterial: 24–72 hours | Redness of eyes, itching, burning of eyes, matted eyelashes | Antibacterial agents, antibiotics, corticosteroids, depending on causative agent |
| Head lice (pediculosis) | Direct contact with infested person; indirect contact is rare | 1 week (**nits**, or eggs, hatch in 1 week, mature in 2 weeks) | Itching of scalp; presence of small, light-gray lice and nits (eggs) at the base of hairs | Topical use of 1% lindane shampoo, lotion, or cream (7–10 days); comb nits from hair; launder washable items in hot water with hottest drying cycle, dry-clean or seal in plastic bags non-washable items (2 weeks); thoroughly vacuum the environment |
| *Haemophilus influenzae* type b Hib (H-flu)* (invasive disease reportable) | Direct and indirect contact and **droplet infection** from respiratory tract | 3+ days | URI symptoms, fever, aches, sleepiness, no appetite; as disease progresses, child is irritable and fussy | Antibiotics, increased fluid intake, antipyretics, rest, analgesics |

*(continues)*

**TABLE 36–1** *(Continued)*

| Disease | Means of Transmission | Incubation | Symptoms | Treatment |
|---|---|---|---|---|
| Hepatitis A* (acute) | Direct contact or by **fecal**-contaminated food or water | 15–50 days, avg. 25–30 days | Slow onset, fever, malaise, loss of appetite, nausea, vomiting, jaundice, joint pain, dark urine, clay-colored stool | Bed rest, increased fluid intake, proper nourishment (no fats or alcohol) |
| Hepatitis B* (acute, chronic, and perinatal) | Contact with infectious blood, semen, and other body fluids primarily through birth to an infected mother, sexual contact with an infected person, sharing of contaminated needles, syringes, other injection drug equipment, or needle sticks or other sharp instrument injuries | 45–160 days, avg. 120 days | Similar to hepatitis A, but onset is rapid and acute | Acute: Same as hepatitis A. Chronic: regular monitoring for signs of liver disease progression; some patients are treated with antiviral drugs |
| Hepatitis C* (acute and chronic; formerly non-A, non-B, or NANB) | Contact with blood of an infected person primarily through sharing of contaminated needles, syringes, or other injection drug equipment. Less commonly through sexual contact with an infected person, birth to an infected mother, needle stick or other sharp injuries | 14–180 days, avg. 45 days | Same as above | Acute: Antiviral drugs and supportive treatment. Chronic: regular monitoring for signs of liver disease progression; some patients are treated with antiviral drugs |
| Herpes simplex virus (HSV) (cold sores, fever blisters) | Direct contact with infected person | 2–14 days, usually 4–6 days | Painful blisters on lips, which turn **pustular** and then form crusted scabs; oral lesions are small ulcerated areas | Topical applications of drying medications; antibiotics for secondary infections |
| H1N1 (Swine Flu)* (associated pediatric mortality) | Direct and indirect contact and by airborne secretions | 1–7 days | Fever, cough, sore throat, runny or stuffy nose, body aches, headache, chills, and fatigue. Some people may have vomiting and diarrhea. Can range from an upper respiratory infection to an acute, life-threatening illness. | Bed rest, increased fluid intake, antipyretics, antiviral drugs. |

| Disease | Means of Transmission | Incubation | Symptoms | Treatment |
|---|---|---|---|---|
| Impetigo | Direct contact with draining sores | 2–10 days | Blister-like lesions (later become crusted), itching | Cleansing of areas with antibacterial soap and water, topical and/or oral antibiotics |
| Influenza* (associated pediatric mortality) | Direct and indirect contact and by airborne secretions | 1–4 days | Sudden onset of fever, chills, headache, sore muscles, malaise (commonly, runny nose, sore throat, and cough) | Bed rest, increased fluid intake, antipyretics |
| Measles* (rubeola) | Direct contact by respiratory droplets from an infected person sneezing or coughing | 7–18 days | Blotchy rash, fever, cough, runny nose, red watery eyes, malaise, tiny white spots with bluish-white centers found inside the mouth (Koplik's spots) | No treatment; however, measures can be taken to protect individuals exposed to the virus, such as post-exposure vaccination, immune serum globulin, analgesics to relieve the fever, and antibiotics if the person develops a bacterial infection while he or she has the measles |
| Meningitis* (bacterial) *Haemophilus* and meningococcal | Direct contact and droplet infection from respiratory tract | 1–10 days, usually 3–7 days | Sudden onset of fever, intense headache, nausea, vomiting; sometimes **petechial** rash, irritability, sluggishness (possible **seizures** or **coma**) | Antibiotics by intravenous and/or oral administration |
| Meningitis* (viral) | Direct contact, fecal-oral route, and respiratory secretions | Symptoms can appear quickly, or they can take several days to appear, usually after a cold or runny nose, diarrhea, vomiting, or other signs of infection show up. | Symptoms in adults may differ from those in children. Common in infants: Fever, irritability, poor eating, hard to awaken. Common in older children and adults: high fever, severe headache, stiff neck, sensitivity to bright light, sleepiness or trouble waking up, nausea, vomiting, lack of appetite | There is no specific treatment for viral meningitis. Most patients completely recover on their own within 2 weeks. Bed rest, plenty of fluids, and analgesics to relieve fever and headache. |

*(continues)*

**TABLE 36–1** *(Continued)*

| Disease | Means of Transmission | Incubation | Symptoms | Treatment |
|---|---|---|---|---|
| MRSA (Methicillin-resistant *Staphylococcus aureus*) | Direct contact or indirect contact. Skin-to-skin contact or shared items, such as towels, razors, and bandages | 1–10 days | Skin infections that may look like pimples or boils and can be read, swollen, painful, and full of pus | Antibiotic vancomycin is used to treat resistant germs. In some cases, antibiotics are not necessary, and the superficial abscess can be drained by the physician. |
| Mumps* | Direct or indirect contact by droplets from the nose or throat of an infected person, usually when they cough or sneeze | 12–25 days | Fever, headache, muscle aches, tiredness, loss of appetite, swollen and tender salivary glands under the ears on one or both sides | No specific treatment. Supportive care is needed. |
| Pertussis* (whooping cough; *Bordetella pertussis*) | Direct contact with discharges from respiratory mucous membranes of infected persons. | 7–10 days | Sneezing, runny nose, low-grade fever, and a mild cough. Within two weeks, the cough becomes more severe and is characterized by episodes of many rapid coughs followed by a crowing or high pitched whoop. Thick, clear mucus may be discharged. | Antibiotics such as azithromycin and erythromycin |
| Pinworms (*Enterobius vermicularis*) | Direct transfer of eggs from anus to mouth; indirect contact with eggs in clothing, bedding | 3 weeks–3 months | Anal itching, insomnia, irritability | Anthelmintics, initiate scrupulous personal hygiene, shorten fingernails; launder washable items in hottest or boiled water |
| Pneumonia | Direct and indirect contact | Abrupt onset | High fever, shaking, chills, productive cough | Antibiotics, liquids, rest, antipyretics |
| Rubella* (German measles) | Direct contact by respiratory droplets from an infected person coughing and sneezing | 12–23 days | Rash and fever for 2–3 days | No specific treatment for this disease; patients can take acetaminophen to reduce fever |
| Scabies | Direct contact or indirect contact with infested clothing/bedding | 2–6 weeks | Intense itching of small, raised areas of skin that contain fluid or tiny burrows under the skin, resembling a line—may be anywhere on the body | Topical scabicide, oral antihistamines, and salicylates to reduce itching |

| Disease | Means of Transmission | Incubation | Symptoms | Treatment |
|---|---|---|---|---|
| Strep throat | Direct contact | 1–3 days | Fever, red and sore throat, pus spots on back of throat, tender and swollen glands of neck | Antibiotics, analgesics, antipyretics, increase fluid intake |
| Scarlet fever (*scarlatina*) (streptococcal) | Direct or indirect contact | 1–7 days | Same as above, plus strawberry tongue, rash on skin and inside mouth, high fever, nausea, and vomiting | Same as above, plus bed rest |
| VRE (Vancomycin-Resistant Enterococci) | Direct and indirect contact. Person-to-person contact or contact with contaminated surfaces | 24 hours | For a skin infection, area may be red and tender. For a urinary tract infection (UTI), possible back pain; a burning sensation when urinating or a need to urinate more often; possible diarrhea, fever, chills; weakness or sick feeling | If no symptoms are present, no treatment is usually needed. Other antibiotics can be used than vancomycin if the VRE infection is in the bladder and a urinary catheter is being used, removal of the catheter can help get rid of the infection |

*Diseases represented with the (*) must be reported to the National Notifiable Diseases Surveillance System of the CDC, through your local state or county health department. Visit the CDC website at www.cdc.gov/ncphi/disss/nndss/phs/infdis.htm for a comprehensive list of all reportable diseases. Refer also to "Sexually Transmitted Diseases" in Unit 11, Chapter 35.*

prevention and protection. You can be instrumental in the interruption of the cycle by being **vigilant** in, and actively making efforts against, the transmission of disease. Breaking the infection cycle helps prevent the spread of disease.

## Infectious Agents

Infections occur when a pathogen (infectious agent, the first link in the chain of infection) finds a body (a reservoir or source, the second link) that offers it the conditions necessary for growth. Common infectious agents are microorganisms that are classified as **bacteria**,**viruses**, **fungi**, **parasites**, and **rickettsiae**. Infection control practices such as sanitization, disinfection, and sterilization are methods to break these links in the chain of infection and are discussed later in this chapter.

### Bacteria

Bacteria are microorganisms that vary in their **morphology**. Bacteria in the body do not indicate that disease is present; many types are beneficial. However, when it gets into the wrong area of the body such as the bloodstream or becomes overpopulated, it can feed on the body's vital nutrients while releasing toxins, causing problems to the body due to the invasion. These single-celled microorganisms are different from all other organisms because they lack a nucleus and organelles (mitrochondria, chloroplasts, and lysosomes; refer to Chapter 23 to review information about cells). Bacteria reproduce by cell division approximately every 20 minutes. Figure 36–2, A through C, shows the various forms of bacteria. Many species of bacteria are pathogenic to humans and animals. For example, *Escherichia coli* causes urinary tract infections (among other illnesses) in humans; *Bordetella pertussis* causes whooping cough, which is transmitted by droplet infection; and *Vibrio cholerae* causes cholera in humans who ingest contaminated food and water.

### Viruses

Viruses, which are the smallest of the microorganisms, may be viewed only by an electron microscope. Figure 36–3 shows a magnified view of a virus. Viruses are classified by the type of DNA or RNA (the type of

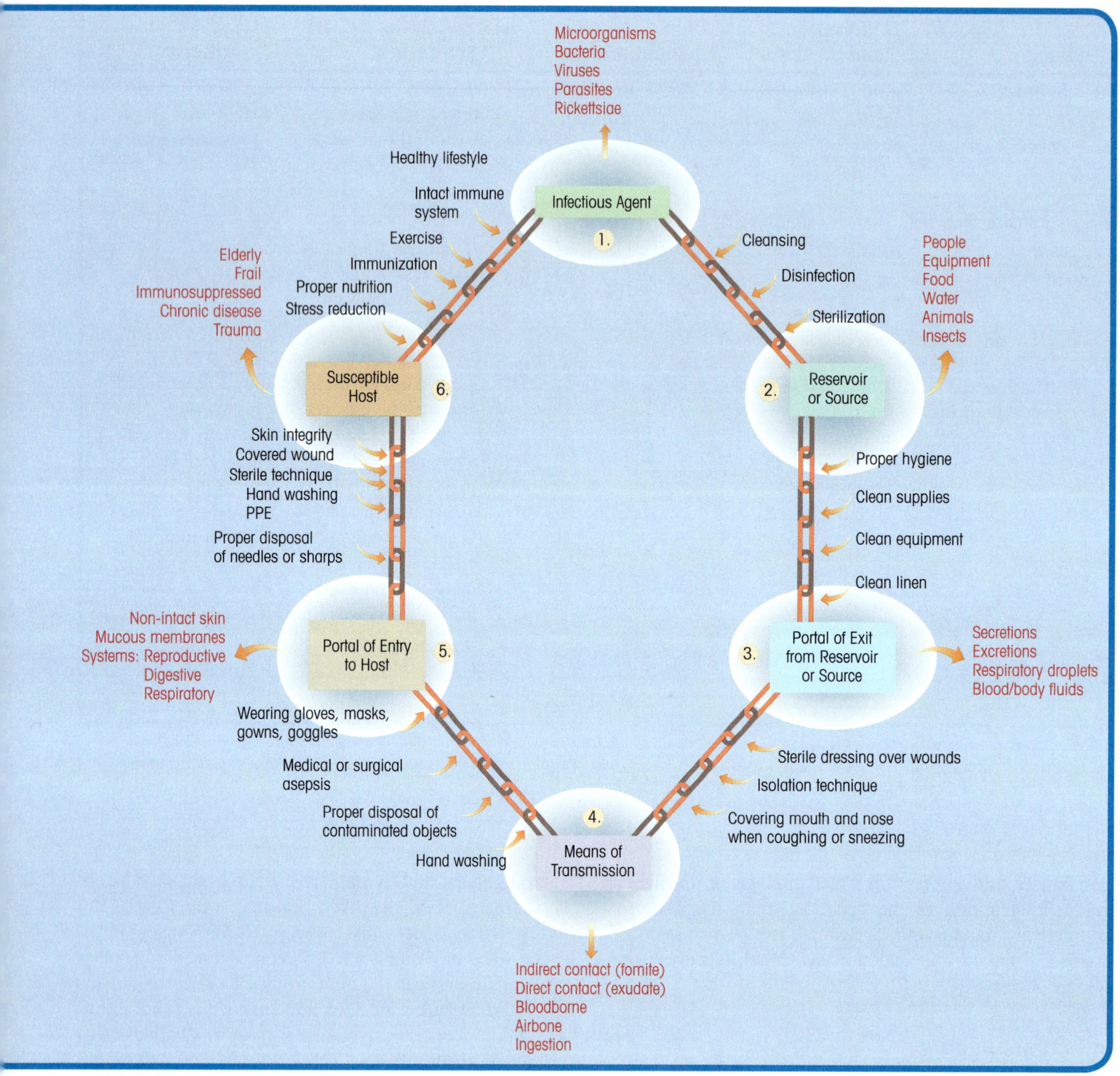


**Figure 36–1:** The chain of infection. *Delmar/Cengage Learning.*

nucleic acid core) they have or by their clinical properties. Viruses can reproduce themselves only within a host, by attaching itself to a cell and taking over the cell's nucleus. It then uses the hostage cell to self-replicate the virus, often destroying the host cell. Commonly known viruses include HIV/AIDS, herpes, chicken pox, hepatitis, the common cold, and influenza.

## Fungi

Fungi are simple parasitic plants that depend on other life forms for a nutritional source. Molds (multicelled) fungi can be found both indoors and outdoors and grow best in warm, damp, and humid conditions. Molds spread and reproduce by spore formation, which is a mode of reproduction in which the organism breaks up into a number of pieces. Mold spores can survive harsh environmental conditions, such as dry conditions, that do not support normal mold growth. Yeasts (single-celled) fungi consist of oval or round cells found in soils and on plant surfaces, in sugary mediums such as flower nectar and fruits, and as mild to dangerous pathogens in humans. The multiplication of yeast cells occurs by

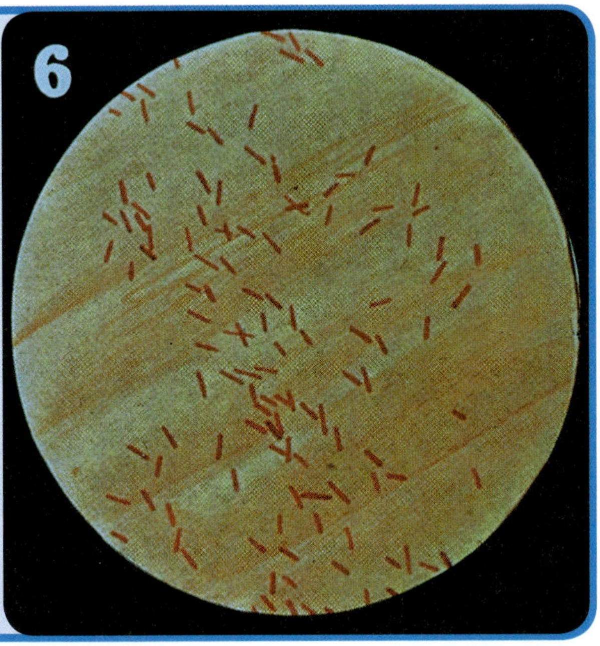


**Figure 36–2A:** Escherichia coli. *Centers for Disease Control and Prevention.*

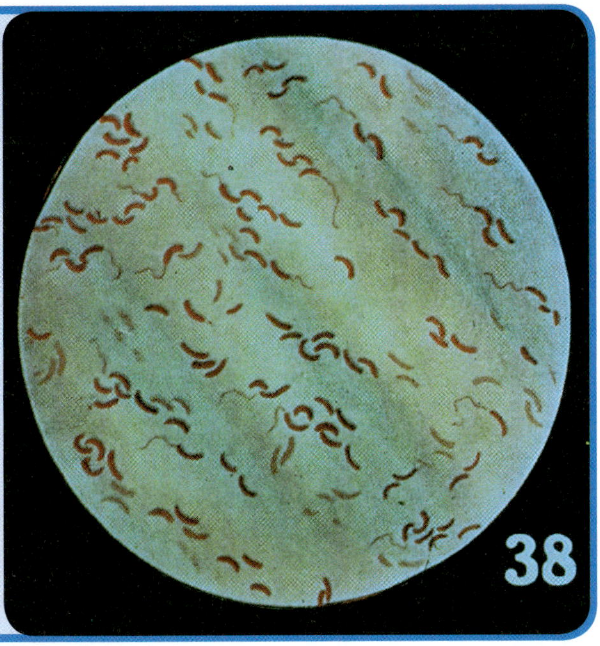


**Figure 36–2B:** Haemophilus pertussis. *Centers for Disease Control and Prevention.*

a budding process, by the formation of cross walls or fission, and sometimes by a combination of these two processes. Roughly 100 types of fungi are common in humans; approximately only 10 of these are pathogenic. Some examples of pathogenic fungal conditions are histoplasmosis (a lung infection passed on by the droppings of certain birds and bats), *Candida albicans* (yeast infection), and *Tinea pedis* (athlete's foot, see Figure 36–4).

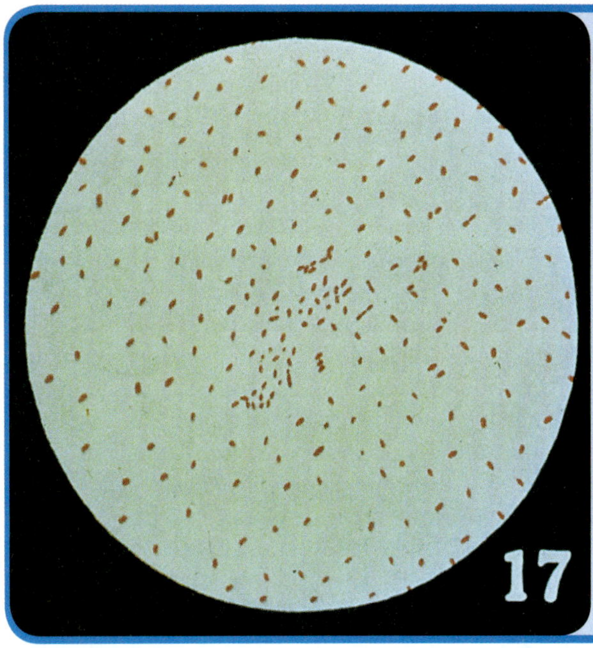


**Figure 36–2C:** *Vibrio cholerae. Centers for Disease Control and Prevention.*

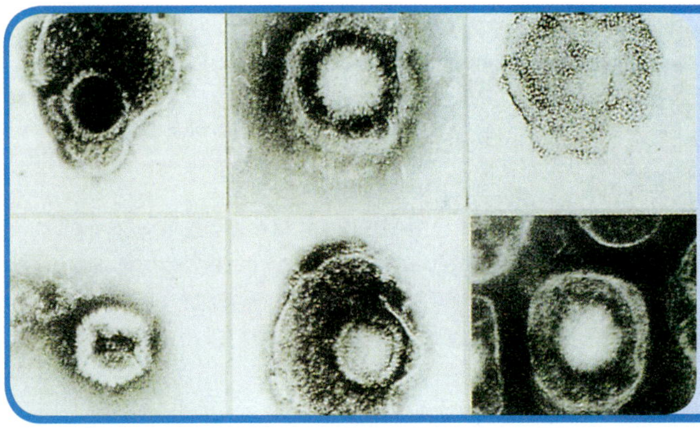

**Figure 36–3:** Electron micrographs of the various types of *Herpes simplex* virus. *Centers for Disease Control and Prevention.*

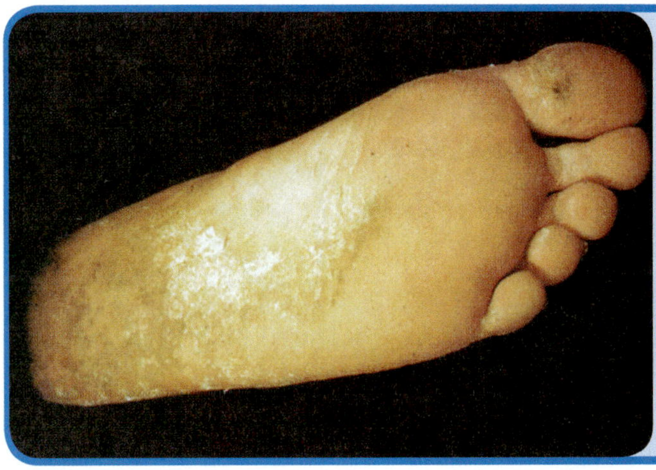

**Figure 36–4:** *Tinea pedis*, more commonly known as athlete's foot. *Centers for Disease Control and Prevention.*

## Parasites

Parasites are organisms that depend on another living organism for nourishment. Parasites are classified as **protozoa**, metazoa, and ectoparasite.

- Protozoa are single-celled internal parasites that have a true nucleus and survive on living matter. Characteristics such as hair-like projections (flagella) and tails determine the classification for these organisms by determining how they move. Common diseases caused by these organisms include malaria, toxoplasmosis, and *Trichomonas vaginalis.* Diarrhea, bowel infection, and inflammation of the brain are some of the symptoms that can be caused by protozoa (Figure 36–5).
- Metazoa are multicellular organisms that cause pinworms, hookworms (Figure 36–6), and tapeworms. Symptoms from these organisms vary but can include diarrhea, itching and rash at site, malaise, and abdominal cramps.
- Ectoparasites, also multicellular parasites, live on the surface of a host and include scabies and lice (Figure 36–7). Intense itching at the site and red, dry, scaly, irritated skin are common symptoms experienced by persons infested by these parasites.

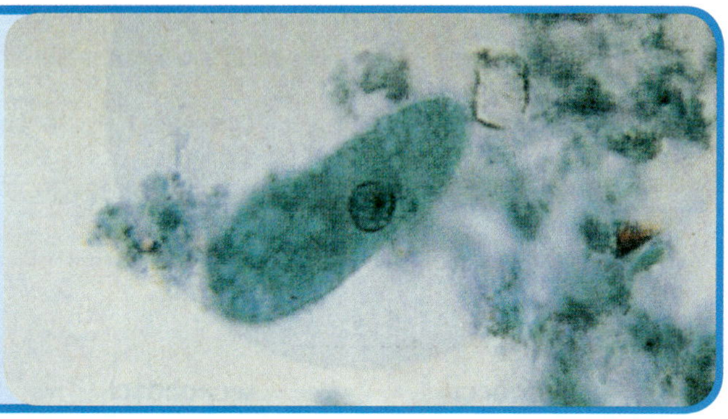

**Figure 36–5:** Intestinal protozoa *Entamoeba coli. Centers for Disease Control and Prevention.*

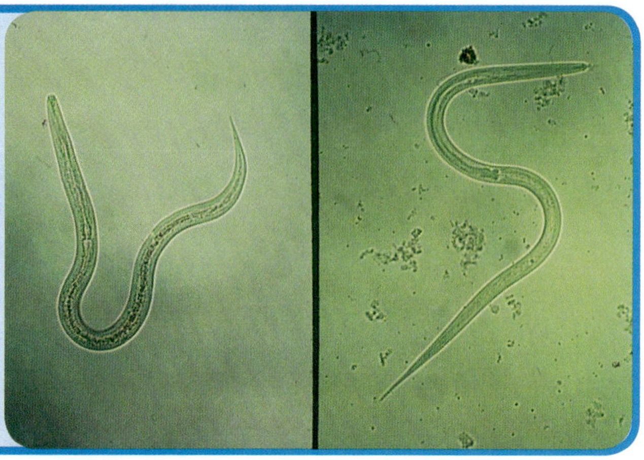

**Figure 36–6:** Strongyloides—filariform larvae of hookworm and strongyloides. *Centers for Disease Control and Prevention.*

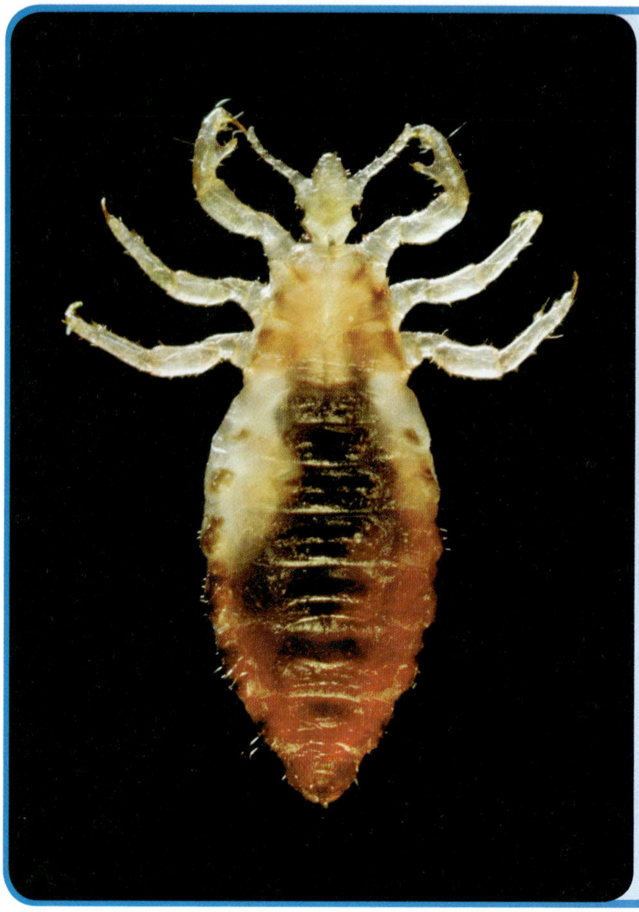

**Figure 36–7:** Lice. *Centers for Disease Control and Prevention.*

## Rickettsiae

Rickettsiae are known as **obligate** parasites because they depend completely on their host for survival. Rickettsiae are larger than viruses and can be seen under conventional microscopes after staining procedures. Most rickettsial pathogens are transmitted by ectoparasites such as fleas, lice, mites, and ticks (Figure 36–8) during blood-feeding or from scarification of infectious feces from these vectors that may be deposited on the skin. Examples of this type of infection include Lyme disease (Figure 36–9), Rocky Mountain spotted fever, and typhus. Different rickettsial infections cause similar symptoms, including fever, severe headache, a characteristic rash, and malaise.

## Reservoir or Source

The reservoir is the place where conditions are ripe for replication. This can be a person or object. Sometimes, a human reservoir is called a carrier because the pathogen can survive, grow, and multiply here. Examples include people, equipment, food, water, animals, and insects. Methods to break this link in the chain of infection

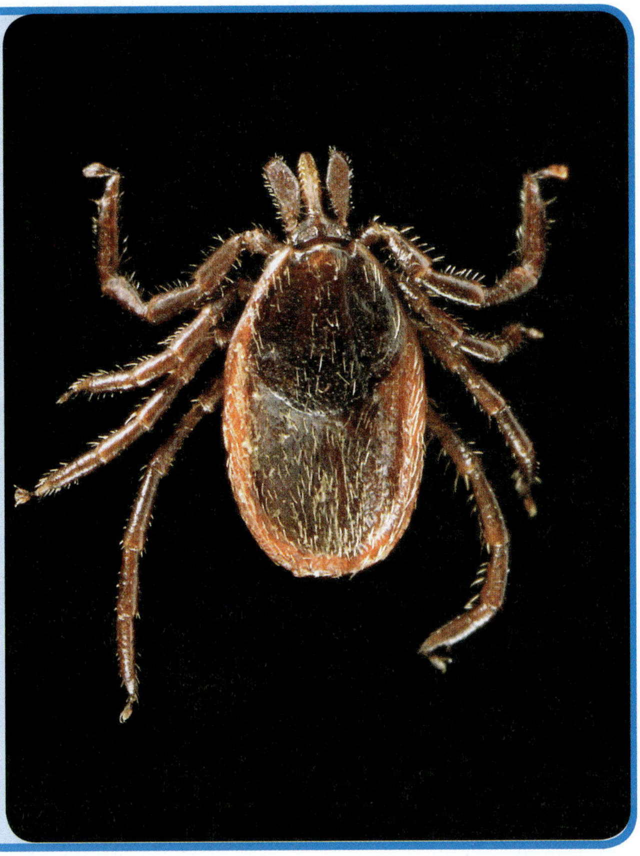

**Figure 36–8:** Deer tick. *Centers for Disease Control and Prevention.*

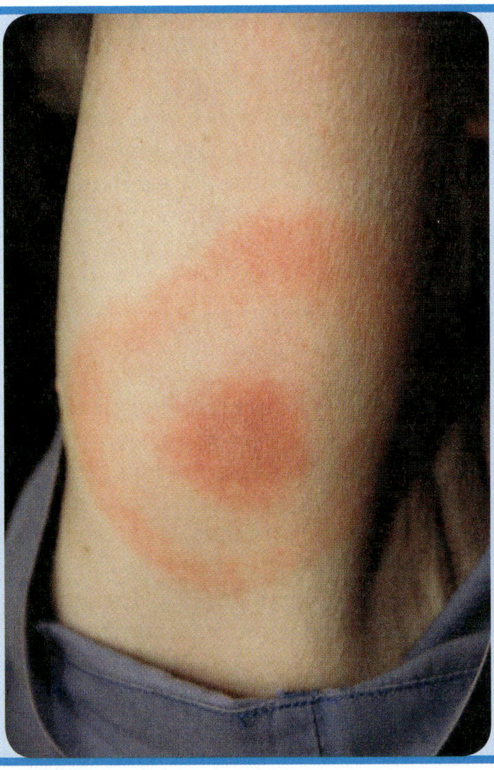

**Figure 36–9:** Lyme disease rash. *Centers for Disease Control and Prevention.*

include proper hygiene and proper cleaning of supplies, equipment, and linen.

## Portal of Exit from Reservoir or Source

The next step in the chain of infection is the portal of exit, how the pathogen departs the reservoir or source to another by way of body openings. The microorganisms leave the reservoir or source through the discharge of body secretions, excretions, respiratory droplets, and blood/body fluids and make either direct or indirect contact with another host. Methods to break this link in the chain include isolation techniques, covering the mouth and nose when coughing or sneezing, and using sterile dressings when applying to wounds.

## Means of Transmission

The next step, means of transmission, refers to how the microorganism travels from the reservoir and portal of exit to a susceptible individual. Diseases can be transmitted in different ways, and it is important for you to recognize the ways in which the infectious agent travels to realize and understand the potential danger that an infected person can have.

Direct contact means there is actual contact with the infected person or body fluids, including **blood-borne** transmission, which is acquired when the infected blood enters the susceptible host through blood or body fluids. Direct contact includes eating, drinking, touching, kissing, and sexual intimacy. Indirect contact means that you can contract the disease from inhaling the contaminated air (such as following a cough or sneeze of an infected person), or by handling a **fomite** (such as soiled tissues, piece of equipment, or door knob) that an infected person touched. When a person with a cold coughs or sneezes, the vapor containing the microorganism that is causing the illness can travel up to 3 feet (however, it does not remain suspended in the air for long periods of time). This is known as a droplet infection.

> **CLINICAL PEARL**
>
> When you are around a person who is sick, you should not inhale deeply when you breathe, or you can subject yourself to an even greater risk of contracting the disease.

A similar means of transmission, airborne transmission, involves tiny drops of vapor (moisture) from the person's breath, which, depending on the force of the breath, can carry droplets quite far, possibly projecting them up to 20 feet or more. Ingestion, the consumption of contaminated food or water, and **vector** transmission (transmission by a disease-carrying insect, usually a mosquito or a tick) are additional examples of indirect contact.

Methods to break this link in the chain of infection include hand washing, wearing gloves, masks, gowns, and goggles, medical and surgical asepsis, and proper disposal of contaminated objects.

### Portals of Entry

The way the pathogen enters the host is the next link in the chain. Portals of entry include the mouth, nose, throat, ears, eyes, intestinal tract, urinary tract, reproductive tract, or open wounds and breaks in the skin. Methods to break this link include hand washing, wearing **personal protective equipment (PPE)**, using sterile technique, proper disposal of needles or sharps, ensuring skin integrity, and covering wounds.

### Susceptible Host

The susceptible host is one who is capable of being infected by the pathogen. The resistance or ability to fight off disease of the host is low, which could be because of poor health, poor nutritional habits, or poor hygiene. Populations that have low resistance and increased susceptibility include the elderly, frail, or immunosuppressive or those with chronic disease, trauma, or both. Methods to break this link include living a healthy lifestyle (exercise, proper nutrition, and stress reduction), maintaining intact immune systems, and immunization.

## INFECTIOUS DISEASE PROCESS

After an individual is exposed to a disease-producing pathogen, a series of stages from exposure to recovery from the condition occur. The stages generally occur in order, and each has its own distinctiveness. This can be useful for providing patient education and assisting the physician with the patient's care and treatment.

- *The incubation stage.* This stage is considered the silent stage because often it is not known when the pathogen gains entry into the host and starts replicating. The length of the incubation period depends on the disease; some are very short, whereas others are lengthy. The stage ends when the first signs and symptoms of the disease appear.
- *The prodromal stage.* The first onset of signs and symptoms occur (malaise, runny nose, itchy and dry eyes, and so on). This stage generally lasts about one to two days and is considered to be the time when symptoms show that a disease process is taking place.
- *The acute stage.* The disease reaches its highest point of development (severe aches, chills, vomiting, and so on). The symptoms during this stage can help determine one disease from another.
- *The declining stage.* The symptoms start to subside; the infection is still present, but the patient's health starts to return to normal.
- *The convalescent stage.* The symptoms have all but completely vanished, and the pathogen has been mostly eliminated. The patient begins to regain strength and return to his or her original state of health.

## DEFENSE MECHANISMS

The body's immune system has amazing abilities. Immunity is best when the body is in a state of good physical, emotional, and mental condition. Essentially, this means that defense against disease can be maintained most efficiently by practicing the good health habits of proper exercise, adequate rest, good nutrition, and proper hygiene. Exercise is most helpful in resisting disease because it promotes circulation, encourages nutrition, and reduces stress. Following the food pyramid guidelines and developing good eating habits help keep energy levels at a maximum. Getting enough rest according to individual need gives the body time to restore strength and vitality.

The body also has specialized defense mechanisms. The respiratory tract contains hair-like cilia that filter out invading pathogens. Coughing and sneezing are reflexes that rid the body of invaders. Body secretions (such as tears, sweat, urine, and mucus) wash pathogens from the body. These body secretions have a low pH, which discourages bacterial growth. Hydrochloric acid found naturally in the digestive tract has a low pH and discourages growth. Refer to Chapter 31 for more information about the various types of immunity and the immune system.

## INFECTION CONTROL AND DISEASE PREVENTION

You can play a useful role in preventing disease transmission and help provide a safe and comfortable environment for staff and patients. For example, when a patient presents with an infectious disease, as a medical assistant, it will be your responsibility to remove the infected individual from the waiting room immediately to prevent others from being infected. Providing patient education is important in breaking the infection cycle. Offer the patient instruction on coughing and sneezing into tissues you provide and show the patient where to deposit the waste. After the patient leaves, it is good practice to follow the patient's steps with a spray disinfectant to help contain the germs. If you do not clean up after the patient carefully (by gloving to pick up used tissues, for example), there is a risk that you and others might contract the same illness. In severe infectious disease cases, it is wise to wear a face mask that covers the mouth and nose. The physician usually suggests this for protection against disease. As you continue reading this chapter, you will learn many more ways to ensure the health and safety of yourself and others.

## Universal Precautions

Universal precautions, as defined by the CDC, are a set of precautions designed to prevent transmission of human immunodeficiency virus (HIV), hepatitis B virus (HBV), and other blood-borne pathogens when providing first aid or health care. Under universal precautions, blood and body fluids of all patients are considered potentially infectious for HIV, HBV, and other blood-borne pathogens.

## Standard Precautions

In addition to protecting patients from infectious diseases, health care workers are responsible for self-protection. **Standard Precautions** (Figure 36–10) have been recommended by the Centers for Disease Control and Prevention (CDC) since 1987 to provide for the safety and welfare of both health care providers and the public, regarding health care standards.

It recommends using standard blood and body fluid precautions when working with all patients, especially when the infection status of the patient is unknown. Appropriate protection against exposure to blood and body fluids should be routine practice for all health care workers.

Follow these general guidelines for disease prevention and safety:

1. Perform proper hand washing before and after every procedure and before and after gloving. This must become a habit for all health care workers for self-protection from disease transmission. Immediately washing *any* skin surface thoroughly that has been contaminated with any blood or body fluid is vital.
2. Gloves should be worn when in contact (direct or indirect) with blood or any body fluids, mucous membranes, or non-intact skin; in handling items or surfaces soiled with blood or body fluid; and when performing venipuncture or any other surgical procedure. After each patient contact, gloves should be changed and hands washed. If you find that you are allergic to latex gloves, gloves made from other materials are available and can be supplied with or without powder.
3. Bandage all scratches, paper cuts, or any breaks in the skin after hand washing and before gloving for self-protection against possible contamination.
4. Refrain from direct patient care if you have an **exudative** skin condition or laceration (or other contagious disease) until the condition clears up. An appropriate bandage should be worn, and the affected person should follow proper gloving procedures to keep the condition contained.
5. When you are working, never eat, drink, chew gum, smoke, place hands or fingers to the mouth (including nail-biting), or place any item in your mouth (such as a pen or pencil).
6. Wear PPE (protective gloves, masks, face shields, gowns or aprons, and goggles) when splashing of any blood or body fluid is possible while you are working to prevent contact with mucous membranes, blood, or any body fluid of any patient (Figure 36–11A and B).
7. Always recap or close bottles, jars, and tubes immediately after desired amounts are obtained to avoid spills, waste, and accidents.
8. Clean up spills immediately to avoid accidents (Figures 36–12A and B). Spilled blood or any body fluid should be flooded with a liquid germicide or bleach solution with a 1:10 ratio before cleaning up with paper towels (wearing latex or vinyl gloves). Commercial spill kits may also be used to solidify liquids, which makes cleanup easier.
9. Work in a well-lit, properly ventilated, uncluttered, and quiet area for better concentration.
10. Immediately discard all disposable sharp instruments, lancets, syringes, and needles (intact) in proper biohazard, puncture-proof containers (Figure 36–13). *Never* break needles off, handle needles after they are used, or reuse needles. Never put the needle cover between your teeth to remove it when giving an injection.
11. Package broken glass or any sharp, unusable items in a puncture-proof container marked "Caution—Broken glass" to discard in the proper waste receptacle. This protects unsuspecting custodial personnel from injury.
12. Discard *all* hazardous waste in proper containers (Figure 36–14).
13. Place reusable metal instruments in a disinfectant solution after rinsing in cold water in preparation for proper cleaning and sterilization.
14. Use disposable equipment in mouth-to-mouth resuscitation procedures, such as mouthpieces, **resuscitation** bags, or any other ventilation supplies necessary for emergency use.
15. Especially strict adherence to safety precautions should be practiced during pregnancy.

If you or a coworker is sick or feverish, it is wise to refrain from contact with patients. Stay home and take care of yourself until you are well and return to work only after you have been fever-free for at least 24 hours. Working as a cooperative team helps solve these types

# STANDARD PRECAUTIONS

**Assume that every person is potentially infected or colonized with an organism that could be transmitted in the healthcare setting.**

## Hand Hygiene

Avoid unnecessary touching of surfaces in close proximity to the patient.

When hands are visibly dirty, contaminated with proteinaceous material, or visibly soiled with blood or body fluids, wash hands with soap and water.

If hands are not visibly soiled, or after removing visible material with soap and water, decontaminate hands with an alcohol-based hand rub. Alternatively, hands may be washed with an antimicrobial soap and water.

Perform hand hygiene:

- Before having direct contact with patients.
- After contact with blood, body fluids or excretions, mucous membranes, nonintact skin, or wound dressings.
- After contact with a patient's intact skin (e.g., when taking a pulse or blood pressure or lifting a patient).
- If hands will be moving from a contaminated-body site to a clean-body site during patient care.
- After contact with inanimate objects (including medical equipment) in the immediate vicinity of the patient.
- After removing gloves.

## Personal protective equipment (PPE)

Wear PPE when the nature of the anticipated patient interaction indicates that contact with blood or body fluids may occur.

Before leaving the patient's room or cubicle, remove and discard PPE.

### Gloves

Wear gloves when contact with blood or other potentially infectious materials, mucous membranes, nonintact skin, or potentially contaminated intact skin (e.g., of a patient incontinent of stool or urine) could occur.

Remove gloves after contact with a patient and/or the surrounding environment using proper technique to prevent hand contamination. Do not wear the same pair of gloves for the care of more than one patient.

Change gloves during patient care if the hands will move from a contaminated body-site (e.g., perineal area) to a clean body-site (e.g., face).

### Gowns

Wear a gown to protect skin and prevent soiling or contamination of clothing during procedures and patient-care activities when contact with blood, body fluids, secretions, or excretions is anticipated.

Wear a gown for direct patient contact if the patient has uncontained secretions or excretions.

Remove gown and perform hand hygiene before leaving the patient's environment.

### Mouth, nose, eye protection

Use PPE to protect the mucous membranes of the eyes, nose and mouth during procedures and patient-care activities that are likely to generate splashes or sprays of blood, body fluids, secretions and excretions.

During aerosol-generating procedures wear one of the following: a face shield that fully covers the front and sides of the face, a mask with attached shield, or a mask and goggles.

## Respiratory Hygiene/Cough Etiquette

Educate healthcare personnel to contain respiratory secretions to prevent droplet and fomite transmission of respiratory pathogens, especially during seasonal outbreaks of viral respiratory tract infections.

Offer masks to coughing patients and other symptomatic persons (e.g., persons who accompany ill patients) upon entry into the facility.

## Patient-care equipment and instruments/devices

Wear PPE (e.g., gloves, gown), according to the level of anticipated contamination, when handling patient-care equipment and instruments/devices that are visibly soiled or may have been in contact with blood or body fluids.

## Care of the environment

Include multi-use electronic equipment in policies and procedures for preventing contamination and for cleaning and disinfection, especially those items that are used by patients, those used during delivery of patient care, and mobile devices that are moved in and out of patient rooms frequently (e.g., daily).

## Textiles and laundry

Handle used textiles and fabrics with minimum agitation to avoid contamination of air, surfaces and persons.

SPR



**Figure 36–10:** A poster such as this one should be posted in the physician's office laboratory to comply with the Standard Precautions and to remind employees of safety precautions. *Courtesy of the Brevis Corp.*

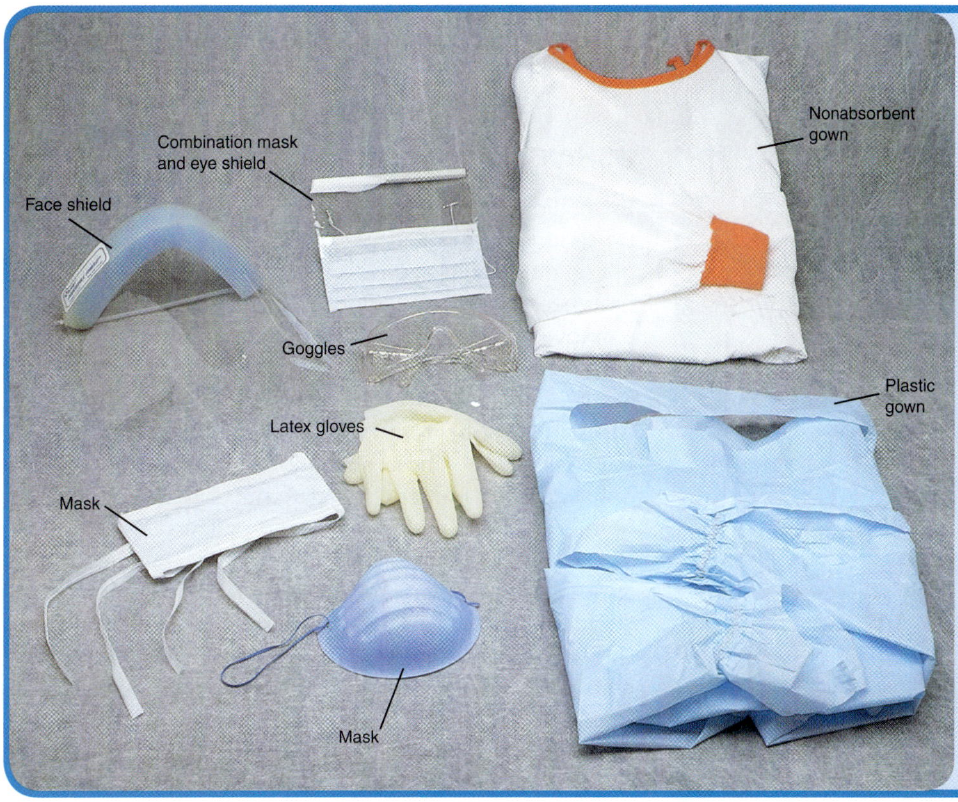


**Figure 36–11A:** Personal protective equipment (PPE). *Delmar/Cengage Learning.*

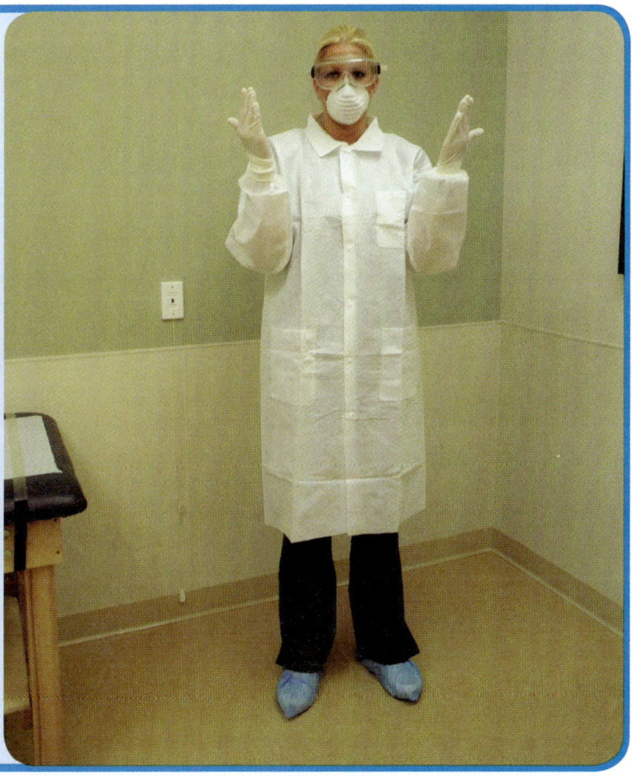

**Figure 36–11B:** The medical assistant is wearing PPE: goggles, mask, gown, and gloves. *Delmar/Cengage Learning.*

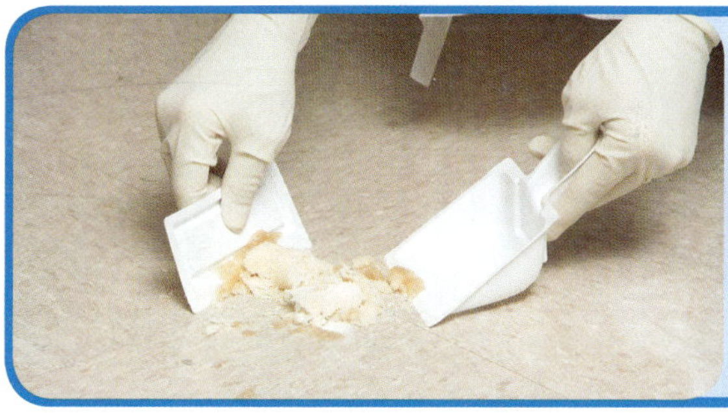

**Figure 36–12A:** Wear gloves to clean up a spill. *Delmar/Cengage Learning.*

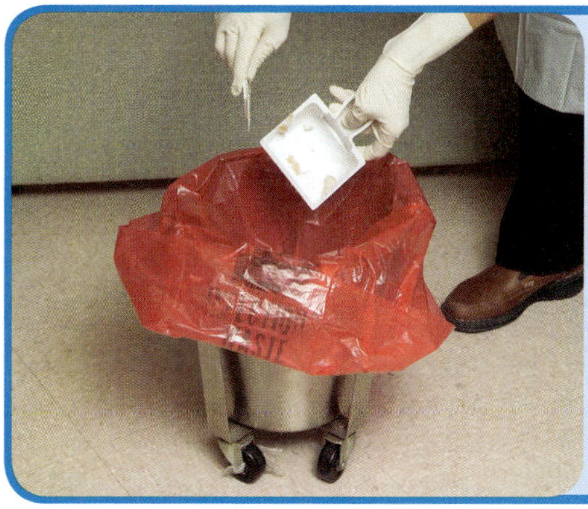

**Figure 36–12B:** All materials used to clean up the spill are placed in a biohazard waste bag. *Delmar/Cengage Learning.*

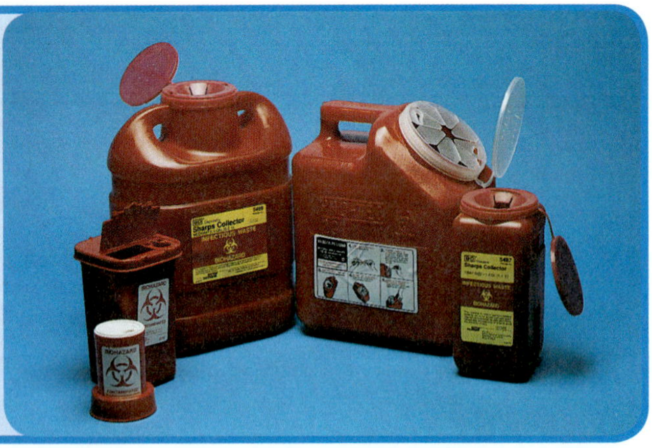

**Figure 36–13:** Various sizes of sharps containers. *Delmar/Cengage Learning.*

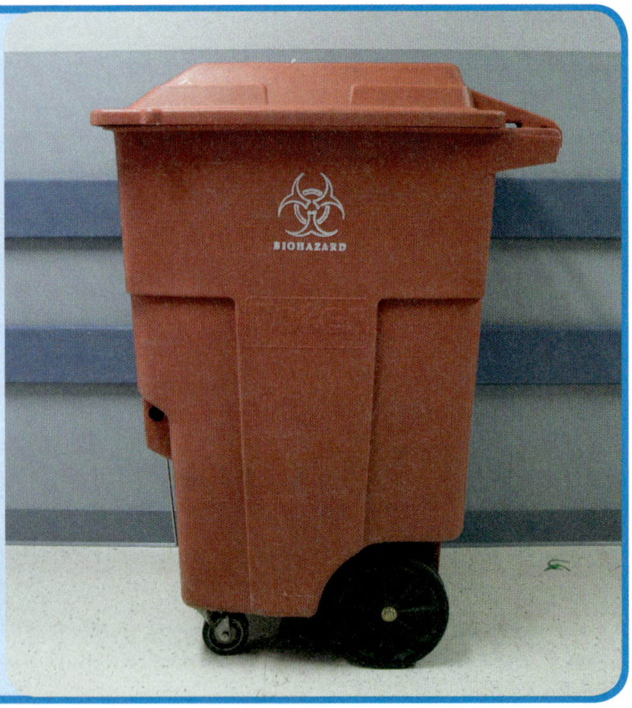


**Figure 36–14:** Properly dispose of hazardous waste. *Delmar/Cengage Learning.*

of problems, which can and do happen from time to time. Remember that the multiskilled medical assistant is a well-prepared team member who can fill in when other staff members are absent.

Further guidelines are discussed in the next section, regarding mandatory **Occupational Safety and Health Administration (OSHA)** regulations. It is up to each person working in the health care field to be honest and credible about following these guidelines. Remember: Some diseases are dangerous and can be fatal. You have a legal, moral, and ethical responsibility to protect yourself and others from such preventable problems. The best way to do this is to establish a routine and stick to it. It is far better and easier to learn good habits from the start than to break established bad habits.

## OSHA Guidelines

In medical care facilities, infection control policies and procedures are put in place to control the transmission of communicable diseases. Regulatory agencies and laws have been established to provide standards for all who are employed with managed care of the public to ensure quality care. Two of the most prominent are the Occupational Safety and Health Administration (OSHA), and the **Clinical Laboratory Improvement Amendments (CLIA)** of 1988. These regulations must be followed not only because of federal mandate but, foremost, to protect both health care professionals and patients.

In each medical office, a posted statement must appear in writing that agrees with compliance of Standard Precautions and other OSHA regulations, as shown in Figure 36–15. Medical offices and employees who do not follow these regulations will be fined by OSHA. Having this statement in clear view provides a constant reminder to all health care personnel to be alert in their duties that they may be exposed to blood or other biohazardous body fluids or infectious waste on a daily basis. Each employee must have this statement explained when he or she is hired and have evidence of this explanation in writing with his or her signature in a permanent file. This statement must be signed and dated by the employer as well.

### The Blood-Borne Pathogen Standard

The blood-borne pathogen standard, published by OSHA in 1991, was established to reduce the risk for occupational exposure. As outlined by the CDC, health

**Standard Precautions**

All employees in this medical practice must follow standard precautions at all times in performing procedures that may expose them to bloodborne pathogens possibly contained in the blood and body fluids from any patient regardless of the patient's health status. All employees must wear protective barriers that are appropriate for the procedure being performed to prevent possible infection. Employees who work with direct patient contact must have HBV vaccine. Any accidental needle sticks, other injuries, or contacts with a potentially infectious body fluid must be reported to the physician at once for treatment and documentation.

**Figure 36–15:** A statement regarding compliance with Standard Precautions, like this one, should be posted in clear view. *Delmar/Cengage Learning.*

care personnel are at risk for occupational exposure to blood-borne pathogens, including hepatitis B virus (HBV), hepatitis C virus (HCV), and human immunodeficiency virus (HIV). Exposures can occur through needlesticks, cuts from other sharp instruments contaminated with an infected patient's blood, or through contact of the eye, nose, mouth, or skin with a patient's blood. To comply with this standard, employers must have a written exposure control plan to protect workers whose employment puts them at an increased risk of contracting a blood-borne pathogen exposure. Documentation of employee input must be included in the exposure control plan.

In 2001, in response to the Needlestick Safety and Prevention Act, OSHA revised the blood-borne pathogens standard. The revised standard clarifies the need for employers to select safer needle devices and to involve employees in the selection process.

## Exposure Control Plan

Employers must update their exposure control plan annually to reflect technological changes that will help eliminate or reduce exposure to blood-borne pathogens. OSHA checks for compliance with this provision during inspections by questioning employees to determine whether and how their input was requested. The plan must include:

- *Engineering controls.* These are devices that isolate or remove the blood-borne pathogen hazard from the workplace. They include sharps disposal containers, self-sheathing needles, and safer medical devices such as sharps with engineered sharps-injury protection and needleless systems.
- *Work practice controls.* These are practices that reduce the likelihood of exposure by changing the way a task is performed. They include appropriate procedures for hand washing, sharps disposing, lab specimen packaging, laundry handling, and contaminated material cleaning.
- *PPE.* Employers must provide PPE such as gloves, gowns, and masks. Employers must clean, repair, and replace this equipment as needed.
- *Hepatitis B vaccinations.* Hepatitis B vaccinations must be available to all employees with occupational exposure to blood-borne pathogens within 10 days of employment, with no cost to the employee. Documentation of the immunization offer must be filed in the employee's record. If the person has already had the vaccine or refuses to be given the vaccine, documentation must be filed in the employee record.
- *Post-exposure follow-up.* Employers must provide post-exposure follow-up to any worker who experiences an exposure incident, at no cost to the worker. This includes conducting laboratory tests; providing confidential medical evaluation; identifying and testing the source individual, if feasible; testing the exposed employee's blood if the worker consents; performing post-exposure prophylaxis; offering counseling; and evaluating reported illnesses. All diagnoses must remain confidential.
- *Labels and signs to communicate hazards.* The standard requires warning labels affixed to containers of regulated waste, refrigerators and freezers, and other containers used to store or transplant blood or other potentially infectious materials. Facilities may use red bags or containers instead of labels (Figure 36–16). Employers also must post signs to identify restricted areas.
- *Information and training to employees.* Employers must ensure that their workers receive regular training that covers the dangers of blood-borne pathogens, preventive practices, and post-exposure procedures. Employers must offer this training on initial assignment and annually thereafter.
- *Documented employee medical and training records.* Medical and training records must be maintained for each employee. The employer also must maintain a log of occupational injuries and illnesses as well as a Sharps Injury Log unless classified as an exempt industry under OSHA's standard on Recording and Reporting Occupational Injuries and Illnesses.

### BIOHAZARD LABELS

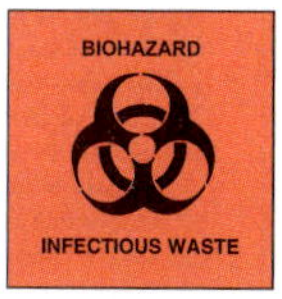


Containers that hold biohazardous materials must be properly labeled. Biohazardous materials include blood and body fluids as well as garments, gloves, masks, needles, gauze, wipes, aprons, and so on that may be contaminated with blood or other potentially contaminated body fluids. Labels shall be used to identify the presence of an actual or potential biological hazard.

**CONSIDERATIONS:**

- Labels shall be fluorescent orange or orange-red, with lettering or symbols in a contrasting color.
- Labels should be affixed onto or as close as feasible to the container by adhesive, string, wire, or other method.
- Red bags or red containers may be substituted for labels.
- If blood or control serum is stored in a refrigerator, the refrigerator shall be marked with a biohazard label.
- If blood is stored in a refrigerator for transport or same-day shipment, it does not need to be labeled but should be put in containment bags.

**Figure 36–16:** Biohazard labels. *Delmar/Cengage Learning.*

**Reporting Exposure Incidents** Your employer should have in place a system for reporting exposures to evaluate quickly the risk of infection, inform you about the treatments available to help prevent infection, and determine whether infection occurs. The CDC recommends the following steps to be taken immediately following an exposure to blood:

- Wash needlesticks and cuts with soap and water.
- Flush splashes to the nose, mouth, or skin with water.
- Irrigate eyes with clean water, saline, or sterile irrigation.

Additionally, the exposure needs to be reported to the appropriate supervisor or person responsible for managing exposures. The steps required after an incident of exposure are covered in Procedure 36–1. Figure 36-17 shows an example of an incident exposure report form.

**Needlesticks and Other Sharps** The greatest risk of exposure to blood-borne pathogens occurs when handling contaminated sharps; OSHA estimates approximately 500,000 exposures occur each year. At all times, health care workers must use extreme caution when handling needles, scalpels, and other sharp instruments to avoid self-injury.

To prevent possible self-injury, it is recommended that needles should never be recapped, broken off, or removed from disposable syringes by hand after use. They should be placed carefully in puncture-proof containers after engaging the safety guard over the needle. Always dispose of the entire used needle intact with the syringe to prevent injury. If it becomes necessary to re-cover a needle prior to performing an injection, a one-handed scoop method should be used. (See Chapter 53 for this procedure.)

Many medical devices have been developed to reduce the risk of needlesticks and other sharps injuries. These safer medical devices replace sharps with a non-needle sharp or a needle device used for withdrawing body fluids, accessing a vein or artery, or administering medications or other fluids, with a built-in safety feature or mechanism that effectively reduces the risk of an exposure incident.

Used needles, lancets, capillary tubes, and glass slides should be properly disposed of in a sharps container. These containers are leak-proof and puncture-proof and are usually red in color to identify the contents as biohazard. Some containers are clear or white in color to make it easier to realize when they are full. A biohazardous warning label must be present on all sharps

OSHA's Form 301
**Injury and Illness Incident Report**

**Attention:** This form contains information relating to employee health and must be used in a manner that protects the confidentiality of employees to the extent possible while the information is being used for occupational safety and health purposes.

**U.S. Department of Labor**
**Occupational Safety and Health Administration**

Form approved OMB no. 1218-0176

This *Injury and Illness Incident Report* is one of the first forms you must fill out when a recordable work-related injury or illness has occurred. Together with the *Log of Work-Related Injuries and Illnesses* and the accompanying *Summary*, these forms help the employer and OSHA develop a picture of the extent and severity of work-related incidents.

Within 7 calendar days after you receive information that a recordable work-related injury or illness has occurred, you must fill out this form or an equivalent. Some state workers' compensation, insurance, or other reports may be acceptable substitutes. To be considered an equivalent form, any substitute must contain all the information asked for on this form.

According to Public Law 91-596 and 29 CFR 1904, OSHA's recordkeeping rule, you must keep this form on file for 5 years following the year to which it pertains.

If you need additional copies of this form, you may photocopy and use as many as you need.

Completed by ______

Title ______

Phone (____)____-______ Date ___/___/___

***Information about the employee***

1) Full name ______

2) Street ______

City ______ State ____ ZIP ____

3) Date of birth ___/___/___

4) Date hired ___/___/___

5) ☐ Male
☐ Female

***Information about the physician or other health care professional***

6) Name of physician or other health care professional ______

7) If treatment was given away from the worksite, where was it given?

Facility ______

Street ______

City ______ State ____ ZIP ____

8) Was employee treated in an emergency room?
☐ Yes
☐ No

9) Was employee hospitalized overnight as an in-patient?
☐ Yes
☐ No

***Information about the case***

10) Case number from the *Log* ______ *(Transfer the case number from the Log after you record the case.)*

11) Date of injury or illness ___/___/___

12) Time employee began work ______ AM / PM

13) Time of event ______ AM / PM ☐ Check if time cannot be determined

14) ***What was the employee doing just before the incident occurred?*** Describe the activity, as well as the tools, equipment, or material the employee was using. Be specific. *Examples:* "climbing a ladder while carrying roofing materials"; "spraying chlorine from hand sprayer"; "daily computer key-entry."

15) ***What happened?*** Tell us how the injury occurred. *Examples:* "When ladder slipped on wet floor, worker fell 20 feet"; "Worker was sprayed with chlorine when gasket broke during replacement"; "Worker developed soreness in wrist over time."

16) ***What was the injury or illness?*** Tell us the part of the body that was affected and how it was affected; be more specific than "hurt," "pain," or sore." *Examples:* "strained back"; "chemical burn, hand"; "carpal tunnel syndrome."

17) ***What object or substance directly harmed the employee?*** *Examples:* "concrete floor"; "chlorine"; "radial arm saw." *If this question does not apply to the incident, leave it blank.*

18) ***If the employee died, when did death occur?*** Date of death ___/___/___

Public reporting burden for this collection of information is estimated to average 22 minutes per response, including time for reviewing instructions, searching existing data sources, gathering and maintaining the data needed, and completing and reviewing the collection of information. Persons are not required to respond to the collection of information unless it displays a current valid OMB control number. If you have any comments about this estimate or any other aspects of this data collection, including suggestions for reducing this burden, contact: US Department of Labor, OSHA Office of Statistical Analysis, Room N-3644, 200 Constitution Avenue, NW, Washington, DC 20210. Do not send the completed forms to this office.

**Figure 36–17:** OSHA's Injury and Illness incident report. This form can be downloaded and printed from OSHA's website, www.osha.gov/recordkeeping/RKforms.html. *United States Department of Labor, Occupational Safety and Health Administration. www.osha.gov.*

## PROCEDURE 36–1 Complete an Incident Report

**PURPOSE:** To provide documentation required by OSHA in the event an employee becomes injured or is exposed to blood or body fluids. A post-exposure plan must be followed, and an incident report must be filled out.

**EQUIPMENT:** OSHA's Form 301 (Injury and Illness Incident Report), pen.

**S SKILL:** Demonstrate the proper procedure for completing an incident exposure report form.

| Procedure Steps | Detailed Instructions and/or *Rationales* |
|---|---|
| 1. Report the incident immediately to a supervisor for documentation. | *This helps determine whether a recordable, work-related injury occurred and the proper protocol according to your facility can be followed. In some cases, post-exposure treatment may be needed and should be started as soon as possible after the exposure.* |
| 2. Assemble equipment. | |
| 3. Fill in the demographic information about the employee. | This includes the full name, address, date of birth, date hired, and sex of the employee. |
| 4. Fill in the information about the physician or other health care professional. | This includes the name of the physician or other health care professional, if treatment was given away from the worksite, and where, if the employee was treated in an emergency room, and if the employee was hospitalized overnight as an inpatient. |
| 5. Complete the section regarding information about the case. | This includes the case number from the log, date of injury or illness, time the employee began work and the time of event (check box provided if a time cannot be determined). |
| 6. Fill in what the employee was doing just before the incident occurred. | Describe the activity as well as the tools, equipment, or material the employee was using. Be specific. Examples: "giving a patient an injection," "drawing blood from the patient," and "cleaning a wound." |
| 7. In the space provided, explain what happened. | Describe how the injury occurred. Examples: "Worker was poked with the needle while removing it from the patient's arm"; "Worker was splashed in the eye while irrigating the patient's wound." |
| 8. Explain what the injury or illness was. | Describe what part of the body was affected and how it was affected; be more specific than "hurt, "pain," or "sore." Example: "punctured left hand." |
| 9. Explain what object or substance directly harmed the employee. | Examples: "blood," "body fluid" |
| 10. If the employee died, fill in the section concerned with when the death occurred. | |

containers to recognize the hazardous materials that are contained in them. The containers must be sealed and or locked when they are full and disposed of according to EPA regulation as biohazardous waste.

Care must also be taken when handling broken glassware, which might be contaminated. Broken glassware is not to be picked up directly with the hands; instead it should be cleaned up using mechanical means, such as with a brush and dust pan, tongs, or forceps.

**Blood Spill Clean Up and Disposal of Hazardous Waste Materials** OSHA standards require all contaminated surfaces to be cleaned by a 1:10 bleach solution or an EPA- (Environmental Protection Agency) approved disinfectant. Some contaminants are not visible; therefore, all work areas must be thoroughly disinfected after each use.

All infectious waste must be disposed of by placing each contaminated item in its appropriate hazardous waste container provided by your employer. Any disposable material that has even a trace of human tissue, blood, or other body fluid on it is considered infectious and must be treated with extreme caution. Latex or vinyl gloves must be worn when handling any contaminated item to reduce the possibility of disease transmission, especially the human immunodeficiency virus (HIV), hepatitis B virus (HBV), and hepatitis C virus (HCV).

**Regulated Waste and Infectious Laundry** According to the blood-borne pathogen standard, any item contaminated with blood, body fluids, or other potentially infectious materials (OPIM) is considered medical or regulated waste. By OSHA standards, regulated waste would contain liquid or semiliquid blood or OPIM that would release blood or OPIM in a liquid or semiliquid state if compressed. Therefore, any contaminated waste that would fall under this category must be disposed of in a red biohazard bag with a biohazard label.

Laundry such as linen, lab coats, and towels can occasionally become contaminated with microorganisms. Although the risk for transmission is minimal, a process must be in place for how to handle the laundry with minimal agitation to prevent contamination into the air as well as of the person handling it. Gloves and other appropriate PPE should be worn during this process. All soiled laundry should be removed and bagged in the area in which it was contaminated and transported to the properly labeled leak-proof biohazard bin to await pickup from the laundry service.

**Incineration** **Incineration** is a method to completely destroy disposable items by flame. Items that will be treated in this way must be properly bagged for the procedure so that anyone handling the contaminated articles will not be affected.

## MEDICAL ASEPSIS

Medical asepsis is a type of infection control that decreases the risk of spreading infection by decreasing the number of pathogenic microorganisms and their spread after they leave the body. Techniques mentioned earlier in this chapter such as practicing standard and universal precautions and using PPE barriers are ways to practice medical asepsis. Other forms of medical asepsis include hand washing, sanitization, and disinfection and sterilization techniques. In addition to practicing medical asepsis in the facility, educating patients should also be part of your daily routine to combat the spread of infection.

### Hand Washing

Practicing proper hand washing and developing good habits is essential in infection control and eliminating the potential of contracting diseases. The very best way to prevent the transfer of microorganisms is by regularly washing your hands. This one task alone could help eliminate many diseases before they even begin. Hand washing, according to the CDC standards, should be done vigorously for at least 15 seconds before and after seeing each patient, before and after eating, before and after using the restroom, before and after handling specimens or any soiled or contaminated materials, and after removing gloves. Proper basic hand washing helps remove microorganisms from the skin and from under fingernails. Minimal or no jewelry should be worn because it is impossible to eliminate all pathogens from the crevices of jewelry items.

Hand washing performed before gloving for a surgical procedure, known as a surgical scrub, includes a 2- to 6-minute scrub (or the length of time recommended by the antimicrobial soap manufacturer). Surgical scrubs are covered in more detail in Chapter 49.

**CLINICAL PEARL**

Lotion may be applied to the hands to prevent dry skin. If you are putting latex gloves on after hand washing, it is important to avoid using lotions that have a petroleum or mineral oil content because they can break down the latex and could intensify a latex allergic reaction. Those who are allergic to latex should use vinyl gloves. To be safe, it is a good practice to use a water-based lotion without perfume.

When a sink is not readily available for hand washing or if hands are not visibly soiled between patients (such as in an area designated for allergy injections or blood pressure readings), a practical way to cleanse the hands is by using an alcohol-based hand-rub preparation. This preparation is a gel or foam applied and spread over the hands in the same manner as you would use soap and water. It dries in approximately one minute. Due to the alcohol in the product, your hands can become dry and chapped; therefore, a supply of hand cream should be readily available. Treating chapped skin with soothing lotions can help prevent a possible infection of the hands.

Learning the correct way to wash the hands thoroughly is outlined in Procedure 36–2. Carefully adhere to each hand-washing step to prevent disease transmission. Even though the hand-washing procedure may seem extensive, it takes only a couple of minutes to complete, and it is done to prevent the spread of disease. Acquiring this important habit is necessary for your well-being and that of others.

## PROCEDURE 36–2 Hand Washing for Medical Asepsis

**PURPOSE:** To reduce pathogens on the hands and wrists, thereby decreasing direct and indirect transmission of infectious microorganisms. Average duration is a vigorous 15-second scrub following each patient contact. (Some facilities might recommend two minutes at the start of your work day, before beginning to work with patients.) Standard precautions recommend proper hand washing to avoid the transfer of microorganisms to other patients, yourself, or the environment.

**EQUIPMENT:** Sink (preferably with foot-operated controls), antimicrobial soap, nail stick or brush, disposable paper towels, lotion, and a waste receptacle.

**S SKILL:** Demonstrate proper hand washing.

| Procedure Steps | Detailed Instructions and/or *Rationales* |
|---|---|
| 1. Assemble equipment. | |
| 2. Remove all jewelry. | Remove all jewelry, including bracelets and rings. (Wedding rings may be left on but must be scrubbed.) *Jewelry harbors microorganisms.* |
| 3. Use a paper towel to turn on faucet and adjust water temperature to lukewarm (Figure 36–18A). | Stand at the sink and turn faucets on, using a paper towel to avoid direct contact with faucets. Adjust water temperature to moderately warm. Leave water running at desired temperature. *Once the procedure is begun, the faucets cannot be touched because the sink and faucets are considered contaminated.* |
| 4. Discard paper towel. | |
| 5. Wet hands and apply soap, use friction and work into lather, being sure to cover all parts of the hands, including the wrists (Figures 36–18B and C). | Wet hands and press the soap dispenser with the heel of your hand to obtain approximately 1 teaspoon of soap in the palm of one hand. Work soap into a lather and distribute soap over both palms and backs of hands in circular motions constantly and vigorously for 15 seconds. *Circular motion and friction are more effective.* |
| 6. Rinse well, hands pointed down; be sure not to touch the inside of the sink. | Keep hands lower than forearms. Rinse well, being careful not to touch the inside of the sink or faucets during the procedure. *Removed soil and water flows into sink. The inside of the sink and faucets harbor microorganisms.* |

*(continues)*

*(continued)*

| Procedure Steps | Detailed Instructions and/or *Rationales* |
|---|---|
| 7. If the first hand cleansing of the day, use a nail stick or a nail brush on the nails and cuticles and repeat steps 5 and 6 (Figure 36–18D). | Use the nail brush or stick to dislodge microorganisms around cuticles and under nails. |
| 8. Use paper towels to dry hands with a blotting method from hands to elbows discarding each towel after one use (Figure 36–18E). | Rinse hands thoroughly. Leave water running and reach for sufficient paper towels to dry hands completely. |
| 9. Turn faucet off with a clean paper towel and discard (Figure 36–18F). | *Touching the faucet contaminates clean hands.* |
| 10. Apply lotion. | Hand lotion may be applied to prevent skin from becoming dry and chafed. |

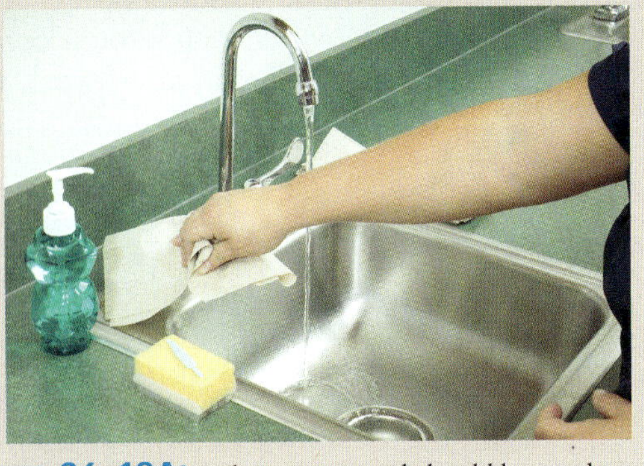

**Figure 36–18A:** A dry paper towel should be used to turn the faucet on (if not lever-operated). *Delmar/Cengage Learning.*

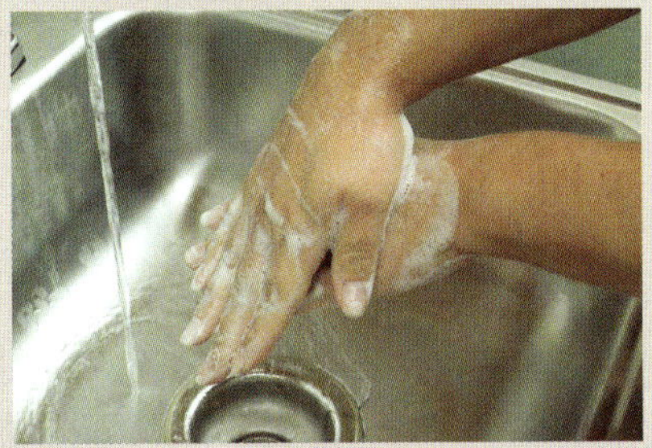

**Figure 36–18B:** Fingertips should be pointed down while washing hands. Use the palm of one hand to clean the back of the other hand. *Delmar/Cengage Learning.*

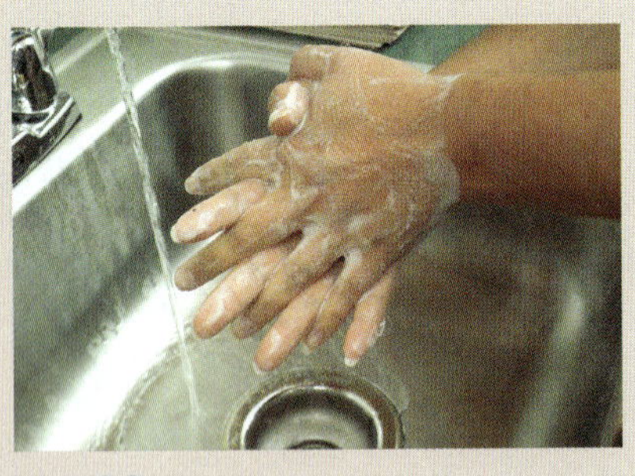

**Figure 36–18C:** Interlace the fingers to clean between them. *Delmar/Cengage Learning.*

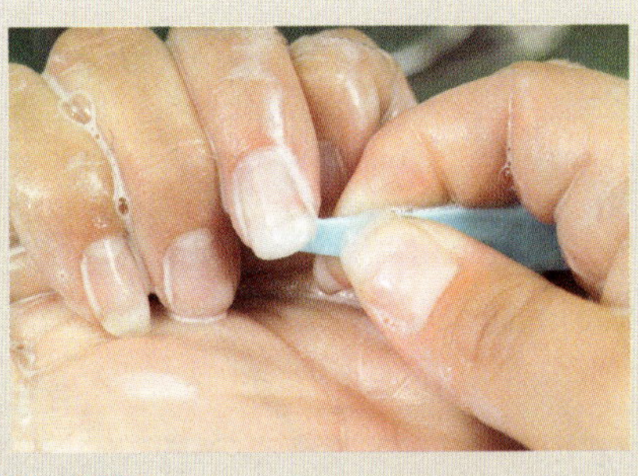

**Figure 36–18D:** Clean under the fingernails. *Delmar/Cengage Learning.*

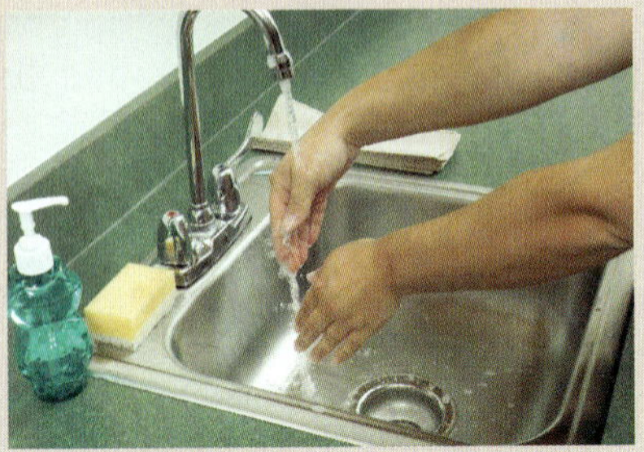

**Figure 36–18E:** Rinse the hands thoroughly with the fingertips down. *Delmar/Cengage Learning.*

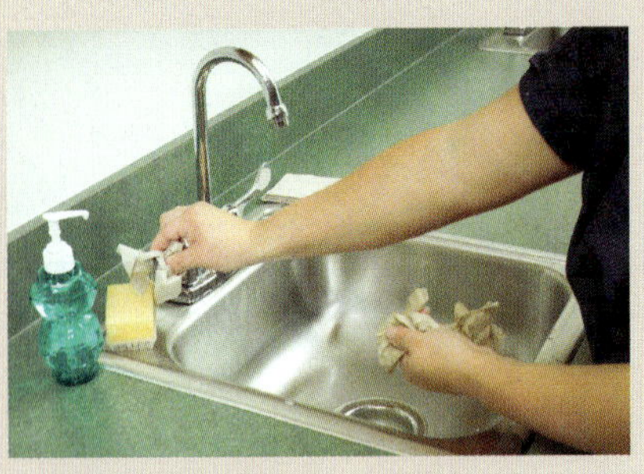

**Figure 36–18F:** Use paper towels to dry the hands and turn off the faucet (if not lever-operated). *Delmar/Cengage Learning.*

## Gloving

Wearing gloves is necessary when cleaning up blood or bodily fluid in the reception area and in the examination or treatment room. Following are three very important reasons latex or vinyl gloves are worn:

1. To provide protection as a barrier and prevent contamination of the hands when touching any blood or body fluid;
2. To reduce the possibility that any pathogens present on your hands will be transferred to another;
3. To diminish the chance of any pathogens being transmitted from you to patients as you go from one patient to another.

Wearing gloves is not a substitute for hand washing. Because gloves can have imperfections, such as small holes or tears, or if gloves are ill-fitting, hand washing is a must before and after wearing them. The risk also exists of becoming contaminated during the removal of soiled gloves. Always remember to protect yourself and follow the proper procedure for removing gloves as outlined in Procedure 36–3.

## PROCEDURE 36–3 Remove Non-Sterile Gloves

**PURPOSE:** To remove and dispose of contaminated gloves without exposing surroundings to contamination.

**EQUIPMENT:** Biohazard waste container, contaminated gloves, hand-washing equipment.

**S SKILL:** Demonstrate proper removal of non-sterile gloves.

| Procedure Steps | Detailed Instructions and/or *Rationales* |
|---|---|
| 1. Hold hands down and away from the body. | *This helps prevent contaminant exposure.* |
| 2. Grasp the used glove by the palm of the non-dominant hand with the dominant hand and remove it by turning the glove inside out (Figure 36–19A–C). | Take care not to touch bare skin on contaminated glove. *This helps prevent contaminant exposure by keeping the contaminants isolated.* |
| 3. Holding the glove that has been removed in the dominant gloved hand, insert three fingers inside the back of the contaminated glove and turn it inside out over the other (Figures 36–19D–F). | *This keeps the contaminants on the inside of the gloves, preventing contaminant exposure.* |
| 4. Dispose of gloves into biohazard waste container. | *Items exposed with blood or body fluids must be disposed of by placing them in the appropriate biohazard container.* |
| 5. Wash hands thoroughly. | *This is an added precaution to prevent exposure.* |

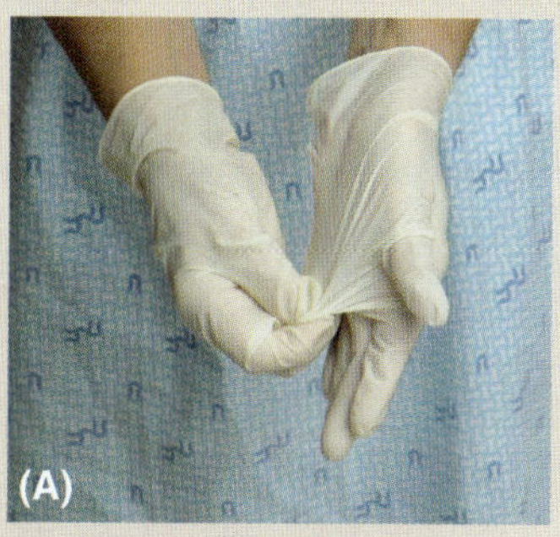


**Figure 36–19A:** Grasp the palm of the used glove with the right hand. *Delmar/Cengage Learning.*

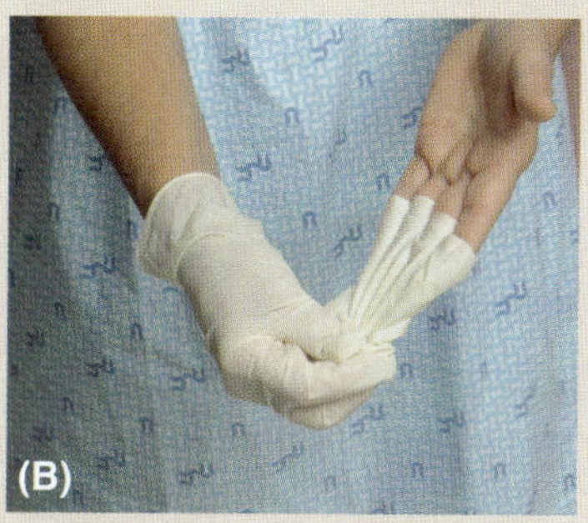


**Figure 36–19B:** Begin removing the first glove. *Delmar/Cengage Learning.*

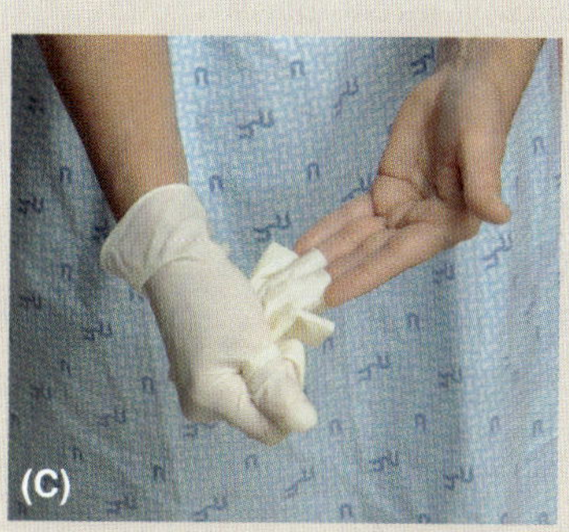


**Figure 36–19C:** Glove is turned inside out as it is being removed. Take care to not touch bare skin on the contaminated glove. *Delmar/Cengage Learning.*

*(continues)*

*(continued)*

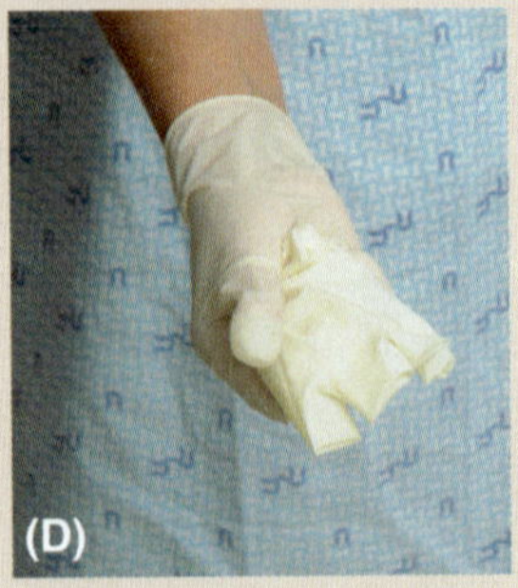


**Figure 36–19D:** Inverted glove is completely removed into the contaminated glove. *Delmar/Cengage Learning.*

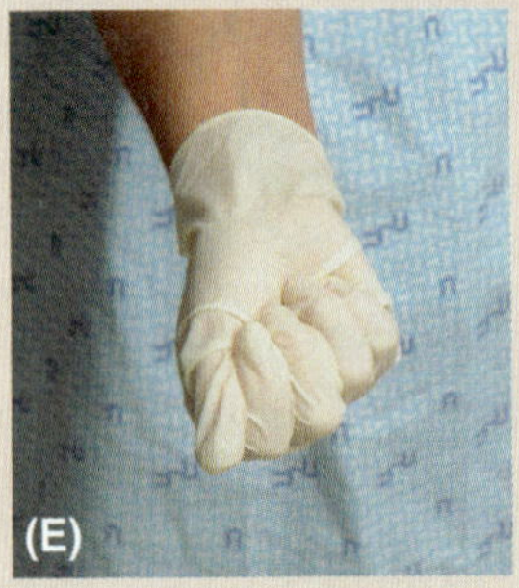


**Figure 36–19E:** Contain the inverted glove completed in the gloved hand. *Delmar/Cengage Learning.*

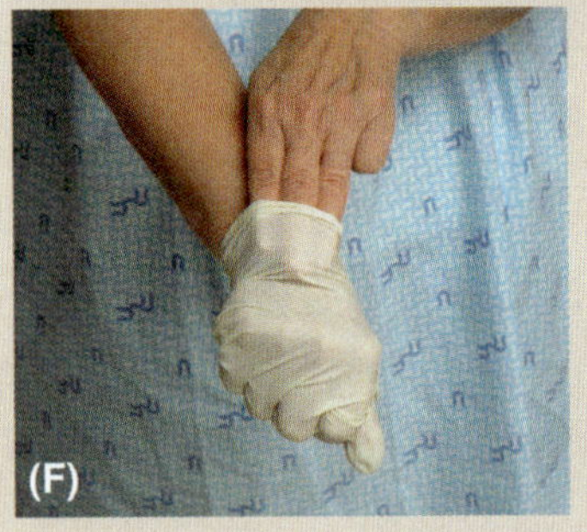


**Figure 36–19F:** Insert three fingers of the ungloved hand inside the back of the contaminated glove and turn it inside out of the other. *Delmar/Cengage Learning.*

Many of the patients you will serve and possibly some of your coworkers may be highly allergic to latex. Although many health care facilities are phasing out the use of latex and going to a latex-free environment, some products are still in use. Be sure when questioning patients about allergies they may have that latex is included. A practical way to care for patients with this sensitivity is to make one of the examination rooms free of all latex products. When latex-allergic patients are treated in this way, they can be less likely to have an allergic episode when visiting your office.

## Applying PPE

Personal protective equipment (PPE) is protective wear required by OSHA and protects health care employees from coming in contact with blood, body fluids, and other potentially infected material. Knowing the appropriate PPE to wear due to the potential exposure is critical for safety. Gloves are generally worn for any direct hand contact exposure. Gowns or lab coats would be worn to protect against any potential splash and sprays or when dealing with large amounts of infectious materials. Safety glasses or face shields should be worn to protect against splashes, sprays, and droplets, and masks against airborne transmission. Refer to Procedure 36–4 for a step-by-step process of choosing, applying, and removing appropriate personal protective equipment.

## Sanitization

Processing items and instruments for use in procedures that are **invasive** is a vital responsibility. When handling any of the instruments or articles that need to be sanitized, disinfected, or prepared for sterilization, always wear gloves to protect you from becoming contaminated with any possible lingering microorganisms on the item and the item from any possible contamination from your hands. Whenever you have a cold or the sniffles, wear gloves and a mask to avoid disease transmission. Never sneeze or cough on or over any items you are preparing for any procedure. Always follow standard precautions in performing procedures with patient contact.

## PROCEDURE 36–4 Choose, Apply, and Remove Appropriate Personal Protective Equipment (PPE)

**PURPOSE:** To provide protection from infectious contamination.

**EQUIPMENT:** Disposable gown, cap, mask, gloves, safety glasses, hand-washing equipment, and biohazard waste receptacle and/or laundry bag.

**S SKILL:** Demonstrate application and removal of appropriate personal protective equipment (PPE) when working in potentially infectious situations.

| Procedure Steps | Detailed Instructions and/or *Rationales* |
|---|---|
| 1. Review provider orders and facility protocols relative to the type of infectious exposure. | *Protocols may vary from facility to facility, depending on the type of exposure.* |
| 2. Choose and place appropriate PPE to be applied in a designated area for application. | *Some facilities have a designated area for applying and removing PPE used for infectious exposures to contain the contaminants.* |
| 3. Remove jewelry, lab coat, and other items not necessary in providing patient care or cleanup process. | *Decreases exposure to microorganisms.* |
| 4. Wash hands, apply safety glasses if necessary, and prepare to apply PPE. | *PPE provides a barrier that prevents the transmission of microorganisms to the medical assistant.* |
| 5. Apply cap if necessary to cover hair and ears completely. | |
| 6. Apply mask if necessary. | Place the top of the mask over the bridge of your nose (top part of the mask has a metal strip) and pinch the metal strip to fit snuggly against nose. Hook straps behind the ears. If using a tie mask, firmly tie the mask at the top and bottom of the back of the head so it covers the nose and mouth entirely. *This protects the mouth and nose from exposures when performing procedures that have the potential for spraying or splashing blood or OPIM.* |
| 7. Apply gown if necessary and tie securely to cover outer garments completely (Figures 36–20A and C). | |
| 8. Apply gloves if necessary and pull over the cuff of the gown to ensure that no skin is exposed. | |
| 9. Enter exposure area and clean up the contaminants following facility protocol. | *Some facilities use specialized kits for cleanup, depending on the type of contaminant.* |
| 10. Dispose of contaminated articles into biohazard bag. If any reusable equipment is involved, transport to appropriate area, following protocol for proper cleaning. | *This prevents transmission and exposure to the contaminant.* |
| 11. Remove contaminated gown (Figures 36–20D and F). | *Untie the gown, pinch a fold in the front of the gown, and pull away from yourself; slide arms out, being careful to turn entire gown inside out and roll into a ball. If disposable, place in biohazard bag; if reusable, place in biohazard laundry bag. By turning the gown inside out, the contaminants remain on the inside, preventing exposure to yourself.* |
| 12. Remove contaminated gloves; place in biohazard bag and wash hands. | |
| 13. Remove safety glasses, mask, and hair covering; dispose of properly. (If they are contaminated, you must reapply new gloves first before removing.) | *This prevents transmission and exposure to the contaminant.* |
| 14. Wash hands. | |

*(continues)*

*(continued)*

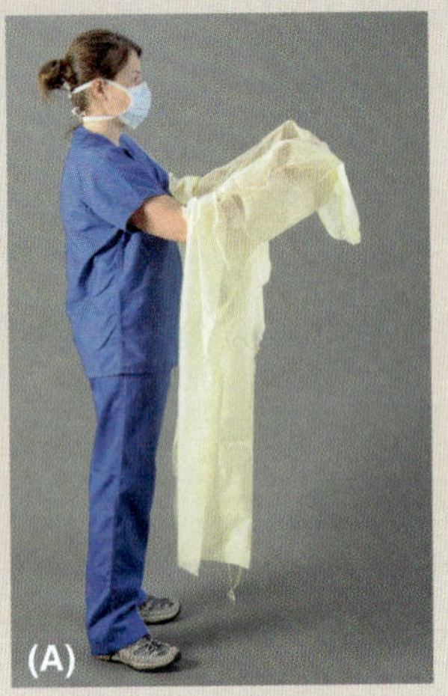


**Figure 36–20A:** The medical assistant has put on a mask and is applying the gown, pulling on the sleeves. *Delmar/Cengage Learning.*

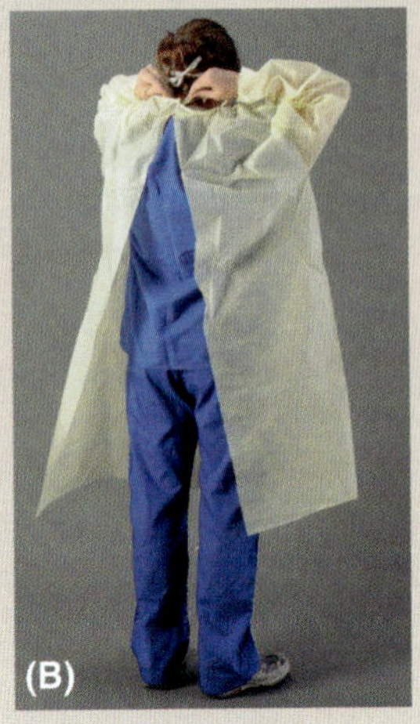


**Figure 36–20B:** The neck of the gown is secured first. *Delmar/Cengage Learning.*

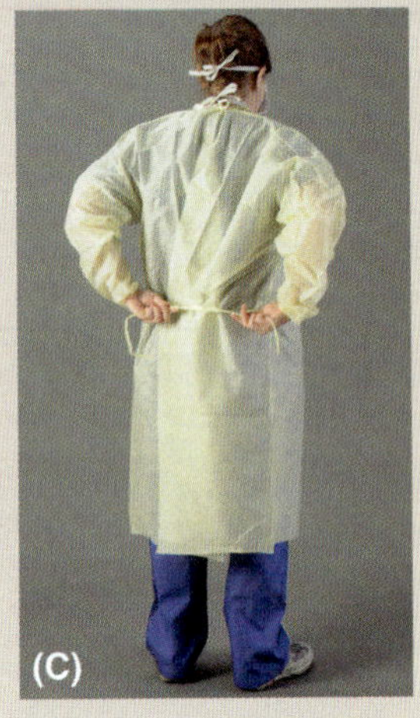


**Figure 36–20C:** The back of the gown is secured last. *Delmar/Cengage Learning.*

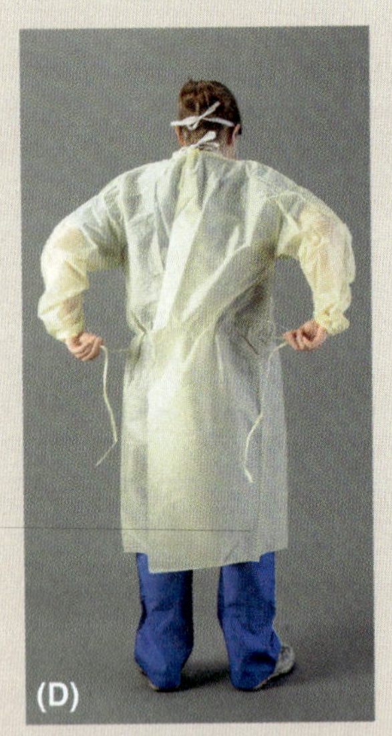


**Figure 36–20D:** When finished with cleaning of contaminants, the medical assistant removes PPE by untying the gown. *Delmar/Cengage Learning.*

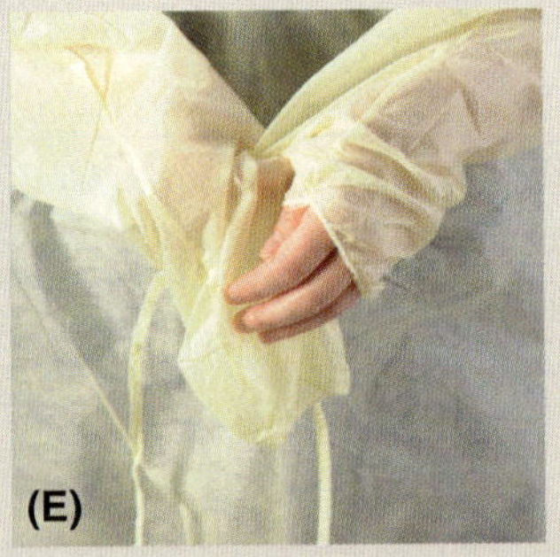


**Figure 36–20E:** Using the hand covered by the gown, pull down the gown over the other hand. *Delmar/Cengage Learning.*

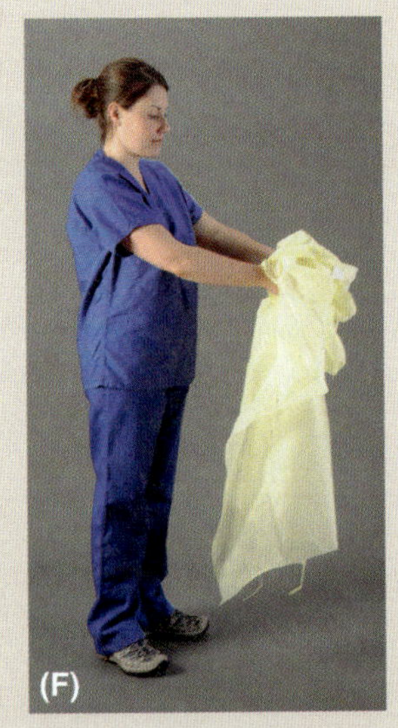


**Figure 36–20F:** Pinch the gown in the center and pull off the body and roll into a ball with the contaminated side of the gown on the inside. *Delmar/Cengage Learning.*

**Sanitization** is the process of washing and scrubbing to remove materials such as body tissue, blood, or other body fluids. Wear latex or vinyl gloves, double-gloving as necessary. Additionally, utility gloves are recommended during the process of sanitization of items and equipment to protect your hands from any possibility of contamination and injury from the articles that you handle (Figure 36–21). As you will practice in Procedure 36–5, items should be rinsed in cool water, soaked in a warm detergent solution for about 20 minutes, washed, and scrubbed thoroughly with a brush, being sure to include all **serrations**, grooves, and hinges, rinsed in warm to hot water to remove the detergent, and dried completely. During this process, the gloves also serve to protect your hands from the harshness of repeated contact with soap and water,

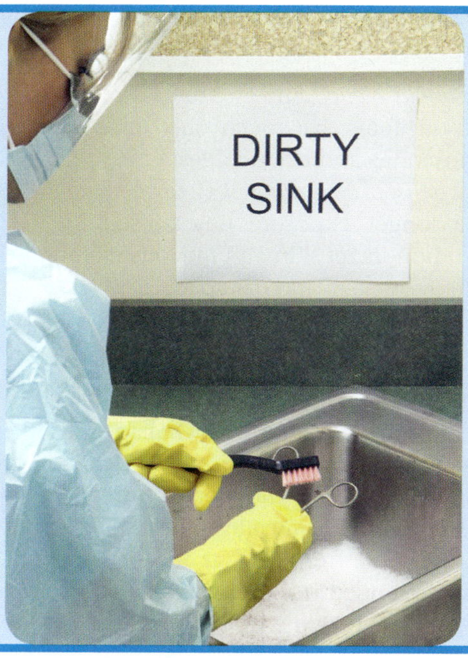


**Figure 36–21:** Medical assistant sanitizing an instrument. *Delmar/Cengage Learning.*

which can result in chafing and cracking of the skin and possibly lead to infection. Remember to wash your hands before and after gloving and use a soothing hand lotion routinely to help prevent dryness.

## Disinfection

**Disinfection** is a process by which disease-producing microorganisms, or pathogens, are killed; however, disinfectants do not always kill **spores**. Spores are thick-walled, hard capsules formed by some bacteria that allow them to remain dormant until conditions for growth are good (Figure 36–22). When the proper growth conditions are present, the bacteria break out of the capsule, grow, and multiply, starting infection. An example of bacteria that produce spores is *Clostridum tetani*, the cause of tetanus, or lockjaw. The only way to be sure spores are eliminated is to sterilize them.

The term *disinfect* pertains to a chemical or physical means of destroying bacteria. It is sometimes referred to as a germicide or bactericide. Disinfectants are used on objects, not on people, and are used mainly for large

## PROCEDURE 36–5 Sanitize Instruments

**PURPOSE:** To properly clean instruments to remove all tissue and debris.

**EQUIPMENT:** Sink with running water, sanitizing agent with enzymatic action, soft brush, towels, disposable paper towels, protective plastic apron, heavy-duty gloves, and goggles.

**S SKILL:** Demonstrate sanitization procedures.

| Procedure Steps | Detailed Instructions and/or *Rationales* |
|---|---|
| 1. Apply PPE: Goggles, apron, and heavy-duty gloves. | *This equipment protects you and your clothing from exposure to blood and body fluids through contact, splashing, or punctures.* |
| 2. If instruments need to be transported from one place to another, place the instrument in a container labeled "Biohazard." | *Following standard precautions, keep contaminated items contained to prevent exposure.* |
| 3. Rinse instruments in cool water and place in disinfectant solution. | *This removes any tissue or debris that might dry onto instruments.* |
| 4. Scrub each instrument well with detergent and water (be sure to include inside edges, serrations, grooves, hinges, and all surfaces); scrub under running water. | *This ensures that all debris has been removed prior to sterilization.* |
| 5. Rinse instruments with hot water. | *This removes any residue left behind from the disinfectant solution.* |
| 6. Place instruments on a clean towel and dry thoroughly with disposable paper towels. | *This prevents the instruments from rusting or corroding.* |
| 7. Remove PPE and wash hands. | |

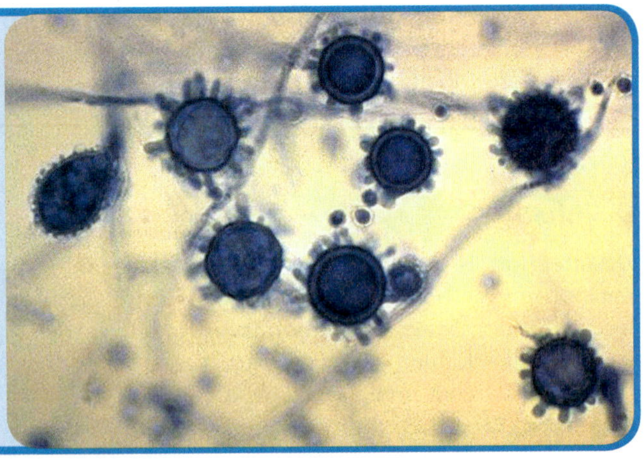

**Figure 36–22:** This picture shows the tough outer wall of spores, which explains their resistance to disinfectants. *Centers for Disease Control and Prevention.*

instruments, scopes, and heat-sensitive items that can't withstand the autoclaving process. Three levels of disinfecting solutions (low, intermediate, and high) may be used in medical facilities. The level used depends on the item or object being disinfected and its function. Common disinfectants include:

- *Household bleach* and *isopropyl alcohol* (low-level), used on items that touch only intact skin, such as stethoscopes and exam tables
- *Ethyl or isopropyl alcohol* (intermediate when used for a longer exposure time), used on items that touch non-intact skin and mucous membranes, such as thermometers and ear speculas
- *Glutaraldehyde-based formulas* (high), used on endoscopes and laryngoscopes.

Disinfectants that are registered as sterilants with the EPA or cleared for marketing by the FDA can be used as high-level disinfectants or for sterilization, depending on the recommended time per the manufacturer. The chemical solutions used for disinfecting must be changed often, depending on the frequency of use of the container, to ensure the intended effect. Always follow the manufacturer's directions for time of exposure and how often to change the solution. Procedure 36–6 gives the high-level steps to follow to disinfect an endoscope.

## PROCEDURE 36–6 Disinfect (Chemical "Cold" Sterilization) Endoscopes

**PURPOSE:** To sterilize heat-sensitive items such as endoscopes by using appropriate chemical disinfectant (glutaraldehyde-based) solution. (This procedure may also be used for delicate cutting instruments.)

**EQUIPMENT:** Chemical disinfectant, timer, sterile water, airtight container, heavy-duty gloves, sterile gloves, poly-lined towels, and sterile towels.

**S SKILL:** Demonstrate disinfection procedures.

| Procedure Steps | Detailed Instructions and/or *Rationales* |
|---|---|
| 1. Ensure that the endoscope has been sanitized thoroughly and dried prior to chemical disinfecting (sterilization). | *All debris must be thoroughly removed before sterilization procedure is performed.* |
| 2. Read manufacturer's instructions for preparation of solution. | *Preparation instructions vary depending on the brand of product being used.* |
| 3. Apply PPE. | *Chemical disinfectants are caustic and can be harmful if exposed to the skin.* |
| 4. Prepare solution and pour into a container with an airtight lid, being careful not to splash the chemical (Figure 36–23A). | *If the lid is not airtight, evaporation can occur, causing the product to lose its potency. Splashing can lead to serious injury to the skin and mucous membranes.* |
| 5. Place items into solution and completely submerge (Figure 36–23B). | *Exposed components of the items will not achieve sterility.* |
| 6. Close the lid securely and label the outside of the container with the name of solution, date, and time required according to the manufacturer for sterilization procedure (Figure 36–23C). | *Exposure time must be precise to ensure sterility.* |
| 7. When required processing time is completed, lift lid and remove endoscope, using sterile gloves. | *Item must remain sterile.* |

| Procedure Steps | Detailed Instructions and/or *Rationales* |
|---|---|
| 8. Rinse scope thoroughly inside and out with sterile water and drain remainder water from scope by holding in an upright position. | *This will remove any chemical that has remained on or inside the scope.* |
| 9. Place scope on sterile poly-lined towels and dry completely, using sterile towels. | *The poly-lined towel acts as a barrier for the sterile scope and prevents contamination while drying.* |
| 10. Place scope in storage container or area until next use. | |
| 11. Remove PPE and dispose of properly. | |
| 12. Wash hands. | |

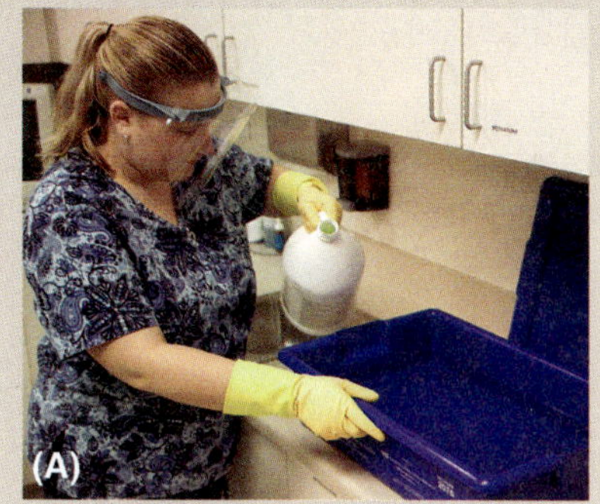


**Figure 36–23A:** Prepare solution and pour into a container with an airtight lid, being careful not to splash the chemical. *Delmar/Cengage Learning.*

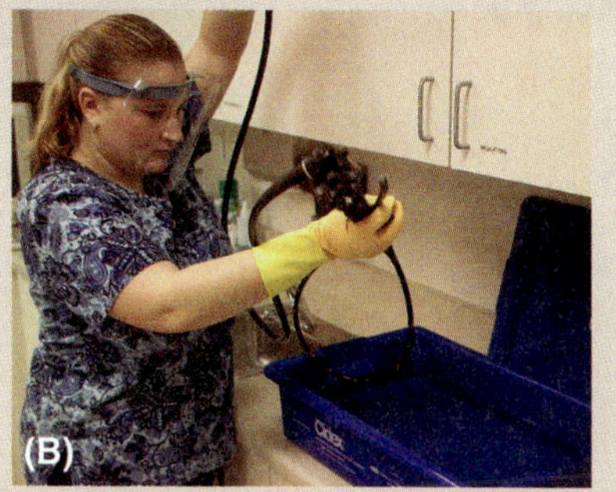


**Figure 36–23B:** Place items into solution and completely submerge. *Delmar/Cengage Learning.*

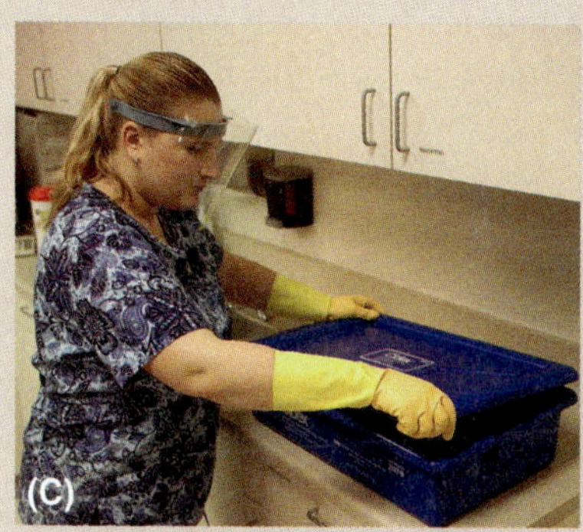


**Figure 36–23C:** Close the lid securely and label the outside of the container with the name of solution, date, and time required according to the manufacturer for sterilization procedure. *Delmar/Cengage Learning.*

## Sterilization

**Sterilization** is the process that destroys all forms of living organisms. Following the sterilization procedure, which is generally performed by **autoclaving**, the item remains sterile for 30 days if its packaging is kept dry and intact. This period is referred to as **shelf life**.

Many medical practices have an autoclave for sterilization of instruments by steam under pressure, which is a method that guarantees the destruction of spores. After the items are removed from the autoclave, exam and procedure rooms must be restocked. Make sure to place the newly sterilized items in the back of the storage area, behind other previously stored items to ensure that your current stock is up to date and save you time by preventing the need to re-sterilize items. Pay attention to the expiration date on all packages to ensure that the contents are sterile. Do not use any sterile package if it is beyond the expiration date (or more than 30 days from the time it was sterilized). If the package is labeled with just the date, it denotes when it was autoclaved. Autoclaved packages can also be labeled with "expiration date, 3-10-XX," which is the last date you could use the contents and be assured that they are sterile. If the packaging is torn or punctured, has signs of having been wet (watermarks), or is wet, this is an indication that the sterility of the contents has been lost. Microorganisms can enter wrapped or enveloped articles through moisture.

## Wrapping Items for Autoclaving

Carefully study and practice the procedure of wrapping items for autoclaving in Procedure 36–7. Articles to be autoclaved must first be sanitized and then wrapped in a double thickness special porous autoclave paper or cloth wrap. Several items may be wrapped together if separated by a gauze square. Items that are up against others during sterilization do not permit the steam to flow properly, and the items do not become sterile. Wrap each package snugly, but not too tight or too loose. If the package is too tight, the steam flow will not be able to get through the package or around each item sufficiently. Packages that are too loose or leave gaps could threaten the sterility of the contents, and they may even come apart.

Envelope packaging is manufactured for some instruments (Figure 36–24), such as scissors, and Figure 36–25 shows a medical assistant inserting an instrument into an envelope type of packaging in preparation for autoclaving. A section on the paper envelope permits recording of the instrument name, the date, and the initials of the person who sterilized it. Sterilization and biological indicators register proper and complete sterilization. Autoclave tape has an indicator stripe that changes color when the proper temperature has been maintained for a long enough time for sterilization to have taken place (Figure 36–26A and B).

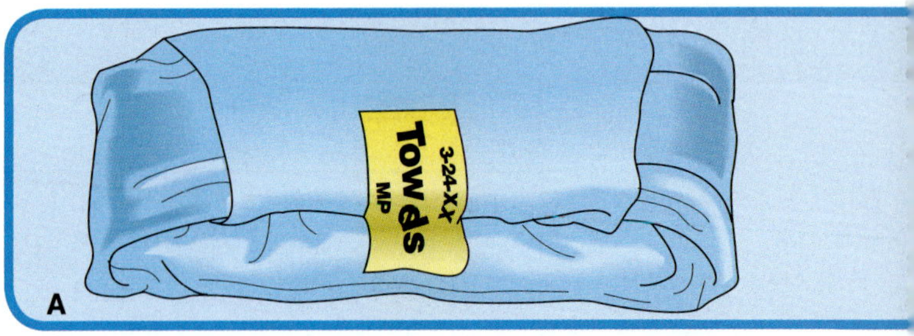


**Figure 36–26A:** Packaging of towels before autoclaving. *Delmar/Cengage Learning.*

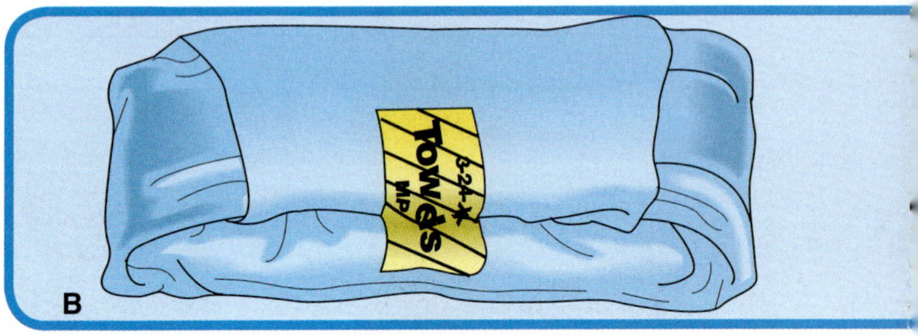


**Figure 36–26B:** Packaging of towels after autoclaving. *Delmar/Cengage Learning.*

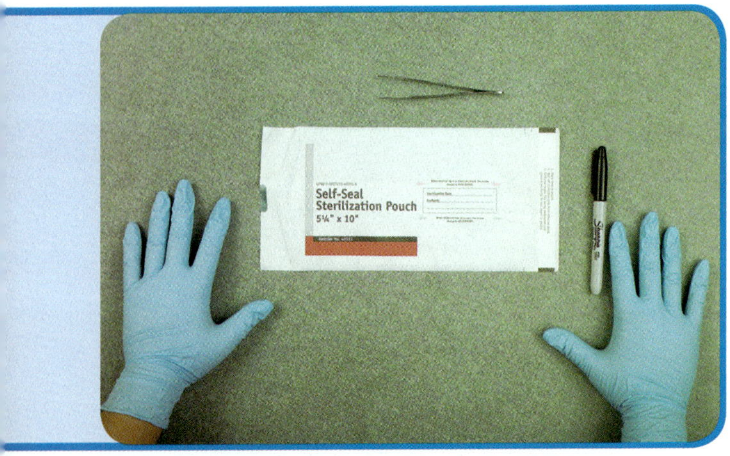


**Figure 36–24:** Envelope-type packaging for autoclaves. *Delmar/Cengage Learning.*

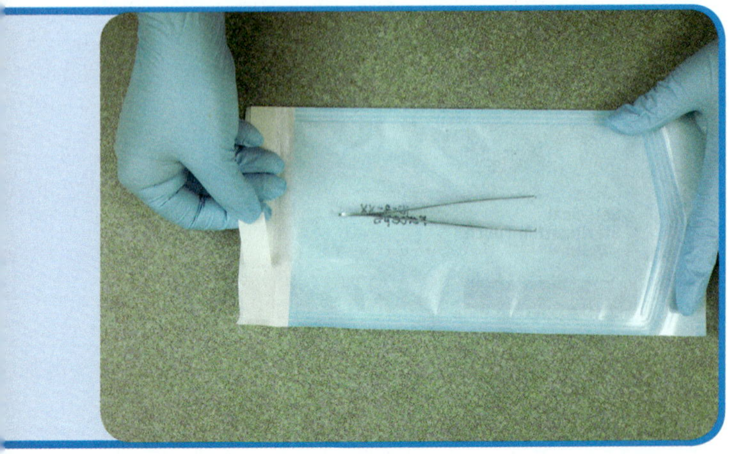

**Figure 36–25:** Placing a single instrument into the autoclave pouch. *Delmar/Cengage Learning.*

The same principle applies to indicators placed inside the wrapped package. Be aware that gas sterilizers and steam autoclaves require different indicator tapes. There are also envelopes for both types of sterilizers. The manufacturer can inform you of the proper indicator tape to use when you purchase a sterilizer or can tell you which one(s) to use with your present equipment. Biological indicators are used as a quality control method to validate that sterilization has been achieved. A common type is a vial that contains bacterial spores that will be killed when the autoclave is functioning properly. You should also clean the sterilizer routinely according to the manufacturer's recommendations.

## Using the Autoclave

The manufacturer's instructions should be followed for the operation and care of the autoclave. Instructions are usually printed either on top of the machine or on a tray that pulls out underneath it. It is important for the desired temperature of the sterilizer to be maintained for the proper time. Temperatures and pressure requirements will vary depending on the type and model of the autoclave as well as on the contents in the load. Following the manufacturer's guidelines ensures that sterility has been achieved. Refer to Procedure 36–7 for the most commonly used articles and the general desired exposure times for sterilization. In the process of sterilization, the autoclave exerts approximately 15 to 30 pounds of steam pressure per square inch at a temperature between

## PROCEDURE 36–7 Wrap Items for Autoclaving

**MEDIA LINK:** Go to the Premium Website and view the Media Link for this chapter: "Wrap Items for Autoclaving."

**PURPOSE:** To wrap items to be autoclaved so that they will be protected from contamination after the sterilization process is completed for storage and handling.

**EQUIPMENT:** Autoclave paper or cloth, disposable plastic sealed pouches, autoclave tape, items to be sterilized or autoclaved, sterilization indicators, gauze, tip protectors, indelible pen.

**S SKILL:** Demonstrate the proper procedure for preparing and wrapping instruments to be autoclaved.

| Procedure Steps | Detailed Instructions and/or *Rationales* |
|---|---|
| 1. Wash hands and assemble all necessary items. (Figure 36–27A). | *Some offices may require the use of gloves in performing this procedure. Check your office's policy.* |
| 2. Ensure that items have been sanitized before wrapping for autoclave process. | |
| 3. Check items for flaws and make sure they function properly. | *Instruments must be working properly, and materials must be in usable condition.* |
| 4. Place two squares of autoclave paper adequate in size to wrap item(s) on a clean, flat surface in a diamond shape with one corner of the paper facing toward you; place item(s) as well as a sterilization indicator in the center of the paper (Figure 36–27B). | *Placing a sterilization indicator on the inside of the package ensures sterility of the contents, which is required for quality control.* |
| 5. Place a cotton ball between any hinged instruments and keep all ratchets open during the sterilization process (Figure 36–27B). | All sharp tips on the instruments must be protected with tip protectors or gauze. *Keeping the instruments open ensures that all parts of the instrument are sterilized, and covering the sharp tips prevents the packages from being punctured.* |
| 6. Wrap item(s), using the first square by folding the corner of the paper toward the center and turning a small corner back toward you (Figure 36–27C). | |
| 7. Continue wrapping the items by folding one side toward the center, leaving a small corner toward the back on itself, and then do the same with the other side (Figure 36–27D and E). | |
| 8. Fold the package up from the bottom and secure, folding the last corner back on itself (Figure 36–27F and G). | |
| 9. Wrap the package in the second square of paper using the same technique; be sure there is no opening and seal with autoclave tape. Wrap item(s) snugly (Figure 36–27H). | *Double thickness and complete enclosure prevent exposures to pathogens. The autoclave tape, which is heat sensitive, serves as a sterilization indicator and should be placed over the final tab for ease in opening wrapped packages after autoclaving by taping 1 to 2 inches of tape to the edge of the package.* |

*(continues)*

*(continued)*

| Procedure Steps | Detailed Instructions and/or *Rationales* |
|---|---|
| 10. Label the contents and write the date and your initials on the tape (Figure 36–27I). | *This is required to identify the contents and ensures accountability and responsibility. Sterilized packages are considered sterile for 30 days from the date of sterilization; if you are not sterilizing the packages immediately, wait to adhere a date until the day of processing.* |
| 11. If using a plastic pouch for sterilization, place item into the pouch, seal, and label. | Items suitable for plastic autoclave pouches include but are not limited to forceps, hemostats, needle holders, and towel clamps. Remember that all hinged instruments must be autoclaved open. *The sterilizing process must reach all parts of the instruments.* |
| 12. Place wrapped instruments in the autoclave for sterilizing and return all unused supplies to the proper storage area when finished. | |
| 13. Wash hands. | |

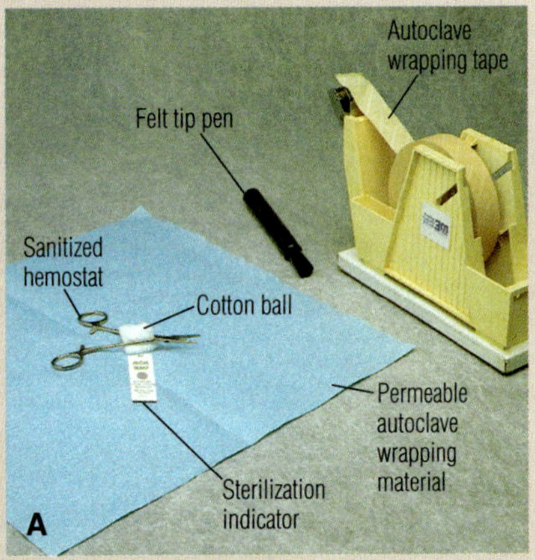


**Figure 36–27A:** Equipment needed to wrap surgical instruments or equipment for sterilization in an autoclave. *Delmar/Cengage Learning.*

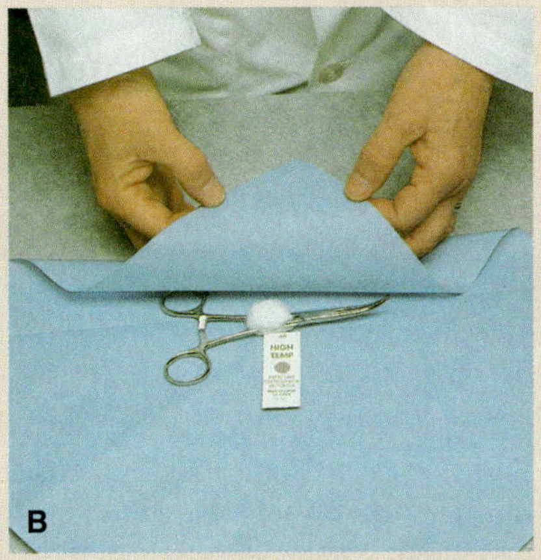


**Figure 36–27B:** Place a cotton ball between any hinged instruments and keep all ratchets open during the sterilization process. Put a sterilization indicator in with the instruments to be wrapped. *Delmar/Cengage Learning.*

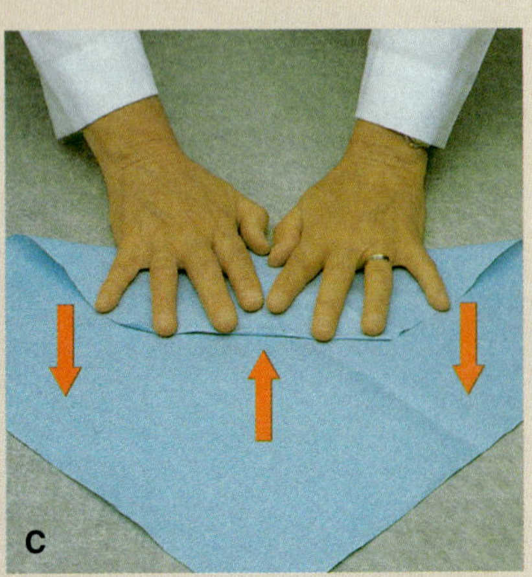


**Figure 36–27C:** Wrap item(s), using the first square by folding the corner of the paper toward the center and turning a small corner back toward you. *Delmar/Cengage Learning.*

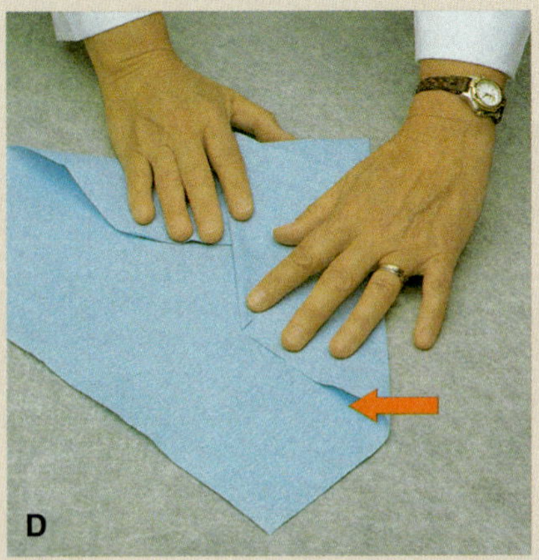


**Figure 36–27D:** Fold the other side toward center, leaving a small corner turned back on itself. *Delmar/Cengage Learning.*

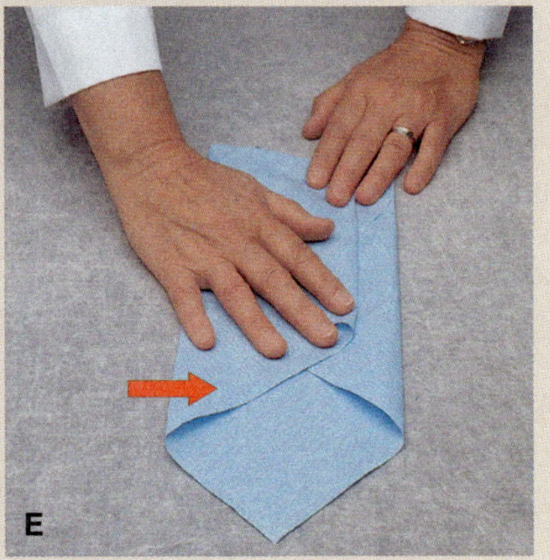


**Figure 36–27E:** Continue wrapping the items by folding one side toward the center, leaving a small corner toward you back on itself and then do the same with the other side. *Delmar/Cengage Learning.*

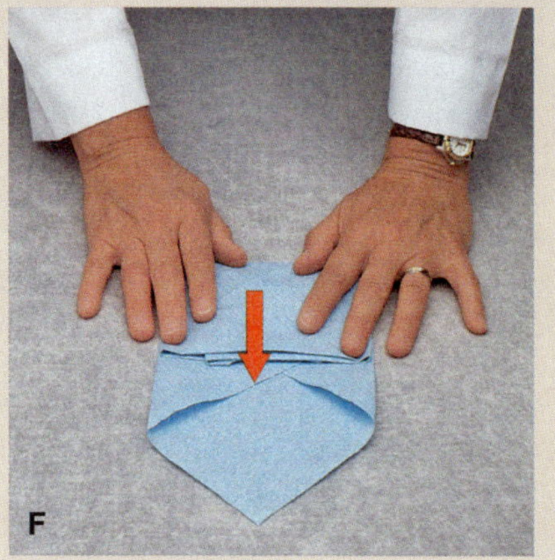


**Figure 36–27F:** The package is folded up from the bottom, leaving the last corner out. *Delmar/Cengage Learning.*

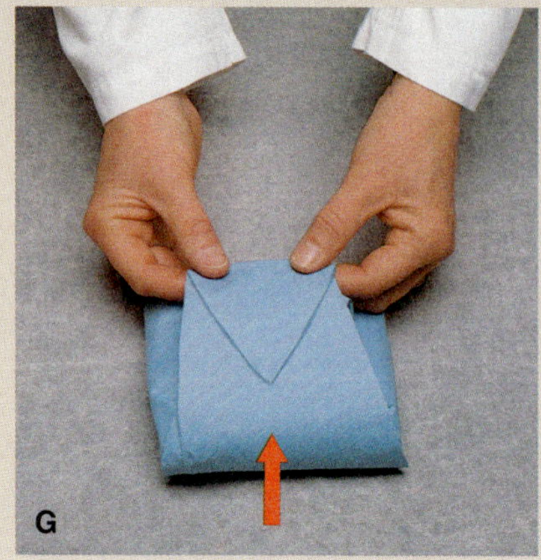


**Figure 36–27G:** Fold the package up from the bottom and secure, folding the last corner back on itself. *Delmar/Cengage Learning.*

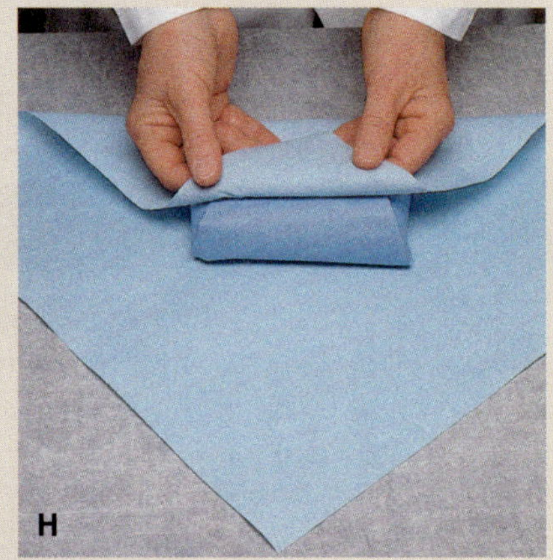


**Figure 36–27H:** Wrap the package in the second square of paper using the same technique; be sure there is no opening and seal with autoclave tape. Wrap item(s) snugly. *Delmar/Cengage Learning.*

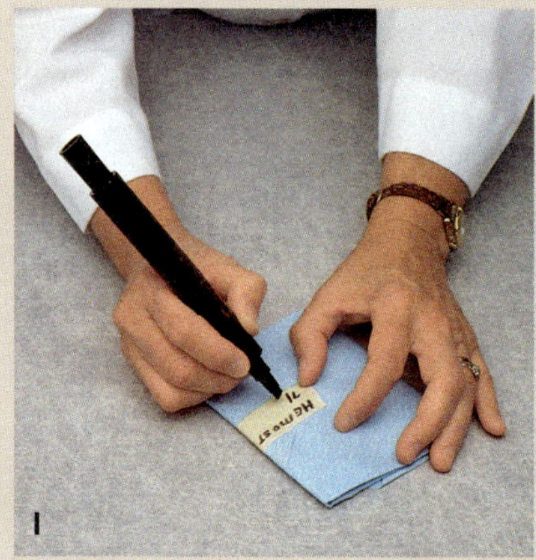


**Figure 36–27I:** Label the contents and write the date and your initials on the tape. *Delmar/Cengage Learning.*

250°F/121° C and 270°F/132°C. The steam flows through the items and destroys all microorganisms and spores (Figures 36–28A, B, and C).

Special care should be taken to avoid touching the autoclave to prevent an accidental burn while sterilization is in progress. It is a good practice to alert the staff

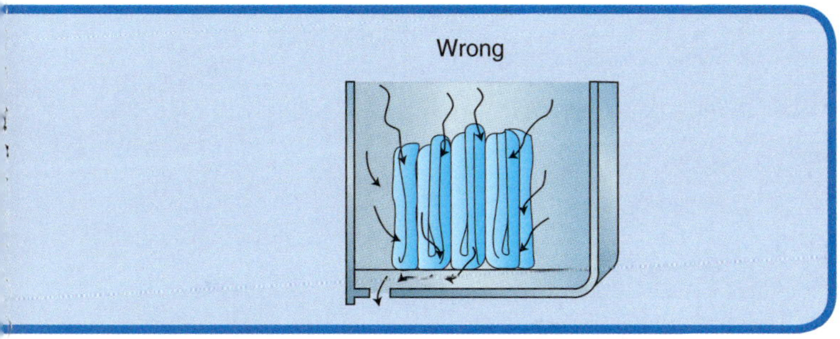


**Figure 36–28A:** Incorrect method of loading packages. *Delmar/Cengage Learning.*

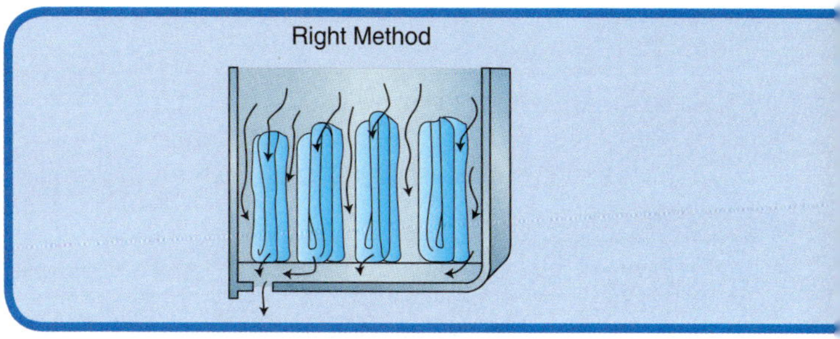


**Figure 36–28B:** Correct method of loading packages. *Delmar/Cengage Learning.*

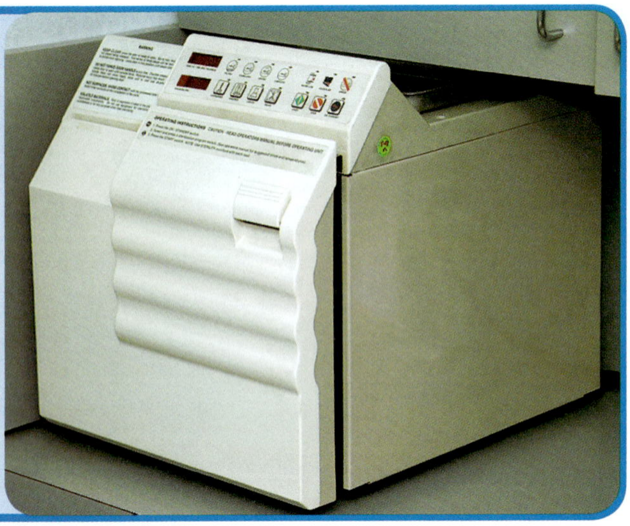

**Figure 36–28C:** Autoclave. *Delmar/Cengage Learning.*

when the sterilizer is operating so that they will also be cautious. When opening the autoclave door after the temperature and pressure are lowered, step to the side to avoid the possibility of a steam burn to the face and upper body. Use caution with any type of sterilizer. You should leave the items in the autoclave with the door partially opened so that the packages can dry. Allow adequate time for the packaging and contents to cool and dry before handling. If packs are touched before they are thoroughly dry, they are subject to contamination because microorganisms may enter through the wrap by the moisture.

Some offices or medical centers use the autoclaving service of a hospital. In this case, minimum cleaning is all that is necessary because all items are properly sanitized before autoclaving.

Study Procedure 36–8 to learn the basic operational steps for use of an autoclave for sterilization.

### Chemical Sterilization

Although the most common method of sterilization is autoclaving, other types of sterilization techniques might need to be used in the medical practice. Because sharp instruments become dull from autoclaving and rubber or vinyl articles are damaged by the intense heat of autoclaving, an alternative method for these items is autoclaving (refer to Procedure 36–8). In this method, the item is placed in a chemical sterilant (a high-level disinfectant

## PROCEDURE 36–8: Perform Autoclave Sterilization

**PURPOSE:** To sterilize instruments or supplies that will penetrate a patient's skin or come in contact with otherwise sterile areas of a patient's body.

**EQUIPMENT:** Items properly sanitized and wrapped or sealed in pouches, disposable gloves, protective mitts, sterile transfer forceps

**S SKILL:** Demonstrate the proper procedure for sterilization of instruments by use of an autoclave.

| Procedure Steps | Detailed Instructions and/or *Rationales* |
|---|---|
| 1. Check the water level in the reservoir and add distilled water to the fill line if required. | |
| 2. Any quality control procedures required must be performed with the load to be sterilized and documented. | *This ensures that the autoclave is performing accurately.* |
| 3. Wash your hands and apply gloves. | *This prevents contamination.* |
| 4. Load the wrapped or pouched items in the autoclave, allowing adequate space around the packs to ensure that steam will reach all the areas (Figure 36–29A). | *If the items are compacted, sterilization might not take place.* |
| 5. Remove gloves and wash hands. | |
| 6. Select the appropriate sterilization cycle, depending on the contents loaded, and press the start button. | Follow the manufacturer's guidelines. *Cycles can vary depending on the type and manufacturer of the autoclave.* |

| Procedure Steps | Detailed Instructions and/or *Rationales* |
|---|---|
| 7. After the cycle has ended, the autoclave will vent on its own. Open the autoclave door to allow the packs to dry before removing them from the autoclave (Figure 36–29B). The door should be ajar only slightly, ¼ to ½ inch. | Check the manufacturer's guidelines regarding opening the door; some models don't require opening during the drying cycle. *Opening the door more than ½ inch causes cold air to enter the autoclave; this can cause excessive condensation in the chamber, preventing the articles from drying completely.* |
| 8. After the drying cycle is completed, wear protective mitts to unload the items, making sure not to unload any packs that are damp (Figure 36–29C). | *Items may still be hot, and the mitts will protect you from getting burned. Organisms can be absorbed through the wet packaging, resulting in contamination.* |
| 9. Check the items to be sure that the stripes on the autoclave tape or indicators on the plastic pouches turned the appropriate color (Figure 36–29D). | *If the stripes or indicators have not changed to the appropriate color, sterilization cannot be guaranteed.* |
| 10. If any individual items have been placed in the autoclave unwrapped, sterile transfer forceps must be used to remove the item and placed in the appropriate storage area (Figure 36–29E). | *This prevents contamination.* |
| 11. Remove the mitts and wash your hands. | |

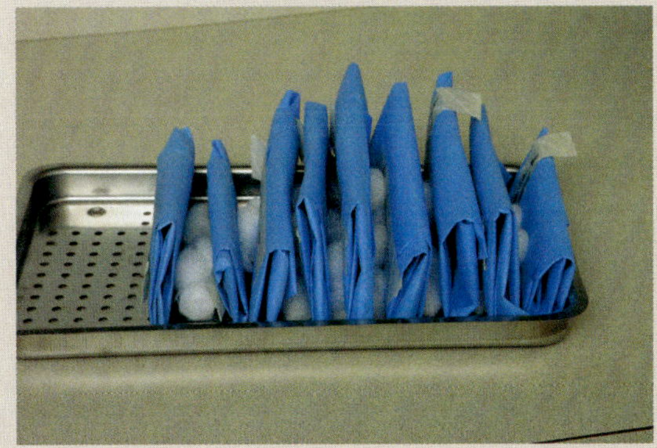

**Figure 36–29A:** Allow adequate space around the packs to ensure that steam will reach all the areas. *Delmar/Cengage Learning.*

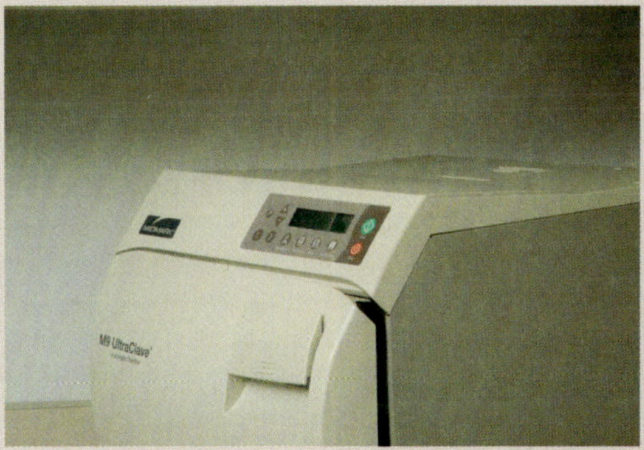

**Figure 36–29B:** Allow the packs to dry before removing them from the autoclave. *Delmar/Cengage Learning.*

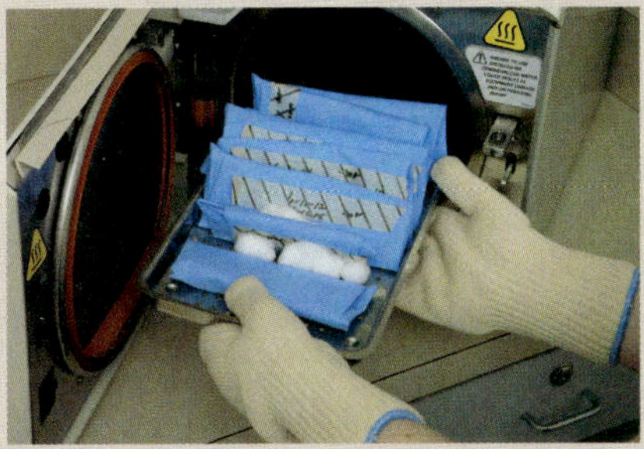

**Figure 36–29C:** Wear protective mitts to unload the items from the autoclave, making sure not to unload any packs that are damp. *Delmar/Cengage Learning.*

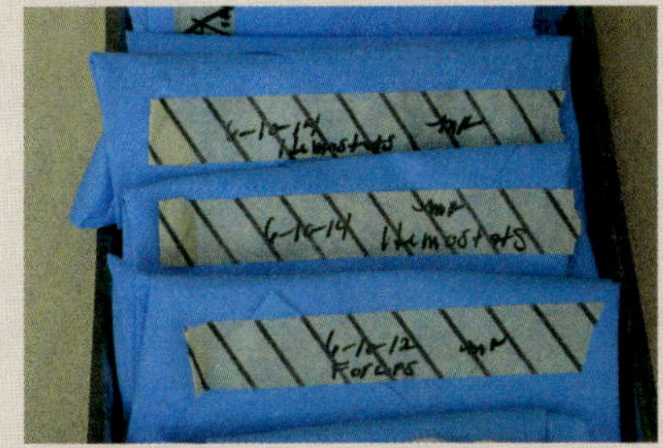

**Figure 36–29D:** Inspect the items and ensure that the stripes on the autoclave tape or indicators on the plastic pouches have turned the appropriate color. *Delmar/Cengage Learning.*

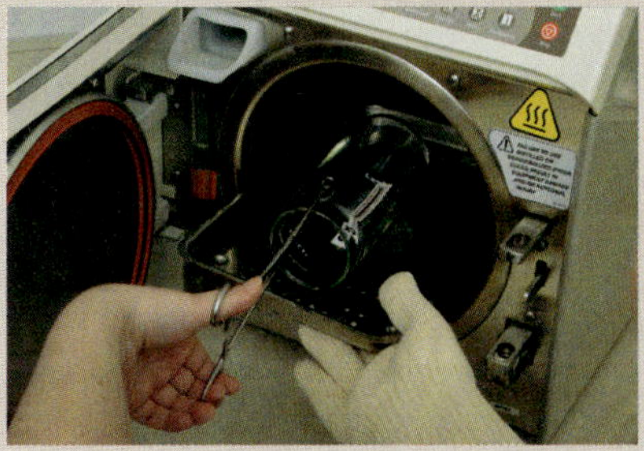

**Figure 36–29E:** Use sterile transfer forceps to remove items that have been placed in the autoclave unwrapped. *Delmar/Cengage Learning.*

solution) and remains in the solution for an exposure time recommended by the manufacturer to achieve sterility. All instruments must be thoroughly cleaned in a detergent (specifically made for this purpose), brushed, and thoroughly dried before placing them into the sterilant. The hinges and handles of instruments should be kept open to allow all parts to be exposed to the solution. A cover over the sterilant container prevents the evaporation of the solution and keeps the vapor from being inhaled by members of the health care team. This sterilizing solution must completely cover the instruments to be effective. Follow the manufacturer's recommendations regarding sterilant strength, proper disposal, and the frequency of how often the solution must be changed.

## Dry Heat Sterilization

Still another method of sterilization is the dry heat oven. Instruments with sharp blades, such as scissors or scalpels, are sometimes sterilized in this way. It is not the most desirable sterilization method for general items because it is time consuming, and spores can still be a threat with this method. The process takes one to two hours at a temperature of 350°F/176.6°C, depending on the article. It is *not* a way to sterilize items made of rubber, which are damaged by the intense heat.

## CHAPTER SUMMARY

- It is important to be familiar with transmission means, symptoms, and treatments of communicable diseases and the reporting regulations regarding them.
- The chain of infection shows how easily diseases can be transferred from one person to another. This chain can be broken by a variety of infection control practices such as sanitization, disinfection, and sterilization. Breaking the chain prevents the transmission of contaminants.
- Common infectious agents are microorganisms that are classified as bacteria, viruses, fungi, parasites, and rickettsiae.
- Diseases can be transmitted through direct contact by eating, drinking, touching, kissing, and sexual intimacy or by indirect contact such as inhaling contaminated air or handling items an infected person has had contact with.
- Stages of infection that occur when an individual is exposed to a disease producing pathogen include the incubation, prodromal, acute, declining, and convalescent stages.
- Microorganisms that are the cause of diseases are called pathogens and have certain requirements for growth and multiplication. If steps are taken to interrupt and prevent their growth, disease transmission can be reduced.
- Strict adherence to universal and standard precautions while treating all patients is essential in preventing the spread of infection.
- The greatest risk of exposure to blood-borne pathogens occurs when handling contaminated sharps. Used needles, lancets, capillary tubes, glass slides, and other sharp instruments should be disposed of properly in an appropriately labeled, leak-proof, puncture-proof container.
- The medical assistant's role and responsibilities in maintaining personal safety and well-being of staff and patients can be achieved by assessing their understanding of risk for infection, educating them on steps to eliminate an infection and methods to control the spread of infection.
- Medical asepsis is a type of infection control that decreases the risk of spreading infection by destroying microorganisms after they leave the body. This can be achieved by wearing the appropriate PPE and practicing proper hand washing, sanitization, disinfecting, and sterilizing techniques.
- Acquiring the Hepatitis B vaccination and following standard and universal precautions are preventive measures health care professionals should use to protect against this virus.

- Sanitization is the process of washing and scrubbing to remove materials such as body tissue, blood, or other body contaminants. Disinfection is a process by which disease-producing microorganisms or pathogens (not always their spores) are killed. Sterilization is the process that destroys all forms of living organisms.
- Autoclaves sterilize instruments and other medical supplies by using steam under pressure. Safety must be maintained by wearing proper PPE and following the manufacture's guidelines for use.
- Sterilization and biological indicators are quality control methods used to register proper and complete sterilization of equipment and should be used according to the autoclave manufacturer's guidelines.

## STUDY TOOLS

| | |
|---|---|
| **Workbook** | Activities for Chapter 36 |
| **Premium Website** | |
| MEDIA LINK | View these **Media Links** for Chapter 36:<br>• Wrap Items for Autoclaving |
| StudyWARE | Activities and Quizzes on the **StudyWARE™ Software** for Chapter 36 |
| | Complete the following **Competency Challenge 2.0** activity:<br>• Tuesday, 8:00 AM, Perform General Clinical Practices |
| | **Audio Library** of medical terms |
| | Online access to the **Critical Thinking Challenge 2.0** |
| **CourseMate** | Activities and Quizzes for Chapter 36 |
| **WebTutor** | Activities and Quizzes for Chapter 36 |

## CHECK YOUR KNOWLEDGE

1. An example of a disease that must be reported to the National Notifiable Diseases Surveillance System of the CDC is:
   a. *herpes simplex* virus.
   b. impetigo.
   c. pediculosis.
   d. meningitis.
2. When the infection cycle is broken:
   a. an individual becomes susceptible.
   b. the spread of disease is prevented.
   c. an individual becomes infected.
   d. disease can be transferred from one person to another.
3. An infectious agent that can be viewed only with an electron microscope and can reproduce itself only within a host is known as:
   a. bacteria.
   b. a virus.
   c. fungi.
   d. a parasite.
4. The stage of infection when the first onset of signs and symptoms of infection occur is the:
   a. incubation stage.
   b. prodromal stage.
   c. acute stage.
   d. convalescent stage.
5. Which of the following organizations established the Blood-Borne Pathogen Standard?
   a. OSHA
   b. CDC
   c. CLIA
   d. EPA
6. Contaminated surfaces must be cleaned with a _____ bleach solution.
   a. 1:100
   b. 100:1
   c. 1:10
   d. 10:1

7. Standard precautions should be used:
   a. only if the infectious status of the patient is unknown.
   b. only if the patient is known to have HIV.
   c. with all patients at all times.
   d. for self-protection rather than for protection of the patient.
8. An exposure control plan should include:
   a. engineering controls.
   b. work practice controls.
   c. PPE.
   d. All of the above
9. Sharps containers should be:
   a. odor-proof.
   b. puncture-proof.
   c. white in color.
   d. red in color.
10. According to CDC standards, vigorous hand washing should be done for at least _____ before and after seeing each patient.
   a. 15 minutes
   b. 30 seconds
   c. 15 seconds
   d. 60 seconds
11. Gloves are worn to:
   a. prevent contamination of the hands when touching blood or body fluids.
   b. increase the possibility of transferring pathogens on your hands to another.
   c. protect hands by reducing the amount of hand washing needed.
   d. all of the above
12. The process that destroys all forms of microorganisms is known as:
   a. disinfection.
   b. sterilization.
   c. sanitization.
   d. Both a and b are correct.
13. Autoclaved items have a shelf life of _____ days if items are kept dried and intact.
   a. 10
   b. 20
   c. 30
   d. 45

## WEB LINKS

Centers for Disease Control and Prevention: www.cdc.gov

Occupational Safety & Health Administration: www.osha.gov

## RESOURCES


Heller, M., and Veach, L. (2009). *Clinical Medical Assisting: A Professional, Field Smart Approach to the Workplace.* Clifton Park, NY: Delmar, Cengage Learning.

Kennamer, M. (2007). *Basic Infection Control for Health Care Providers* (2nd ed.). Clifton Park, NY: Delmar, Cengage Learning.

Lindh, W., Pooler, M., Tamparo, C., and Dahl, B. (2010). *Delmar's Comprehensive Medical Assisting Administrative and Clinical Competencies* (4th ed.). Clifton Park, NY: Delmar Cengage Learning.

Neighbors, M., and Jones, R. T. (2006). *Human Diseases* (2nd ed.). Clifton Park, NY: Delmar, Cengage Learning.

U.S. Department of Health and Human Services, Centers for Disease Control and Prevention. (2003). *Exposure to Blood: What Healthcare Personnel Need to Know.* Retrieved October 19, 2009, from www.cdc.gov/ncidod/dhqp/pdf/bbp/Exp_to_Blood.pdf.

U.S. Department of Health and Human Services, Centers for Disease Control and Prevention. (2008). *Guideline for Disinfection and Sterilization in Healthcare Facilities, 2008.* Retrieved January 10, 2010, from www.cdc.gov/hicpac/pdf/guidelines/Disinfection_Nov_2008.pdf.

U.S. Department of Labor, Occupational Safety and Health Administration. (2009). *Bloodborne Pathogens and Needlestick Prevention.* Retrieved November 16, 2009, from www.osha.gov/SLTC/bloodbornepathogens/index.html.

Venes, D., (ed.) (2009). *Taber's Cyclopedic Medical Dictionary* (21st ed.). Philadelphia: F. A. Davis.

CHAPTER 1

# Infection Control and Medical Asepsis

## Words to Know Challenge

**Spelling: Each line contains three spellings of a word. Underline the correctly spelled word.**

| | | |
|---|---|---|
| 1. obligate | abligate | oblegate |
| 2. susceptable | susseptible | susceptible |
| 3. rickettsiae | ricettsiae | rickettcia |
| 4. anirobes | anaerobes | anerobes |
| 5. pathagens | pathogens | pathegins |
| 6. acepcis | accepses | asepsis |
| 7. exudative | xudative | exudadiv |
| 8. malaize | malaisia | malaise |
| 9. petechial | petikial | patechial |
| 10. higene | hygiene | hyjiene |

**Matching: Match the term in column I to its definition in column II.**

| | COLUMN I | COLUMN II |
|---|---|---|
| J | 1. Bacteria | A. Pressurized device used to sterilize |
| H | 2. Communicable | B. The eggs of a louse or other parasitic insect |
| E | 3. Virus | C. Single-celled animal |
| G | 4. Pruritic | D. Organism or substance that poses a threat to human health |
| B | 5. Nits | E. Unicellular microorganism; disease-causing agent |
| I | 6. Aerobe | F. Involving entry into living tissue |
| D | 7. Biohazardous | G. Pertaining to an itching sensation |
| A | 8. Autoclave | H. Transmitted from one person to another |
| C | 9. Protozoa | I. Lives and grows only in the presence of oxygen |
| F | 10. Invasive | J. Microorganisms capable of replicating within living cells |

Chapter

# 2

# The Medical History and Patient Screening

## CHAPTER OBJECTIVES

In this chapter, you will learn the following:

### KB KNOWLEDGE BASE

1. Spell and define, using the glossary at the back of this text, all the Words to Know in this chapter.
2. Explain the purpose of screening in today's medical office.
3. Describe the process for screening and determining the urgency of a patient's condition.
4. Identify the skills necessary to conduct a patient interview.
5. List the characteristics of the patient's chief complaint and the present illness.
6. Explain the purpose of obtaining a health history.
7. Identify the components of the health history form and their documentation.
8. Compare and contrast the patient's medical, family, and social and occupational histories.
9. Discuss the genogram and explain why it is useful.
10. Explain how the review of systems is obtained and documented.

### S SKILLS

1. Perform in-person screening.
2. Obtain and record a patient health history.

### B BEHAVIORS

1. Demonstrate professionalism by being courteous and diplomatic; showing respect, empathy, and cultural sensitivity; maintaining privacy and confidentiality; and adapting to change.
2. Apply critical thinking skills in performing patient assessment and care.
3. Use language and verbal skills that enable patients' understanding and appropriate, congruent body language and other nonverbal skills.
4. Apply active listening skills.
5. Demonstrate awareness of the territorial boundaries of the person with whom communicating.
6. Demonstrate recognition of the patient's level of understanding in communications.
7. Analyze communications in providing appropriate responses and feedback.
8. Recognize and protect personal boundaries in communicating with others.
9. Demonstrate sensitivity to patient rights.
10. Use time management and anticipation skills.

## WORDS TO KNOW

allergies
biases
chief complaint (CC)
clinical diagnosis
emergent
familial
genogram
interview
objective
over-the-counter (OTC)
patronizing
prioritizing
remedies
screening
subjective
symptoms
triage

## PATIENT SCREENING

**Screening** is the process of obtaining information from patients to determine who will be the most beneficial to handle their needs. As a medical assistant, one of your responsibilities is to perform both incoming phone call screening (covered in Chapter 9) and in-person screening. Phone screening occurs in some form every time a patient calls into the medical facility, whereas in-person screening occurs in the office every time the patient is seen to identify the **chief complaint (CC)** presented as well as secondary conditions. A more intense form of this process was originated during wartimes and was referred to as **triage**, a concept developed by the military and particularly applicable to trauma and disaster situations. It referred to the sorting and assessment of soldiers' injuries. The French word *triage* means "to sort." After the medics made a decision regarding the seriousness of the wounds, the soldier was taken as soon as possible for treatment. Those in charge of treatment had a clear description of the nature of the wounds from the initial triage.

In addition, triage is a term also used in **prioritizing** the conditions of the injured following a disaster. The injured were separated into groups according to the seriousness of their needs. Usually, they were tagged with a particular color-coded tape or cloth so that the other members of the emergency medical team would know which victims required immediate attention. As discussed more in Unit 18, the rules regarding those who have **emergent** conditions should be given first priority. Conditions that are not life threatening can wait a short time.

Many of the emergent conditions are rarely (if ever) seen initially in the physician's office in metropolitan areas due to the presence of emergency medical services and hospital emergency rooms. The word *screening* has replaced the term *triage* because it is more appropriate for the process used in the medical office.

When conducting the screening process, you must communicate in the most efficient and effective manner for each individual. Patients may be shy or embarrassed by their problems or questions and may not ask and answer direct questions. Therefore, excellent listening skills are vital to understanding what the patient is trying to convey. Be familiar with information about the patient before proceeding with an explanation. This will help determine how to communicate best with each individual.

### CLINICAL PEARL

Never assume that a patient already knows the information you are conveying. Sometimes a patient will state that he or she understands something to keep from being embarrassed. If you sense that this is the situation, you should briefly repeat the information to ensure that you are receiving the information accurately.

## IN-PERSON SCREENING

In-person screening is the first step taken between the patient and you to make their experience at the office beneficial. Talking to patients one on one and asking questions about their condition requires professional communication skills and the assurance of privacy. Some offices may have a private area specifically for screening (Figure 37–1). Other offices conduct the screening and **interview** in the privacy of the examination room. It is important to remember that all of the data obtained is subject to legal and ethical considerations and must remain confidential. Patients are entitled to certain rights, and these rights must be enforced. (Refer to "Patient Bill of Rights" in Unit 3.) Your ability to obtain and accurately record information received from the patient is crucial. Your goal is to determine why the patient is seeking health care; what he or she sees as the main problem; any other concerns he or she may have; and what, if anything, he or she has done about it.

The purpose of the screening is to help patients focus on their main concern, the CC, and its related **symptoms**. After this is established, it may be necessary to continue the screening to obtain and record other health concerns. For example, a work-in patient whose chief complaint is severe muscle spasms of the back may also express concern because of occasional irregular heartbeats and an increasing need to take antacids for indigestion. These complaints need to be recorded and will probably require an additional visit to address, depending on the severity of the symptoms due to previous patient scheduling.

The patient's initial visit will require varying amounts of questioning depending upon the reason for the visit. Someone requesting a complete physical, but who has no complaints, will not require the in-depth inquiry that someone would who has complaints of intermittent pain, fever, and fatigue for the past two weeks. Face-

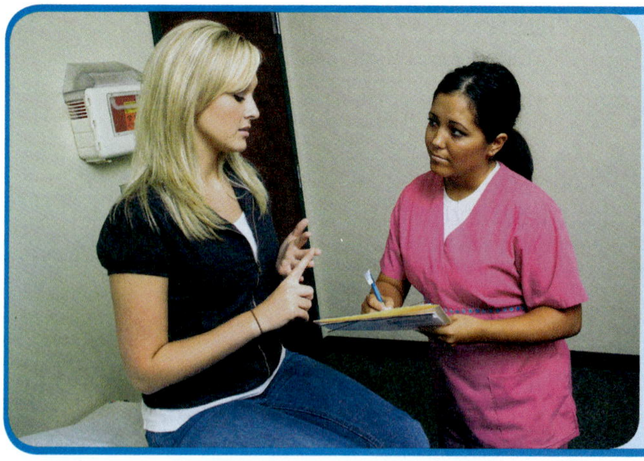

**Figure 37–1:** A medical assistant and patient are in a private area discussing symptoms and assessing the patient's condition. This is called in-person screening. *Delmar/Cengage Learning.*

to-face screening is also required when patients return for follow-up visits. The line of questioning then is to determine how they have felt since the last office visit. Establishing an accurate database is a very important duty because it is the beginning of the patient's medical record with the physician.

When patients are called into the office, the medical assistant makes the initial personal contact to begin gathering the information that relates to their reason for the office visit. It is important to not appear rushed or as if just performing a routine task. Because this is the patients' first visit, they may be naturally ill at ease and nervous about seeing a new provider, especially if they fear they may have a serious condition. This in-person screening procedure requires a professional approach and is critical to the patient's perception of the practice.

Following the determination of a clear reason the patient is there, it is generally customary on the patient's first visit to obtain an accurate and comprehensive personal and family health history. A complete history is very revealing and a great aid in diagnosing conditions.

**CLINICAL PEARL**

To follow HIPAA privacy standards, be sure to get the patient's approval to involve another person in the discussion of his or her private health information. Document the permission; without documentation, it is considered "not permitted." For more information about HIPAA, refer to Unit 4.

## Factors Influencing Screening

Successfully conducting the first interview with a new patient establishes a favorable relationship among the patient, you, and the practice. Many factors must be considered to make that experience as beneficial as possible. The following gives you some things to remember when you are talking with the patient.

- *Ensure privacy*: Not only in the setting, but also assure the patient that the information you are gathering will be protected within the privacy policy of the office.
- *Be aware of your* **biases**: Our beliefs and behaviors tend to influence how we view others. All patients must be treated with respect without evaluating them based on their race, religion, sexual orientation, cultural or ethnic origin, or socioeconomic or educational status. Take care that your value system does not interfere with what you hear or observe.
- *Establish a non-threatening, relaxed atmosphere*:
    - Greet the patient by name.
    - State your name.
    - Explain what you would like to do.
    - You may say something like this: "Mrs. Green, I am Ginny, Dr. Long's medical assistant. I would like to ask you a few questions about what brought you to the office today. Would you be willing to share this information with me?"
- *Be aware of your own nonverbal messages*: Be attentive and give eye contact so the patient can tell you are interested in who he or she is and what he or she has to say. Do not be overly involved with note taking or watching the time.
- *Be sure the patient understands*: Using medical terminology is not appropriate for most patients. Pay attention to their expressions as you talk. Is there a hearing problem or a lack of understanding? Responses to questions will usually indicate any difficulty. Repeating or restating the question will probably be sufficient. If there is a language barrier, it may be necessary to enlist help from an approved translator. Someone who is hearing or speech impaired will require a person who can sign your questions and speak for them (Figure 37–2).
- *Allow the patient to do most of the talking*: Remember, you are trying to learn about his or her condition and concerns.
- *Listen attentively to what the patient says*: Be an active listener; ask questions to be sure you understand what was said. You can repeat what you think the patient stated to see whether he or she agrees.
- *Nonverbal communication*: Watch the patient's body language; does it agree with what he or she is saying? This may take some experience. For example, if the patient does not look at you when answering personal questions, is it because of embarrassment or is he or she not being truthful? For example, a married

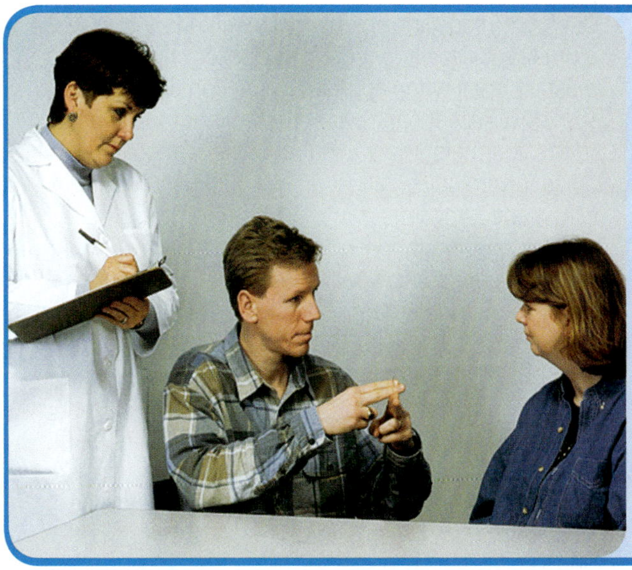

**Figure 37–2:** A person who can sign may be needed to assist with the patient interview. *Delmar/Cengage Learning.*

person seeking care because of a sexually transmitted disease acquired from an affair may be reluctant to tell anyone other than the provider. Additionally, it may be none of these but rather due to a cultural difference.

- *Use open-ended questions*: These ask for more than a yes or no answer and provide the opportunity for additional information. Asking, "How would you describe your pain?" will get you more information than asking, "Do you have pain now?"
- *Focus on the interview*: Do not allow the conversation to go off course.
- *Conclude the screening portion of the interview with a summary*: State to the patient what has been identified and recorded as the chief complaint and any additional concerns in decreasing order of importance. With the patient's agreement, record the CC and other data.

## Conducting the In-Person Screening

What is done by the medical assistant during the in-person screening will be determined by the employing provider. Some providers prefer the medical assistant to do only the chief complaint, and the providers conduct the in-depth interview so they have the advantage of getting the information personally. Other providers want all preliminary questioning done by the medical assistant so they can review it briefly and begin their examination. Detailed information is provided later in the chapter regarding the health history form, the components, and what information is obtained in each section.

### CLINICAL PEARL

One very important aspect of patient care is your attitude toward the patient. The medical assistant must be open when approaching patients. This means you must accept each patient as an individual who needs your help. There is no room in the medical office for prejudice. All patients should be treated with respect regardless of their financial status, race, religion, age, or station in life. Remember, your job is to provide assistance. Calling patients by pet names or terms of endearment (e.g., Honey, Hon, and Dear) may be taken as **patronizing**, especially if your attitude is questionable. It is more respectful to patients if you call them by their titles (i.e., Mr. or Ms.) or their full names. The patient will let you know if a first-name basis is all right with him or her. If the patient senses any negative feelings on your part, he or she will be less likely to pay attention to your instructions and suggestions.

## Developing the Chief Complaint

After introducing yourself to the new patient, establishing a comfortable environment, and requesting the patient's assistance, it is time to start the interview. Begin by asking what brought the patient to the office today, the CC. Record the CC in the patient's own words on the chart or electronic medical record (EMR) and then add other descriptive information given by the patient. By asking the patient to describe certain characteristics regarding the symptoms, you can ensure that the chief complaint is documented thoroughly. The following are examples of aspects to have the patient consider:

- *Location:* Where is the symptom located?
- *Radiation:* What area does the symptom cover?
- *Quality:* Describe the characteristic of the symptom, for instance, "dull ache," "throbbing," "tingling," and so on.
- *Severity:* Describe the pain associated with the symptom. (A pain scale such as the one in Figure 37–3 can be used.)
- *Associated symptoms:* Describe other minor symptoms in addition to the CC.
- *Aggravating factors:* Describe what makes symptoms worse.
- *Alleviating factors:* Describe what makes the symptoms better.
- *Setting and timing:* Describe when the symptoms started and what the patient was doing at the time.

When the patient has identified all the complaints and together you have determined the specifics of the symptoms, you can summarize the results of your screening. Read to the patient what you have written on the chart or entered into the EMR and ask whether there is anything else to add. The finished statement may read something like this:

| | |
|---|---|
| 8/6/XX<br>11:30 am | CC: "I have a pain in my stomach." RLQ, Pain level 4, intermittent ×3 days, nausea, no vomiting or diarrhea. Some relief by lying down.<br>G. Jenks, RMA(AMT) |

Procedure 37–1 provides a generic guide for in-person screening of a patient.

After obtaining this initial information, you are ready to proceed with interviewing and reviewing the patient's health history. Completing both these tasks establishes a good basis for not only diagnosing and treating the patient's current condition but also understanding the patient's and the family's past health conditions, which might have some bearing on the present.

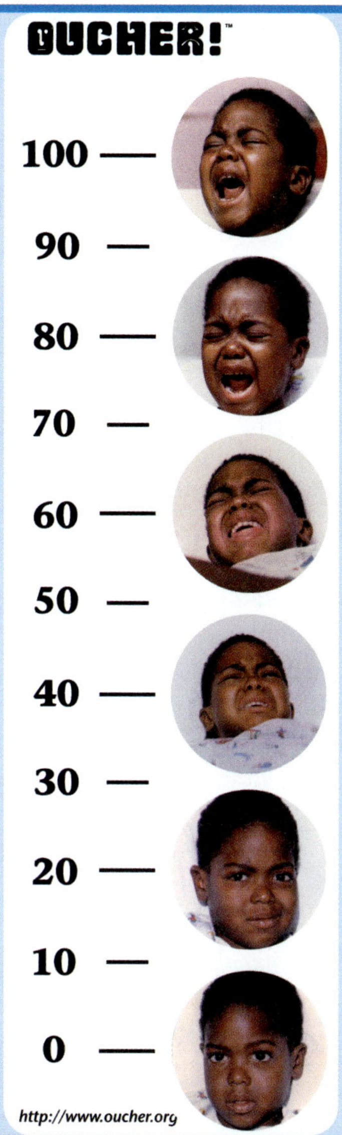


**Figure 37–3:** The OUCHER! pain scale. *Courtesy of the Pain Associates of Nursing, www.oucher.org.*

**CLINICAL PEARL**

Pain assessment can be challenging because patients may experience a comparable condition or surgical procedure; however, their pain response can vary considerably. Individuals of every age and culture experience pain, and many practitioners consider pain a fifth vital sign. Because pain is **subjective**, it is whatever the experiencing person says it is and exists whenever the experiencing person says it does. Today, health care providers are more perceptive to pain and recognize that unrelieved pain can have both physiological and psychological effects on patients. Constant pain can slow recovery, create hassles for patients and their families, and increase the cost of care.

## THE HEALTH HISTORY

A patient's health history is a comprehensive medical history that includes information about the patient and the patient's family. Information incorporated in the history includes previous illnesses, medications, allergies, and surgical history. The health history is the basis for all treatment given by the provider and is a guide for future treatment of the patient. The history is helpful for patients and providers when patients are seen by a provider who is not their primary provider or when referred to a specialist. This information gives them useful information about past and present health concerns and saves them time from not having to collect that data again. In addition to providing the patient comprehensive health information for the provider, health histories can also provide statistical data to research companies and the health department as well as insurance data.

The health history is acquired when the patient is new to the facility. In general, before extensive care is provided to new patients, a complete physical exam is performed and a complete and thorough medical history is obtained so the providers have a good idea of the patient's current and past health status as well as any family conditions that might factor into the patient's health. All patients are asked to complete a health history form at their initial visit to a provider's office. Some are mailed prior to the appointment, depending on the provider's preference, and others are completed in the office prior to the provider's examination. The standard paper health history form can vary, depending on the type of practice, from short and concise to fairly comprehensive (Figure 37–4). Notice at the end of the comprehensive form a statement regarding errors or omissions. The absence of pertinent information could result in a misdiagnosis, a consequence that this form addresses.

As part of your duties as a medical assistant, you may need to assist in the completion of the history. Refer to Procedure 37–2 to help you practice interviewing a patient. With a copy of a history form or the one included in the workbook, proceed through the form, asking clarifying questions and recording patient information. Include any significant additional remarks in your notes on the patient's chart. If you have access to a computer with office practice software, proceed through the form and enter the patient's responses directly into the EMR.

The patient might need help with some unfamiliar medical terms and some confusing questions. Language, literacy, cultural, and other barriers can prevent completion. Assist these patients with respect and without judgment. Some providers may wish to interview and complete the form themselves as a means to gain insight into the patient's condition. You will need to be familiar with the individual provider's preference.

## PROCEDURE 37–1 Perform In-Person Screening

**MEDIA LINK:** View the video for this chapter, "Developing a Chief Complaint," on the Premium Website.

**PURPOSE:** To conduct an in-person screening to identify and accurately record the patient's chief complaint (CC) and related symptoms in the patient's medical record.

**EQUIPMENT:** Patient's chart or computer with appropriate software, pen, any supplies or equipment needed to set up the room according to the reason for the patient being seen.

**S SKILL:** Perform In-Person Screening

| | Procedure Steps | Detailed Instructions and/or *Rationales* |
|---|---|---|
| B | 1. ***Select a private location for the interview.*** | *Talking to patients one on one and asking questions about their personal condition requires professional communication skills and the assurance of privacy and confidentiality.* |
| | 2. Review any completed office forms, including the HIPAA authorization agreement. | *This saves time and helps the medical assistant identify why the patient is there and determine whether any assistance is needed.* |
| B | 3. ***Call the patient by name from the reception room.*** | The general rule is to use the patient's full name unless the patient has requested something different. |
| B | 4. ***Take the patient to the interview area and make the patient comfortable.*** | Sitting face to face to begin the interview allows for eye contact with the patient. |
| | 5. Restate the patient's name and introduce yourself. | *This helps build rapport.* |
| B | 6. ***Explain what you will be doing and request participation.*** | *This shows respect for the patient and provides helpful information for the provider.* |
| | 7. Ask what brings the person to the office today. | |
| | 8. Use questioning to focus on the CC, its characteristics, and any related symptoms. | *Certain characteristics should be obtained for a complete understanding of why the patient is being seen.* |
| | 9. Identify and record any secondary concerns. | *Due to the allotted time for the appointment, these might need to be addressed at a future appointment, depending on the severity.* |
| | 10. Ask the patient whether he or she is taking any medications. | *Be sure to include prescription, over-the-counter (OTC), and herbal supplements. Include the dosages and reason for taking them.* |
| | 11. Ask the patient whether he or she has any allergies. | Be sure to include all medications, food, and environmental allergies. |
| | 12. Reconfirm the CC, symptoms, and any other concerns with the patient. | *This clarifies that the information you obtained is accurate.* |
| | 13. Record the CC statement and related information on the chart or EMR. | Concise documentation is essential in providing an accurate account of the patient's visit. *Documentation identifies the person responsible for providing the screening.* |
| B | 14. ***Set up the room according to the patient's complaint, demonstrating time management and anticipation skills.*** | *This enhances the patient's visit by saving time for the provider, making the visit more efficient.* |

| Procedure Steps | Detailed Instructions and/or *Rationales* |
|---|---|
| B 15. ***Dismiss yourself in a professional manner and indicate to the patient the approximate wait time.*** | *This is provided as a courtesy to the patient so he or she can anticipate the wait time.* |
| 16. Notify the provider that the patient is ready to be seen. | |

**Charting Example**

| | |
|---|---|
| 8/6/XX 11:30 am | CC, "I have a pain in my stomach." RLQ, pain level 6, intermittent, ×3 days, nausea, no vomiting or diarrhea. Some relief from lying down. Patient not on any medications at this time. Patient has NKDA. G. Jenks, RMA(AMT) |

With electronic health records (EHR) software becoming more abundant in the medical office, another common way to collect the history data is electronically. Some facilities enter the data obtained from the paper copy or scan the paper copy the patient fills out into the system. Other systems allow the patient to fill out the forms ahead of time via a patient portal, either in the comfort of his or her home with access to a computer or by a kiosk inside of the facility prior to the appointment. Most of the electronic versions of the health history forms have drop-down lists within the system, making it quicker and easier for the patient to fill in the information. These systems are also easier to update if changes need to be made rather than having the patient fill out an annual paper form. Figure 37–5 shows a screen shot of a completed patient medical history (PMH) form from an EHR program. Whichever technique is used, it may be your responsibility as a medical assistant to review the history with the patient to be certain that all of the data collected is accurate. Before calling the patient in for the in-person screening, if the patient has completed the form ahead of time, you should obtain the form from the receptionist and review its contents.

## Reviewing the Patient's Health History

As mentioned earlier, even if the patient has completed the form in its entirety, you must still review all the information for omission and clarity. For instance, if a patient checks "hazardous substances" under occupational concerns, it would be important to identify what those substances are. Another question might arise about who is a "blood relative." You must be thoroughly familiar with the form used by your employer and be prepared to answer any questions. In the sample form in Figure 37–4, notice that not only the patient but also the person reviewing the form must sign and date the document. The validity of this baseline document can become very important later in the patient's course of treatment.

**CLINICAL PEARL**

Note that if the form is not completed, the patient may have a language barrier or reading problem. If this is the case, the patient may be very sensitive about his or her inability to read and write. It may be necessary for you to ask the questions and help complete the form for such a patient. Use tact when asking whether a patient needs assistance with the form.

## Sections of the Health History

Most medical facilities have a standard health history form, or electronic template if using EHR, that will be used for all patients. A four-page history form developed for an oncology practice is included in the workbook to provide you with an interview experience. Regardless of the specific form used, some information requests are standard and are elaborated in the next sections.

### Chief Complaint

The chief complaint (CC) is why the patient is being seen currently in the office. It should be short and written with precision and conciseness and should contain the subjective and objective data that the patient discusses. Information you receive from patients is subjective, meaning it is based upon symptoms they feel. Subjective symptoms or sensations are those that only the patient can perceive, such as pain, dizziness, itching, or numbness. Information or symptoms that can be observed (that are perceptible to other people), such as swelling, bruising, vital signs, and physical examination findings, are known as **objective** findings. It is important for you to know the difference. These two distinctions become necessary when you proceed with recording information

## CONFIDENTIAL HEALTH HISTORY

Name: ______________________ Date: __________

Birthdate: __________ Age: ______ Date of last physical examination: __________

Occupation: ______________________

Reason for visit today: ______________________

| **MEDICATIONS** List all medications you are currently taking | **ALLERGIES** List all allergies |
|---|---|
| | |
| | |
| | |
| | |

**SYMPTOMS** Check ( ✓ ) symptoms you currently have or have had in the past year.

**GENERAL**

- ☐ Chills
- ☐ Depression
- ☐ Dizziness
- ☐ Fainting
- ☐ Fever
- ☐ Forgetfulness
- ☐ Headache
- ☐ Loss of sleep
- ☐ Loss of weight
- ☐ Nervousness
- ☐ Numbness
- ☐ Sweats

**MUSCLE/JOINT/BONE**

Pain, weakness, numbness in:

- ☐ Arms
- ☐ Hips
- ☐ Back
- ☐ Legs
- ☐ Feet
- ☐ Neck
- ☐ Hands
- ☐ Shoulders

**GENITO-URINARY**

- ☐ Blood in urine
- ☐ Frequent urination
- ☐ Lack of bladder control
- ☐ Painful urination

**GASTROINTESTINAL**

- ☐ Appetite poor
- ☐ Bloating
- ☐ Bowel changes
- ☐ Constipation
- ☐ Diarrhea
- ☐ Excessive hunger
- ☐ Excessive thirst
- ☐ Gas
- ☐ Hemorrhoids
- ☐ Indigestion
- ☐ Nausea
- ☐ Rectal bleeding
- ☐ Stomach pain
- ☐ Vomiting
- ☐ Vomiting blood

**CARDIOVASCULAR**

- ☐ Chest pain
- ☐ High blood pressure
- ☐ Irregular heart beat
- ☐ Low blood pressure
- ☐ Poor circulation
- ☐ Rapid heart beat
- ☐ Swelling of ankles
- ☐ Varicose veins

**EYE, EAR, NOSE, THROAT**

- ☐ Bleeding gums
- ☐ Blurred vision
- ☐ Crossed eyes
- ☐ Difficulty swallowing
- ☐ Double vision
- ☐ Earache
- ☐ Ear discharge
- ☐ Hay fever
- ☐ Hoarseness
- ☐ Loss of hearing
- ☐ Nosebleeds
- ☐ Persistent cough
- ☐ Ringing in ears
- ☐ Sinus problems
- ☐ Vision - Flashes
- ☐ Vision - Halos

**SKIN**

- ☐ Bruise easily
- ☐ Hives
- ☐ Itching
- ☐ Change in moles
- ☐ Rash
- ☐ Scars
- ☐ Sores that won't heal

**MEN only**

- ☐ Breast lump
- ☐ Erection difficulties
- ☐ Lump in testicles
- ☐ Penis discharge
- ☐ Sore on penis
- ☐ Other

**WOMEN only**

- ☐ Abnormal Pap Smear
- ☐ Bleeding between periods
- ☐ Breast lump
- ☐ Extreme menstrual pain
- ☐ Hot flashes
- ☐ Nipple discharge
- ☐ Painful intercourse
- ☐ Vaginal discharge
- ☐ Other

Date of last menstrual period __________

Date of last Pap Smear __________

Have you had a mammogram? __________

Are you pregnant? __________

Number of children __________

**MEDICAL HISTORY** Check ( ✓ ) the medical conditions you have or have had in the past.

- ☐ AIDS
- ☐ Alcoholism
- ☐ Anemia
- ☐ Anorexia
- ☐ Appendicitis
- ☐ Arthritis
- ☐ Asthma
- ☐ Bleeding Disorders
- ☐ Breast Lump
- ☐ Bronchitis
- ☐ Bulimia
- ☐ Cancer
- ☐ Cataracts
- ☐ Chemical Dependency
- ☐ Chicken Pox
- ☐ Diabetes
- ☐ Emphysema
- ☐ Epilepsy
- ☐ Gall Bladder Disease
- ☐ Glaucoma
- ☐ Goiter
- ☐ Gonorrhea
- ☐ Gout
- ☐ Heart Disease
- ☐ Hepatitis
- ☐ Hernia
- ☐ Herpes
- ☐ High Cholesterol
- ☐ HIV Positive
- ☐ Kidney Disease
- ☐ Liver Disease
- ☐ Measles
- ☐ Migraine Headaches
- ☐ Miscarriage
- ☐ Mononucleosis
- ☐ Multiple Sclerosis
- ☐ Mumps
- ☐ Pacemaker
- ☐ Pneumonia
- ☐ Polio
- ☐ Prostate Problem
- ☐ Psychiatric Care
- ☐ Rheumatic Fever
- ☐ Scarlet Fever
- ☐ Stroke
- ☐ Suicide Attempt
- ☐ Thyroid Problems
- ☐ Tonsillitis
- ☐ Tuberculosis
- ☐ Typhoid Fever
- ☐ Ulcers
- ☐ Vaginal Infections
- ☐ Venereal Disease

CONFIDENTIAL HEALTH HISTORY

**Figure 37–4:** Comprehensive Health History form. *Delmar/Cengage Learning.*

**HOSPITALIZATIONS**

| Year | Hospital | Reason for Hospitalization and Outcome |
| --- | --- | --- |
| | | |
| | | |
| | | |
| | | |
| | | |
| | | |
| | | |

**Have you ever had a blood transfusion?** ☐ Yes ☐ No

If yes, please give approximate dates: ______

| OCCUPATIONAL CONCERNS Check (✓) if your work exposes you to the following: | HEALTH HABITS Check (✓) which substances you use and indicate how much you use per day/week. | PREGNANCY HISTORY Year of Birth | Sex of Birth | Complications if any |
| --- | --- | --- | --- | --- |
| ☐ Stress | ☐ Caffeine | | | |
| ☐ Hazardous Substances | ☐ Tobacco | | | |
| ☐ Heavy Lifting | ☐ Drugs | | | |
| ☐ Other | ☐ Alcohol | | | |

| SERIOUS ILLNESS/INJURIES | DATE | OUTCOME |
| --- | --- | --- |
| | | |
| | | |
| | | |
| | | |

**FAMILY HISTORY** Fill in health information about your family.

| Relation | Age | State of Health | Age at Death | Cause of Death | Check (✓) if your blood relatives had any of the following Disease | Relationship to you |
| --- | --- | --- | --- | --- | --- | --- |
| Father | | | | | ☐ Arthritis, Gout | |
| Mother | | | | | ☐ Asthma, Hay Fever | |
| Brothers | | | | | ☐ Cancer | |
| | | | | | ☐ Chemical Dependency | |
| | | | | | ☐ Diabetes | |
| | | | | | ☐ Heart Disease, Strokes | |
| Sisters | | | | | ☐ High Blood Pressure | |
| | | | | | ☐ Kidney Disease | |
| | | | | | ☐ Tuberculosis | |
| | | | | | ☐ Other | |

I certify that the above information is correct to the best of my knowledge. I will not hold my doctor or any members of his/her staff responsible for any errors or ommisions that I may have made in the completion of this form.

______ Signature ______ Date

______ Reviewed By ______ Date

## PATIENT EDUCATION

The medical assistant is often involved in patient education, which can include supplying information about diseases and disorders, explaining diagnostic tests, and providing instruction in health care procedures. Recording the patient's health history may identify areas in which educational materials can be helpful. Your office policy may make it appropriate for you to mention these resources. To instruct a patient properly, the medical assistant must know the material. Be prepared to answer any questions from the patient. If you cannot answer one of the patient's questions, tell the patient that you do not know the answer but will ask the physician. Never try to answer a question that you are not prepared to discuss. You could give incorrect information that could harm the patient's well-being. Never give information that is beyond your scope of practice. In teaching a patient about health care and all that is involved in medical well-being, the primary goal of the medical assistant should be good communication. Refer to Chapter 8 for more on patient education and detailed information about instructing patients according to their needs.

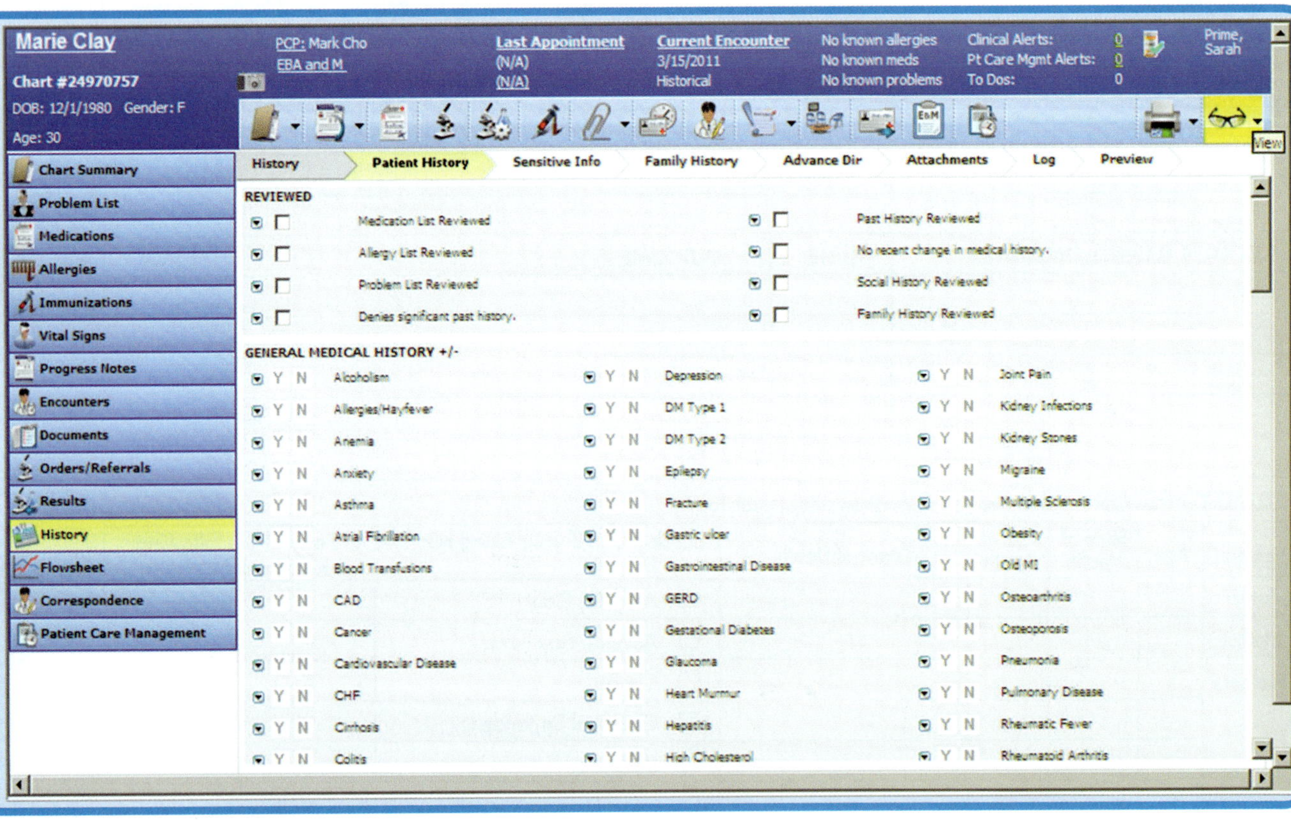

**Figure 37–5:** Screen shot of a completed patient medical history (PMH) within an EMR health history. *Courtesy of Ingenix CareTracker.*

on the chart. As discussed in Chapter 13, many providers use a method called SOAP (subjective, objective, assessment, and plan) for recording data regarding the patient's office visit. The assessment is made by the provider upon examination, and the plan refers to what course or courses of action will be taken.

### Present Illness

The patient will be asked to elaborate on the present illness (PI) or history of present illness (HPI), which will include detailed information about the chief complaint, including when the problem started, concerns on what the patient has done for the condition, and whether any treatment was attempted (such as **over-the-counter [OTC]** medications, vitamins and herbal supplements, or home **remedies**) and, if so, what they were and whether they were effective.

### Medical History

The past history (PH) or past medical history (PMH) section identifies all health problems, illnesses, or disorders ever diagnosed and surgeries. In the example, the sections are divided into symptoms during the past year and the history, which refers to present and past *diseases* and *disorders*. Usual childhood diseases (UCHD) are also included in the medical history section, which can help patients remember previous illnesses or symptoms they may have forgotten. Notice some questions are gender specific, and others deal with serious illnesses and hospitalizations. The hospitalization section should include all hospitalizations and any surgeries the patient has had.

If not included in the present illness section, two very important sections within the history list current medications being taken, including dosages and the reason the patient is taking them and a listing of any **allergies** the patient may have. In addition to the health history form, medications and allergies should be discussed with the patient at every visit. Drug reactions and interactions, from both prescribed and OTC medications, can cause significant symptoms. Some offices identify allergies with red ink or separate labels attached to the chart. Always question the patient about any allergies to drugs, including OTC and herbal supplements, food, or environmental factors because true allergic reactions can be very serious, even life-threatening. If the patient indicates he or she does not have any allergies, enter "No known drug allergies" (NKDA) on the form and in the initial charting to indicate the question was addressed and not overlooked.

## Family Health History

Most forms also request information about the health status of the immediate family members. These data, in addition to the physical examination, assist the provider with not only the information necessary to arrive at a diagnosis and treatment for the current complaint but also perhaps to forewarn and possibly prevent future conditions that tend to develop within families. The family history (FH) section asks for ages and status of health or age and cause of death for immediate family members. Family members should include siblings, parents, grandparents (maternal and paternal), aunts, uncles, and children. Some forms ask about the incidence of specific diseases among blood relatives and or provide space to add any other conditions.

Providers who treat **familial** disorders and diseases may also use another type of history form called a **genogram**. Figure 37–6 illustrates a family's medical history. Most genograms include at least three generations. This provides visual information to the provider that is helpful in determining the patient's chances of developing a disease that has genetic tendencies.

## Social/Occupational History

It is also necessary to determine the patient's personal or lifestyle habits. A patient's lifestyle can have a huge impact on the prevention or creation of certain diseases or conditions. Patients may not want to answer questions pertaining to some of the sensitive subjects in this area and may need to be asked again later by the provider. The excessive use of some prescribed drugs can lead to a dependency the same as with illegal drugs. Alcohol and tobacco are commonly abused substances and may require assistance to control. If any habits are problematic, they may be addressed by the provider. You may be instructed to provide the patient with educational materials related to the problem and to make him or her aware of any community resources or office-sponsored meetings related to the habit.

Work history for the patient is also conducted in this area. Certain occupations may contribute to industrial diseases by exposure to harmful chemicals such as asbestos, coal, and pesticides. Noise level from certain factories can also be problematic. Questioning the patient about the hazardous occupation and how long he or she was employed in that occupation can help in determining illnesses that may have been associated from this or could result in the future.

Additional questioning about the patient's living environment, firearm practices, hobbies, sexual practices, diet, and exercise can also provide insight into his or her health history and give the provider greater detail about the patient's health status and direction.

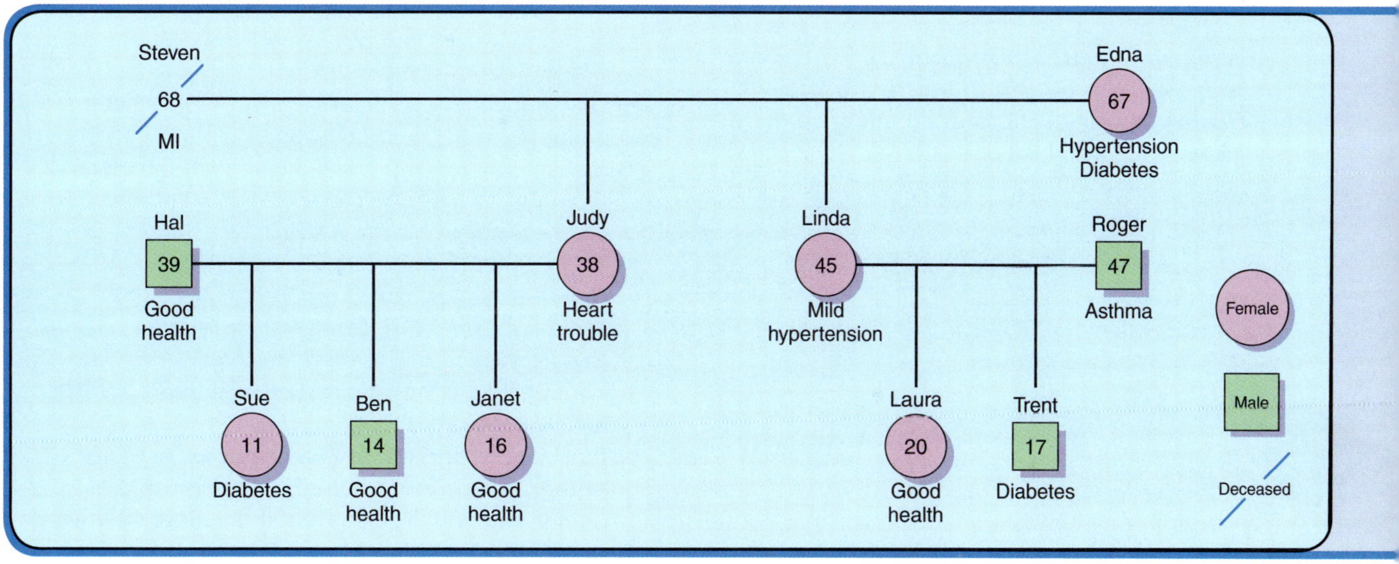


**Figure 37–6:** Example of a genogram tracing a family's medical history. *Delmar/Cengage Learning.*

## PROCEDURE 37–2 Obtain and Record a Patient Health History

**MEDIA LINK:** View the video for this chapter, "Reviewing a Patient's Health History," on the Premium Website.

**PURPOSE:** To obtain and record a comprehensive health history of a patient, including family, occupational, and social factors; to facilitate the diagnosis and health care plan for the patient.

**EQUIPMENT:** Health history form, and pen or computer with appropriate software. Using the computer or copies of a medical history form and a pen, obtain and record a medical history by interviewing a person and reviewing the completed form. Allergies are identified or "NKDA" stated. All areas must be addressed and the form signed as appropriate.

S **SKILL:** Obtain and Record a Patient Health History

| Procedure Steps | Detailed Instructions and/or *Rationales* |
|---|---|
| 1. If using a paper system, obtain the medical history form and pen. | |
| B 2. ***Escort the patient to a private area where you can both sit comfortably.*** | *Obtaining a history from the patient can be time consuming; you want to ensure the patient's comfort at all times.* |
| B 3. ***Sit opposite patient.*** | *Allows you to establish eye contact.* |
| B 4. ***Explain the purpose of the health history and inform the patient that all the information obtained is confidential.*** | *Helps the patient understand why the information is necessary and allows him or her to be more at ease to discuss sensitive information.* |
| B 5. If the patient completed the form prior to the visit, review the information with the patient, clarifying information and ensuring no omissions. ***Use reflection, restatement, and clarification techniques to obtain an accurate patient history.*** | *Patients may not understand what the questions are asking, omitting some of the data. Reviewing the information also allows them to elaborate on YES answers, saving time for the provider.* |
| B 6. If you are completing the form with the patient, be sure to ask all necessary questions and record or enter answers neatly and accurately. ***Use reflection, restatement, and clarification techniques to obtain an accurate patient history.*** If using EHR software, bring up the patient's medical history section on the screen and enter the information appropriately. | Following these protocols will make the interview flow smoothly and save time for the provider:<br>• Speak in a clear and distinct voice so that the patient can understand you easily.<br>• Give the patient adequate time to answer before going on to the next question.<br>• Explain any terms the patient may not understand. *A patient cannot give correct answers to inquiries he or she does not understand.*<br>• Avoid getting off the subject and discussing irrelevant topics. *This is inappropriate, unprofessional, and wastes time unless it is obvious that the patient needs to vent feelings.*<br>• List the chief complaint and characteristics for today's visit.<br>• Properly expand on all YES responses in the past history section. Be sure to list concise name of disease or condition, onset and duration, treatment, current status, and resolution if applicable. |

| Procedure Steps | Detailed Instructions and/or *Rationales* |
|---|---|
| | • Properly expand on all YES responses in the family and social or occupational sections.<br>• Ensure that all medications (including dosages and reason for taking) and allergies are identified and recorded on the chart as instructed.<br>• Be sure to include all hospitalizations and surgeries on the form. |
| 7. When finished with the form or entering the data, summarize and clarify the information with the patient. | *Helps confirm that the information is concise and accurate.* |
| B 8. ***Thank the patient and explain the next step in the examination. Ensure that the patient is comfortable and explain whether there will be a wait.*** | *This is provided as a courtesy to the patient so he or she can anticipate any wait time that might occur.* |
| 9. Chart a summary of the findings on the patient's chart or EMR. Highlight significant information as instructed. | *Allows the provider to point out any pertinent information easily that needs to be addressed with the patient.* |
| B 10. Assemble all necessary forms into the patient's chart or templates within EHR software to have them ready for the provider to use during the examination, ***demonstrating time management and anticipation skills.*** | |

## Review of Systems

After the history is completed and appropriate notations are made on the form and on the chart or in the EMR, the patient is weighed and measured and the vital signs are obtained and recorded. This completes the baseline data, and the patient is ready for the provider's examination. With the areas of concern identified, you may have an indication of what type of examination the provider will need to do. According to the office policy, you might begin preparing the patient. This could include partial or complete disrobing and putting on a gown, obtaining a urine specimen, or having the female patient empty her bladder in preparation for a pelvic exam. However, some providers feel it is preferable to meet the patient initially while she is still clothed. They will review the history form and make notations on the chart or in the EMR and conduct a brief screening conversation and then indicate which examination they will be performing.

Whichever procedure is followed, after the history is completed and the baseline measurements and vital signs recorded, express your appreciation to patients for their cooperation and indicate to them what follows next. Be sure to ask whether they have any questions. If there is apt to be a waiting period, try to estimate the time involved and offer reading materials to occupy their time. After the data are accurately recorded on the patient's chart or EMR, it is time for the provider to greet the patient and begin the medical discussion and examination.

The Review of Systems (ROS) is performed by the provider during the physical examination. An orderly and systematic check of each of the body systems is recorded. The ROS can provide information that will be essential in the current diagnostic state of the patient as well as information used as a baseline for subsequent visits. Providers' preference of how the ROS will be performed can vary; however, all the body systems as mentioned in Unit 11 are generally covered.

The provider will document all findings during the ROS, whether positive or negative, on the health history form. If the patient responds positively to an area, the provider will then ask the patient to elaborate. Using the information obtained from the health history, physical exam, ROS, and any laboratory tests completed can help the provider determine a **clinical diagnosis** for the patient. All the sections of the patient's health history must be complete to determine the patient's health condition. With a little experience, you will be able to perform an in-person screening and an interview with confidence.

## CHAPTER SUMMARY

- Screening is the process of obtaining information from patients to determine who will be the most beneficial to handle their needs. As a medical assistant, one of your responsibilities is to perform both incoming phone call screening and in-person screening.
- *Triage* is a term used in prioritizing the conditions of the injured following a disaster. The injured are separated into groups according to the seriousness of their needs. Those who have emergent conditions should be given first priority. Conditions that are not life-threatening can wait a short time.
- When conducting the screening process, you must communicate in the most efficient and effective manner for each individual. Patients may be shy or embarrassed by their problems or questions and may not ask or answer direct questions. Therefore, excellent listening skills are vital to understanding what the patient is trying to convey.
- In-person screening is the first step taken between the patient and you to make his or her experience at the office beneficial. Talking to patients one on one and asking questions about their personal condition requires professional communication skills and the assurance of privacy.
- The purpose of the screening is to help patients focus on their main concern, called the chief complaint (CC), and its related symptoms. It should be short and written with precision and conciseness and contain the subjective and objective data that the patient discusses.
- The present illness (PI) or history of present illness (HPI) includes detailed information about the chief complaint, including when the problem started, concerns on about what the patient has done for the condition, whether any over-the-counter (OTC) medications or home remedies were tried, and, if so, what they were and whether they were effective.
- Successfully conducting the first interview with a new patient establishes a favorable relationship among the patient, you, and the practice. Many factors need to be considered to make that experience as beneficial as possible.
- A patient's health history is a comprehensive medical history that includes information about the patient and the patient's family. Information incorporated in the history includes information about previous illnesses, medications, allergies, and surgical history. The health history is the basis for all treatment given by the provider and is used as a guide for future treatment of the patient.
- The past history (PH) or past medical history (PMH) section identifies all surgeries as well as health problems, illnesses, or disorders ever diagnosed.
- Most forms also request information about the health status of the immediate family members. These data, in addition to the physical examination, assist the provider with not only the information necessary to arrive at a diagnosis and treatment for the current complaint but also perhaps to forewarn and possibly prevent future conditions that tend to develop within families.
- It is also necessary to determine the patient's personal or lifestyle habits. A patient's lifestyle can have a huge impact on the prevention or creation of certain diseases or conditions.
- Providers who treat familial disorders and diseases may also use another type of history form called a genogram, which illustrates a family's medical history. Most genograms include at least three generations. This provides visual information to the provider that is helpful in determining the patient's chances of developing a disease that has genetic tendencies.
- The Review of Systems (ROS) is performed by the provider during the physical examination. An orderly and systematic check of each of the body systems is recorded. The ROS can provide information that will be essential in the current diagnostic state of the patient as well as information used as a baseline for subsequent visits.

## STUDY TOOLS

| | |
|---|---|
| **Workbook** | Activities for Chapter 37 |
| **Premium Website** | |
| MEDIA LINK | View the following **Media Link** for this chapter:<br>• Developing the Chief Complaint<br>• Reviewing the Patient's Health History |
| StudyWARE | Activities and Quizzes on the **StudyWARE™ Software** for Chapter 37 |
| | **Audio Library** of medical terms |
| | Online access to **Critical Thinking Challenge 2.0** |

| | |
|---|---|
| **CourseMate** | Activities and Quizzes for Chapter 37 |
| **WebTutor** | Activities and Quizzes for Chapter 37 |

## CHECK YOUR KNOWLEDGE

1. The purpose of screening in today's medical office is to:
   a. prioritize the condition of the injured following a disaster.
   b. tag the victims requiring immediate attention.
   c. sort and assess soldiers' injury.
   d. determine who will be the most beneficial to handle the patient's needs.
2. An example of an open-ended question would be:
   a. "How long have you had the pain?"
   b. "Does strenuous activity increase your symptoms?"
   c. "How would you describe your pain?"
   d. "Do you have pain now?"
3. Information collected in the health history includes:
   a. medications.
   b. allergies.
   c. previous illness.
   d. all of the above.
4. When a medical office has the patient fill out the health history form, areas that are incomplete may indicate the following:
   a. laziness
   b. language problem
   c. reading problem
   d. both b and c
5. A genogram determines genetic tendencies and covers how many generations?
   a. Three
   b. Four
   c. Two
   d. Five
6. Questions regarding alcohol and tobacco use would be found under the following section of the health history form:
   a. family health history
   b. review of systems
   c. social or occupational
   d. medical history
7. Where on the health history form is a systematic check of all the body systems recorded?
   a. Medical history
   b. ROS
   c. EHR
   d. Present illness
8. Having the patient elaborate on his or her present illness by asking him or her, "What makes the symptoms better?" would cover the following aspect while the screening the chief complaint.
   a. Aggravating factors
   b. Alleviating factors
   c. Associated symptoms
   d. Severity

## WEB LINK

American Medical Association: **www.ama-assn.org**

## RESOURCES

Brasin, G.A., & Favreau, C.R. (2010). *The Total Practice Management Workbook: Using e-Medsys*. Clifton Park, NY: Delmar Cengage Learning.

Estes, M. E. Z. (2010). *Health Assessment & Physical Examination* (4th ed.). Clifton Park, NY: Delmar Cengage Learning.

Heller, M., and Veach, L. (2009). *Clinical Medical Assisting: A Professional, Field Smart Approach to the Workplace*. Clifton Park, NY: Delmar Cengage Learning.

Lindh, W., Pooler, M., Tamparo, C., and Dahl, B. (2010). *Delmar's Comprehensive Medical Assisting Administrative and Clinical Competencies* (4th ed.). Clifton Park, NY: Delmar Cengage Learning.

Maki, S. E., and Petterson, B. (2008). *Using the Electronic Health Record in the Health Care Provider Practice*. Clifton Park, NY: Delmar Cengage Learning.

CHAPTER 2

# The Medical History and Patient Screening

## Words to Know Challenge

**Spelling: Each line contains three spellings of a word. Underline the correctly spelled word.**

| | | |
|---|---|---|
| 1. emergant | emergent | emirgent |
| 2. familiel | femelial | familial |
| 3. genogram | geneogram | jeanogram |
| 4. treage | triage | treeage |
| 5. clinical diagnoses | clinical diagnosis | clinicle diagnosis |
| 6. alergies | allergys | allergies |
| 7. objective | abjective | objectiev |
| 8. sabjective | subjactive | subjective |
| 9. patronizing | patranizing | peitronizing |
| 10. remadies | remedies | remedys |

**Matching: Match the term in column I to its definition in column II.**

| | COLUMN I | COLUMN II |
|---|---|---|
| ___ | 1. Screening | A. Symptoms that can be observed |
| ___ | 2. Triage | B. Referring to accessible, nonprescription drugs |
| ___ | 3. Chief complaint (CC) | C. Beliefs that influence observations |
| ___ | 4. Interview | D. Any perceptible change in the body that indicates disease |
| ___ | 5. Over-the-counter | E. Process of obtaining information from patient |
| ___ | 6. Prioritizing | F. Main reason for office visit |
| ___ | 7. Symptoms | G. Talking to patients one on one and asking questions |
| ___ | 8. Objective | H. Sort and assess injury |
| ___ | 9. Biases | I. Arranging in order of importance |

Chapter

# 3 Body Measurements and Vital Signs

## CHAPTER OBJECTIVES

In this chapter, you will learn the following:

### KB KNOWLEDGE BASE

1. Spell and define, using the glossary at the back of the text, all the Words to Know in this chapter.
2. Name five types of mensurations.
3. Explain why and when a patient's height and weight is measured.
4. Identify the four vital signs and the body functions they measure.
5. Identify the average normal temperature for aural, axillary, oral, temporal, and rectal measurement.
6. Demonstrate knowledge of basic math calculations by being able to calculate the following: foot and inch measurement conversions, weight and BMI conversions, and Celsius and Fahrenheit temperature conversions.
7. Identify normal pulse rates, describing five factors that affect the rate.
8. Identify and locate five pulse sites and explain the appropriate use of each.
9. Explain indications for apical pulse measurement.
10. Describe normal respiration and explain abnormal breathing patterns.
11. Explain what blood pressure measures.
12. Describe the appropriate equipment for obtaining a blood pressure.
13. Name the two phases of blood pressure; describe the corresponding action that occurs and the relative amount of pressure with each phase.
14. Identify normal and abnormal blood pressure, including factors affecting blood pressure.

### S SKILLS

1. Measure and record height and weight.
2. Measure and record oral temperature with an electronic thermometer.
3. Measure and record rectal temperature with an electronic thermometer.
4. Measure and record axillary temperature with an electronic thermometer.
5. Measure and record core body temperature with a tympanic (aural) thermometer.
6. Measure and record temperature with a temporal artery thermometer.
7. Measure and record radial pulse rate and respirations.
8. Measure and record apical pulse rate.
9. Measure and record blood pressure.

### B BEHAVIOR

1. Demonstrate professionalism by being courteous and diplomatic; showing respect, empathy, and cultural sensitivity; maintaining privacy and confidentiality; and adapting to change.
2. Use language/verbal skills that enable patients' understanding and appropriate, congruent body language and other nonverbal skills.
3. Apply critical thinking skills in performing patient assessment and care.

## WORDS TO KNOW

| | | | |
|---|---|---|---|
| afebrile | bradypnea | idiopathic | rectal |
| aneroid | carotid | infrared | respiration |
| antecubital | Cheyne-Stokes | inhale | rhythm |
| apex | diastole | mensuration | sphygmomanometer |
| apical | dorsalis pedis | oral | stethoscope |
| apnea | dyspnea | orthostatic | systole |
| arrhythmia | essential | palpate | tachycardia |
| aural | exhale | popliteal | tachypnea |
| auscultate | fatal | pulse | temperature |
| axillary | febrile | pulse pressure | thermometer |
| blood pressure | femoral | pyrogen | thready |
| body mass index (BMI) | groin | radial | vital signs |
| brachial | hyperventilation | rales | volume |
| bradycardia | | | |

## BODY MEASUREMENTS

Body measurements are sometimes referred to as **mensuration**, meaning the process of measuring. When used in connection with patient care, it refers to body measurements such as height and weight; length of extremities; and the circumference of head, chest, or abdomen with infants. The initial measurements are usually taken before or after the vital signs are obtained and become the baseline for all measurements that follow. Precise measurements are extremely important with infants and children to ensure that there is proper growth and development. (Refer to Chapter 42 for details about infant and child measurements.) For adults, abnormal changes could indicate the presence of a disease or disorder such as osteoporosis or fluid retention.

Measurements can also provide information concerning treatment. Some diagnostic testing relies on a patient's measurements for correct interpretation. Certain medication dosages are determined by the patient's weight (see Unit 16).

Measurements are obtained at the beginning of the patient's visit, prior to seeing the provider and usually follow the completion of recording the patient history with new patients to complete the initial base information. Any follow-up visit measurement policy will be determined by the provider. Weight may be measured at each visit and height for adults may be monitored only occasionally unless a disease condition warrants more frequent measurement. The measurement performed and the frequency of that measurement will be determined largely by the patient's condition.

### Height and Weight Measurements

Measurements are important to patients for many reasons:

- A young adult may be very interested in his height, especially those who wish to play certain sports.
- An elderly patient may be concerned about the loss of height.
- Athletes may have to gain or lose a certain amount of weight to meet regulations or goals.
- People of all ages may be interested in losing excess pounds and achieving a healthier weight range.

Measurement of height and weight are very familiar to patients, and most understand their implications. The accurate measurement of height and weight is best done on a balance beam scale (Figure 38–1). Scales should be balanced frequently and properly maintained to ensure accuracy. The scale should also sit on a firm surface. Figure 38–2 shows an electronic scale. The patient stands on the platform and the weight is displayed in the window of the unit. Many of these electronic scales have the capacity to convert units from pounds to kilograms if needed.

#### Height

Most of the balance beam scales have a height apparatus attached to them; however, there are also stand-alone devices that can be mounted to a wall. On a balance beam scale, the height bar is calibrated in inches by quarter-inch markings. When the height bar is lowered to touch the patient's head, the extension bar will indicate the height in inches on the calibrated height bar. The height should be measured to the nearest quarter of an inch. Height can be recorded in total inches or

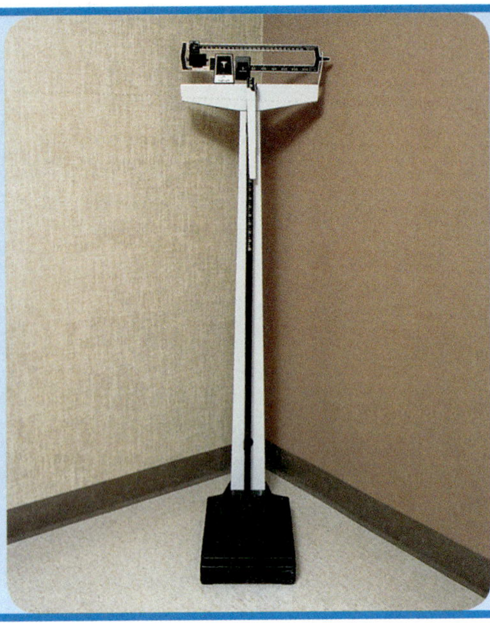

**Figure 38–1:** The traditional balance beam scales with measuring bar. *Delmar/Cengage Learning.*

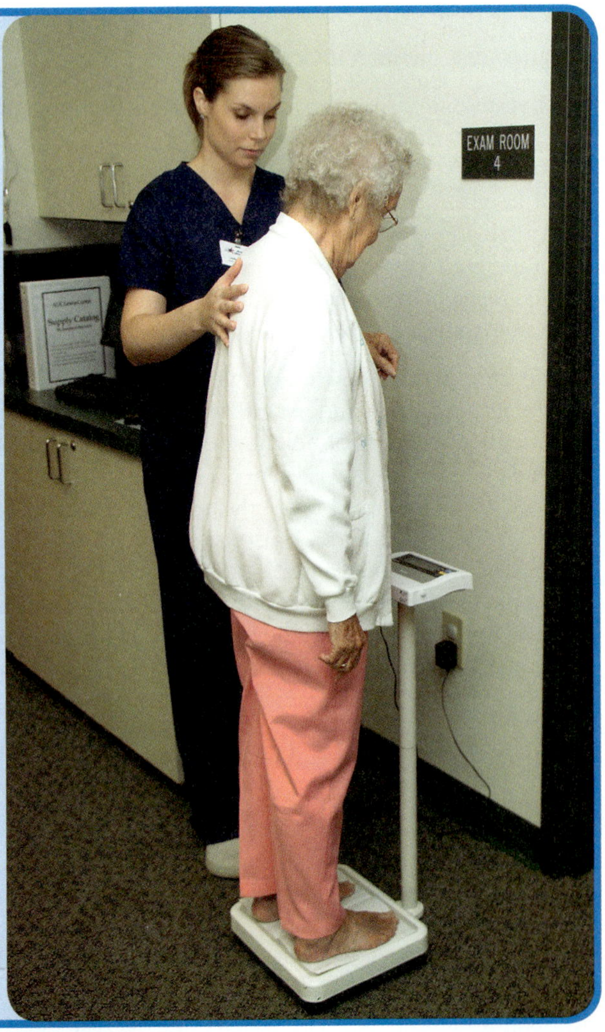


**Figure 38–2:** An electronic scale. *Delmar/Cengage Learning.*

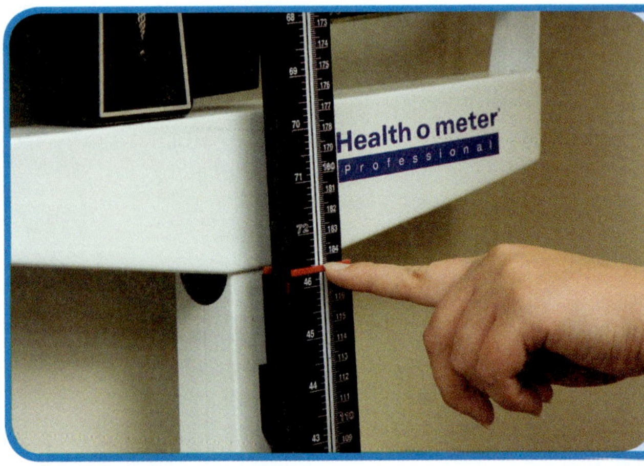


**Figure 38–3:** The height is read at the movable point on the ruler, where the two sections of the height bar meet. The bars are measured in quarter inches. *Delmar/Cengage Learning.*

converted to feet and inches, obtained by dividing the inches by the number 12 because there are 12 inches in 1 foot. The height bar in Figure 38–3 indicates where the height is read.

## Weight

Obtaining the patient's weight by using a balance beam scale requires you to manipulate the two weights on the balance bar until the pointer rests in the middle of the rectangle at the end of the frame. Before an accurate weight can be measured, you must be sure that the scale is calibrated. This is performed by setting both of the weights at zero and making sure that the pointer floats in the middle of the rectangle at the end of the frame. Some scales have a screw at the end that can be adjusted to get the scale to balance. The bottom large weight slides along the balance bar that is calibrated in 50-pound increments. Place the large weight into the groove you estimate closest to the weight of the patient without going over it. The balance beam should indicate an inadequate weight amount by the pointer's position above the center of the rectangle. Move the smaller weight on the top of the balance beam until you have added enough weight for the beam to balance in the center of the rectangle. The top calibration is in full pounds divided into quarters (Figure 38–4). If your large weight estimation was too low, you will need to move that weight to the next higher 50-pound increment and readjust the smaller weight to balance. If you estimated too high, move the large weight one groove lower and then adjust the top. When the beam balances, add the two measurements together and record the patient's weight.

## Measuring and Weighing the Patient

After calling the patient into the back office, tell him or her you are going to measure his or her height and weight; instruct the patient to remove his or her shoes.

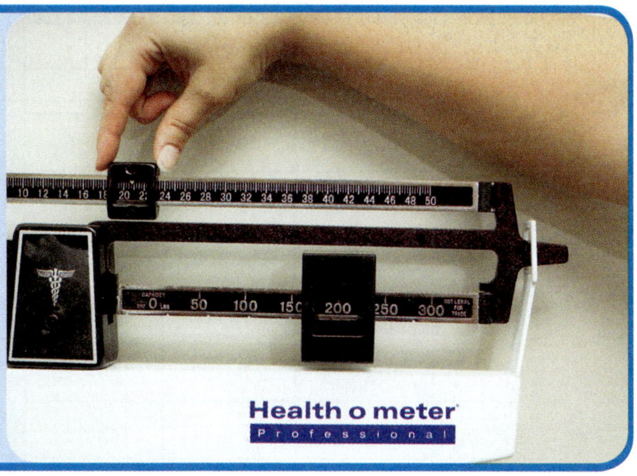


**Figure 38–4:** The balance bar reads 220¾ pounds. *Delmar/ Cengage Learning.*

## PATIENT EDUCATION

Patients may be asked to monitor their weight at home when they have certain conditions that can cause fluid retention, such as cardiac or kidney diseases, or for a weight gain or loss program. Remind them to weigh at about the same time each day, since weight varies throughout the day, and to wear clothing of about the same weight. A suggestion to weigh each morning before eating while still in night clothing would provide consistent variables for a more accurate assessment of weight trends.

Remind patients that handbags and items in pockets, such as keys and coin purses, should be put aside. While they are getting ready, check to ensure that the scale is calibrated correctly and reads 0 (zero). If not, make a slight adjustment of the scale as mentioned previously until it does.

Raise the height bar *above* the patient's estimated height and extend the measuring bar. Place a paper towel on the scale base to provide a clean surface. Follow the steps in Procedure 38–1 to obtain the patient's height.

Please note that some providers indicate that the patient should face away from the scale with his or her back to the height bar to ensure that he or she is standing up straight. However, if you are measuring height and weight together, many patients want to face the bar so they can watch you balancing the scale to get their accurate weight. Facing the height bar initially eliminates the need to get off, turn, and get back on or prevents patients from trying to turn around on the narrow scale base, which could result in a fall. It is also more difficult for elderly patients to get on the scale backward. They normally grasp the scale base to aid them when stepping on. Check with your employer to see which technique is used in your office.

While the patient is still on the scale, proceed with Procedure 38–1 to obtain the weight. If there is room to position the scale away from the wall, it is often easier from the other side, where the patient is not in the way. Note that the height bar can remain lowered when you are only measuring the patient's weight. Accurately record your findings on the patient's chart.

## CLINICAL PEARL

Most people are very interested in their measurements. Because some may be sensitive about their weight, be careful about any remarks you make. If they are on a weight-gain or weight-loss program and show even a small change, give them praise and encouragement. Some might question what they should weigh for their height. Different weight charts are available, and one should be posted near the scale as a patient education tool. Some charts differentiate by age, whereas others use gender or both. Figure 38–5 is gender-specific and considers relative frame size. These are only guidelines because the composition of the body tissue has an effect on the weight.

## Body Mass Index

Another common measurement in the medical office today is the **body mass index (BMI)**. This is a numerical correlation between a patient's height and weight. Many providers prefer the BMI to be calculated by the medical assistant and documented in the patient's record along with the height and weight. There are a number of ways to determine the patient's BMI. You can use the following formula, which is:

- Multiply the patient's weight in pounds by 703.
- Divide this total by the patient's height in inches.
- Divide this total by the patient's height in inches again and then round to the nearest whole number.

## EXAMPLE

**Calculate the BMI of a patient weighing 140 pounds, and measuring 5'4" (64 inches).**

Step 1: 140 × 703 = 98420
Step 2: 98420/64 = 1537.81
Step 3: 1537.81/64 = 24.03

Rounded to the nearest whole number = 24

| MEN | | | |
|---|---|---|---|
| Height | Small | Medium | Large |
| 5'2" | 128–134 | 131–141 | 138–150 |
| 5'3" | 130–136 | 133–143 | 140–153 |
| 5'4" | 132–138 | 135–145 | 142–156 |
| 5'5" | 134–140 | 137–148 | 144–160 |
| 5'6" | 136–142 | 139–151 | 146–164 |
| 5'7" | 138–146 | 142–154 | 149–168 |
| 5'8" | 140–148 | 145–157 | 152–172 |
| 5'9" | 142–151 | 148–160 | 155–176 |
| 5'10" | 144–154 | 151–163 | 158–180 |
| 5'11" | 146–157 | 154–166 | 161–184 |
| 6'0" | 149–160 | 157–170 | 164–188 |
| 6'1" | 152–164 | 160–174 | 168–192 |
| 6'2" | 155–168 | 164–178 | 172–197 |
| 6'3" | 158–172 | 167–182 | 176–202 |
| 6'4" | 162–176 | 171–187 | 181–207 |

| WOMEN | | | |
|---|---|---|---|
| Height | Small | Medium | Large |
| 4'10" | 102–111 | 109–121 | 118–131 |
| 4'11" | 103–113 | 111–123 | 120–134 |
| 5'0" | 104–115 | 113–126 | 122–137 |
| 5'1" | 106–118 | 115–129 | 125–140 |
| 5'2" | 108–121 | 118–132 | 128–143 |
| 5'3" | 111–124 | 121–135 | 131–147 |
| 5'4" | 114–127 | 124–138 | 134–151 |
| 5'5" | 117–130 | 127–141 | 137–155 |
| 5'6" | 120–133 | 130–144 | 140–159 |
| 5'7" | 123–136 | 133–147 | 143–163 |
| 5'8" | 128–139 | 138–150 | 146–167 |
| 5'9" | 129–142 | 139–153 | 149–170 |
| 5'10" | 132–146 | 142–156 | 152–173 |
| 5'11" | 135–148 | 145–159 | 155–176 |
| 6'0" | 138–151 | 148–162 | 158–179 |

**FIGURE 38–5:** Chart of desirable weight for men and women. *Delmar/Cengage Learning.*

## PROCEDURE 38–1 Measure Height and Weight Using a Balance Beam Scale

**PURPOSE:** To obtain an accurate measurement of a patient's height and weight.

**EQUIPMENT:** Balance beam scale with extension measuring bar, paper towel, patient's chart or computer with EHR software, pen.

**S SKILL:** Measure and record height and weight.

| Procedure Steps | Detailed Instructions and/or *Rationales* |
|---|---|
| 1. Wash hands. | |
| 2. Identify the patient and introduce yourself. | *Ensures that you are performing the procedure on the correct patient.* |

| Procedure Steps | Detailed Instructions and/or *Rationales* |
|---|---|
| B 3. Explain the procedure, ***using language the patient can understand,*** and instruct the patient to remove shoes and any heavy clothing. | *Ensures understanding, consent, and cooperation from the patient. Accurate measurement cannot be obtained if shoes or heavy clothing are worn.* |
| 4. Place a paper towel on the scale platform (Figure 38–6A). | *Provides a clean surface for the shoeless foot.* |
| 5. Assist patient to the center of the scale (Figure 38–6B). | Make sure the patient is in the center of the platform. Ask the patient to stand still while you adjust the balance and read the weight. Remind the patient not to hold on to the scale. *Holding on to any part of the scale will cause a lighter, inaccurate measurement.* |
| 6. Move the lower weight bar (measured in 50-pound increments) to the estimated number and slowly slide the upper bar until the balance beam point is centered (Figure 38–6C). | You may want to ask the patient for an approximate weight. |
| 7. Read the weight by adding the upper bar measurement to the lower bar measurement. Round to the nearest ¼ pound. | |
| 8. Raise the measuring bar beyond the patient's height and lift the extension (Figure 38–6D). | *Avoids the possibility of striking the patient if the bar is raised after the patient steps on the scale.* |
| 9. Lower measuring bar until firmly resting on top of patient's head (Figure 38–6E). | Measurement of height is from the top of the head, not from the hair. |
| 10. Assist patient off the scale and allow the patient to sit and put on shoes. | Help the patient from the scale and discard the paper towel. Tell the patient to put his or her shoes back on unless ready for a physical exam. |
| 11. Read line where measurement falls. Round to the nearest ¼ inch (Figure 38–6F). | |

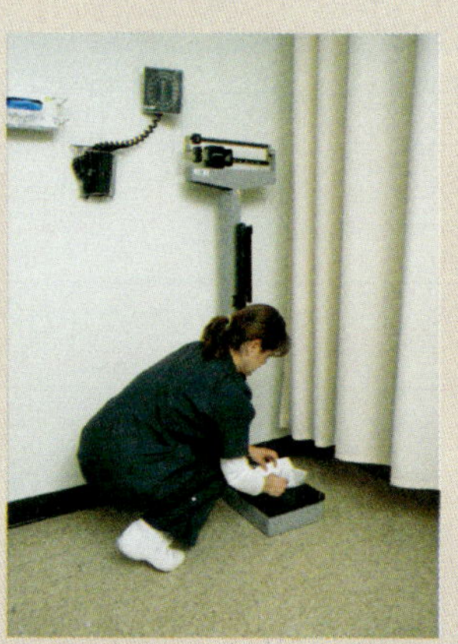

**FIGURE 38–6A:** Prepare the scale to measure the patient's weight and height by placing a paper towel on the scale platform. *Delmar/Cengage Learning.*

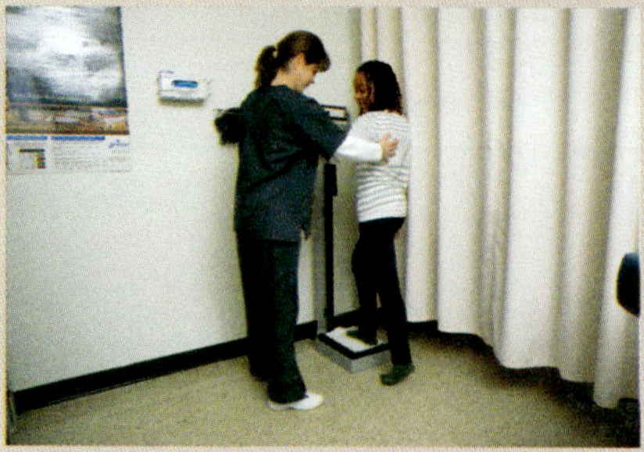

**Figure 38–6B:** Assist the patient to the center of the scale. *Delmar/Cengage Learning.*

*(continues)*

*(continued)*

| Procedure Steps | Detailed Instructions and/or *Rationales* |
|---|---|
| 12. Lower measuring bar to its original position and return the weights to zero. | |
| 13. Document in the patient's chart. | Record the weight and height on the patient's chart or in the EMR. Be sure to record whether the patient was wearing street clothing or a gown. |

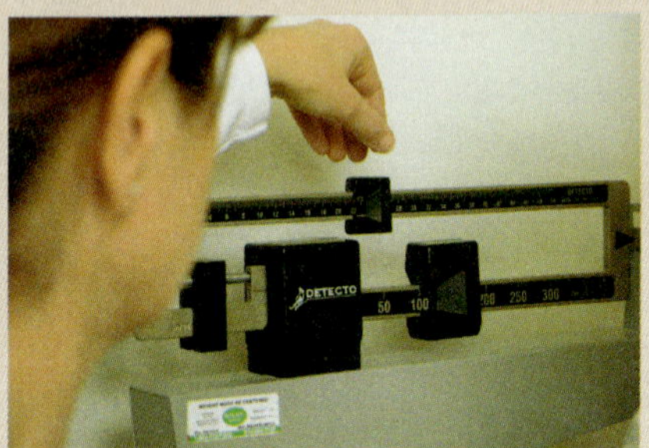


**Figure 38–6C:** Move the lower weight bar to the estimated number and slowly slide the upper bar until the balance beam point is centered. Read the resulting weight, rounding to the nearest quarter pound. *Delmar/Cengage Learning.*

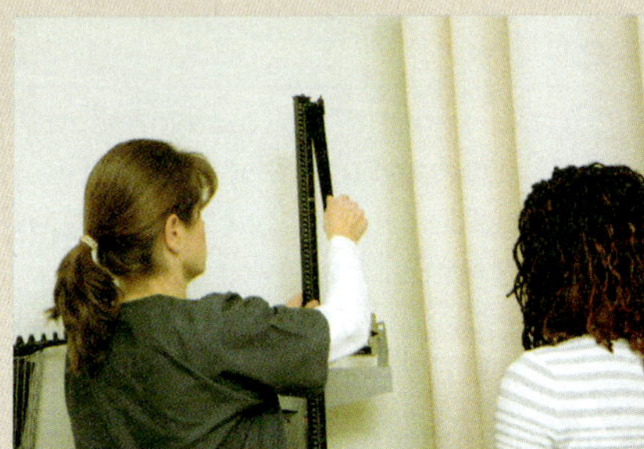

**Figure 38–6D:** Raise the measuring bar beyond the patient's height and lift the extension. *Delmar/Cengage Learning.*

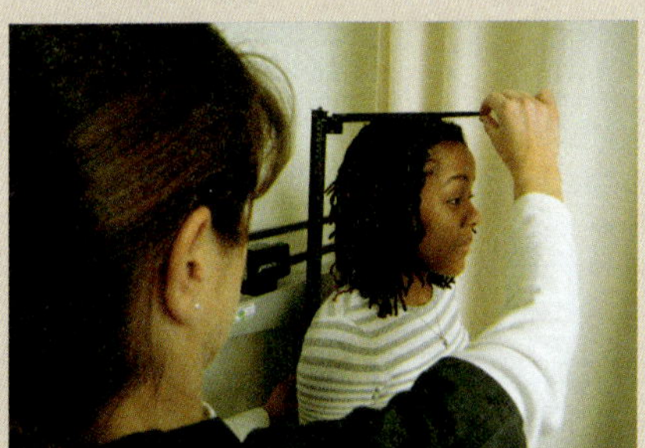

**Figure 38–6E:** Lower the measuring bar until firmly resting on top of patient's head. Then, assist patient off the scale. *Delmar/Cengage Learning.*

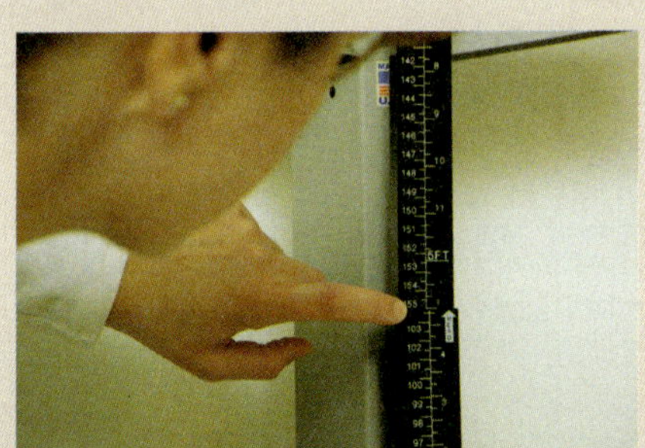

**Figure 38–6F:** Read the line where the measurement falls, rounding to the nearest quarter inch. *Delmar/Cengage Learning.*

## Charting Example

| | |
|---|---|
| 5-12-XX<br>11:30 am | Wt. 147# (147 lbs) without shoes, in street clothing. Ht. 68". J. Rivera, CMA(AAMA) |

Many websites provide a free electronic BMI measurement, and many EHR systems automatically calculate BMI. The National Institutes of Health has published a BMI index chart that is easy to use (Figure 38–7), and many providers prefer to have this chart posted near the scale and in the exam rooms. You can access a copy of this chart on their website at www.nih.gov.

## VITAL SIGNS

The term **vital signs** is used by health care personnel to identify the measurement of body functions that are essential to life. The four vital indicators are **temperature**, **pulse**, **respiration**, and **blood pressure**, commonly referred to as TPR and B/P. They indicate

**FIGURE 38–7:** Body Mass Index table. (Adapted from *Clinical Guidelines on the Identification, Evaluation, and Treatment of Overweight and Obesity in Adults: The Evidence Report*. National Institutes of Health, www.nih.gov.)

**Body Mass Index Table**

| | Normal | | | | | | Overweight | | | | | Obese | | | | | | | | | | Extreme Obesity | | | | | | | | | | | | | | |
|---|---|---|---|---|---|---|---|---|---|---|---|---|---|---|---|---|---|---|---|---|---|---|---|---|---|---|---|---|---|---|---|---|---|---|---|---|
| BMI | 19 | 20 | 21 | 22 | 23 | 24 | 25 | 26 | 27 | 28 | 29 | 30 | 31 | 32 | 33 | 34 | 35 | 36 | 37 | 38 | 39 | 40 | 41 | 42 | 43 | 44 | 45 | 46 | 47 | 48 | 49 | 50 | 51 | 52 | 53 | 54 |
| Height (inches) | Body Weight (pounds) | | | | | | | | | | | | | | | | | | | | | | | | | | | | | | | | | | | |
| 58 | 91 | 96 | 100 | 105 | 110 | 115 | 119 | 124 | 129 | 134 | 138 | 143 | 148 | 153 | 158 | 162 | 167 | 172 | 177 | 181 | 186 | 191 | 196 | 201 | 205 | 210 | 215 | 220 | 224 | 229 | 234 | 239 | 244 | 248 | 253 | 258 |
| 59 | 94 | 99 | 104 | 109 | 114 | 119 | 124 | 128 | 133 | 138 | 143 | 148 | 153 | 158 | 163 | 168 | 173 | 178 | 183 | 188 | 193 | 198 | 203 | 208 | 212 | 217 | 222 | 227 | 232 | 237 | 242 | 247 | 252 | 257 | 262 | 267 |
| 60 | 97 | 102 | 107 | 112 | 118 | 123 | 128 | 133 | 138 | 143 | 148 | 153 | 158 | 163 | 168 | 174 | 179 | 184 | 189 | 194 | 199 | 204 | 209 | 215 | 220 | 225 | 230 | 235 | 240 | 245 | 250 | 255 | 261 | 266 | 271 | 276 |
| 61 | 100 | 106 | 111 | 116 | 122 | 127 | 132 | 137 | 143 | 148 | 153 | 158 | 164 | 169 | 174 | 180 | 185 | 190 | 195 | 201 | 206 | 211 | 217 | 222 | 227 | 232 | 238 | 243 | 248 | 254 | 259 | 264 | 269 | 275 | 280 | 285 |
| 62 | 104 | 109 | 115 | 120 | 126 | 131 | 136 | 142 | 147 | 153 | 158 | 164 | 169 | 175 | 180 | 186 | 191 | 196 | 202 | 207 | 213 | 218 | 224 | 229 | 235 | 240 | 246 | 251 | 256 | 262 | 267 | 273 | 278 | 284 | 289 | 295 |
| 63 | 107 | 113 | 118 | 124 | 130 | 135 | 141 | 146 | 152 | 158 | 163 | 169 | 175 | 180 | 186 | 191 | 197 | 203 | 208 | 214 | 220 | 225 | 231 | 237 | 242 | 248 | 254 | 259 | 265 | 270 | 278 | 282 | 287 | 293 | 299 | 304 |
| 64 | 110 | 116 | 122 | 128 | 134 | 140 | 145 | 151 | 157 | 163 | 169 | 174 | 180 | 186 | 192 | 197 | 204 | 209 | 215 | 221 | 227 | 232 | 238 | 244 | 250 | 256 | 262 | 267 | 273 | 279 | 285 | 291 | 296 | 302 | 308 | 314 |
| 65 | 114 | 120 | 126 | 132 | 138 | 144 | 150 | 156 | 162 | 168 | 174 | 180 | 186 | 192 | 198 | 204 | 210 | 216 | 222 | 228 | 234 | 240 | 246 | 252 | 258 | 264 | 270 | 276 | 282 | 288 | 294 | 300 | 306 | 312 | 318 | 324 |
| 66 | 118 | 124 | 130 | 136 | 142 | 148 | 155 | 161 | 167 | 173 | 179 | 186 | 192 | 198 | 204 | 210 | 216 | 223 | 229 | 235 | 241 | 247 | 253 | 260 | 266 | 272 | 278 | 284 | 291 | 297 | 303 | 309 | 315 | 322 | 328 | 334 |
| 67 | 121 | 127 | 134 | 140 | 146 | 153 | 159 | 166 | 172 | 178 | 185 | 191 | 198 | 204 | 211 | 217 | 223 | 230 | 236 | 242 | 249 | 255 | 261 | 268 | 274 | 280 | 287 | 293 | 299 | 306 | 312 | 319 | 325 | 331 | 338 | 344 |
| 68 | 125 | 131 | 138 | 144 | 151 | 158 | 164 | 171 | 177 | 184 | 190 | 197 | 203 | 210 | 216 | 223 | 230 | 236 | 243 | 249 | 256 | 262 | 269 | 276 | 282 | 289 | 295 | 302 | 308 | 315 | 322 | 328 | 335 | 341 | 348 | 354 |
| 69 | 128 | 135 | 142 | 149 | 155 | 162 | 169 | 176 | 182 | 189 | 196 | 203 | 209 | 216 | 223 | 230 | 236 | 243 | 250 | 257 | 263 | 270 | 277 | 284 | 291 | 297 | 304 | 311 | 318 | 324 | 331 | 338 | 345 | 351 | 358 | 365 |
| 70 | 132 | 139 | 146 | 153 | 160 | 167 | 174 | 181 | 188 | 195 | 202 | 209 | 216 | 222 | 229 | 236 | 243 | 250 | 257 | 264 | 271 | 278 | 285 | 292 | 299 | 306 | 313 | 320 | 327 | 334 | 341 | 348 | 355 | 362 | 369 | 376 |
| 71 | 136 | 143 | 150 | 157 | 165 | 172 | 179 | 186 | 193 | 200 | 208 | 215 | 222 | 229 | 236 | 243 | 250 | 257 | 265 | 272 | 279 | 286 | 293 | 301 | 308 | 315 | 322 | 329 | 338 | 343 | 351 | 358 | 365 | 372 | 379 | 386 |
| 72 | 140 | 147 | 154 | 162 | 169 | 177 | 184 | 191 | 199 | 206 | 213 | 221 | 228 | 235 | 242 | 250 | 258 | 265 | 272 | 279 | 287 | 294 | 302 | 309 | 316 | 324 | 331 | 338 | 346 | 353 | 361 | 368 | 375 | 383 | 390 | 397 |
| 73 | 144 | 151 | 159 | 166 | 174 | 182 | 189 | 197 | 204 | 212 | 219 | 227 | 235 | 242 | 250 | 257 | 265 | 272 | 280 | 288 | 295 | 302 | 310 | 318 | 325 | 333 | 340 | 348 | 355 | 363 | 371 | 378 | 386 | 393 | 401 | 408 |
| 74 | 148 | 155 | 163 | 171 | 179 | 186 | 194 | 202 | 210 | 218 | 225 | 233 | 241 | 249 | 256 | 264 | 272 | 280 | 287 | 295 | 303 | 311 | 319 | 326 | 334 | 342 | 350 | 358 | 365 | 373 | 381 | 389 | 396 | 404 | 412 | 420 |
| 75 | 152 | 160 | 168 | 176 | 184 | 192 | 200 | 208 | 216 | 224 | 232 | 240 | 248 | 256 | 264 | 272 | 279 | 287 | 295 | 303 | 311 | 319 | 327 | 335 | 343 | 351 | 359 | 367 | 375 | 383 | 391 | 399 | 407 | 415 | 423 | 431 |
| 76 | 156 | 164 | 172 | 180 | 189 | 197 | 205 | 213 | 221 | 230 | 238 | 246 | 254 | 263 | 271 | 279 | 287 | 295 | 304 | 312 | 320 | 328 | 336 | 344 | 353 | 361 | 369 | 377 | 385 | 394 | 402 | 410 | 418 | 426 | 435 | 443 |

Source: Adapted from *Clinical Guidelines on the Identification, Evaluation, and Treatment of Overweight and Obesity in Adults: The Evidence Report.*

the body's ability to control heat; the rate, volume, and rhythm of the heart; the rate and quality of breathing; and the force of the heart and condition of the blood vessels. The vital signs give the provider an assessment of the status of the brain, the autonomic nervous system, the heart, and the lungs. Additionally, it is worth noting here that some providers are also considering pain a fifth vital as discussed in Chapter 37.

The correct measurement of vital signs is extremely important. Proper technique are essential. Findings should be recorded immediately following measurement to avoid a memory error. Always repeat the procedure if you think you might have made a mistake in measuring or recording. Occasionally, you may have a problem measuring a vital sign because a patient's unusual physical condition makes measurement difficult. Inform the provider of your problem and follow the course of action advised. Avoid alarming the patient. *Never* estimate the measurement. The provider's choice of treatment and medication is often based on the findings; therefore, they must be accurate.

## Temperature

The temperature of the body indicates the amount of heat produced by the activity of changing food into energy. The body loses heat through perspiration, breathing, and the elimination of body wastes. The balance between heat production and heat loss determines the body's temperature.

Conditions affecting body heat include metabolic rate, time of day, and amount of activity. Body temperature is usually lower in the morning following a period of rest. In the afternoon and evening, body temperature rises because of the heat produced by activity and the metabolism of food. These activities warm the blood that circulates through the body. "Normal" body temperature for an individual is that temperature at which his body systems function most effectively. An *average* normal oral temperature is 37°C (centigrade) or 98.6°F (Fahrenheit), but normal temperatures can vary from 36.5°C to 37.5°C (97.6°F to 99.6°F) (see Table 38–1). A person with a temperature above normal is said to be **febrile** or to have a temperature elevation. A person with a temperature that is normal or subnormal is said to be **afebrile**.

## Controlling Body Temperature

The temperature-regulating center in the body is located in the hypothalamus of the brain (Figure 38–8). The action of the hypothalamus can be compared with a thermostat that turns the furnace in your home off and on to keep the room temperature at the set number of degrees. As discussed in Unit 11, the brain, autonomic nervous system, blood vessels, and skin cooperate to regulate temperature through a feedback mechanism from temperature receptors. In the body, the hot and cold peripheral receptors in the skin send messages to the hypothalamus about the environment surrounding the body. Temperature receptors in the spinal cord, abdomen, and other internal structures send messages about the internal body temperature. One section of the hypothalamus also has many heat-sensitive neurons, which increase their output of impulses when temperature rises and decrease their output when it drops. The signals from this section of the hypothalamus merge with those received in another section, along with the internal and skin receptors, to evaluate the situation and send signals to control heat loss or heat production. Therefore, this central center is referred to as the *hypothalamic thermostat*.

The hypothalamic thermostat is very effective. When receptors sense the body is too warm, they send a message to the brain, which in turn acts on the sweat glands of the skin to produce moisture. The moisture evaporates from the skin's surface and cools the body. At the same time, nerve impulses are sent to the surface blood vessels

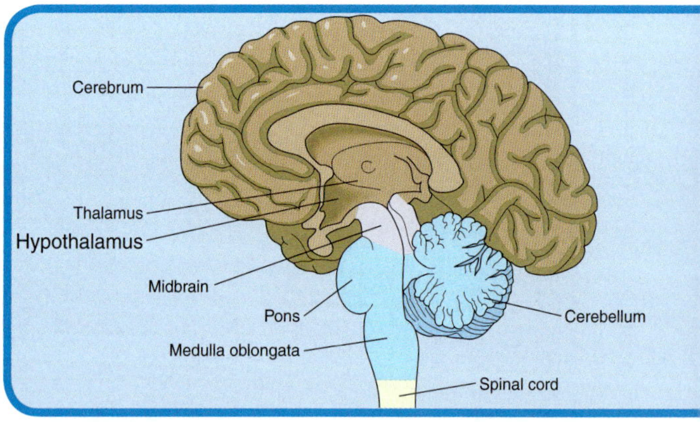


**Figure 38–8:** The hypothalamus regulates body temperature. *Delmar/Cengage Learning.*

**TABLE 38–1 Temperature Variations Considered Normal**

| | Oral | Axillary | Rectal |
|---|---|---|---|
| Average | 98.6°F | 97.6°F | 99.6°F |
| Normal temperature | (37°C) | (36.5°C) | (37.5°C) |
| Range | 97.6–99.6°F | 96.6–98.6°F | 98.6–100.6°F |
| | (36.5–37.5°C) | (36–37°C) | (37–38.1°C) |

to dilate, which brings more blood in contact with the surface of the skin. The blood gives up heat, which cools the blood within the vessels and therefore cools the body.

When the body senses coolness, the opposite activities occur. Surface blood vessels constrict to keep the blood away from the surface of the skin and prevent the loss of heat. Impulses to the sweat glands are stopped when temperature falls below normal, and small papillary muscles around the hair follicles contract, causing goose bumps on the skin. Heat is produced by the activity of the papillary muscles, thereby helping warm the body. In addition, a portion of the hypothalamus becomes active when cold signals are received. Now hypothalamic messages are sent to skeletal muscles throughout the body, causing increased muscle tone that produces heat. When the muscle tone rises above a certain level, shivering results and heat production is raised dramatically. This is evident with an infectious process such as influenza. Microorganisms cause the patient to experience chills and shivering until the temperature rises to warm the body and a fever develops.

During an infectious process, the presence of microorganisms causes **pyrogens** to be secreted, which raise the set point of the hypothalamic thermostat. Pyrogens are toxins from bacteria or a by-product of degenerating tissues. When the set point is higher than normal, the body's heat production and conservation processes are activated. Surface blood vessels constrict, causing the person to feel cold even though the temperature is above normal. No sweat is secreted. Increased white blood cell activity from fighting bacterial invasion also produces heat. Chills and shivering begin and continue until the temperature reaches the higher set point, at which the hypothalamus will continue to operate until the infectious process is reversed. After this occurs, the hypothalamic thermostat is reset to a lower or normal value, and the body's temperature-reduction process results in profuse sweating and hot, red skin from general vasodilation. After this onset reaction, the temperature will begin to fall.

The extent of the infection determines the amount of heat (fever) generated. A mild infection might cause the temperature to rise to 37.7°C (100°F). A moderate infection can elevate the temperature to 38.8°C (102°F). Fevers are categorized by the degree of body heat as slight, moderate, severe, dangerous, or **fatal** (Table 38–2).

**TABLE 38–2 Classification of Fevers**

| | Fahrenheit | Celsius |
|---|---|---|
| Slight | 99.6°–101.0° | 37.5°–38.3° |
| Moderate | 101.0°–102.0° | 38.3°–38.8° |
| Severe | 102.0°–104.0° | 38.8°–40.0° |
| Dangerous | 104.0°–105.0° | 40.0°–40.5 |
| Fatal | over 106.0° | 41.1° |

**PATIENT EDUCATION**

Instruct the patient to inform the provider of any significant changes in temperature. Advise the patient at what point an oral temperature should be reported to the provider. Caution the patient that a fever should not be "watched" to see how high it will go. Prolonged high fever can cause seizures, brain damage, and, ultimately, death.

Fatality-associated elevated temperature depends on the extent of time the fever is present. Fevers of short duration well above 41.1°C (106.0°F) have not proved fatal, but immediate measures to reduce body temperature must be administered. Temperatures below normal are called subnormal. Collapse will occur at about 35.5°C (96.0°F), and death follows if temperature goes below 33.8°C (93.0°F) more than briefly.

## Thermometer Types and Designs

Body temperature is measured by means of a **thermometer** in scales of Fahrenheit or the metric system equivalent, Celsius. Thermometers are of the following main types: disposable, in the form of plastic strips; battery-operated electronic; self-contained digital; tympanic **infrared**; and temporal artery. The mouth (**oral**), underarm (**axillary**), rectum (**rectal**), ear (**aural** or tympanic membrane), or the temporal area of the forehead may be used to measure body temperature. The large variety of thermometers, each with its own advantages and disadvantages, allows for personal preference in equipment selection for the physician's office. Table 38–3 briefly outlines the main advantages and disadvantages for each type.

### Disposable Thermometers

Chemical disposable thermometers can be used by the oral or axillary route (Figure 38–9A and B). When using with the oral route, care must be taken to avoid touching the dot matrix portion, which is placed in the patient's mouth. The dots can be placed up or down. The thermometer must be held under the tongue as far back as possible in the heat pocket, with the tongue pressed against the end and the mouth closed on the stem for the allotted time. The heat in the mouth causes a reaction on the heat-sensitive dots printed on the surface of the plastic strip. The thermometer is then removed and the dots observed for color change. Read the results by counting the number of dots that change color within a degree grouping. The last changed dot on the matrix indicates the correct temperature. Record the temperature and discard the thermometer in a waste container.

## TABLE 38–3 Comparison of Thermometer Types

| Type | Advantage | Disadvantage |
|---|---|---|
| Plastic disposable | Single use avoids cross-contamination, no cleaning, relatively fast | Must protect from heat, somewhat unpleasant for patient, storage and inventory costs |
| Digital | Quick, signals when registered, easily read, self-contained | Moderate initial cost, plastic cover, and battery expenses |
| Electronic probe | Quick, signals when registered, easily read, self-contained | Fairly expensive, cumbersome cord, requires recharging, probe cover costs, may cause inaccurate readings if patient bites too hard on probe |
| Tympanic infrared | Instant results, easily read, core temperature, individualized probe cover, eliminates mucous membrane concerns | Expensive, probe cover costs, replacement battery costs. An improper seal in the ear canal, the presence of cerumen, or an infection of the middle ear can cause inaccurate readings |
| Temporal artery | Instant results, easily read, as accurate as rectal, noninvasive, no mucous membrane concerns | Expensive, requires probe cover or cleaning when used, requires environmental acclimation, somewhat delicate |

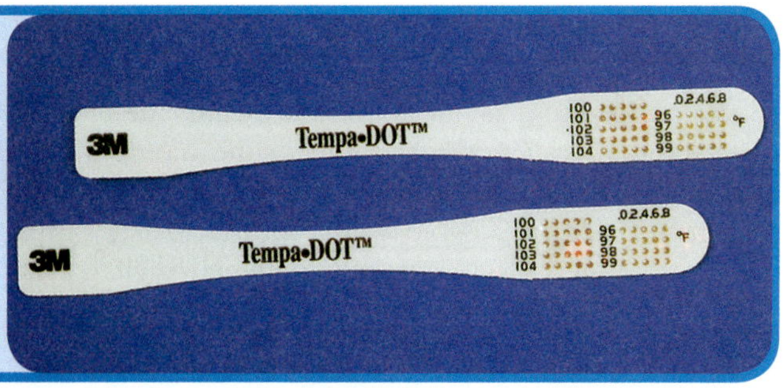


**Figure 38–9A:** Disposable chemical thermometer. *Delmar/Cengage Learning.*

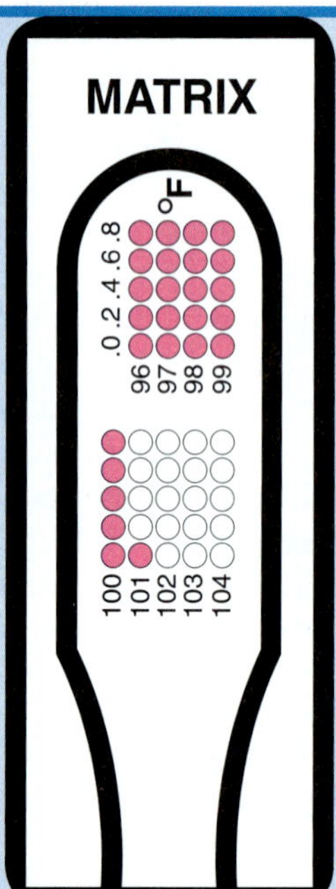


**FIGURE 38–9B:** The matrix reads 101°F. *Delmar/Cengage Learning.*

When measuring the axillary temperature, the dot matrix portion is placed next to the body, deep in the axillary space, with the handle extending straight down the patient's side. The arm must be held tightly at the side. After time recommended by the manufacturer, remove the thermometer; read and record the temperature.

### Electronic Thermometers

The use of electronic thermometers is very common in the medical office. A small, battery-operated unit with a digital read-out window is capable of measuring a temperature within a few seconds (Figure 38–10A). A color-coded probe, blue for oral, red for rectal, is attached by a cord to the battery unit. A disposable cover slips over the probe to provide each patient with an individual barrier for the thermometer. The covered probe is inserted in

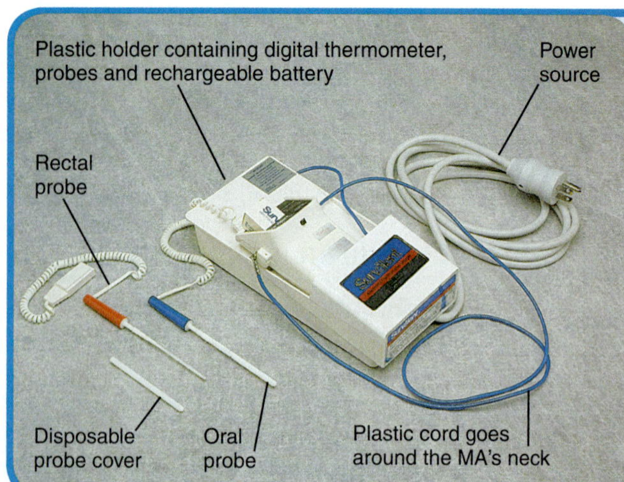


**Figure 38–10:** Electronic thermometer with labeled parts. *Delmar/Cengage Learning.*

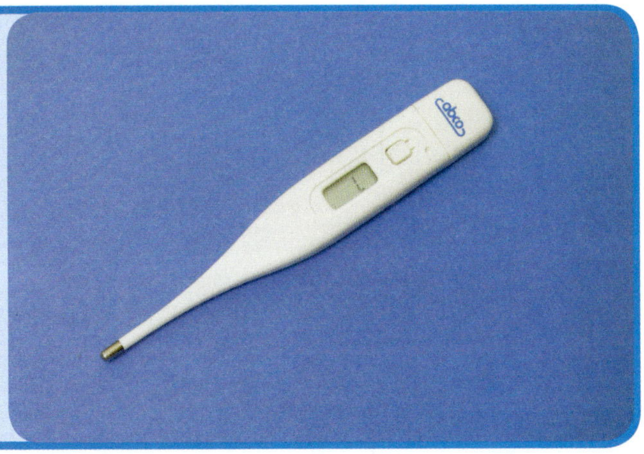

**Figure 38–11:** Electronic digital thermometer that is excellent for home use. *Delmar/Cengage Learning.*

the patient's mouth. As soon as the temperature level has been reached, the unit will sound a signal and the final reading will appear in the window of the unit. The probe cover is then discarded into a waste container. Refer to Procedure 38–2 for a step-by-step guide on obtaining an oral temperature with this type of thermometer.

Another electronic thermometer that is simple and self-contained is a digital thermometer that is excellent for home use (Figure 38–11). The thermometer registers the temperature in about one to two minutes on an easy-to-read LCD panel that shows the temperature in tenths of degrees. The thermometer can be cleaned with soap and water and sanitized with a disinfectant. Probe covers are available for office or home use. It may be used for oral, axillary, or rectal measurement. Some models have a beeper that sounds when the maximum temperature is reached. This feature is especially appealing to children.

## Tympanic Membrane Thermometers

Another method for temperature measurement is the instantaneous tympanic membrane (aural) thermometer (Figure 38–12). The thermometer operates by the principle of measuring the strength of the infrared heat waves generated by the tympanic membrane and digitally displays that temperature in fewer than two seconds. Because the tympanic membrane shares the same blood supply as the hypothalamus, it is believed the auditory canal is an ideal site for obtaining an accurate assessment of the body's core temperature. Studies conducted with temperature-sensing devices placed internally in a large blood vessel have shown strong correlation in results.

Although its greatest asset is the instant result, it is also very easy to use and has become a real benefit to health care professionals in hospital emergency rooms, labor and delivery rooms, and pediatric units because it does not involve contact with mucous membranes and because the site is so easily accessible. Another advantage is that the readings are not affected by hot or cold liquids or smoking, as are oral methods. In addition, the patient does not even need to be conscious. There are a few instances when inaccurate readings can result, including if the probe is not properly sealed in the ear canal, if the beam is not directed toward the eardrum, if cerumen is present, or if there is an infection of the middle ear.

## Temporal Artery Thermometers

The latest thermometer to be developed is the temporal scanner or, as it is commonly called, the temporal artery thermometer (TAT) (Figure 38–13). Both home and clinical models are available. The TAT determines body temperature by measuring the temperature of the skin over the temporal artery (TA) of the forehead where the artery is less than 2 mm below the surface of the skin. The probe of the thermometer has a sensor that assesses the infrared heat in the artery. The TAT has another unique feature. If the forehead is not an appropriate site for measurement, temperature can be measured in alternative sites. Temperatures can be taken over the femoral artery or lateral thoracic or axillary areas.

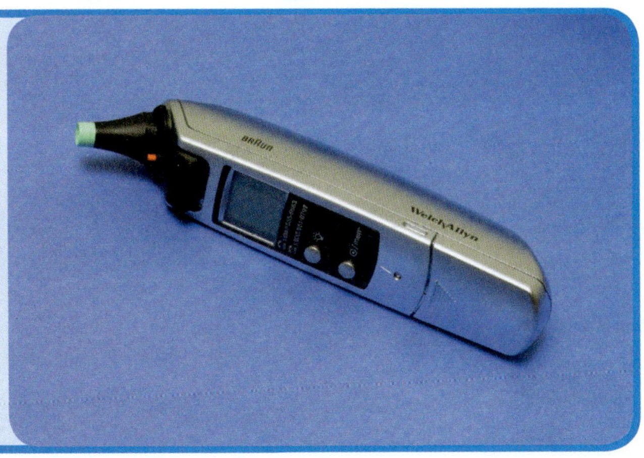


**FIGURE 38–12:** Tympanic (aural) thermometer. *Delmar/Cengage Learning.*

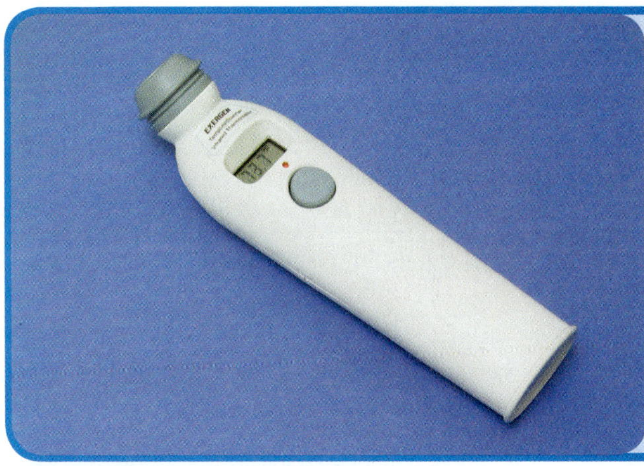


**Figure 38–13:** Temporal artery thermometer. *Delmar/Cengage Learning.*

It is important for the probe lens and cone to be very clean so the thermometer can register the heat accurately. Follow the manufacturer's instructions for the cleaning process for the specific model you are using. A variety of disposable probe covers, caps, or sheaths can be used instead of cleaning if desired.

## Measuring Oral Temperatures

Measuring body temperature by mouth is convenient, quick, fairly accurate, and relatively inexpensive. Refer to Procedure 38–2 for detailed steps for measuring an oral temperature. Remember that oral temperature requires contact with mucous membranes, so a thermometer must either be disposable or require a barrier cover. Some factors also influence the accurate measurement:

- The thermometer must be place sublingually into the heat pocket (Figure 38–14).
- Patients must not have smoked or had anything hot or cold by mouth for at least 15 minutes prior to measuring.
- Patients must be able to maintain the thermometer in place appropriately for the required period of time.

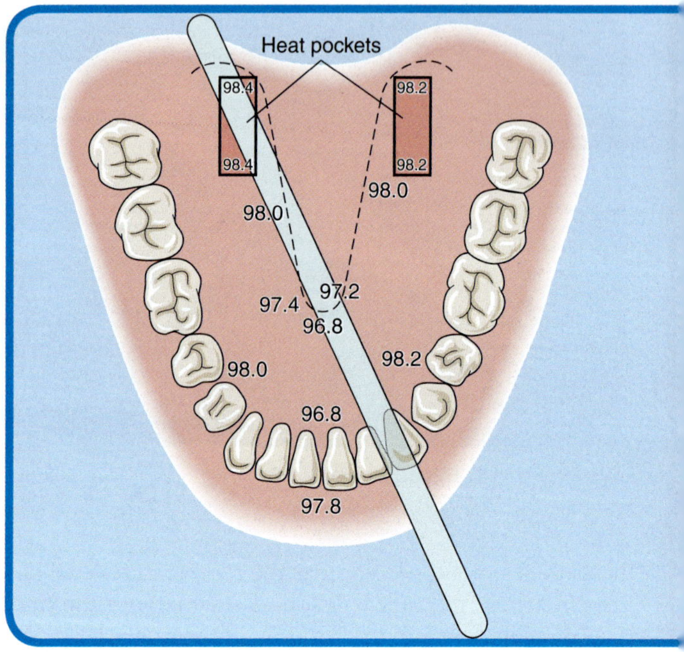


**FIGURE 38–14:** Placement of an oral thermometer. When taking an oral temperature, place the thermometer under the tongue to the side of the mouth into the heat pockets as shown here. *Courtesy of 3M Healthcare.*

## PROCEDURE 38–2 Measure and Record Oral Temperature with an Electronic Thermometer

**PURPOSE:** To determine a patient's oral temperature with an electronic thermometer

**EQUIPMENT:** Electronic thermometer unit, oral probe, probe cover, waste container, patient chart or EHR, pen

S **SKILL:** Measure and record oral temperature with an electronic thermometer.

| Procedure Steps | Detailed Instructions and/or *Rationales* |
|---|---|
| 1. Wash hands; assemble equipment. | |
| 2. Identify the patient and introduce yourself. | *Ensures that you are performing the procedure on the correct patient.* |
| B 3. Explain the procedure, ***using language the patient can understand.*** | *Ensures understanding, consent, and cooperation from the patient.* |
| 4. Ensure that the patient has not smoked or consumed anything hot or cold in past 15 minutes. | *Smoking or consuming hot or cold substances can increase or decrease temperature.* |
| 5. Correctly prepare the thermometer. | a. Be sure the blue probe connector is plugged into the receptacle of the unit base. *The blue probe is used for oral temperatures.*<br>b. Remove probe from the stored position.<br>c. Insert the probe firmly into the probe cover (Figure 38–15A). |

| Procedure Steps | Detailed Instructions and/or *Rationales* |
|---|---|
| 6. Insert the covered probe into the patient's mouth. Instruct the patient to keep his or her lips pursed around the probe and not to bite down. Maintain the covered probe in position until the unit signals, approximately 10 to 15 seconds (Figure 38–15B). | The probe and connecting cord are rather heavy and cumbersome. It may be necessary to hold the thermometer steady in place. *Early removal results in inaccurate measurement.* |
| 7. Remove the probe from the patient. Do not touch the probe cover. | *Probe is contaminated with patient's saliva.* |
| 8. Read the temperature, noting the temperature. | Temperature is displayed digitally in the window of the unit. |
| 9. Press the eject button to discard the used probe cover into the waste container. | *All materials coming in contact with bodily secretions are deposited in a waste container.* |
| 10. Return the probe to the stored position in the unit and store the unit in the charging stand. | The thermometer display will read zero and shut off. *The unit should remain in the stand so it is fully charged and ready for use.* |
| 11. Wash hands. | |
| 12. Document in the patient's chart. | |

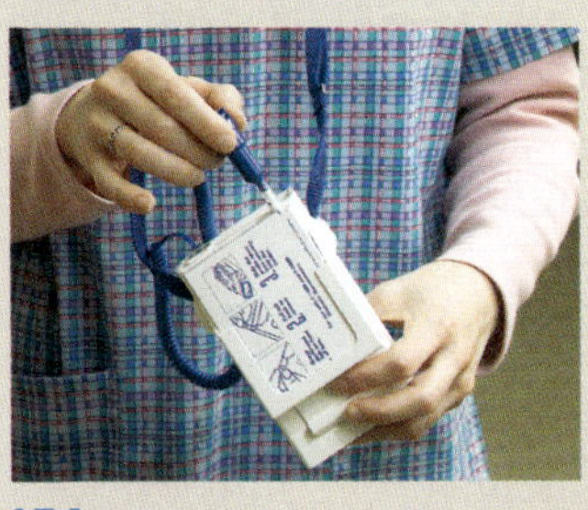

**FIGURE 38–15A:** Slide the probe into the disposable cover. *Delmar/Cengage Learning.*

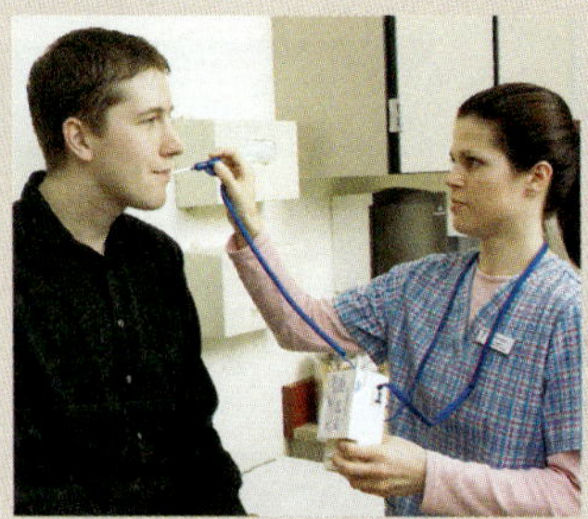

**FIGURE 38–15B:** The medical assistant holds the probe of the electronic thermometer in the patient's mouth until it signals completion. *Delmar/Cengage Learning.*

**Charting Example**

| | |
|---|---|
| 5/10/XX 11:30 am | T. 99.8 B. Davis, RMA (AMT) |

However, oral temperature measurement is not always the method of choice. Temperature must be measured by an axillary, rectal, tympanic, or temporal method in the following situations:

- Infants and young children
- Patients with respiratory complications that result in mouth breathing or use of supplemental oxygen
- Confused, disoriented, or emotionally unstable patients
- Patients with oral injuries or dental problems such as diseased gums or abscesses
- Patients with recent oral surgery
- Patients with facial paralysis
- Patients with nasal obstruction, sinus congestion, or colds

## Measuring Rectal Temperatures

Rectal temperature is a very accurate measurement simply because it is taken internally. Rectal measurement is appropriate with babies and young children who have not yet learned how to keep an oral thermometer in place. Children may complain about having a rectal temperature taken when they think they are "too big." The provider usually has a policy concerning the age limit and recommendations for rectal temperatures, which you must follow.

Electronic thermometers may be used to measure rectal temperature. Gloves must always be worn. Use the rectal (red) probe to take a rectal temperature (refer back to Figure 38–10). Remove the rectal probe from its holder and attach a probe cover. The probe is inserted into the rectum approximately 1 inch for adults and ½ inch for infants and small children. The use of lubricant is optional. After the reading is registered, remove the probe and discard the cover in a waste container.

When measuring the temperature of infants, they may be positioned on the stomach or the back. If positioning on the back, unfasten the diaper to expose the anus. Grasp the ankles securely with one hand, flexing the knees to the abdomen. With the other hand, insert the thermometer into the anal canal. Hold the thermometer securely in place. Maintain your grasp on the ankles so the infant cannot turn over. Be prepared for the procedure to initiate urination or expelling of stool. It would be wise to cover the male infant's penis with a diaper to absorb the urine stream. If positioning prone on a table, be certain to maintain control of the infant or child's position to prevent turning over and causing injury to the rectum from the inserted thermometer probe. Older children can be positioned either on their abdomen or side (lateral or Sims position, Chapter 39), whichever is preferred. Adults would be positioned on their side (lateral or Sims position), generally the left side because the rectum is angled in that direction and draped with a sheet for privacy.

When recording a rectal measurement, place the letter *R* in parentheses following the reading. Normal rectal temperature is 37.5°C or 99.6°F, one full degree above normal oral temperature. Temperature must never be measured rectally if the patient has had recent rectal surgery; it is possible to damage the operative site or perforate newly sutured lines. The rectal route also should not be used in patients with chronic diarrhea. Refer to Procedure 38–3 for detailed steps for measuring a rectal temperature using a digital thermometer.

## PROCEDURE 38–3 Measure Rectal Temperature with an Electronic Thermometer

**PURPOSE:** To determine a patient's rectal temperature using a electronic thermometer

**EQUIPMENT:** Mannequin (if simulated), electronic thermometer, rectal probe, probe cover, drape (if adult), gloves, lubricant, tissues, waste container, patient chart or EHR, pen

S **SKILL:** Measure and record rectal temperature with an electronic thermometer.

| Procedure Steps | Detailed Instructions and/or *Rationales* |
|---|---|
| 1. Wash hands, assemble equipment, and put on gloves. | *Protects you from microorganism contamination.* |
| 2. Identify the patient and introduce yourself. | *Ensures that you are performing the procedure on the correct patient.* |
| B 3. Explain the procedure, ***using language the patient can understand,*** and instruct the patient to remove appropriate clothing, assisting as needed. | *Ensures understanding, consent, and cooperation from the patient. Provide privacy when patient is removing clothing.* |
| B 4. Assist the adult patient onto the examining table, position the patient on his or her side (lateral or Sims position) and cover with a drape, ***displaying sensitivity to patient privacy***. | When performing the procedure on infants or small children, ask the parent or accompanying adult to prepare the child while you prepare the thermometer. Position the infant according to the parent's or physician's preference. Ensure safety during the procedure by maintaining control of the infant's or child's position. (A parent can be instructed to assist you, especially if it comforts the child.) |

| Procedure Steps | Detailed Instructions and/or *Rationales* |
|---|---|
| 5. Place a small amount of lubricant onto a tissue and place it within reach. | |
| 6. Correctly prepare the thermometer. | a. Place the red probe connector into the receptacle of the unit base. *The red probe is used for rectal temperatures.*<br>b. Remove probe from the stored position.<br>c. Insert the red probe firmly into the probe cover. *Check to make sure it is properly seated.* |
| 7. Apply lubricant to the end of the probe cover. | *This eases the insertion.* |
| 8. Arrange the drape to expose the buttocks, raise the upper buttock to expose the anus, and carefully insert the lubricated thermometer probe into the anal canal approximately 1 inch for adults and ½ inch for infants and children. Hold the thermometer in place until the unit signals. | Angle the probe slightly to ensure contact with mucosa. Do not force the thermometer. Rotating will often facilitate insertion. If opening is not apparent, ask the patient to bear down slightly; this will usually expose the opening. |
| 9. Withdraw the thermometer. Eject the probe cover into the waste container. | *All materials coming into contact with bodily secretions are deposited in a waste container.* |
| 10. Read the thermometer, noting the temperature. | Temperature is displayed digitally in the window of the unit. |
| 11. Replace the probe in the unit and return the thermometer to the charging stand. | The thermometer display will read zero and shut off. *The unit should remain in the stand so it is fully charged and ready for use.* |
| 12. Remove any excess lubricant from the anal area with a tissue. | Wipe from front to back. |
| 13. If the patient is an adult, assist the adult patient from the examining table and instruct him or her to dress.<br>If the patient is a child, ask the parent or accompanying adult to dress an infant or child. | Provide privacy as appropriate for adult patients. |
| 14. Remove and discard gloves in the waste container. | |
| 15. Wash hands. | |
| 16. Document the temperature in the patient's chart, placing an (R) after the finding. | |

### Charting Example

| | |
|---|---|
| 3-6-XX<br>11:30 am | T. 100.2 (R) B. Davis, RMA(AMT) |

## Measuring Axillary Temperatures

Temperature can be measured by placing the electronic or digital thermometer in the axilla (armpit). This method is the least accurate. Axillary measurement is appropriate when oral and rectal temperatures are undesirable or contraindicated. Normal axillary temperature is 36.4°C or 97.6°F, one full degree *below* normal oral temperature. When recording the axillary temperature, place the letters *Ax* in parentheses following the reading.

Some electronic thermometers can change the reading mode to axillary and read the temperature by adding one degree; consult the instructional booklet with your equipment to determine whether your model has this. Apply a probe cover to the probe (unless otherwise indicated, use the oral probe) and insert the tip well into the axillary space with the probe extending down and slightly forward along the patient's side. Press gently into the space to establish good tissue contact. Have the patient lower his or her arm over the probe. Hold the probe in position to maintain good contact. Remove and read after the unit signals completion.

Axillary temperature can also be taken using the digital thermometer. The tip of the thermometer is placed into the axillary space and supported in place. The arm is held tight against the body until the signal is heard. Refer to Procedure 38–4 for detailed steps on measuring an axillary temperature.

## Measuring Tympanic (Aural) Temperatures

The normal tympanic (aural) temperature is 99.1 degrees, generally 0.5 degrees higher than the normal oral temperature of 98.6 degrees. Tympanic membrane thermometers are easy, safe, fast to use, and fairly common in many medical offices. You simply remove the thermometer from its charging cradle and apply a disposable sheath. Position the covered plastic tip properly inside the auditory canal by pulling up and back on the ear for adults and down and back for children. Be sure the probe fits snuggly and press the scan button; an infrared beam measures the heat waves. The results are displayed digitally on the screen. A release button ejects the probe cover, and in 10 seconds, another temperature can be taken. The units operate on batteries and will measure approximately 10,000 temperatures before the batteries need to be replaced. Be sure to follow the manufacturer's instructions for the model you are using because each model varies somewhat. Procedure 38–5 provides step-by-step directions for obtaining a temperature by using a tympanic thermometer.

## Measuring Temporal Artery Temperatures

Temperature is measured by scanning (gently sliding) the probe of the handheld thermometer across the forehead, halfway between the eyebrow and the hairline, from the midline to the side hairline. As long as the button is depressed and the scanner is moved

## PROCEDURE 38–4 Measure Axillary Temperature

**PURPOSE:** To determine a patient's axillary temperature with an electronic thermometer

**EQUIPMENT:** Electronic thermometer, probe, probe cover, tissues, waste container, patient chart or EHR, pen

S **SKILL:** Measure and record axillary temperature with an electronic thermometer.

| Procedure Steps | Detailed Instructions and/or *Rationales* |
|---|---|
| 1. Wash hands; assemble equipment. | |
| 2. Identify the patient and introduce yourself. | *Ensures that you are performing the procedure on the correct patient.* |
| B 3. Explain the procedure, ***using language the patient can understand.*** | *Ensures understanding, consent, and cooperation from the patient.* |
| 4. Assist the patient, as necessary, to expose the axilla. Pat the axillary space with a tissue to remove perspiration. | Perspiration prevents the probe from coming into direct contact with skin. |
| 5. Correctly prepare the thermometer. | If using an electronic thermometer:<br>a. Be sure the blue probe connector is plugged into the receptacle of the unit base. *The blue probe is used for axillary temperatures.*<br>b. Remove probe from the stored position.<br>c. Insert the probe firmly into the probe cover. |

| Procedure Steps | Detailed Instructions and/or *Rationales* |
|---|---|
| 6. Insert the covered probe deep in the axillary space. | Position so that it is in direct contact with the top of the axillary space, with the probe extending down and slightly forward. |
| 7. Hold the arm tightly against the body. Maintain the covered probe in position until the thermometer unit signals, approximately 10 to 15 seconds (Figure 38–16). | *Early removal results in inaccurate measurement.* |
| 8. Remove the probe from the patient. (Do not touch the probe cover) and discard the used probe cover into the waste container. | *Probe is contaminated with patient's sweat.* If using an electronic thermometer, press the eject button to discard the probe cover.<br><br>If using a digital thermometer, a*ll materials coming into contact with bodily secretions are deposited in a waste container.* |
| 9. Read and note the temperature. | Temperature is displayed digitally in the window of the unit. |
| 10. Disinfect thermometer and return the probe to the stored position in the unit. Store the unit in the charging stand. | The thermometer display will read zero and shut off. *The unit should remain in the stand so it is fully charged and ready for use.* |
| 11. Help the patient replace his or her clothing. | |
| 12. Wash hands. | |
| 13. Document the temperature in the patient's chart, placing an (Ax) after the finding. | |

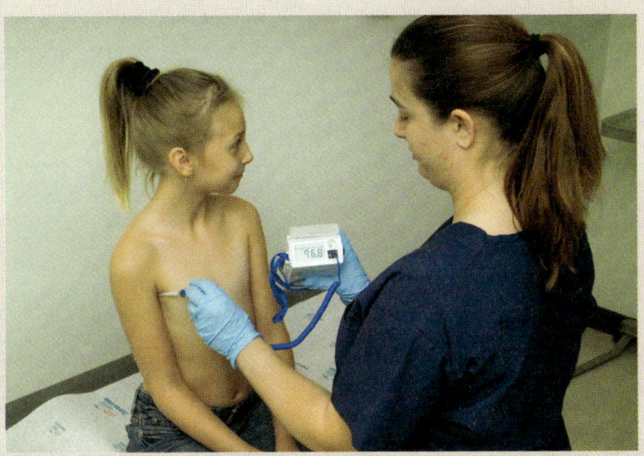

**FIGURE 38–16:** Measuring axillary temperature with an electronic thermometer. *Delmar/Cengage Learning.*

## Charting Example

| | |
|---|---|
| 3-6-XX<br>11:30 am | T. 97.2 (ax) B. Davis, RMA(AMT) |

## PROCEDURE 38–5 Measure Core Body Temperature with a Tympanic (Aural) Thermometer

**PURPOSE:** To determine a patient's core body temperature by using an infrared tympanic thermometer

**EQUIPMENT:** Tympanic thermometer unit, probe cover, waste container, patient chart or EHR, pen

**S SKILL:** Measure core body temperature with a tympanic (aural) thermometer

| Procedure Steps | Detailed Instructions and/or *Rationales* |
|---|---|
| 1. Wash hands; assemble equipment. | |
| 2. Identify the patient and introduce yourself. | *Ensures that you are performing the procedure on the correct patient.* |
| **B** 3. Explain the procedure, ***using language the patient can understand.*** | *Ensures understanding, consent, and cooperation from the patient.* |
| 4. Correctly prepare the thermometer. | a. Remove the thermometer from the base.<br>b. Attach a disposable probe cover firmly to the ear piece. The display should read "ready." |
| 5. Insert the covered probe into the ear canal, sealing the opening. | Pull up and back on the ear for adults (Figure 38–17 A) and down and back for children (Figure 38–17 B). *Air leaks will occur if the ear canal is not sealed.* |
| 6. Press the scan button to activate the thermometer. Wait until the temperature reading is displayed on the screen. | |
| 7. Withdraw the thermometer. Observe the display window, noting the temperature. | |
| 8. Press the release button on the thermometer to eject the probe cover into a waste container and return the thermometer to the base. | |
| 9. Document the temperature in the patient's chart, using (T) or (Tym) to indicate tympanic temperature. | |

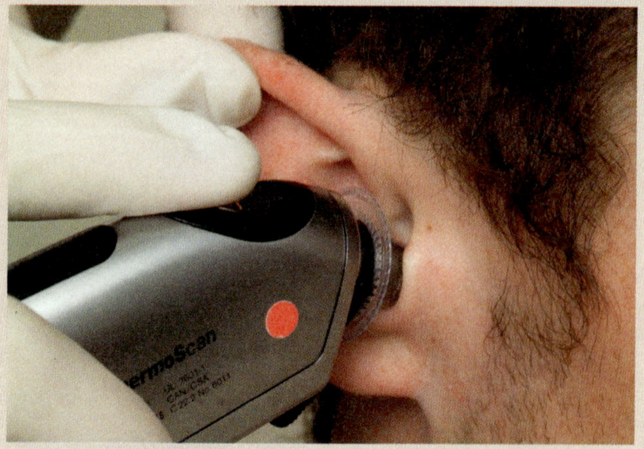

**FIGURE 38–17A:** For adults, pull up and back on the ear. *Delmar/Cengage Learning.*

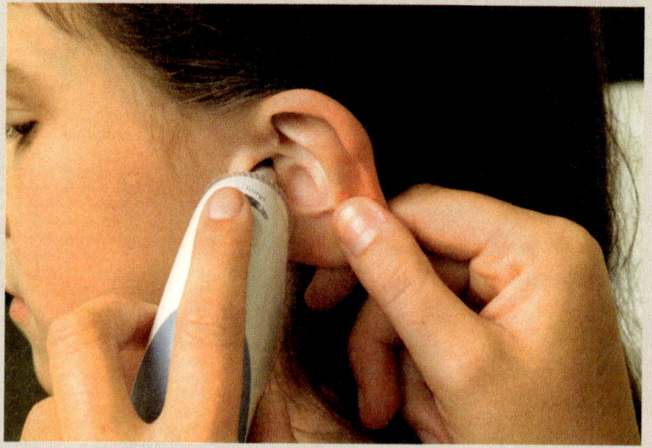

**FIGURE 38–17B:** For children, pull down and back on the ear. *Delmar/Cengage Learning.*

### Charting Example

| | |
|---|---|
| 5/10/XX<br>11:30 am | T. 100.3 (T or Tym) J. Cook, CMA(AAMA) |

slowly, it continually samples and records to measure the highest temperature. Multiple readings can cool the skin, so another immediate measurement may be slightly lower.

Clinical studies have shown TA measurement provides results more closely related to the true internal body temperature measured in a major artery than any other method. The normal TA measurement is equivalent to a rectal temperature; therefore, it is approximately one degree higher than oral measurement. *Note*: When recording on the chart, put (TA) after the temperature to indicate the method used. Measuring temperature by using a TA thermometer has several advantages:

- Appropriate for all ages, infants through elderly
- Convenient, easily accessible, and fast
- Comfortable and safe for the patient
- Proven highly accurate
- No danger from contact with mucous membranes
- Reading is not affected by oral factors such as hot and cold fluids, mouth breathing, oral surgery, or injury.
- Can be sanitized between patients like a stethoscope, with an antiseptic wipe, or clinical models have covers, caps, and sheaths if desired

Temperature of the skin is affected by the temperature of the surroundings. The sensor in the probe performs two processes when temperature is measured. At 1,000 times per second, it reads the infrared heat within the artery and measures the temperature in the immediate environment. The interior software performs calculations to determine the patient's temperature in relation to the surroundings. A few factors, however, affect the accurate measurement:

- Do not glide the probe over burns, open sores, abrasions, or scars.
- The forehead side measured must have been exposed to the environment with no hats, bangs, or bandages to trap heat.
- If there is perspiration on the forehead, measurement will be inaccurate. You must follow TA measurement with placing the probe against the neck behind the earlobe to obtain accurate assessment.
- The TAT must be in the same ambient temperature as the patient. It must be acclimated to the room temperature before it is used if it is moved from a hot to cold area or vice versa (e.g., window ledge exposed to hot sun or in line of air conditioning). Each 10° degree difference can cause a 1° error.
- Some models cannot be used near aerosol products or when oxygen is being administered.

Be sure to follow the manufacturer's guidelines for any additional factors. Procedure 38–6 lists the step-by-step details on how to obtain a temporal artery temperature.

**PATIENT EDUCATION**

Often, the provider will suggest that a patient should monitor his or her temperature at home. It can be the medical assistant's responsibility to instruct the patient about using a thermometer and how to record the temperature. The provider will name a certain elevated temperature level at which, if reached, the patient should call the office. Many types of less expensive but easy-to-use temperature measuring devices are available for home use in addition to the ones discussed in this unit and are available at most large chain pharmacies and children's stores.

## Temperature Conversions

Temperature can be converted from one scale to another by a mathematical calculation:

- To convert from Celsius to Fahrenheit, multiply the degrees by 9/5 and add 32 ([C × 9/5] + 32 = F).
- To change from Fahrenheit to Celsius, subtract 32 and multiply by 5/9 ([F − 32] × 5/9 = C).

## PROCEDURE 38–6 Measure Temperature with a Temporal Artery Thermometer

**PURPOSE:** Measure a patient's temperature with a temporal artery thermometer

**EQUIPMENT:** Temporal artery thermometer, alcohol wipe or cover, patient chart or EHR, pen

**S SKILL:** Measure and record temperature with a temporal artery thermometer.

| Procedure Steps | Detailed Instructions and/or *Rationales* |
|---|---|
| 1. Wash hands; assemble equipment. Clean the probe with alcohol or attach a cover. | |
| 2. Identify the patient and introduce yourself. | *Ensures that you are performing the procedure on the correct patient.* |

*(continues)*

*(continued)*

| Procedure Steps | Detailed Instructions and/or *Rationales* |
|---|---|
| B 3. Explain the procedure, ***using language the patient can understand***. | *Ensures understanding, consent, and cooperation from the patient.* |
| 4. Observe the forehead for perspiration and exposure to the environment. Adjust as necessary (e.g., remove hat, hold back hair). | *False readings can occur if the skin is cooled from moisture on the forehead or warmed by a hat or hair covering.* |
| 5. Position the probe at the midline of the forehead. | *Probe must be centered properly over the area for an accurate reading.* |
| 6. Keeping the probe flush on the skin, press, and hold the scan button while slowly sliding the thermometer across the forehead until reaching the hairline (Figure 38–18). | If perspiration is present, continue to hold button, lift probe from forehead, and position on neck behind ear lobe. Note: You will hear clicking, indicating a rise to a higher temperature until the maximum is measured. |
| 7. When scanning is completed, release the button and lift the probe from the forehead or neck. Read the temperature on the display and return the thermometer to storage. | The reading will remain on the display until 15 to 30 seconds after the button is released, depending on the model. To turn off the thermometer immediately, depress and quickly release the button. |
| 8. Document the temperature in the patient's chart, using (TA) to indicate temporal artery temperature. | |
| 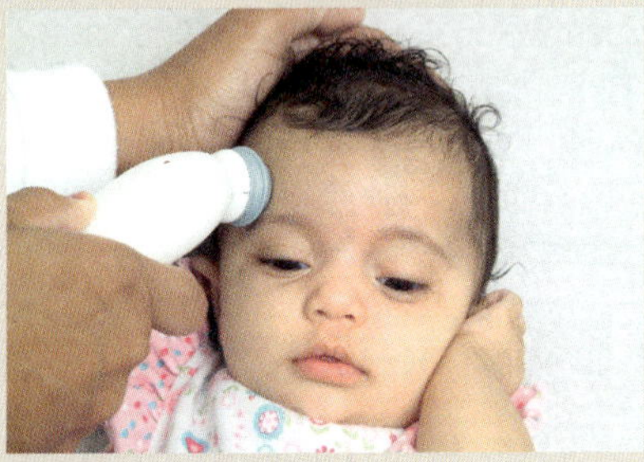 **FIGURE 38–18:** Slide thermometer across forehead. *Delmar/Cengage Learning.* | |

## Charting Example

| | |
|---|---|
| 5/10/XX 11:30 am | T. 99.5 (TA) B. Davis (RMA) |

Another way to convert temperature uses a different mathematical calculation. Some people find this easier to do:

- To convert Celsius to Fahrenheit, the equation is: F = (C × 1.8) + 32.
- To convert Fahrenheit to Celsius, the equation is: C = F − 32/1.8

### EXAMPLE

To convert Celsius to Fahrenheit:
37° C × 9/5(333/5) = 66.6 + 32 = 98.6° F
C × F–32/1.8
C = 98.6–32 = 66.6/1.8 = 37

To convert Fahrenheit to Celsius:
98.6° F–32 = 66.6 × 5/9(333/9) = 37° C
F = (C × 1.8) + 32
F = 37 × 1.8 = 66.6 + 32 = 98.6

**TABLE 38–4 Temperature Conversion and Comparison**

| Comparison | Celsius (C) | Fahrenheit (F) |
|---|---|---|
| Freezing | 0° | 32° |
| Body temperature | 37° | 98.6° |
| Pasteurization | 63° | 145° |
| Boiling | 100° | 212° |
| Sterilizing (autoclave) | 121° | 250.0° |

Table 38–4 compares some common temperatures in Celsius and Fahrenheit.

## PULSE

Each time the heart beats, blood is forced into the aorta, temporarily expanding its walls and initiating a wavelike effect. This wave continues through all the body's arteries, causing the alternating expansion and recoil of the arterial walls (Figure 38–19). This effect can be **palpated** (felt) in the arteries that are close to the body surface and that lie over bone or firm structures. When the artery is pressed against the underlying structure, it is possible to feel the rhythmic pulsation, known as the pulse.

### Pulse Sites

The pulse can be felt in several locations on the body, as shown in Figure 38–20:

- The **radial** pulse is located on the thumb side of the inner surface of the wrist, lying over the radius bone. The radial pulse site is used most frequently when measuring pulse rate.
- The **brachial** artery pulse location is on the inner medial surface of the elbow, at the **antecubital** space (crease of elbow). This site is used to palpate and **auscultate** (listen to) blood pressure.
- The **carotid** pulse can be felt in the carotid artery of the neck when pressure is applied to the area at either side of the trachea. It is the carotid pulse that is palpated during the cardiopulmonary resuscitation (CPR) life-saving maneuver.
- The **femoral** pulse is located midway in the **groin** where the artery begins its descent down the femur.
- The **dorsalis pedis**, on the instep of the foot, and the **popliteal**, at the back ofthe knee, are other sites palpated to evaluate circulation in the lower extremities.

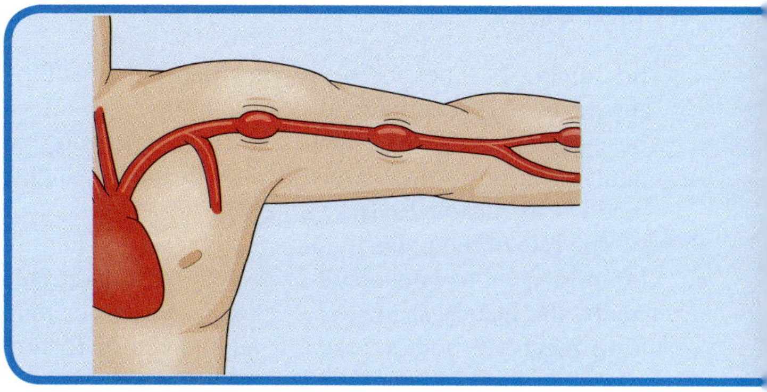

**Figure 38–19:** Blood pumped from the heart causes a wavelike effect in the arteries. *Delmar/Cengage Learning.*

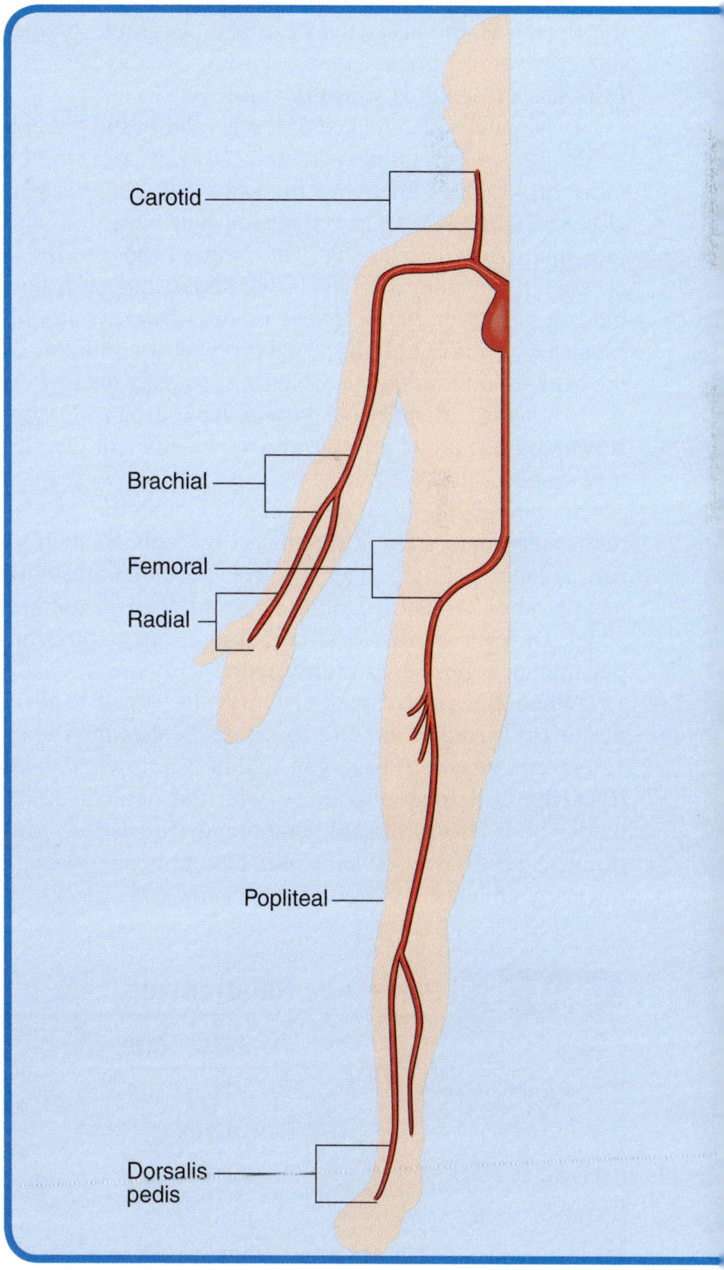


**FIGURE 38–20:** Pulse sites of the upper and lower extremities and the neck. *Delmar/Cengage Learning.*

## Pulse Rate

The number of times the heart beats per minute is typically measured by counting the pulse in the radial artery. The average adult pulse range is 60 to 100 beats per minute. The pulse rate is recorded as beats per minute preceded by a capital *P* (i.e., P. 72).

The rate of the pulse is influenced by several factors. The most obvious is exercise or activity. With increased activity, the heartbeat increases 20 to 30 beats per minute to meet the body's needs. It should return to normal within three minutes after activity has stopped. Of course, the rate of increase will be in proportion to the level of activity.

Pulse rate is directly related to age. The younger the person is, the faster the heartbeat. A sample of age-related average pulse rates according to the National Institutes of Health is shown in Table 38–5.

Pulse rate is also related to the gender of the patient. A female's pulse is approximately 10 beats per minute more rapid than a male's of the same age. Pulse rate is also related to size; a larger person will have a slower rate than a smaller person. The relationship of size is particularly evident in animals. The heart rate of a bird may be well over 200 beats per minute, whereas an elephant has a rate of about 30. The physical condition of the body is another factor. Athletes, especially those who run or engage in strenuous sports, have a considerably slower pulse rate as a result of a more efficient circulatory system.

In general, the heart rate increases when the sympathetic nervous system is stimulated by feelings such as fear, anxiety, pain, or anger. The rate also increases with certain other conditions, such as thyroid disease, anemia, shock, or fever. A consistent rate of more than 100 beats per minute is known as **tachycardia**.

When the parasympathetic nervous system affects the heart, it causes the rate to be much slower. A consistent rate below 60 beats per minute is known as **bradycardia**. This may also occur with the use of certain medications, heart disease, emotional depression, and drugs. A rate below 60 beats per minute is also normal for many athletes.

**TABLE 38–5** Pulse–Age Relationship

| Age | Pulse Rate |
|---|---|
| Less than 1 year | 100–160 |
| 1–10 years | 70-120 |
| 11–Adult years | 60–100 |
| Midlife Adult | 60–100 |
| Older adult | 50–65 |

## Pulse Characteristics

When measuring pulse rate, two other characteristics must also be observed and recorded. The force or strength of the pulse is referred to as its **volume**. Words to describe this quality are *normal*, *full* or *bounding*, *weak*, and **thready** (scarcely perceivable).

The quality of **rhythm** of the pulse refers to its regularity, or the equal spacing of the beats. The term **arrhythmia** refers to a pulse that lacks a regular rhythm. The pulse can be irregular (without a consistent pattern) or regularly irregular (unequally spaced but consistently the same beating pattern). A pulse can also be intermittent and occasionally skip or insert beats. Often, caffeine or nicotine react on the heart to cause irregularity and increased rate.

## Measuring the Radial Pulse

The patient should be completely relaxed and sitting comfortably or lying down when the pulse is measured and evaluated. Ideally, the arm should be well supported, with the wrist near the level of the heart. Place the tips of your fingers at the wrist area, about an inch above the base of the thumb (Figure 38–21). Never use your thumb to measure pulse rate; you might feel and record your own heart rate in your thumb's artery.

An appropriate amount of pressure applied to the artery will permit the pulsations to be felt. Too much pressure will shut off the circulation and therefore eliminate the pulse beat. Too little pressure will not compress the artery sufficiently against the radius. With practice, applying the correct amount of pressure will become routine. The pulse rate may be measured for 30 seconds and multiplied by two; however, if there is any irregularity, the rate should be measured for a full minute. Respirations are often measured at the same time as the

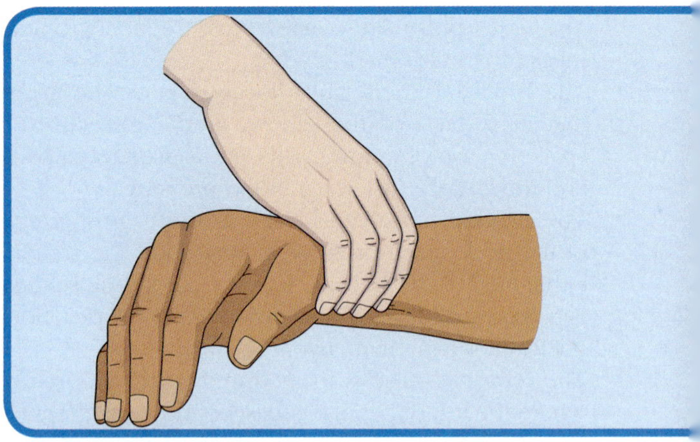

**FIGURE 38–21:** Measuring the radial pulse. *Delmar/Cengage Learning.*

patient's pulse. After you read the section, "Respiration," later in the chapter, refer to Procedure 38–8 for step-by-step details about how to obtain a radial pulse and respiration rate.

## Measuring the Apical Pulse

When measuring heart rate by the radial pulse is not appropriate, it is necessary to listen to the heart at its **apex** with a **stethoscope**. This is a very accurate method of measuring pulse rate. The contraction of the atria and the ventricles will be heard as two closely occurring sounds known as the "lubb dupp"; however, both contraction phases are counted as only one beat. Whenever a pulse rate is measured at a point other than the radial, the location should be noted when recording the rate (e.g., P. 97 [Ap]). Note that an **apical** pulse is counted for a full minute, so it is possible to record an uneven number.

### Apical Indications

Apical pulse measurement is indicated for infants and small children because of their normally rapid rate, which is easier to hear and count than to palpate. Patients with heart conditions, especially if being medicated with cardiac drugs, will require apical measurement for greater accuracy. Apical measurement is always indicated if you have difficulty feeling a radial pulse and believe you may be missing beats. Other indications are an excessively rapid or slow rate or a thready or irregular quality.

### Locating the Apex

The bottom or lower edge of the heart is known as the apex. This is the point of maximum impulse of the heart against the chest wall. It can be palpated at the left fifth intercostal space in line with the middle of the left clavicle. This spot may be located by pressing the fingertips between the ribs and counting down five spaces on the left chest wall (Figure 38–22 A). Often, the beat at the apex can be felt with the fingertips.

Another, quicker method for estimating the location of the apex is to place the outstretched *left* hand on the chest wall with the tip of the middle finger in the suprasternal notch and the thumb at a 45-degree angle (Figure 38–22 B). The end of the thumb will be approximately over the apex. This is only an approximate measurement because the size of the chest and the hand will vary. For a ready reference point, the apex should be just below the left breast. Again, this is variable, particularly in the female, because of the size and placement of the breast. Refer to Procedure 38–7.

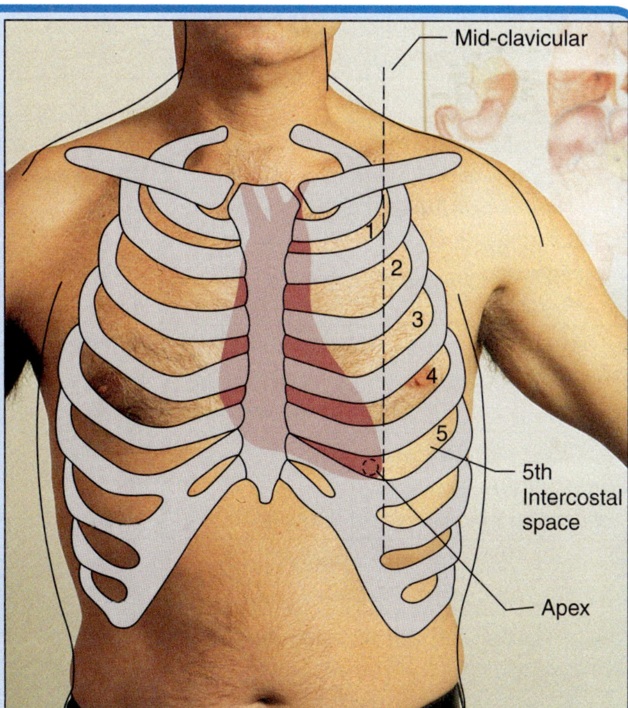


**Figure 38–22A:** Locate the apical pulse by counting intercostal spaces. *Delmar/Cengage Learning.*

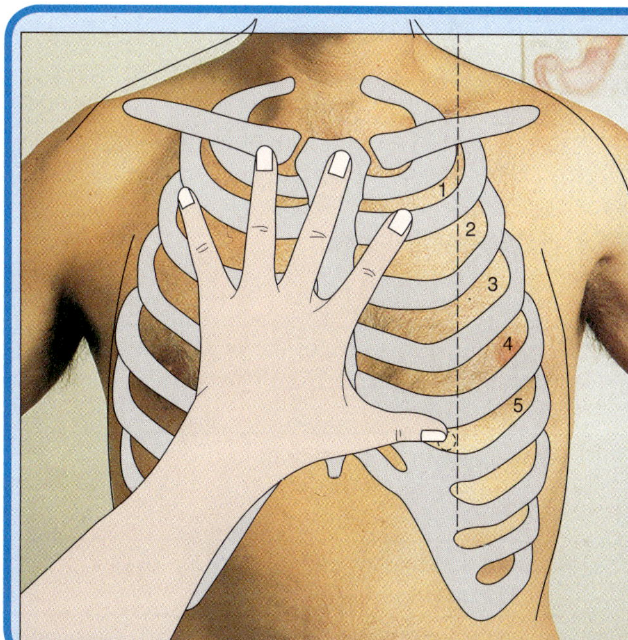


**Figure 38–22B:** Alternative method for locating the apex of the heart. *Delmar/Cengage Learning.*

## PROCEDURE 38–7 Measure the Apical Pulse

**MEDIA LINK:** View the video for this chapter, "Measure an Apical Pulse," on the Premium Website

**PURPOSE:** To determine the rate, rhythm, and quality of a patient's apical pulse

**EQUIPMENT:** Watch with second hand, stethoscope, alcohol wipe, patient chart or EHR, pen

S **SKILL:** Measure and record apical pulse rate.

| Procedure Steps | Detailed Instructions and/or *Rationales* |
|---|---|
| 1. Wash hands; assemble equipment. Clean the stethoscope. | Wipe stethoscope earpieces and chest piece with an alcohol pad to *prevent transfer of organisms.* |
| 2. Identify the patient and introduce yourself. | *Ensures that you are performing the procedure on the correct patient.* |
| B 3. Explain the procedure, ***using language the patient can understand***. | *Ensures understanding, consent, and cooperation from the patient.* |
| B 4. Uncover the left side of the chest. ***Provide privacy and a gown or drape if indicated***. | *Auscultation must be done directly against the skin surface.* |
| 5. Place the stethoscope earpieces in your ears. | The openings in the tips should be forward, entering the auditory canal. |
| 6. Locate the apex. | Palpate to the left fifth intercostal space at the mid-clavicular line. *Note*: If the chest piece does not have a chill ring, warm it in the palm of one hand while locating the apex. *This also prevents accidental striking against a hard surface and the resulting noise in your ears.* |
| 7. Place the chest piece of the stethoscope at the apex. | |
| 8. Count the beats for a full minute. Note the rate. | Observe wristwatch and begin counting rate when second hand is at 3, 6, 9, or 12. *It is easier to measure* one *minute when beginning at one of these four numbers.* Both pulse phases count as one beat. *Apical rates are indicated when quality or rhythm irregularities are present or possible; therefore, full-minute measurement is essential.* |
| 9. Determine the quality of the heart sounds and remove the earpieces from your ears. | Concentrate on rate, rhythm, and volume. *The quality of the beat is significant in evaluation of the heart action. Be certain of sounds and pattern.* |
| 10. Assist or instruct the patient to dress. | *Unless the physician also wishes to assess heart action. Determine this by asking the physician prior to measurement or if your findings indicate the need.* |
| 11. Clean the earpieces and chest piece of the stethoscope. | *This can be done with an alcohol pad; return it to storage.* |
| 12. Document the rate and quality of the heart sounds in the patient's chart. | Indicate that it is apical measurement. *Immediate recording aids in eliminating errors.* |
| 13. Wash hands. | |

### Charting Example

| | |
|---|---|
| 5/10/XX<br>11:30 am | P. 103 (Ap), full but irregular with an extra beat every four beats. C. WILLIAMS, CMA(AAMA)——— |

### Pulse Oximetry

Many of the electronic blood pressure units, which will be discussed later in the chapter, can check blood pressure, pulse, and oxygen saturation all at the same time and are becoming more and more popular in the medical field. Another device that can be used to obtain a patient's pulse and arterial oxygen saturation in the blood is the pulse oximeter machine, a small, handheld unit with a clip attached that is usually applied to the patient's middle finger. The clip uses an infrared light to measure the pulse and oxygen levels. If the pulse is outside of the normal range, it should be taken manually for confirmation. Detailed information along with the procedure on how to perform a pulse oximetry is covered in Chapter 40.

## RESPIRATION

One respiration is the combination of total inspiration (breathing in) and total expiration (breathing out). Other frequently used terms are **inhale** and **exhale**. Respirations are usually measured as one part of total vital signs assessment. Because patients can voluntarily control the depth, rate, and regularity of their breathing to some extent, it is important for them to be unaware that the procedure is being done. To accomplish this, it is common practice to observe and measure respiration immediately after assessing the radial pulse, while maintaining your fingers at the radial pulse site.

### Quality of Respiration

Respirations should be quiet, effortless, and regularly spaced. Breathing should be through the nose with the mouth closed. Excessively fast and deep breathing, commonly associated with hysteria, is called **hyperventilation**. Difficult or labored breathing is called **dyspnea**. Frequently, dyspnea is accompanied by discomfort and an anxious expression, caused by the fear of being unable to breathe. This patient will use the accessory respiratory muscles of the rib cage, neck, shoulders, and back to assist the breathing process.

The presence of **rales** (noisy breathing) usually indicates constricted bronchial passageways or the collection of fluid or exudate. Rales may be present with pneumonia, bronchitis, asthma, and other pulmonary diseases.

Respirations should be observed for the depth of inhalation. Three words are used to describe this quality: normal, shallow, or deep. Depth of inhalation can be determined by watching the rise and fall of the chest. The rhythm of the respirations must also be assessed. This quality can be described as regular or irregular. Absence of breathing is known as **apnea**. A breathing pattern called **Cheyne-Stokes** occurs with acute brain, heart, or lung damage or disease and with intoxicants. It is characterized by slow, shallow breaths that increase in depth and frequency, followed by a few shallow breaths, and then a period of apnea for 10 to 20 seconds and often longer (Figure 38–23). This type of breathing pattern frequently precedes death.

### Respiration Rate

The normal respiration rate for adults is 16 to 20 times per minute. The respiration rate in infants and children has a greater range and fluctuates more during illness, exercise, and emotion than adult rates do. In the newborn, the rate per minute can range from 30 to 60; in early childhood, from 20 to 40; and during late childhood, from 16 to 26. The rate will reach an adult normal range of 16 to 20 by age 16. An abnormally slow rate of respiration is known as **bradypnea**. A faster than normal rate of respiration is known as **tachypnea**.

### Counting Respirations

It is necessary to observe the patient carefully while measuring respiration rate. If the patient is lying on the examination table, position the patient's arm across the upper abdominal area, placing your fingers over the radial pulse site. In this position, you can visualize and feel respiration. With the patient in a sitting position, you need to observe more carefully because you count the respirations. Remember, it is also necessary to keep your watch in view as you observe. With a little practice, you will be able to manage both at the same time.

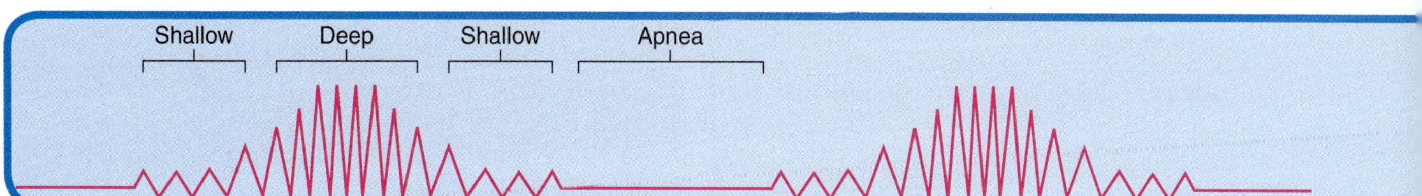


**Figure 38–23:** Cheyne-Stokes breathing pattern. *Delmar/Cengage Learning.*

When counting respirations as part of the TPR assessment, it is very important to remember the number of heartbeats you have just counted. It may help you to use the following method:

1. Assume the pulse measuring position.
2. Observe, determine the characteristics, and describe to yourself the qualities of both the pulse and the respirations.
3. Count the number of heartbeats during the first 30 seconds of the minute.
4. Repeat the pulse rate to yourself as you count the number of respirations during the second 30 seconds.

(*Note*: You *must* use the word "and" between each respiration so you do not accidentally add counts to the pulse rate.)

For example, if your patient's pulse rate after 30 seconds is 40, repeat this number as you count the respirations: "40 and 1, 40 and 2, 40 and 3," and so on, until the second 30-second period is past. At the end of a minute, you will have counted both rates. Multiply the rates by two and record. Procedure 38–8 gives step-by-step instruction for measuring radial pulse and respirations.

## PROCEDURE 38–8 Measure the Radial Pulse and Respirations

**PURPOSE:** To determine the rate, rhythm, and quality of a patient's radial pulse and the rate, rhythm, sound, and depth of a patient's respirations

**EQUIPMENT:** Watch with second hand, patient chart or EHR, pen

S **SKILL:** Measure and record radial pulse rate and respirations.

| Procedure Steps | Detailed Instructions and/or *Rationales* |
|---|---|
| 1. Wash hands; assemble equipment. | |
| 2. Identify the patient and introduce yourself. | *Ensures that you are performing the procedure on the correct patient.* |
| B 3. Explain the procedure, ***using language the patient can understand.*** | *Ensures understanding, consent, and cooperation from the patient.*<br>Note: In this procedure, it is preferable to explain only the pulse measurement and not the respirations. If the patient knows you will be counting respirations, control of breathing is possible, resulting in an inaccurate measurement. |
| 4. Determine the patient's recent activity. | *Exertion within the past three to five minutes will cause a temporary increase in pulse and respiration rate.* |
| 5. Position the patient with the wrist supported on a table or lap. | |
| 6. Locate the radial artery on the thumb side of the wrist (Figure 38–24) and observe the quality of the pulse before beginning to count. Determine whether it is regular, strong, weak, or thready. | Do not use your thumb because it has its own pulse. Place the tips of your fingers lightly over the artery. *Concentration on the quality prior to measurement assists in accurate evaluation.* |
| 7. Count a *regular* pulse for 30 seconds and multiply the results by two. | Check your watch. Begin counting beats when the second hand is at 3, 6, 9, or 12. *This makes 30 seconds easier to observe.* If the pulse is irregular, count for full minute. Do not multiply by 2. |
| 8. Assess respiration quality. | Determine depth, rhythm, and sound. *In certain disease conditions, the presence or absence of quality characteristics is a significant finding.* |

| Procedure Steps | Detailed Instructions and/or *Rationales* |
|---|---|
| 9. Count respirations for 30 seconds and multiply the results by two. | One rise and fall of the chest equals one respiration. Maintain the radial pulse position. Note: If respirations are irregular, count for a full minute and do not multiply results by two. |
| 10. Document the patient's pulse and respiration (including quality characteristics) in the chart. | Record both the pulse and respirations in beats per minute and describe the quality characteristics. |
| 11. Wash hands. | |

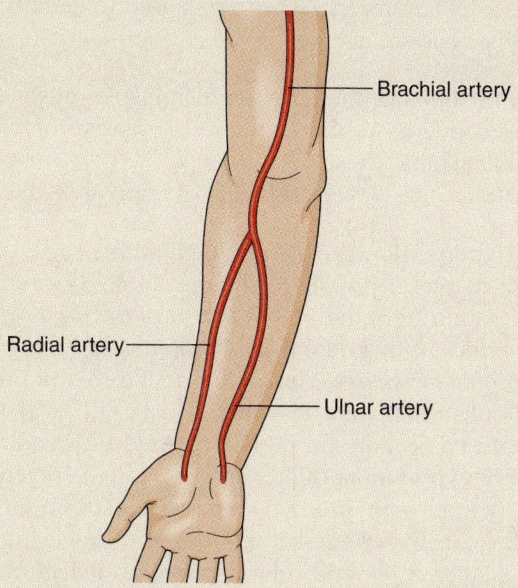


**FIGURE 38–24:** The radial pulse is measured in the radial artery, on the thumb side of the wrist.
*Delmar/Cengage Learning.*

**Charting Example**

| | |
|---|---|
| 5/10/XX<br>11:30 am | P. 96, weak but regular R. 24, rate and rhythm regular B. Davis RMA (AMT)———— |

## BLOOD PRESSURE

Learning to assess blood pressure accurately requires attention to details, careful listening, and correct technique. The term *blood pressure* means the fluctuating pressure the blood exerts against the arterial walls as it alternately contracts and relaxes. The blood pressure reflects the condition of the heart, the amount of blood forced from the heart at contraction, the condition of the arteries, and, to some extent, the volume and viscosity (thickness) of the blood.

Blood pressure is measured in the brachial artery of the arm at the antecubital space (Figure 38–25). It should be measured in both arms, at least initially. There is normally a 5- to 10-mm difference. Subsequent readings should be made on the arm with the higher pressure.

### Maintaining Blood Pressure

Two main factors cooperate to maintain a fairly constant blood pressure. The first is the heart or pump, which exerts pressure on the blood. About 100,000 times a

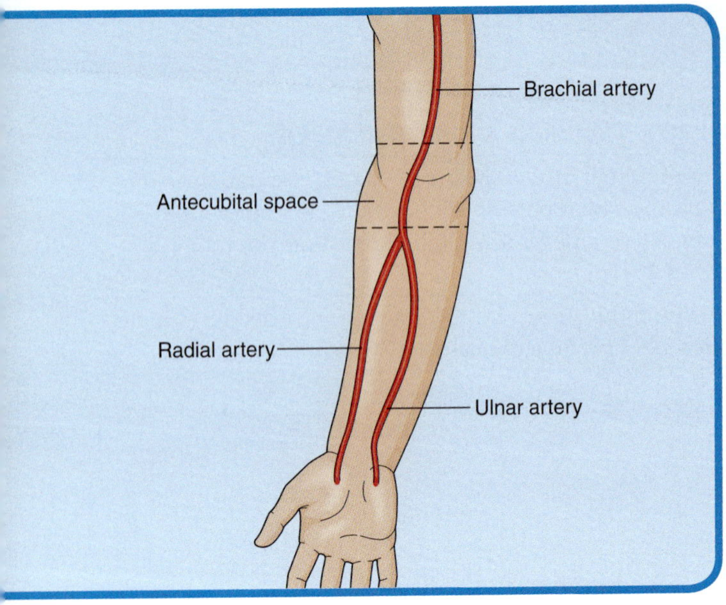


**Figure 38–25:** Blood pressure is measured in the brachial artery at the antecubital space. *Delmar/Cengage Learning.*

day, the heart contracts, forcing blood into the aorta and throughout the blood vessels of the body. Without a strong, effective pump, the blood will not flow, and the pressure will drop.

The second factor is the brain, which controls, through the autonomic nervous system, the rate of the heart and the size of the opening or caliber of the arteries. When sensors in the arteries detect an increase in arterial pressure, a message is sent to the brain, which in turn directs the arteries to dilate slightly (reducing resistance to the flow of blood) and directs the heart to slow down (reducing the amount of blood being forced out). If the pressure drops too far, the message to the brain results in a slightly increased heart action and constriction of the arteries, which cause the pressure to rise. Both actions are needed to maintain homeostasis.

## Blood Pressure Phases

The phases of blood pressure are identical to those of the pulse. A contraction phase, known as **systole**, corresponds to the beat phase of the heart and is the period of greatest pressure. The relaxation phase, known as **diastole**, corresponds to the resting or filling action of the heart and is the period of least pressure.

## Normal Blood Pressure

Blood pressure readings are measurements of systolic and diastolic pressure written as a fraction, for example, B/P 120/80, when 120 represents the systolic and 80 represents the diastolic pressure. An adult should have a systolic pressure less than 120 mm Hg and a diastolic pressure less than 80.

Blood pressure readings persistently in the ranges of 140–159 and 90–99 indicate stage 1 *hypertension* (high blood pressure). Hypertension can result from things such as stress, obesity, high salt intake, sedentary lifestyle, and aging. Physical conditions that cause hypertension are kidney disease; thyroid dysfunction; neurological disorders; and vascular conditions (such as atherosclerosis and arteriosclerosis), which make circulation more difficult, therefore requiring a greater pressure to circulate the blood. An elevated pressure without apparent cause is said to be **idiopathic** or **essential** stage 1 hypertension. Other terms used to identify types of hypertension include:

- Primary—without another identifiable cause
- Secondary—results from renal disease or another identifiable cause
- Malignant—severe, difficult, or impossible to control

Hypertension can also be defined by stages as they relate to blood pressure findings. Table 38–6 contains information from the *Eighth Report of the Joint National Committee on Detection, Evaluation, and Treatment of High Blood Pressure.* The table classifies blood pressure for adults older than 18 years. It is based on the average of two or more properly measured B/P readings on each of two or more office visits. It has been determined that people with pre-hypertension are twice as likely to develop hypertension as those with lower findings. The higher a person's blood pressure, the greater the chance for heart attack, heart failure, stroke, and kidney disease.

A blood pressure consistently below 90/60 indicates *hypotension* (low blood pressure), which may be normal for some persons. Hypotension can be present with heart failure, severe burns, dehydration, deep depression, hemorrhage, and shock. A drop in blood pressure can also occur when a patient changes from a sitting to a standing position. This is known as **orthostatic** hypotension and occurs commonly in elderly patients because of decreased circulation efficiency. It often results in dizziness and sometimes syncope. Certain medications can also be the cause of hypotension. Typically, if blood pressure is measured, it will show a drop of at least 20 mm Hg systolic and 10 mm Hg diastolic. Some providers routinely assess orthostatic pressure on all older patients as part of the physical assessment.

## Pulse Pressure

**Pulse pressure** refers to the difference between the systolic and diastolic reading and is an indicator of the tone of the arterial walls. For example, when the

**TABLE 38–6 Classification and Management of Blood Pressure for Adults**

| | | | | Initial Drug Therapy | |
|---|---|---|---|---|---|
| **Blood Pressure Classification** | **Systolic Blood Pressure (mm Hg)** | **Diastolic Blood Pressure (mm Hg)** | **Lifestyle Modification** | **Without Compelling Indication** | **With Compelling Indications** |
| Normal | <120 | and <80 | Encourage | No antihypertensive drug indicated | Drugs for compelling indications |
| Pre-hypertension | 120–139 | or 80–89 | Yes | No antihypertensive drug indicated | Drugs for compelling indications; other antihypertensive drugs as needed. |
| Stage 1 hypertension | 140–159 | or 90–99 | Yes | Thiazide-type diuretics for most; may consider ACEI, ARB, BB, CCB*, or combination | |
| Stage 2 hypertension | ≥160 | or ≥ 100 | Yes | Two-drug combination for most usually (thiazide-type diuretic and ACEI, ARB, BB, CCB) | |

*ACEI, angiotensin-converting enzyme inhibitor; ARB, angiotensin receptor blocker; BB, beta blocker; CCB, calcium-channel blocker.

Source: *Seventh Report of the Joint National Committee on Detection, Evaluation, and Treatment of High Blood Pressure (JNC 7).*

pressure is 120/80, the pulse pressure is 40, which is a normal finding. A pulse pressure over 50 or less than 30 mm Hg may be considered abnormal. A general rule is that the pulse pressure should be approximately a third of the systolic measurement. If less, the patient may have an auscultatory gap (absence of sound), and the pressure may have been incorrectly measured. This disorder is described later.

## Equipment Factors

Blood pressure is measured using a stethoscope and a **sphygmomanometer** (Figures 38–26 A and B). It is important for sphygmomanometers be in proper working order, correctly calibrated, and serviced regularly.

**Aneroid** models must be checked regularly over the entire pressure range. Studies have shown many aneroid sphygmomanometers used in family practice to be faulty. There are two primary areas of failure. The control valves of the cuffs often result in leakage, and a greater problem with accuracy occurs as a result of dial errors because they are rarely calibrated. Faults in aneroid models have to be corrected by service technicians or the manufacturer. The office should have a maintenance policy whereby all sphygmomanometers are on a scheduled service plan.

Blood pressure cuffs are critical to correct measurement. They are available in different sizes to measure blood pressure in neonates (infants), children, adults, obese adults, and adult thighs (Figure 38–27). If the reading is to be accurate, the cuff must be the appropriate size. If it is too small for the upper arm, the reading will be falsely high; if too large, falsely low. To determine the proper size, compare the cuff width to the width of the upper arm. The cuff should be about 20 percent wider than the arm. When a cuff is too small and you do not have access to a wide adult cuff, measure to the width of the forearm. If the cuff is of adequate size, take the blood pressure reading in the forearm by placing the stethoscope over the radial artery.

An electronic sphygmomanometer is totally automatic and facilitates blood pressure measurement by providing a digital readout in the display window (Figure 38–28). It does not require the use of a stethoscope and should eliminate errors from improper technique or hearing

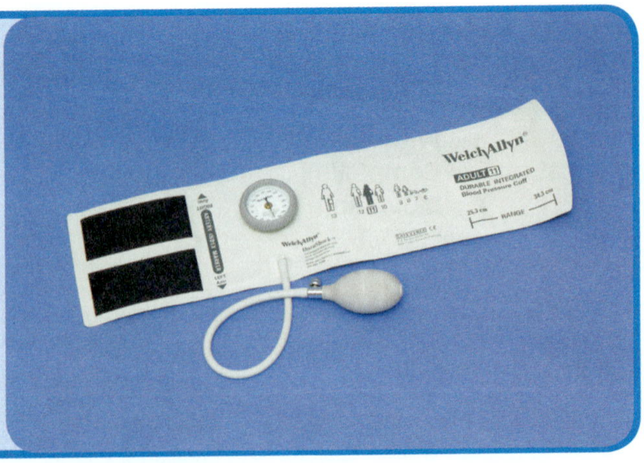

**FIGURE 38–26A:** Aneroid sphygmomanometer. *Delmar/Cengage Learning.*

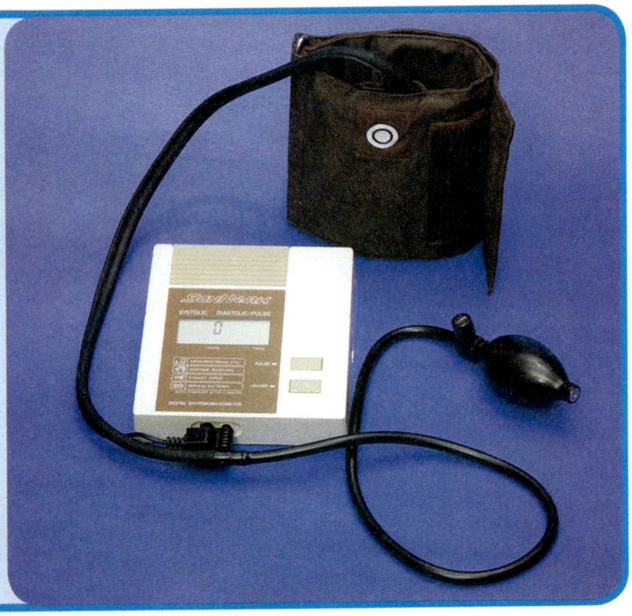

**FIGURE 38–26B:** Digital sphygmomanometer. *Delmar/Cengage Learning.*

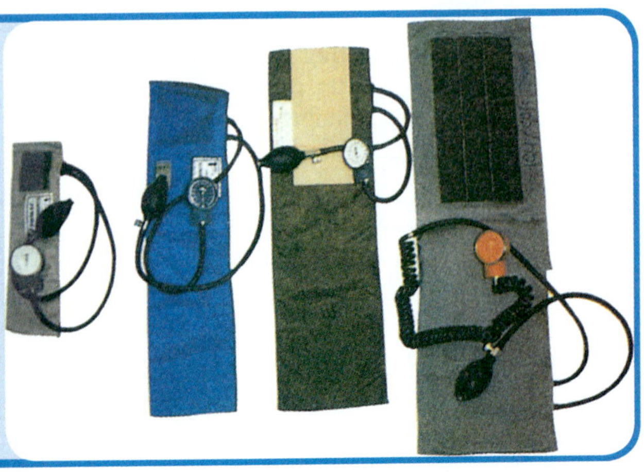

**FIGURE 38–27:** Blood pressure cuffs in different sizes to fit from the arm of a small child up to an adult thigh. *Delmar/Cengage Learning.*

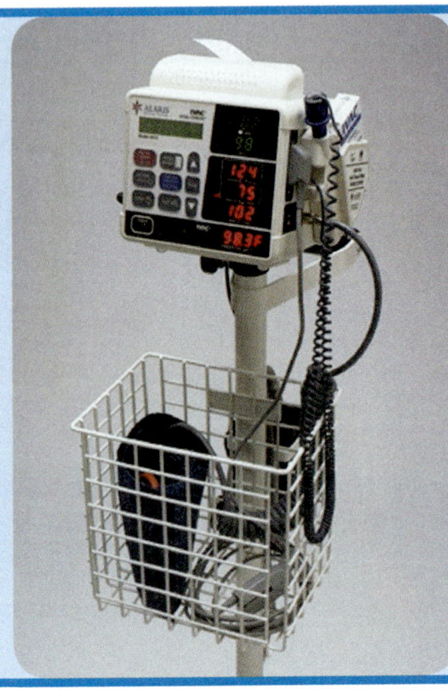

**FIGURE 38–28:** Electronic sphygmomanometer. *Delmar/Cengage Learning.*

difficulties. After the cuff is applied, the operator presses a button and the cuff automatically inflates, releases pressure slowly, and displays the results. The equipment can also be equipped with a pulse oximeter feature, which measures pulse rate and oxygen saturation when the sensor is attached to the finger. As with any piece of mechanical equipment, if the reading seems unlikely, it should be repeated or checked with another piece of equipment.

## Measuring Techniques

Blood pressure readings are critical for the determination of hypertension and for proper medication for managing it; therefore, strict procedure techniques must be followed to ensure the accuracy of the results when using manual equipment.

1. The cuff must be completely deflated when applied.
2. The patient must be comfortable, with the arm slightly flexed at the elbow and the brachial artery on a level with the heart. The arm must be free of a constricting sleeve.
3. The center of the bladder in the cuff must be placed over the brachial artery. Fold the bladder area of the cuff in half to locate the center. Many cuffs have improper artery markings.
4. The manometer must be viewed directly from a distance of not more than 3 feet.
5. A palpatory reading should be taken first to determine proper inflation. This is achieved by placing your fingers on your patient's wrist and slowly opening the valve on the inflation bulb to allow air out at about 5 mm Hg/second. As the brachial artery

**CLINICAL PEARL**

A study at Duke University, reported in the Harvard Medical School's *Heart Letter*, stated that researchers had taken blood pressure measurements through clothing on 36 volunteers to determine whether readings would be inaccurate. One arm was bare, whereas the other was covered with clothing, either a shirt or a shirt with a light sweater. Simultaneous automated blood pressure measurements revealed that findings through light clothing were within 2 mm Hg of the results on bare skin. It was felt that based on this data, patients visiting a physician for a simple blood pressure reading may not need to change into a gown if the clothing covering the arm is light. This decision, however, needs to be made by the employing physician.

becomes less constricted, blood will begin to flow through. The first beat you feel at the radius is the systolic blood pressure. Afterward, deflate the cuff completely by compressing with your hands before reinflation.

6. A minimum of 15 seconds should elapse between inflations (30 is better) to allow blood pressure to normalize.
7. The cuff should be inflated rapidly to 30 mm Hg above the palpatory reading.

To obtain a baseline reading for new patients, it might be desirable to measure the pressure twice in each arm, once while the patient is sitting and once while lying down. As stated earlier, in certain situations, it may be necessary to obtain orthostatic blood pressure measurement in addition to the general measurement. If this is desired, simply follow the regular sitting or prone measurement by having the patient stand and immediately measure and record the results. Observe the patient for signs of dizziness or syncope.

Blood pressure has two phases, both of which must be determined. When the cuff is properly inflated, the valve must be opened carefully to allow deflation at a rate of 2 to 3 mm per beat. Listen for the first sounds of heartbeat and note the reading as the systolic pressure after you have heard at least two consecutive beats. Continue to listen and observe as the cuff is deflated until you hear a sudden change in sound to a softer, muffled tone. Note this reading as the diastolic pressure. Continue to observe the manometer until the sound disappears. Note this reading also, even if 0. To record, for example, you would write: B/P 140/90/70. You should ask the provider for his or her preference about which sound, the change or the absence, you are to record as the diastolic measurement.

Probably the mistake made most often in measuring blood pressure is reinflating the cuff after only partial deflation or too soon after complete deflation. Either error can cause a false reading and will cause difficulty in hearing the sound changes because of venous congestion in the forearm. Procedure 38–9 provides step-by-step details on measuring blood pressure.

## PROCEDURE 38–9 Measure Blood Pressure

**PURPOSE:** To determine a patient's palpatory and auscultatory blood pressure measurements

**EQUIPMENT:** Stethoscope, aneroid manometer, alcohol wipe, patient chart or EHR, pen

S **SKILL:** Measure and record blood pressure.

| Procedure Steps | Detailed Instructions and/or *Rationales* |
|---|---|
| 1. Wash hands; assemble equipment. Clean the earpieces and head of the stethoscope with antiseptic. | *Prevents transfer of organisms.* |
| 2. Identify the patient and introduce yourself. | *Ensures that you are performing the procedure on the correct patient.* |
| B 3. Explain the procedure, ***using language the patient can understand***. | *Ensures understanding, consent, and cooperation from the patient.* |

*(continues)*

*(continued)*

| Procedure Steps | Detailed Instructions and/or *Rationales* |
|---|---|
| 4. Place the patient in a relaxed and comfortable sitting or lying position. Expose the patient's upper arm well above the elbow, extending the arm with the palm up. | The arm may be either bare or covered with light clothing. Remove the arm from a constricting sleeve. Note: *Arm must be relaxed, on a supporting surface, slightly flexed at the elbow,* with the brachial artery approximately at the level of the heart. |
| 5. With the valve of the inflation bulb open, squeeze all air from the bladder and place it over the brachial artery (Figure 38–29 A). Be sure the aneroid dial is in direct view. | The bottom edge of the cuff should be 1 to 2 inches above the elbow. Wrap the cuff smoothly and snugly around the arm, with the deflated bladder centered over the brachial artery. Be certain the dial can be easily viewed and the end of the cuff does not interfere. |
| 6. With *one hand,* close the valve on the bulb, turning clockwise. | *Do not over-tighten the valve, or it will be hard to open.* |
| 7. Position your other hand to palpate the radial pulse (Figure 38–29 B). | |
| 8. While observing the manometer, rapidly inflate the cuff to 30 mm above the level at which radial pulse disappears. | |
| 9. Open the valve, slowly releasing the air until the radial pulse is detected. Observe the dial reading. | *This provides information for auscultatory measurement. This is palpatory systolic pressure, which may be recorded, for example, as B/P 120 (P).* |
| 10. Deflate the cuff rapidly and completely. | Squeeze the cuff with hands to empty. *All the air must be expressed between inflations to obtain accurate results. Adjust the position if necessary.* |
| 11. Position the earpieces of the stethoscope in your ears. | The openings should be entering the ear canals. |
| 12. Palpate the brachial artery at the medial antecubital space with your fingertips (Figure 38–29 C). | |
| 13. Place the head of the stethoscope directly over the palpated pulse (Figure 38–29 D). | The stethoscope head should not touch the cuff (creates static). |
| 14. Close the valve on the bulb and rapidly inflate the cuff to 30 mm above the palpated systolic pressure. | A minimum of 15–30 seconds must have elapsed since the previous inflation. *This is the minimum time required for the normalizing of blood flow through the artery.* |
| 15. Open the valve, slowly deflating the cuff. Note the reading at which you hear the systolic pressure. | Pressure should drop 2 to 3 mm Hg per second. The reading must be at least two consecutive beats. Remember the systolic measurement. |
| 16. Allow the pressure to lower steadily until you note a change in sound to a softer, more muffled sound. Note this as diastolic pressure (if so instructed). | |

| Procedure Steps | Detailed Instructions and/or *Rationales* |
|---|---|
| 17. Continue to release pressure until all sound disappears. Note this point as diastolic pressure (if so instructed). | |
| 18. Remove the stethoscope from your ears and release the remaining air from the cuff. | Squeeze the cuff between your hands. *This removes all the remaining air to make the patient more comfortable and ensures accurate results if re-evaluation is necessary.* |
| 19. Remove the cuff from the patient's arm. Assist the patient with clothing if necessary. | |
| 20. Reevaluate, if indicated, after a minimum of 15 seconds. | |
| 21. Clean the stethoscope. Fold the cuff properly and place it with the manometer and stethoscope in storage. | Use alcohol to disinfect the stethoscope. |
| 22. Wash hands and document the systolic and whichever diastolic reading the provider prefers in the patient's chart. | |

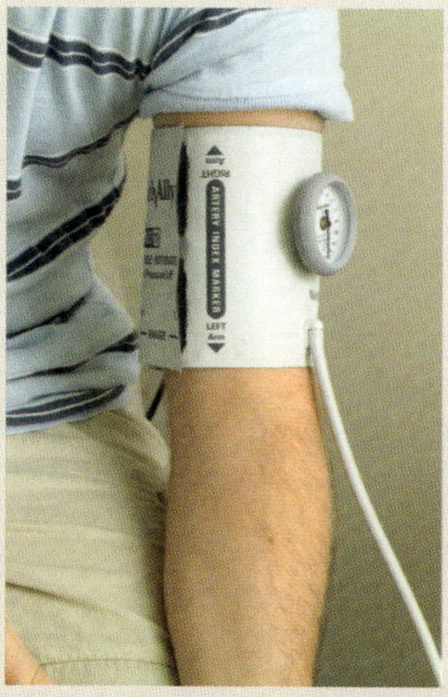

**FIGURE 38–29A:** Ensure that the patient is comfortable, with the arm slightly flexed at the elbow and the brachial artery on a level with the heart. The arm must be free of a constricting sleeve. With the valve of the inflation bulb open, squeeze all air from the bladder and place it over the brachial artery. *Delmar/Cengage Learning.*

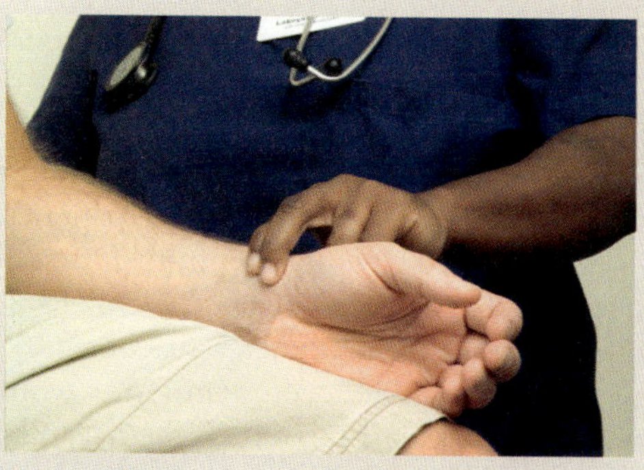

**FIGURE 38–29B:** With *one hand,* close the valve on the bulb, turning clockwise. Then, position your other hand to palpate the radial pulse. *Delmar/Cengage Learning.*

*(continues)*

*(continued)*

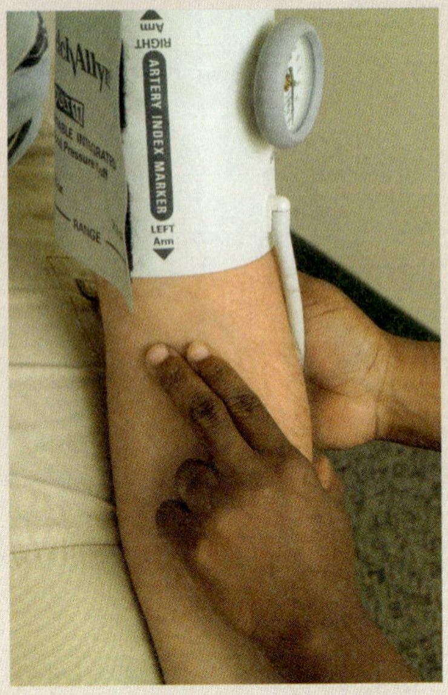


**FIGURE 38–29C:** Palpate the brachial artery at the medial antecubital space with your fingertips. *Delmar/Cengage Learning.*

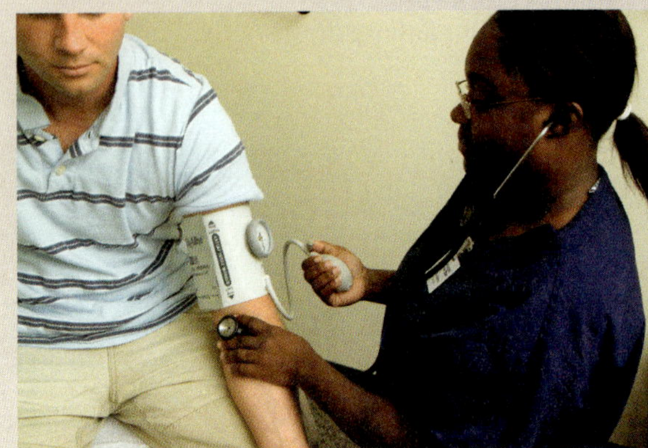

**FIGURE 38–29D:** Place the head of the stethoscope directly over the palpated pulse. *Delmar/Cengage Learning.*

### Charting Example

| | |
|---|---|
| 6-30-XX<br>11:30 am | B/P 186/94 or B/P 186/94/56. A. Ostrosky, CMA(AAMA) |

## Auscultatory Gap

In some patients, usually those who are hypertensive, there is a silent interval between systolic and diastolic pressure, called an *auscultatory gap*. If this is not detected, it may lead to serious under-measurement of the systolic pressure. For example, the patient's actual systolic pressure is 200, with a gap from 170 to 140 and a diastolic of 120/110. You inflate the cuff to 170 and hear nothing until the manometer reaches 140, which you presume is the systolic pressure. You would continue deflation and record 120/110 as the diastolic; therefore, you would have a pulse pressure of only 20 or 30 mm Hg. Keeping in mind the normal range for pulse pressure, however, you would view 20/30 as suspicious. Taking one third of 140 would give you about 47. To be certain you had not missed a portion of the pressure, you would remeasure, palpating the systolic and then inflating the cuff 30 mm above. If sounds were still audible at that point, you would wait 15–30 seconds and reinflate it higher *after complete deflation* until you hear the first sounds of systolic pressure. When recording a blood pressure with an auscultatory gap, list your complete findings (e.g., B/P 200/120/110 with the auscultatory gap from 170 to 140).

## Blood Pressure in Children

The blood pressure of infants and children is often omitted from the physical examination until the child reaches the age of three or older because it is so difficult to obtain. You must check with the provider for the policy at your specific medical office. Variation in blood pressure caused by anxiety and emotional upset make accurate readings very challenging. Basically, the procedure is the same as with adults; however, providers often prefer to do the measurement last after having established some rapport with the child.

The cuff size is important in measuring a child's pressure. It should be appropriate to the size of the arm.

The inflatable bag must entirely encircle the extremity. The level of systolic pressure gradually rises throughout childhood. Normal pressure for a 6-month-old is 70; at 1 year, it is 95; and it rises to 100 at 6 years. By age 16, the systolic pressure will be 120, the adult average. The diastolic pressure reaches 65 by age 1 and does not change appreciably during childhood.

Measurement of vital signs and body measurements provides essential information regarding the patient's overall condition. Monitoring while treatment and medication are being given for diseases and disorders of these systems is very important. The goal of treatment is to maintain the patient within as normal limits as possible.

## CHAPTER SUMMARY

- Body measurements are sometimes referred to as mensuration, meaning the process of measuring. When used in connection with patient care, it refers to body measurements such as height and weight; length of extremities; and the circumference of head, chest, or abdomen with infants.
- Height and weight measurements are important with infants and children to ensure there is proper growth and development. For adults, abnormal changes could indicate the presence of a disease or disorder. Measurements can also provide information regarding treatment, diagnostic testing, and medication dosages.
- The four vital indicators are temperature, pulse, respiration, and blood pressure, commonly referred to as TPR and B/P. They indicate the body's ability to control heat; the rate, volume, and rhythm of the heart; the rate and quality of breathing; and the force of the heart and condition of the blood vessels. Some providers consider pain a fifth vital sign.
- Normal body temperature for an individual is that temperature at which his or her body systems function most effectively. (Refer to Table 38–1 for normal temperature ranges.) All temperature methods have factors that cause inaccuracies; however, the rectal and TA methods are most accurate, and axillary is least accurate.
- The average adult pulse range is 60 to 100 beats per minute. The rate of the pulse is influenced by several factors, including exercise or activity; age; gender; physical condition of the body; and emotions such as fear, anxiety, pain, or anger.
- The radial pulse is used most frequently when measuring pulse rate. The brachial artery is used to palpate and auscultate blood pressure. The carotid pulse is palpated during the CPR life-saving maneuver. The femoral pulse is palpated to evaluate circulation in the lower extremities. Review Figure 38–19 for the locations of these pulse sites.
- Apical pulse measurement is indicated for infants and small children, patients with heart conditions, patients whose radial pulse is difficult to feel or who have an excessively rapid or slow rate or a thready or irregular quality.
- Respirations should be quiet, effortless, and regularly spaced. Abnormalities in respirations can indicate a variety of diseases or disorders.
- The term *blood pressure* means the fluctuating pressure the blood exerts against the arterial walls as the heart alternately contracts and relaxes. The blood pressure reflects the condition of the heart, the amount of blood forced from the heart at contraction, the condition of the arteries, and, to some extent, the volume and viscosity (thickness) of the blood.
- Equipment needed to obtain a blood pressure include a stethoscope; sphygmomanometer; alcohol wipe; blood pressure cuffs available in different sizes to measure blood pressure in neonates (infants), children, adults, obese adults, and adult thighs; or an electronic sphygmomanometer that is totally automatic and facilitates blood pressure measurement by providing a digital readout in the display window.
- An adult should have a systolic pressure less than 120 mm Hg and a diastolic pressure less than 80. Blood pressure readings with a ranges of 140–159 and 90–99 indicate stage 1 hypertension (high blood pressure); above this range indicates stage 2 hypertension.
- Hypertension can result from factors such as stress, obesity, high salt intake, sedentary lifestyle, and aging. Physical conditions that cause hypertension are kidney disease; thyroid dysfunction; neurological disorders; and vascular conditions (such as atherosclerosis and arteriosclerosis).

## STUDY TOOLS

| | |
|---|---|
| **Workbook** | Activities for Chapter 38 |
| **Premium Website** | |
| MEDIA LINK | View this **Media Link** for Chapter 38:<br>• Measure an Apical Pulse |
| StudyWARE | Activities and Quizzes on the **StudyWARE™ Software** for Chapter 38 |
| | Complete the following **Competency Challenge 2.0** activity:<br>• Tuesday, 9:00 AM, Obtain Vital Signs |
| | **Audio Library** of medical terms |
| | Online access to the **Critical Thinking Challenge 2.0** |
| **CourseMate** | Activities and Quizzes for Chapter 38 |
| **WebTutor** | Activities and Quizzes for Chapter 38 |

## CHECK YOUR KNOWLEDGE

1. The process of measuring body measurements is referred to as:
   a. measuration.
   b. menstruation.
   c. mensuration.
   d. ministration.
2. Although the height bar is usually recorded in inches, you might need to convert into feet and inches by dividing the number of total inches by:
   a. 10.
   b. 12.
   c. 6.
   d. 5.
3. The four vital indicators that measure the body functions essential to life include:
   a. height, weight, temperature, and pulse.
   b. temperature, pulse, respiration, and blood pressure.
   c. temperature, pulse, respiration, and weight.
   d. height, weight, pulse, and blood pressure.
4. When measuring the oral temperature using an electronic thermometer, select the following probe:
   a. green.
   b. red.
   c. blue.
   d. black.
5. The radial pulse can be found:
   a. on the thumb side of the inner surface of the wrist, lying over the radius bone.
   b. on the pinkie side of the inner surface of the wrist, lying over the ulna bone.
   c. on the thumb side of the inner surface of the wrist, lying over the ulna bone.
   d. on the pinkie side of the inner surface of the wrist, lying over the radius bone.
6. Normal respiration rate in adults is:
   a. 16–26 times a minute.
   b. 20–40 times a minute.
   c. 16–20 times a minute.
   d. 30–80 times a minute.
7. The term *systole* refers to:
   a. noisy breathing.
   b. resting phase of the heart.
   c. contraction phase of the heart.
   d. absence of breathing.
8. This type of hypertension is caused by renal disease or another identifiable cause:
   a. primary.
   b. secondary.
   c. tertiary.
   d. malignant.

## WEB LINKS

LifeClinic: www.lifeclinic.com

National Institutes of Health: www.nih.gov

## RESOURCES

Exergen Corporation. (2005). *Temporal Scanner Reference Manual*. Watertown, MA.

Heller, M., and Veach, L. (2009). *Clinical Medical Assisting: A Professional, Field Smart Approach to the Workplace*. Clifton Park, NY: Delmar, Cengage Learning.

Lindh, W., Pooler, M., Tamparo, C., and Dahl, B. (2010). *Delmar's Comprehensive Medical Assisting Administrative and Clinical Competencies* (4th ed.). Clifton Park, NY: Delmar Cengage Learning.

Rizzo, D. (2010). *Fundamentals of Anatomy and Physiology* (3rd ed.). Clifton Park, NY: Delmar Cengage Learning.

U.S. Department of Health and Human Services. (2003, December). NIH Publication No. 03-5233. Bethesda, MD: National Institutes of Health.

CHAPTER 3

# Vital Signs and Measurements

## Words to Know Challenge

**Spelling: Each line contains three spellings of a word. Underline the correctly spelled word.**

| | | |
|---|---|---|
| 1. afibrile | afebrile | effebrial |
| 2. aral | oural | aural |
| 3. bradypnea | bradipenia | braedypenia |
| 4. fatil | fatal | fatel |
| 5. ideopathic | idiopathic | edeopathic |
| 6. menstration | menstruation | mensuration |
| 7. orthostatic | orthastatic | orthostatec |
| 8. pirogen | pyragen | pyrogen |
| 9. sphygmomanometer | spygmonometer | spygmomanometer |
| 10. sistole | systole | systoli |

**Matching: Match the term in column I to its definition in column II.**

| | COLUMN I | COLUMN II |
|---|---|---|
| C | 1. Antecubital | A. Excessively slow heart rate |
| H | 2. Apex | B. Feel by touching |
| K | 3. Arrhythmia | C. Inner elbow area |
| I | 4. Auscultate | D. A pulse site at the groin |
| J | 5. Brachial | E. Excessively rapid heart rate |
| A | 6. Bradycardia | F. A pulse site at the inner wrist |
| G | 7. Carotid | G. A pulse site near the trachea |
| D | 8. Femoral | H. Lower edge of the heart |
| B | 9. Palpate | I. To listen |
| E | 10. Tachycardia | J. A pulse site at the inner elbow |
| F | 11. Radial | K. Without a regular pattern of beats |

Chapter 4

# Preparing for Examinations

## OBJECTIVES

In this chapter, you will learn the following:

### KB KNOWLEDGE BASE

1. Spell and define, using the glossary at the back of the text, all the Words to Know in this chapter.
2. List the supplies that should be available in an examination room.
3. Explain the steps necessary to prepare for an exam.
4. Explain examination room cleanup and equipment that may need to be disinfected following a patient examination.
5. Name the examination positions and explain the purpose of each.
6. Explain the technique and purpose of draping the patient for each examination position.

### S SKILLS

1. Prepare and maintain the examination and treatment areas.
2. Transfer a patient from a wheelchair to the examination table.
3. Transfer a patient from the examination table to a wheelchair.
4. Demonstrate positioning a patient for a variety of examinations.

### B BEHAVIOR

1. Demonstrate empathy in communicating with patients, family, and staff.
2. Demonstrate awareness of the territorial boundaries of the person with whom communicating.
3. Apply critical thinking skills in performing patient assessment and care.
4. Use language/verbal skills that enable patients' understanding.

## WORDS TO KNOW

anatomical
anterior
dorsal recumbent
dyspnea
fenestrated
Fowler's
horizontal
incompetent
knee-chest
lithotomy
proctological
prone
recumbent
shock
sigmoidoscopy
Sims'
supine
Trendelenburg
ventral

## PREPARING THE ROOM

Preparation and maintenance of the examination room for an exam is the responsibility of the medical assistant. Before every patient encounter in the room, you must ensure that the room is clean, well-organized, and at a comfortable temperature (Figure 39–1). Patients expect to find exam rooms neat and clean. A clean, well-stocked exam room reflects positively on the provider and the staff.

It is important to know how to operate the examination table to ensure a smooth and efficient examination process. The provider might require the patient to assume certain positions during the examination, some of which necessitate changing the table structure. The exam table in Figure 39–2A is limited to changing the angle of the top half, pulling out the leg rest, and extending the hidden stirrups. The power table in Figure 39–2B can be adjusted for the height of the provider as well as for many examination positions. The desired position can be achieved by pressing a button on the programmed hand control or using the optional plug-in foot control.

All surfaces within the room that might be potentially contaminated should be cleaned with a disinfectant between patient examinations. This would include cabinet and table surfaces where used supplies and instruments may be discarded and the examination table that can have soiled table paper. Refer to Chapter 36 for standard precautions that should be followed when cleaning a room and using disinfectants.

After the examination table is cleaned, new table paper at the proper width to appropriately cover the table is pulled down. The paper is supplied in a roll that is inserted on a dowel under the head of the table. The jagged torn edge of the paper is folded and tucked under the seat section of the table for a neat appearance. It is important to check the amount of paper left on the roll periodically. Some tables accommodate two rolls so a replacement one would be available immediately if you ran out; otherwise, you would need to make a trip to the supply cabinet. The table pillow is covered by a disposable cover or towel that is discarded after each use and replaced with a fresh one.

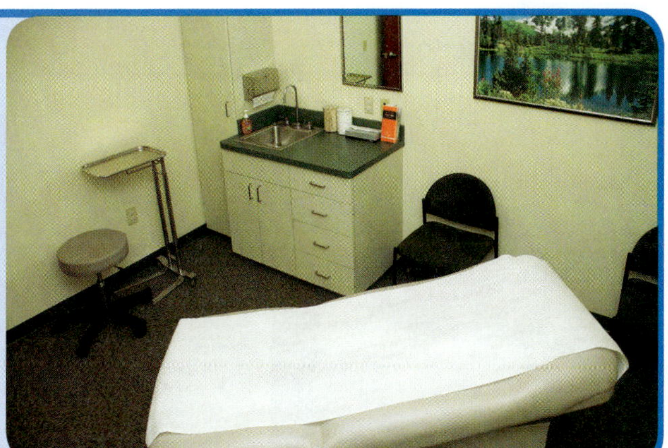

**FIGURE 39–1:** An example of a clean and well-organized exam room. *Delmar/Cengage Learning.*

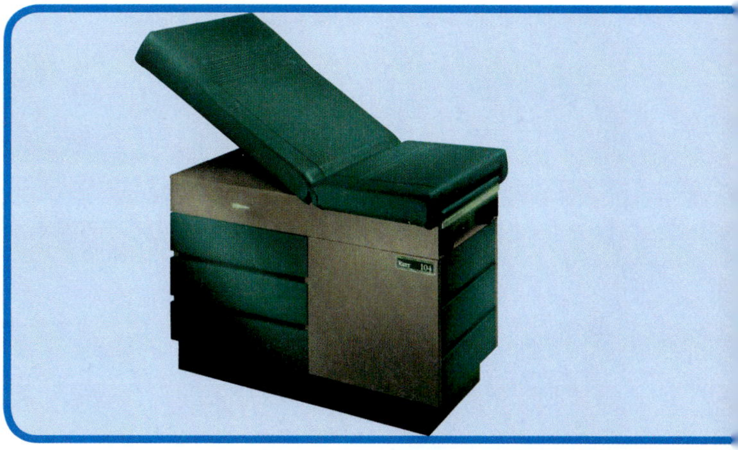

**FIGURE 39–2A:** A manual medical examination table commonly used in medical offices. *Courtesy of Midmark Corp.*

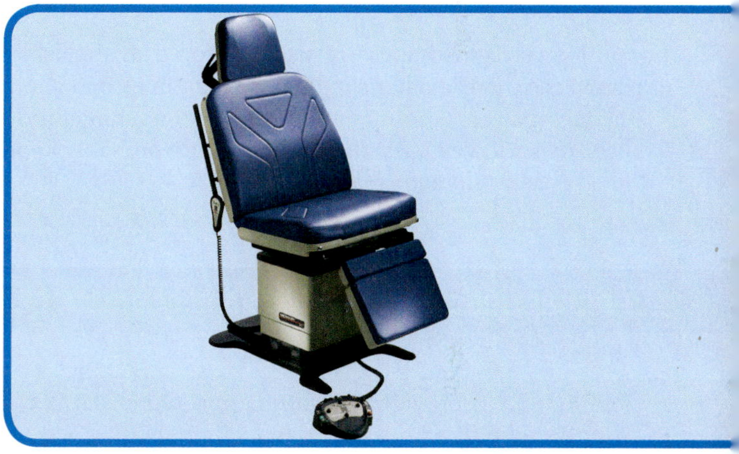

**FIGURE 39–2B:** A power table that can be adjusted by hand or foot controls. *Courtesy of Midmark Corp.*

### Supplies and Equipment

Preparation also includes checking for all the supplies needed within the room, such as:

- A hand-washing product
- Biohazardous waste containers
- Face guards and gloves
- Patient gowns and drapes
- Paper towels, tissues
- A working light source
- Standard examination equipment (tongue blades, speculums, gauze squares, applicators, and so on)

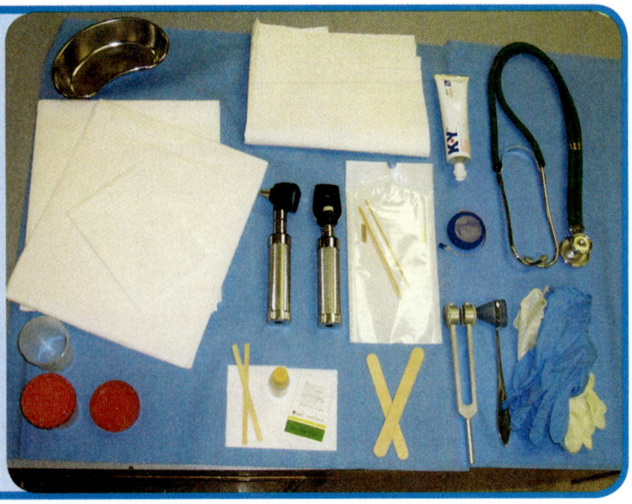

**FIGURE 39–3:** Standard examination equipment. *Delmar/Cengage Learning.*

Gowns and drapes are usually stored in the table drawers, whereas other supplies are kept in examination cabinet drawers or a supply cabinet. Hand-washing products, paper towels, and biohazard bags are probably kept in a separate storage area.

**Table 39–1 Supplies Commonly Used for Patient Examinations**

| | |
|---|---|
| Stethoscope | Penlight |
| Gloves | Otoscope |
| Drapes | Ophthalmoscope |
| Tongue depressor | Lubricant |
| Percussion hammer | Basin |
| Tuning fork | Fecal occult blood test |
| Various specimen collection kits or containers | Tape measure |

You may also need to prepare a tray of routine examination instruments used during the physical examination. The items commonly used for patient examinations are shown in Figure 39–3, and listed in Table 39–1. It is important for you to know the name and function of each item so you can anticipate the need and assist the provider if asked.

Procedure 39–1 provides guidelines on how to prepare and maintain an examination room.

## PROCEDURE 39–1 Prepare and Maintain Examination and Treatment Areas

**PURPOSE:** To provide an examination room that is comfortable and clean and has the usual equipment and supplies necessary ready for an examination

**EQUIPMENT:** Disposable gloves, disinfectant, disposable cloth, exam table, pillow, table paper, patient gowns, drapes, hand-washing liquid, paper towels, gauze squares, examination light, biohazard and regular waste containers, and appropriate supplies and equipment (stethoscope, otoscope, ophthalmoscope, percussion hammer, pin wheel, hemocult supplies, lubricant, pelvic exam supplies, tissues, tape measure).

**S SKILL:** Prepare and maintain examination and treatment areas

| Procedure Steps | Detailed Instructions and/or *Rationales* |
|---|---|
| 1. Assess the room condition, temperature, furniture, and equipment. | Review Figure 39–4, which is an example of a room that is not prepared. 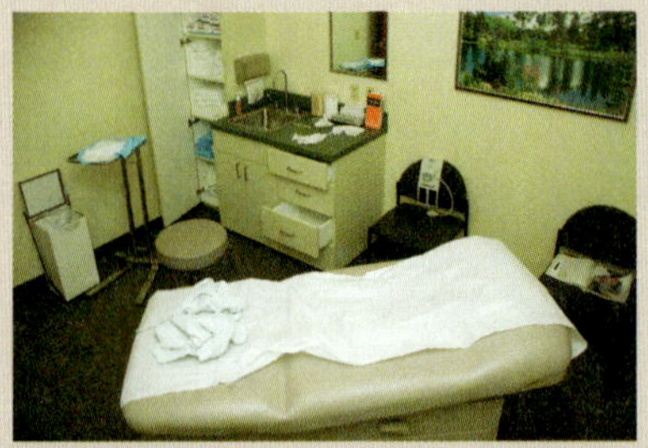 **Figure 39–4:** An example of an exam room that needs to be prepared for the patient. *Delmar/Cengage Learning.* |

| Procedure Steps | Detailed Instructions and/or *Rationales* |
|---|---|
| | *You want to be sure the room is a comfortable environment for the patient. Check all furniture and equipment to be sure everything is in working order.* |
| 2. Wash hands and put on disposable gloves. | |
| 3. Place used supplies and disposable examination equipment in the waste or biohazard container. Check the waste container for space; replace it if the bag is full. | *Depending on the use, supplies and equipment* can *potentially be exposed to microorganisms. Place the used items in the appropriate waste receptacle, depending on exposure, following standard precaution guidelines. Refer to* Chapter 36 *for guideline information.* |
| 4. Tear the table paper near the top and roll it up with the pillow cover. | Dispose of it in the wastebasket unless contaminated with body fluid, then place it in the biohazard container. Be sure to follow standard precaution guidelines. |
| 5. Wipe permanent examination equipment with disposable cloth or gauze squares and disinfectant. | *Prevents microorganism cross-contamination.* |
| 6. Wipe the examination room table tops with disposable cloth and disinfectant if contaminated from discarded examination supplies. Prepare the exam table for the next patient:<br>a. Pull down clean table paper, fold the ragged edge, and place it under the table seat.<br>b. Place a clean cover on the pillow.<br>c. Check the table paper supply, gowns, and drapes. | Prevents microorganism cross-contamination. |
| 7. Wipe any other equipment contaminated by the provider, such as a stool or exam lamp. | *Prevents microorganism cross-contamination.* |
| 8. Disinfect the examination table and dispose of the cloth and gloves in the appropriate container. | |
| 9. Check the hand-washing dispenser and stock the supply. | |
| 10. Check the paper towel dispenser and supply more if needed. | |
| 11. Check the supplies in the cabinet and the examination table drawers and replace as needed. | *This ensures that all supplies needed by the provider are ready and available, preventing any delay in the patient exam.* |
| 12. Make a final visual check of the room. | |
| 13. Remove gloves and wash hands. | |

## PREPARING AND ASSISTING THE PATIENT

Making sure that patients have a good understanding of what they can expect from the visit and are made to feel as comfortable as possible are the first steps in preparing them for any examination. The medical assistant will probably be the main person with whom the patient interacts prior to the examination. It is important for the patient to feel comfortable in the surroundings and with the anticipated medical exam. Having the patient emotionally prepared goes a long way in helping the provider obtain an accurate assessment of a patient's condition.

> **CLINICAL PEARL**
>
> Some examinations can be embarrassing to a patient, but a clear explanation of each procedure can help relax him or her. You can assist the patient greatly by giving empathy and support and answering any questions he or she may have prior to the exam.

Many times, the provider will want the patient to prep prior to the exam in case laboratory testing is performed. Usually, patients are asked to fast so that specific diagnostic blood tests may be drawn. It can also be more comfortable when other procedures are performed if nothing has been eaten before the examination. In general, the fasting process usually begins at midnight the night before the exam and is indicated as (NPO), meaning "nothing by mouth." The patient needs to understand completely that he or she is to have nothing to eat or drink. Most providers allow the patient to have a small amount of water to take any medications that are prescribed to them or to brush their teeth, but other than that, they must refrain from everything else, including chewing gum or breath mints.

After the initial screening and vitals are taken, instruct the patient to empty his or her bladder. Often, the provider will want to obtain a urine specimen from the patient. If this is the case, provide a specimen container and instruct the patient to collect a sample for you to test. Allowing the patient time to empty his or her bladder will also make the examination process more comfortable.

If gowns and drapes are needed to facilitate examination, ask the patient to disrobe and instruct on how to wear a gown and apply the drape per the provider's preference. Patient gowns and drapes are made of cloth or disposable paper. Depending on the type of exam, the patient may be asked to have the gown either open to the front or open to the back.

After the gown and drapes are applied, ask the patient to have a seat on the examination table. Offer assistance with any of the tasks if the patient needs help. Some patients might need assistance when getting up on the examination table. If the examination table is too high for the patient to get on it comfortably, a foot stool should be provided. Never try to lift a patient who obviously weighs more than you can safely handle; have someone help you. (For more information on proper safety techniques with lifting and moving a patient, refer to the body mechanics section in Chapter 56.) If a patient needs help moving on the table, reach under the arm at the shoulder and help the person move up. You should move with the patient. Additionally, a very ill patient or a small child should never be left alone on a table; a member of the family should be asked to sit with him or her if you must leave the room.

If you are a female medical assistant, you may be asked to remain in the room when a female patient is being examined by a male provider (and vice versa). The rationale is that the patient should feel more relaxed, and the provider is protected from lawsuits that could result from patients claiming the provider acted improperly during the examination.

There may be a period of time before the provider enters the room. If the patient is anxious, this is a good time to reiterate the general format of the exam and answer any questions he or she may have. It can also be an excellent opportunity for patient education. Knowing about the pamphlets and other resources available in your office, you can talk with the patient and supply the material after the exam if the provider indicates. There are patient education boxes within this chapter and throughout the text that can give you some ideas upon which to build conversation and that have general information appropriate for discussion. This skill will become easier after you gain knowledge and experience.

> **PATIENT EDUCATION**
>
> To prevent injuries of the face and head:
>
> - In work and recreational environments, wear protective head gear: hard hat at work (construction sites), helmet for sports (motorcycle riding, football).
> - Wear protective face mask or goggles for sports such as football, hockey, and lacrosse to prevent possible eye injuries.
> - Use ear plugs to protect ears from exposure to loud noises (machinery, band concerts) that can lead to possible damage to auditory nerves resulting in hearing loss.

**PATIENT EDUCATION**

To protect the skin:

- Keep skin clean and soft by using mild soap and water for bathing and a moisturizing lotion as necessary.
- Discourage sun worship. Encourage remaining covered in the sun or the use of a sun blocker to prevent damage from ultraviolet rays if one must be in the sun for prolonged periods. Do not use tanning beds.
- Wash hands of (chemical) irritants immediately to prevent caustic burns.

**PATIENT EDUCATION**

To prevent diseases of the respiratory system and other contagious diseases:

- Discourage sharing utensils or drinking out of another person's glass to keep from transmitting viruses and diseases.
- Wash hands after handling items in or from public places (money, doorknobs, and soon).
- Discourage smoking or tobacco use of any kind. (Post antismoking pamphlets or meetings for patients to read.)
- Remind patients of the dangers of drug and alcohol use and abuse. (Display information about Alcoholics Anonymous meetings.)
- Encourage exercise and physical fitness programs with the advice of the provider.
- Promote proper nutrition and weight control by helping patients plan their diets and reminding them to eat well-balanced meals regularly.
- Encourage *safe sex* by providing explicit information to teach patients about the dangers of sexually transmitted diseases, hepatitis, and AIDS.
- Discourage patients from using laxatives and enemas unless specifically ordered by the provider.
- Remind patients about immunizations and encourage compliance.
- Encourage patients to read labels for contents of the products they buy and use for their safety.
- Remind patients to use seat belts.
- Promote regular medical and dental checkups.

## WHEELCHAIR TRANSFERS

If a patient comes to your office in a wheelchair, it is important to know how to help that patient from the wheelchair to the examination table and back to the wheelchair. This is not an easy task to do alone if the patient is unable to support his or her own weight. Always enlist help from coworkers to prevent injury to the patient and yourself. Always remember to position the chair and lock the wheels before trying to help the patient move from the chair to the table. To make it easier to assist the patient to stand or walk, a wide-strap called a gait belt should be placed around the patient's waist. The belt provides a way to hold and support the patient while he or she is being transferred in and out of the wheelchair. The belt is grasped in the front to assist the patient to stand from a sitting position and is held in the back if supporting the patient while walking. Procedures 39–2 and 39–3 detail the steps on transferring a patient from a wheelchair to an exam table and vice versa.

### PROCEDURE 39–2 Transfer a Patient from a Wheelchair to the Examination Table

**PURPOSE:** To move a patient safely from a wheelchair to an examination table

**EQUIPMENT:** Examination table, wheelchair, and gait belt

**S SKILL:** Transfer a patient from a wheelchair to the examination table.

| Procedure Steps | Detailed Instructions and/or *Rationales* |
|---|---|
| 1. Unlock the wheels of the chair and wheel the patient to the examination room. | *Wheelchairs should always be locked in position when sitting still to prevent unexpected movement. This is accomplished by flipping the brake on each wheel.* |

*(continues)*

*(continued)*

| Procedure Steps | Detailed Instructions and/or *Rationales* |
|---|---|
| 2. Position the chair as near as possible to the place you want the patient to sit on the table. Lock the wheels on the chair. | |
| 3. Lower the table to chair level. | Note: If this cannot be done, position a footstool beside the table and determine whether assistance will be needed. |
| 4. Apply the gait belt (Figure 39–5A) and fold the footrests back (Figure 39–5B). | If necessary, assist the patient to move his or her feet. |
| 5. Stand directly in front of the patient with your feet slightly apart. | To give a good base, place one foot forward, between the patient's legs. |
| 6. Bend your knees and have the patient place his or her hands on your shoulders while you place your hands under the gait belt and assist the patient to a standing position. | Pause in this position for a moment before the next step. |
| 7. Maintaining the position of your hands, pivot or side step to a position beside the table (Figure 39–5C). | |
| 8. Place one foot slightly behind you for support and help the patient to a sitting position on the table. | |
| 9. If it is necessary to use a stool, determine the assistance required and enlist the needed help *before* taking the patient from the wheelchair. | |
| 10. While supporting the patient, stabilize the stool by placing your feet on the outside next to the legs and assist the patient to step onto the stool. | Caution: Be certain the patient steps onto the stool squarely to avoid tipping the stool. |

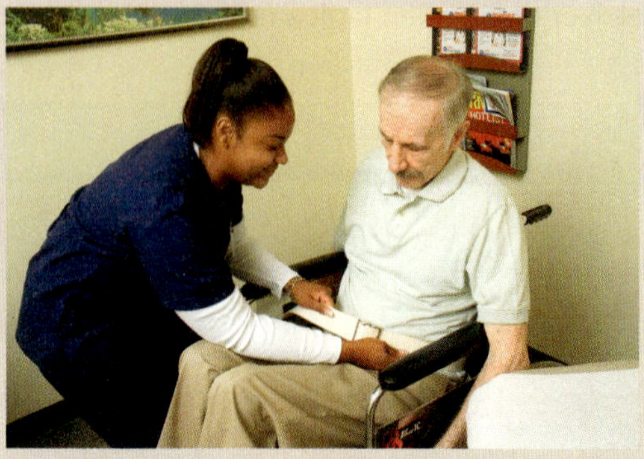

**Figure 39–5A:** A gait belt makes it easier to support the patient when walking.
*Delmar/Cengage Learning.*

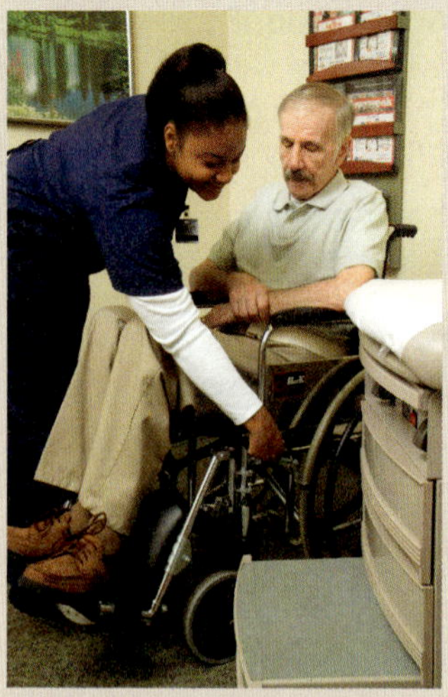

**Figure 39–5B:** Fold the footrests back.
*Delmar/Cengage Learning.*

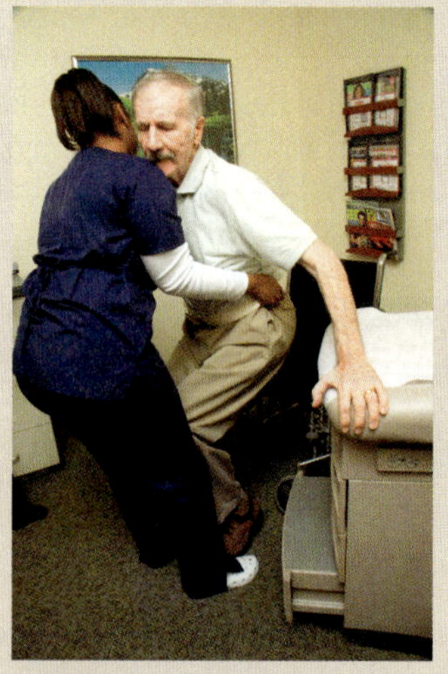

**Figure 39–5C:** Assisting a patient from a wheelchair.
*Delmar/Cengage Learning.*

| Procedure Steps | Detailed Instructions and/or *Rationales* |
|---|---|
| 11. Assist the patient to sit on the table (Figure 39–5D). | |
| 12. If the patient needs assistance to lie down, place one hand around the patient's back. Help the patient raise his or her legs to the table by placing your free arm under the legs and lifting them as the patient turns. | Note: If the patient needs to remove clothing, get someone to help you. One person balances the patient while the other removes necessary clothing. |
| 13. Place a pillow under the patient's head. Drape the patient appropriately. | *Never leave a very ill or weak patient alone on a table. There is danger of a fall.* |
| 14. Unlock the chair wheels and move the chair out of the way. | Note: If the room is small, it may be necessary to place the chair outside the examination room. |

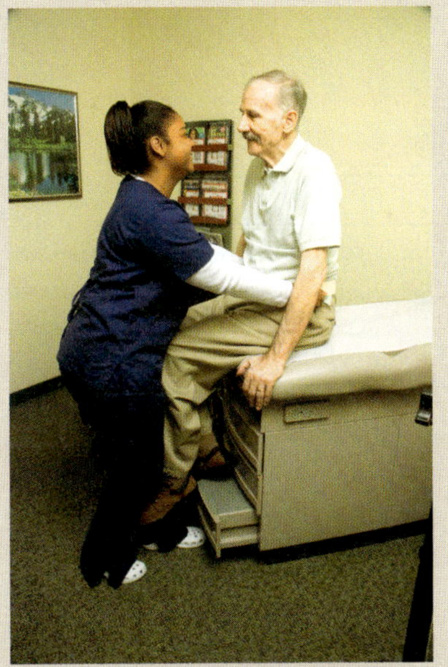

**Figure 39–5D:** Assist the patient to a comfortable sitting position.
*Delmar/Cengage Learning.*

## PROCEDURE 39–3 Transfer a Patient from an Examination Table to a Wheelchair

**MEDIA LINK:** View the video clip for this chapter, "Transferring a patient from an exam table to a wheelchair," on the Premium Website.

**PURPOSE:** To move a patient safely from the examination table to a wheelchair

**EQUIPMENT:** Wheelchair, gait belt, and examination table

S **SKILL:** Transfer a patient from an examination table to a wheelchair.

| Procedure Steps | Detailed Instructions and/or *Rationales* |
|---|---|
| 1. Reposition the chair and lock the wheels. | |
| 2. Assist the patient to a sitting position on the table. | Support the patient's back if necessary. Lift the patient's legs as the patient is turned until his or her feet dangle over the edge of the table. |
| B 3. Explain the procedure to the patient, ***using language the patient can understand, outlining what you will do and enlisting the patient's help.*** Assist the patient to dress if needed. | |
| 4. Apply a gait belt to the patient. | |
| 5. Move so you are directly in front of the patient. Grasp the patient on the sides below the armpits by placing your hands under the gait belt. Plant your feet a shoulder's width apart and bend your knees. Ask the patient to put his or her hands on your shoulders. Assist the patient to step onto the floor (or have a stepstool in place if the table cannot be lowered to chair height.) | Caution: Take special care to ensure that the patient steps squarely on the stool when getting down from the examining table. Place your feet against the legs of the footstool, on the outside, to maintain its position. |
| 6. Support the patient into a standing position on the stool or floor. (If using a stool, help the patient step down from the stool.) Side step or pivot the patient to a position in front of the chair. | |
| B 7. Have the patient reach back to the arms of the chair as you help lower the patient into the chair. ***Ensure that the patient is comfortably seated.*** | |
| 8. Remove the gait belt from the patient and adjust the footrests. | |
| 9. Unlock the wheels and return the patient to the reception room. | |

## EXAMINATION POSITIONS

A patient will be asked to assume certain positions to facilitate examination of the body. During a comprehensive physical examination, several of the standard positions may be used. The medical assistant must know their names and be able to assist the patient into each position. The following is a list of examination positions that will be discussed:

- Anatomical
- Sitting
- Horizontal recumbent (supine)
- Dorsal recumbent

- Prone
- Sims'
- Knee-chest
- Trendelenburg
- Fowler's
- Semi-Fowler's
- Lithotomy
- Jackknife or Kraske

Procedure 39–4 has step-by-step instructions for assisting patients to assume most of the examination positions. Performing this procedure will assist you in becoming familiar with their names, the patient's position, and the relationship between the examination and the position. This information, along with mastery of the skills is necessary before you begin to assist the provider to perform a partial or complete physician examination.

## PATIENT EDUCATION

It is important to instruct the patient about the need for a specific position for the examination to be performed. This information should be included with the instructions on preparing for the examination. The patient should understand that the provider needs to examine certain parts of the body or perform certain procedures and tests, and the patient must be positioned in the most accessible manner.

The provider may begin the examination by asking the patient to assume the **anatomical** position, which means to stand erect, arms at sides with palms pointed forward. This allows a visual inspection of posture and is usually followed by requests to perform several movements (such as range-of-motion exercises). Next, the patient will be asked to sit at the end of the examination table, with the legs hanging down (sitting position). You should assist the patient as needed. If the patient is shorter in stature, it may be necessary to pull out the step from the bottom of the table or use a small stepping stool. Be careful to be sure the patient does not fall. Once seated on the table, a drape should be placed over the lap and legs for privacy and warmth. Several inspections and examinations are done with the patient in sitting position.

The patient will then be asked to lie down on the table. You will assist the patient to lie back and pull out the leg rest at the bottom of the table to support the patient's legs. A small pillow can be placed under the head for comfort. If a power table is used, and it is in the sitting position, press the appropriate button and reassure the patient as the table levels. Patients often feel like their head is lower than their body after being in an upright position. Readjust the drape as needed.

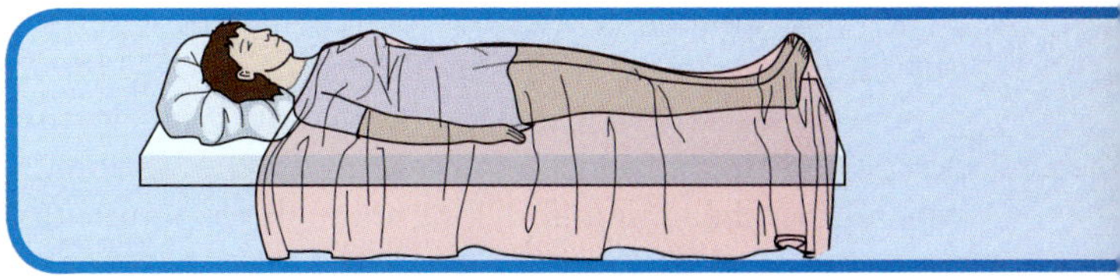

**Figure 39–6:** Horizontal recumbent or supine position. *Delmar/Cengage Learning.*

The **horizontal** recumbent or **supine** position is used for examination and treatment of the **anterior** portion of the body, including the breasts and abdominal organs (Figure 39–6). The term **recumbent** means lying down. The **dorsal recumbent** position indicates that the knees are bent (Figure 39–7), which allows for relaxation of the abdominal muscles and thus easier examination of the abdominal area. This position may also be used for digital vaginal or rectal examination. The gown is open in the front, and a drape sheet of cloth or paper is used to cover the patient from the neck down.

During a complete physical, the provider may request the patient to turn over so the **ventral** surface may be examined. This is called the **prone** position (Figure 39–8) and is used to examine the spine and structures of the back. Assist the patient as necessary to turn over, instructing him or her to turn toward you. Watch to be certain the patient does not get too close to the edge when turning and fall off the table. Instruct the patient to lie face down with his or her arms folded to make a place to rest the head. Because the gown was originally put on with the opening in the front, it will be necessary to pull the gown up to expose the back. Reposition the drape from the upper back to the feet to cover the exposed area. When the ventral surface

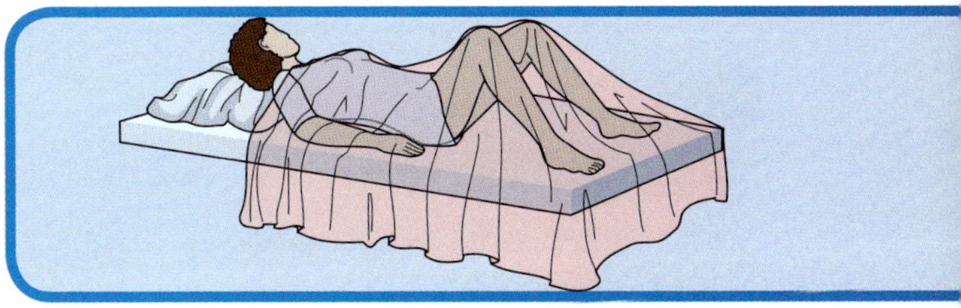

**Figure 39–7:** Dorsal recumbent position. *Delmar/Cengage Learning.*

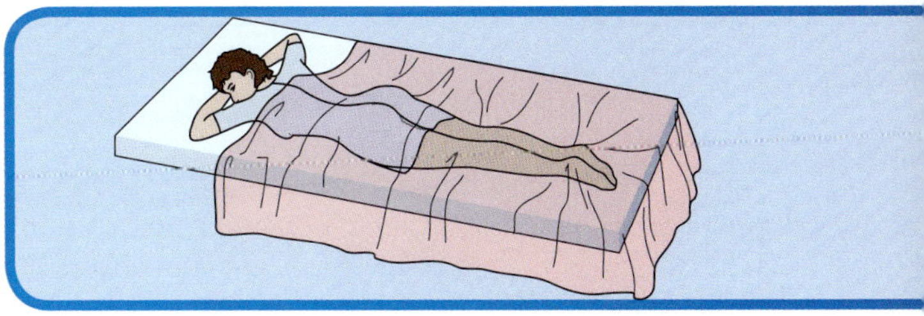

**Figure 39–8:** Prone position. *Delmar/Cengage Learning.*

is being examined alone, the patient is instructed to put on the gown with the opening in the back. Some patients may experience back discomfort lying in this position. Often placing a pillow under the abdomen will relieve the discomfort long enough to permit the examination.

The **Sims'** position is used in examination and treatment of the rectal area and for enemas, rectal temperature, and instilling rectal medications (Figure 39–9). This position may also be used for perineal and some pelvic examinations. This is also referred to as the lateral recumbent position. The patient is positioned on his or her left side with the left arm extended behind the body and the right arm flexed upward. A pillow under the head adds to the comfort of this position. The left leg may be slightly flexed, but the right leg is sharply flexed upward. The drape should cover at least from the axillary area to below the knees. The drape is raised to permit examination or treatment of the rectal area.

The **knee-chest** position (Figure 39–10) is a difficult position for patients to assume. The chest and knees are placed flat against the table with the knees separated. The arms can be crossed under the head or flexed to each side with the head turned to the side. The buttocks extend upward with the back straight. Patients will need support and assistance in assuming and maintaining this position; therefore, you must remain with the patient while he or she is in this position. The patient should not be placed in the position until the provider is ready to do the examination. If the patient cannot get into the knee-chest position, it can be modified to a knee-elbow position, which is easier to assume and maintain.

The knee-chest position is used for rectal or **proctological** examinations and occasionally for a **sigmoidoscopy** if a proctological table is not available. The position causes the intestinal organs to move toward the chest, thereby somewhat straightening the sigmoid colon to facilitate insertion of instruments. The patient is commonly covered with a fenestrated drape, in which a special opening provides access to the area being examined.

The **Fowler's** position is used for patients with respiratory or cardiovascular problems. The patient who is having **dyspnea** must be in a sitting or semi-sitting position to breathe comfortably. This position is also used to examine the trunk of the body (head, neck, and chest area). The patient may simply sit upright at the foot of the table or be supported by the back of the examination table. When the patient's upper body is at a 90-degree angle to the table, it is known as a Fowler's position (refer to Figure 39–11 A). If the patient is resting against the back of the table and it is lowered to a 45-degree angle, it is known as the semi-Fowler's position (refer to Figure 39–11 B). The patient gown should open in the front, and the drape should cover from the axillary area down to the feet. When the high Fowler's position is used, the drape will naturally fall to cover from the top of the legs to over the feet.

The **lithotomy** position is used for vaginal or rectal examination (Figure 39-12). This position can also be used for examination of the male genital area and for catheterization of a female patient. The primary use of the position is for vaginal examinations of the female patient when a speculum is inserted, as when obtaining Pap smears.

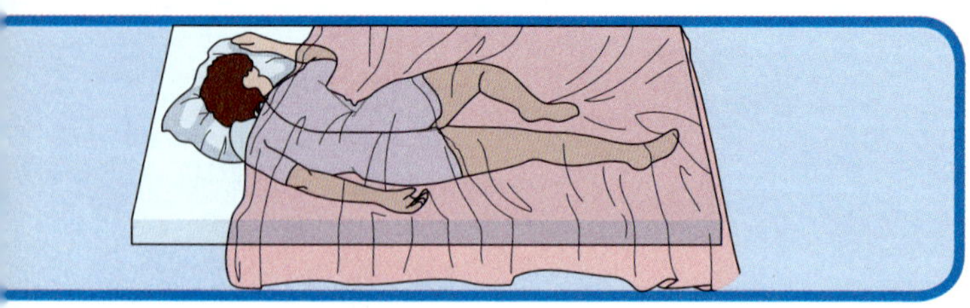

**Figure 39–9:** Sims' position. *Delmar/Cengage Learning.*

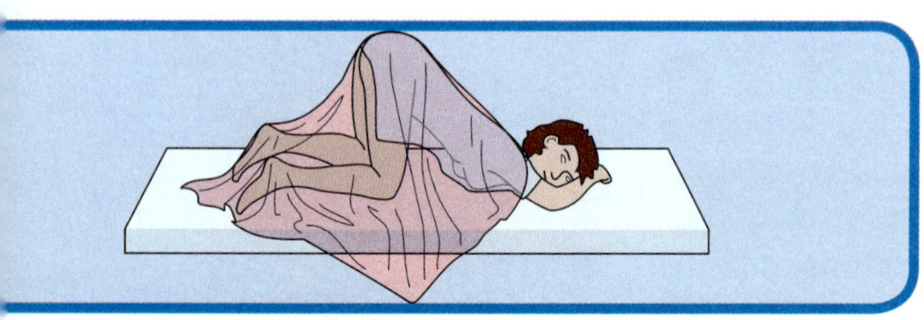

**Figure 39–10:** Knee-chest position. *Delmar/Cengage Learning.*

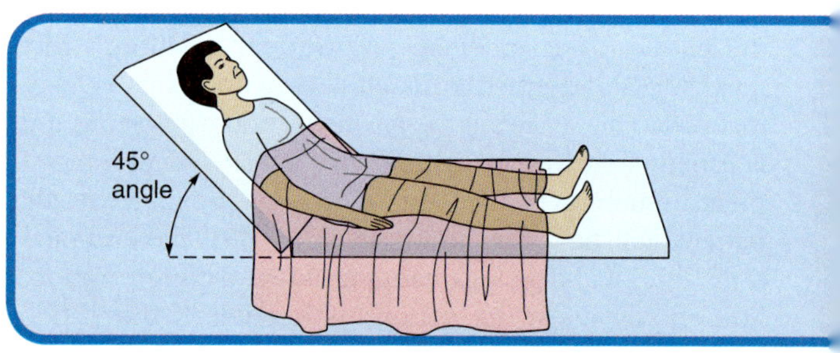


**Figure 39–11A:** Semi-Fowler's position. *Delmar/Cengage Learning.*

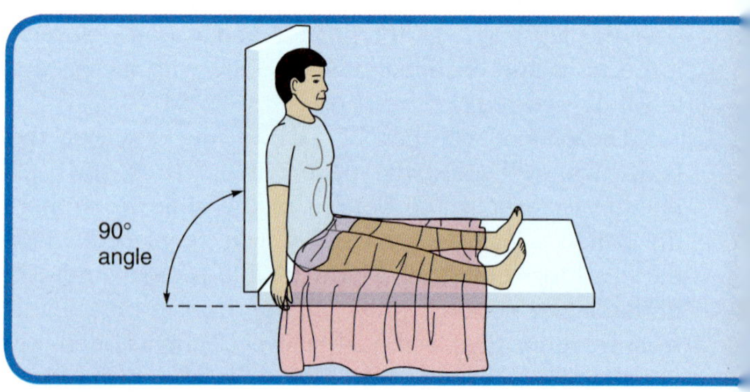


**Figure 39–11B:** Fowler's position. *Delmar/Cengage Learning.*

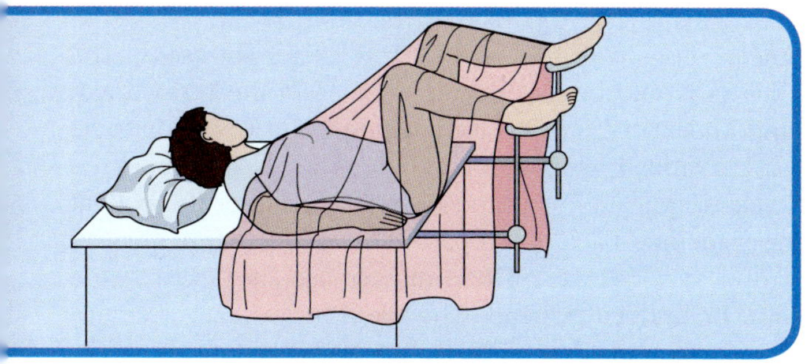

**Figure 39–12:** Lithotomy position. *Delmar/Cengage Learning.*

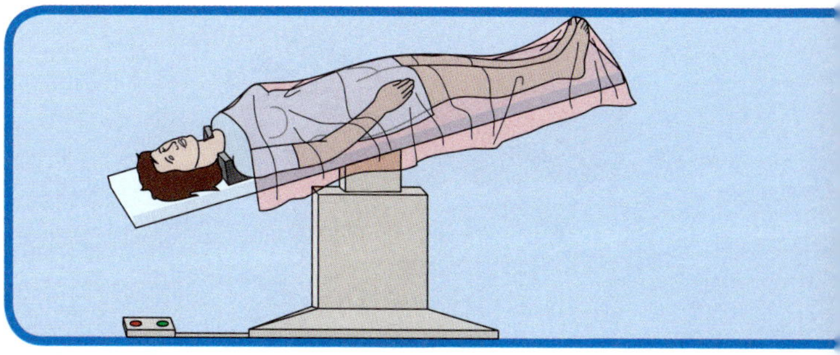

**Figure 39–13A:** Trendelenburg or shock position with power table. *Delmar/Cengage Learning.*

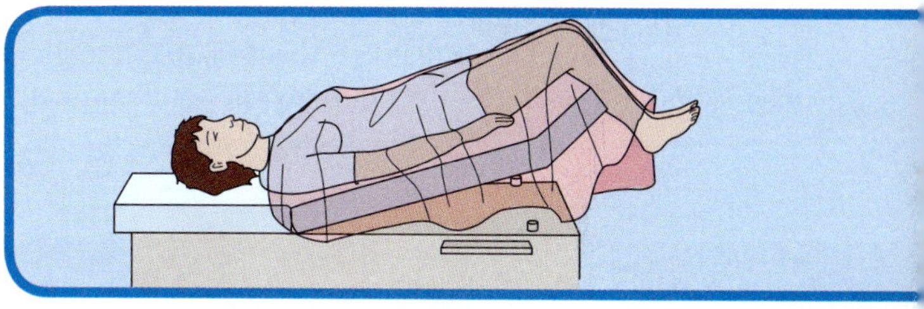

**Figure 39–13B:** Modified Trendelenburg with manual table. *Delmar/Cengage Learning.*

Assisting a patient into the lithotomy position requires her first to sit at the end of the table and then lie back. The leg support may be extended temporarily. A drape is placed over the patient from the chest to the feet, usually in the shape of a diamond. Placing the drape with one corner between the legs will make the exam easier in this position. The stirrups are extended from the table and tightened or secured into position. They should be extended far enough to allow the patient to be comfortable to facilitate abdominal relaxation and prevent leg cramps. The legs are flexed, and the heel of each foot is placed in a stirrup. The patient is instructed to slide down so that the hips are at the edge of the table. A pillow under the head will make the patient more comfortable. The arms may be crossed over the abdomen or placed at the sides. You should ensure that the patient is as comfortable as possible and provide support for the anxious patient.

## Additional Body Positions

Three additional body positions need mentioning but are used infrequently in most providers' offices: the Trendelenburg, the jackknife, and the proctologic. In the **Trendelenburg** or **shock** position, the patient is supine with the feet elevated slightly (Figure 39–13 A). This position may easily be accomplished with a power table. The controls would automatically lower the head of the table while keeping the patient in supine or horizontal recumbent position. With a manual table, the top section can be raised to elevate the thighs and hips, thereby achieving a lower position for the head and a modified Trendelenburg position. The lower legs are bent over the end of the table to maintain the position (Figure 39–13 B). The patient is typically draped from the neck, or the axillary, to the knees. This position would be used if a patient experiences or has symptoms of syncope. Patients may experience difficulty when blood samples are drawn or intravenous therapy is given or with some examinations.

Trendelenburg positioning is frequently used in a critical care facility and by EMS personnel with trauma, hemorrhage, and dangerously low blood pressure. It is also beneficial in certain abdominal and pelvic surgical procedures to displace organs upward. The position can also be used as a simple test for **incompetent** valves in persons with varicose veins. After being placed in straight-line Trendelenburg, the patient is asked to stand, and the provider observes whether the veins fill from above or below.

A special table is needed for the jackknife, or Kraske, position to be comfortable (Figure 39-14). The patient is in a semi-sitting position with the shoulders elevated and the thighs flexed at right angles to the abdomen. This position is especially useful for examination and instrumentation of the male urethra. Draping is from the upper chest to the ankles.

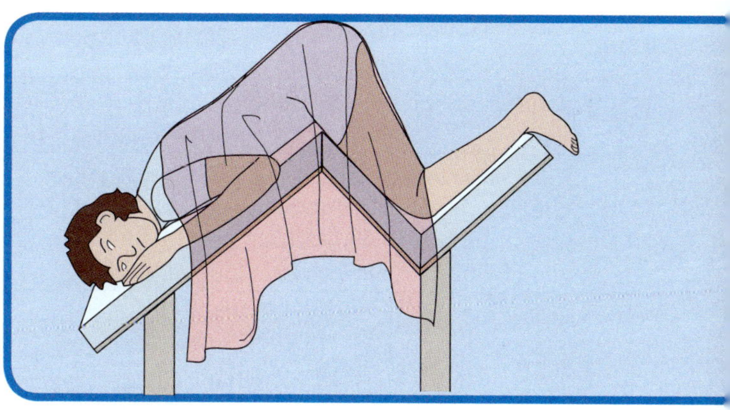

**Figure 39–14:** Jackknife, or Kraske, position. *Delmar/Cengage Learning.*

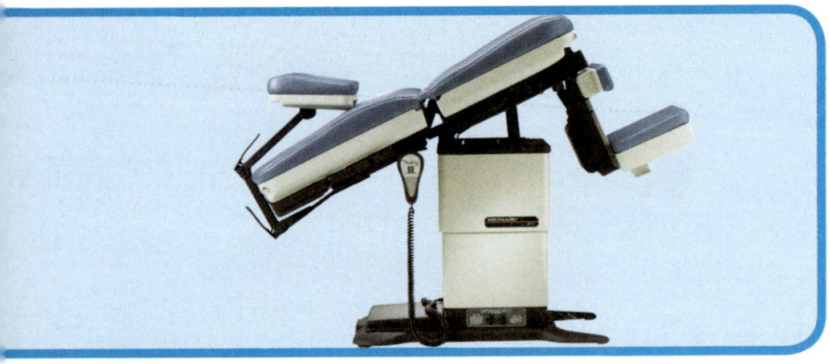

**Figure 39–15:** The Midmark power table in position for specialty exams. *Courtesy of Midmark Corp.*

This position requires a power table (Figure 39–15) or a special manual table that has an attachable kneeling extension and can be upended by a hand-cranking mechanism. The top half of the table is flat, while the leg portion, with the extender, is at a right angle. The patient would be asked to disrobe from the waist down and kneel on the extension, flexing his upper body to lie on the table. If clothing is one piece, a gown open in the back is indicated. A drape is positioned over the patient from the mid-back down past the knees or a **fenestrated** drape may be used. The arms are usually flexed at the side or under the head. The medical assistant operates the controls or cranks the table over until the buttocks are elevated. The head is lower than the body, and the internal abdominal organs move toward the chest. This helps straighten the "S" curve of the sigmoid colon to facilitate sigmoidoscope insertion during a sigmoidoscopy, covered in Chapter 40. The position is also used for examination and treatment of rectal and anal conditions such as thrombosed and internal hemorrhoids.

## PROCEDURE 39–4 Positioning the Patient for an Exam

**MEDIA LINK:** View the video for this chapter, "Positioning the Patient" on the Premium Website.

**PURPOSE:** To assist the patient into a variety of positions used in general physical and other examinations

**EQUIPMENT:** Adjustable examination table, table paper, gown, drape sheet, pillow, disposable pillow cover

S **SKILL:** Demonstrate positioning a patient for a variety of examinations.

| Procedure Steps | Detailed Instructions and/or *Rationales* |
|---|---|
| 1. Check the examination room for cleanliness. | Always have clean paper on the table and a clean pillow cover or clean towel over the pillow. *Every precaution must be maintained to prevent any possible cross-contamination of disease.* |
| 2. Identify the patient and introduce yourself. | *Speaking to the patient by name and checking the chart ensures that you are performing the procedure on the correct patient.* |
| B 3. Explain the procedure to the patient, ***using language the patient can understand.*** | |
| 4. Give clear instructions to the patient regarding the amount of clothing to be removed and where it is to be placed and instruct the patient in use of the gown. | *The procedure to be performed dictates whether the front or back should be open.* |
| 5. Assist the patient with gown if help is needed. | *If no help is needed, respect the privacy and modesty of the patient by leaving the room while the patient changes.* |

| Procedure Steps | Detailed Instructions and/or *Rationales* |
|---|---|
| 6. Assist the patient onto the examination table if help is needed. | |
| 7. Explain to the patient the necessary exam and the position required. | *For some examinations, multiple positions may be needed. Be sure the patient is aware of the position he or she will be assisted into and confirm that he or she is comfortable with this prior to positioning.* |
| 8. Assist the patient into the required position: | A pillow may be used for patient support in any of the positions to aid comfort. |
| a. Anatomical | Patient stands up straight |
| b. Sitting | Patient sits at the edge of the examination table, drape on lap covering legs |
| c. Horizontal recumbent (supine) | Patient lies flat on the back, drape from neck to feet |
| d. Dorsal recumbent | Patient lies face up, flat on back with knees bent, drape from neck to feet |
| e. Prone | Patient lies flat, face down, drape from upper back to feet |
| f. Sims' | Patient lies on left side, leg slightly bent, arm placed behind back, drape from axillary to knees |
| g. Knee-chest | Patient lies on table face down, supporting body with knees and chest, fenestrated drape used, covering area to be examined |
| h. Trendelenburg | Patient is in the supine position on a tilted table with head lower than legs |
| i. Fowler's | Patient lies back on exam table on which head is elevated 90 degrees, drape from waist down |
| j. Semi-Fowler's | Patient lies back on exam table on which head is elevated 45 degrees, drape from chest down |
| k. Lithotomy | Patient lies on back with knees bent and feet in the stirrups, drape diamond shape, chest to feet |
| 9. Drape the sheet evenly over the patient but leave loose on all sides. | |
| 10. Assist the patient from the table when the examination is completed. | Patient may be dizzy from the change in position. Allow him or her to sit upright before standing. Clean the room and replace the supplies. *The examination table surface and base must be thoroughly cleaned with disinfecting cleanser at regular intervals and following any contact with body fluids that may contain blood-borne pathogens.* |

Now that you have been trained in the skills needed for positioning and draping the patient for physical and other examinations, we will continue in the next unit with the examination process as we proceed through a complete physical examination, OB/GYN exam, and pediatric exam.

## CHAPTER SUMMARY

- Supplies used in the preparation of the exam room will vary depending on the provider's preference and the exam being performed; however, common ones include (but are not limited to) hand-washing products; biohazardous and regular waste containers; face guards; gloves; patient gowns; drapes; paper towels; tissues; an examination light source; and standard examination equipment such as tongue blades, speculums, gauze squares, and applicators.
- Preparation and maintenance of the examination room for an exam is also the responsibility of the medical assistant (see Procedure 39–1). Ensure that the room is clean and tidy and at a comfortable temperature.
- Between patient examinations, all surfaces within the room that might be contaminated should be cleaned with a disinfectant between patient examinations. The examination table is cleaned and new table paper and pillow cover is applied. Discard all disposable items into the proper waste receptacle and non-disposables in the laundry bin. Put all reusable supplies in the proper storage area, restock any used items, spray disinfectant or deodorizer if needed.
- Proper transfer techniques for assisting patients from their wheelchair to the exam table and back again is imperative to ensure that injuries don't occur. This is not an easy task to do alone if the patient is unable to support his or her own weight. Always enlist help from coworkers to prevent injury to the patient and yourself.
- Several positions may be incorporated into a patient examination; it may be your responsibility to assist the patient into the various positions appropriate for the provider's examination. Safety and patient comfort must be made a priority in any positioning that occurs. Refer to Procedure 39–4 for a comprehensive list of positions and reasons for their use.
- Draping for the various positions is essential for patient comfort and privacy. Patient gowns and drapes should be positioned so that only the portion of the body being examined is exposed. Positions may frequently change, so be prepared to assist the provider with the changes and keep the patient adequately covered.

## STUDY TOOLS

| | |
|---|---|
| **Workbook** | Activities for Chapter 39 |
| **Premium Website** | |
| MEDIA LINK | View these **Media Links** for Chapter 39:<br>• Transferring a Patient from a Wheelchair<br>• Positioning the Patient |
| StudyWARE | Activities and Quizzes on the **StudyWARE™ Software** for Chapter 39 |
| | Complete the following Competency Challenge 2.0 activity:<br>• Tuesday, 10:00 AM, Prepare Patients for Exams |
| | **Audio Library** of medical terms |
| | Online access to the **Critical Thinking Challenge 2.0** |
| learninglab | Module 17: Preparing for Clinical Procedures |
| **CourseMate** | Activities and Quizzes for Chapter 39 |
| **WebTutor** | Activities and Quizzes for Chapter 39 |

## CHECK YOUR KNOWLEDGE

1. The primary use of this position is for vaginal examinations of the female patient when a speculum is inserted, as when obtaining pap smears.
   a. Trendelenburg
   b. Lithotomy
   c. Fowler's
   d. Semi-Fowler's
2. These supplies are usually stored in the table drawers, whereas other supplies are kept in examination cabinet drawers or a supply cabinet.
   a. Tongue depressors
   b. Gauze squares
   c. Gowns and drapes
   d. Applicators
3. The lateral recumbent position is another term that may be used to describe the following position.
   a. Sims'
   b. Lithotomy
   c. Supine
   d. Prone
4. Which position would be used if a patient experiences or has symptoms of syncope?
   a. Prone
   b. Trendelenburg
   c. Sims'
   d. Anatomical
5. The horizontal recumbent or supine position is used for examination and treatment of the _____ portion of the body, including the breasts and abdominal organs.
   a. posterior
   b. superior
   c. inferior
   d. anterior
6. Which position would be used for patients with respiratory or cardiovascular problems?
   a. Fowler's
   b. Prone
   c. Knee-chest
   d. Jackknife

## WEB LINKS

Occupational Safety and Health Administration: www.osha.gov

## RESOURCES

Corning Metpath Laboratories. (1996). *Patient Education* [Pamphlet]. Columbus, OH: Author.

*Diagnostic tests, nurse's ready reference.* (1991). Springhouse, PA: Springhouse Corporation.

Estes, M. E. Z. (2010). *Health Assessment & Physical Examination.* Clifton Park, NY: Delmar Cengage Learning.

Heller, M., and Veach, L. (2009). *Clinical Medical Assisting: A Professional, Field Smart Approach to the Workplace.* Clifton Park, NY: Delmar, Cengage Learning.

Lindh, W., Pooler, M., Tamparo, C., and Dahl, B. (2010). *Delmar's Comprehensive Medical Assisting Administrative and Clinical Competencies* (4th ed.). Clifton Park, NY: Delmar Cengage Learning.

Venes, D. (ed.). (2009). *Taber's Cyclopedic Medical Dictionary* (21st ed.). Philadelphia: F. A. Davis.

**Labeling: Label the following illustrations, indicating the various examination positions.**

1.
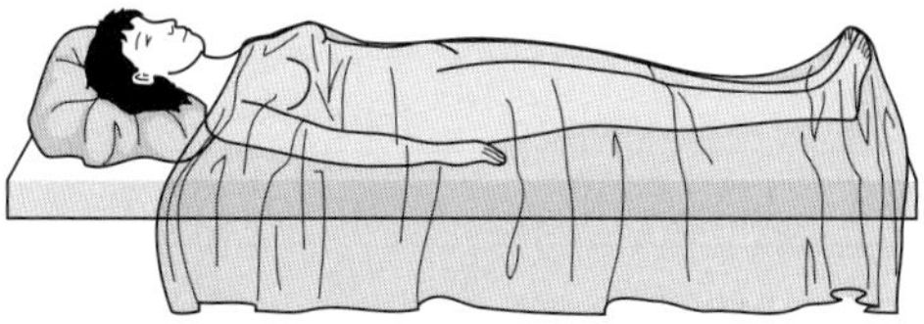

2.
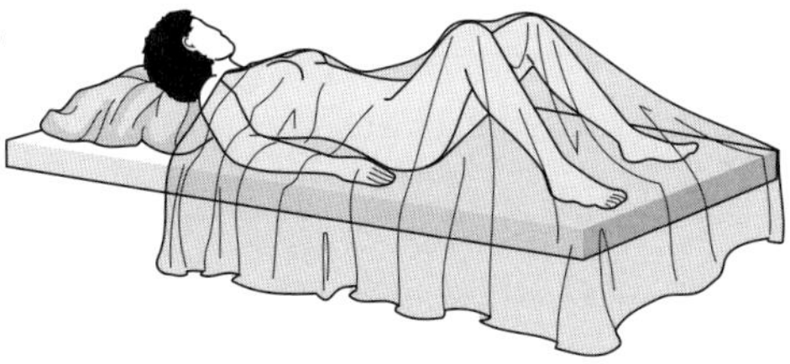

3.
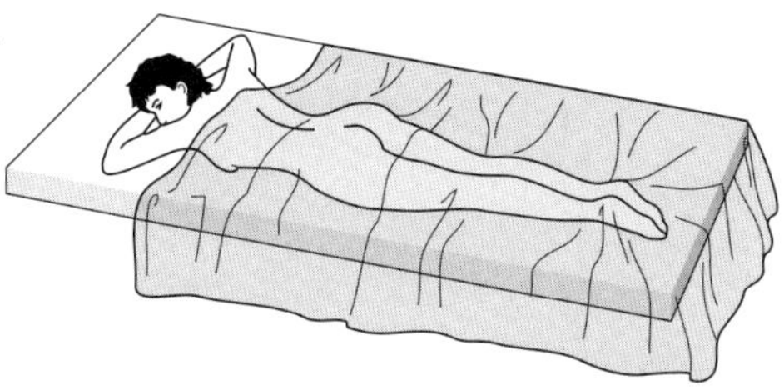

4.
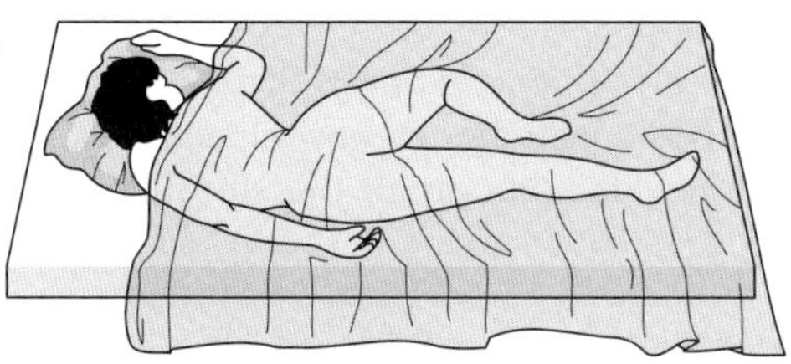

5.
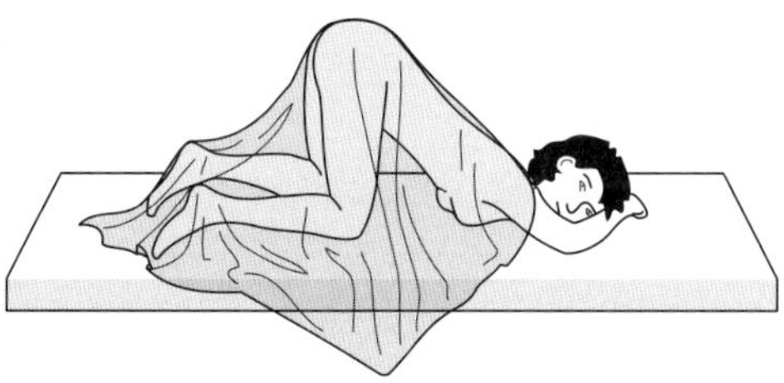

6.
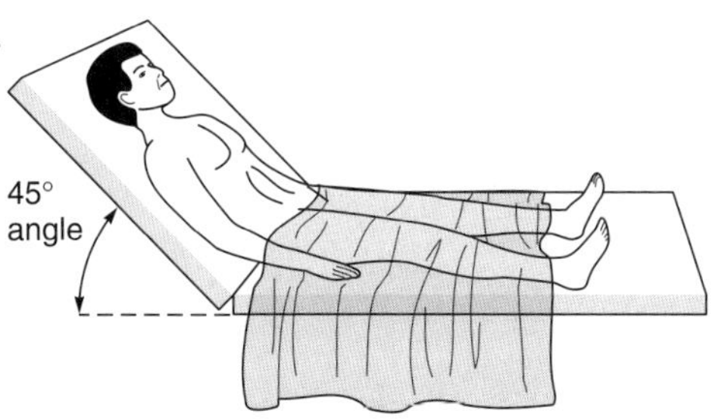


7.
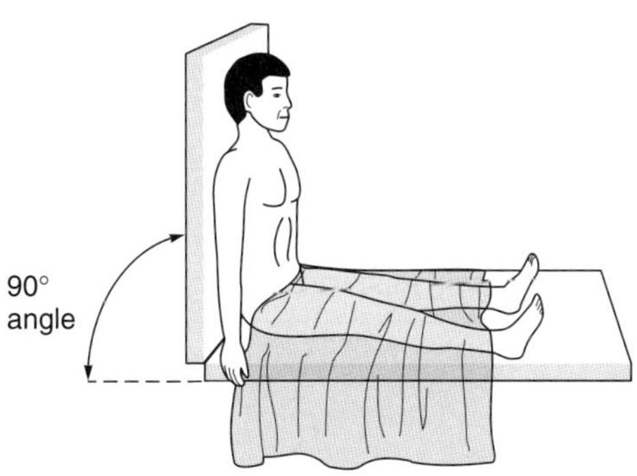


8.
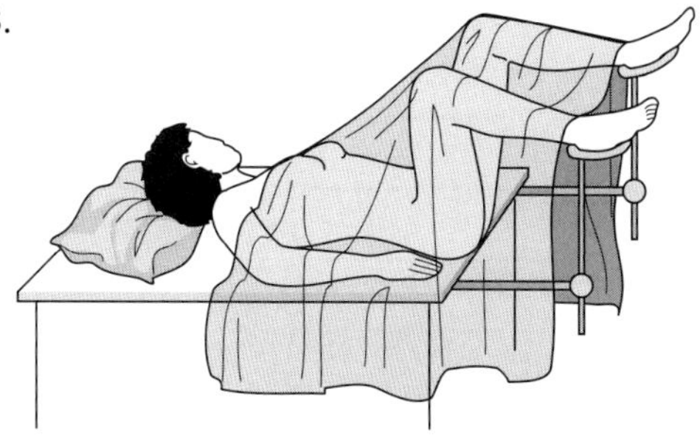

9.
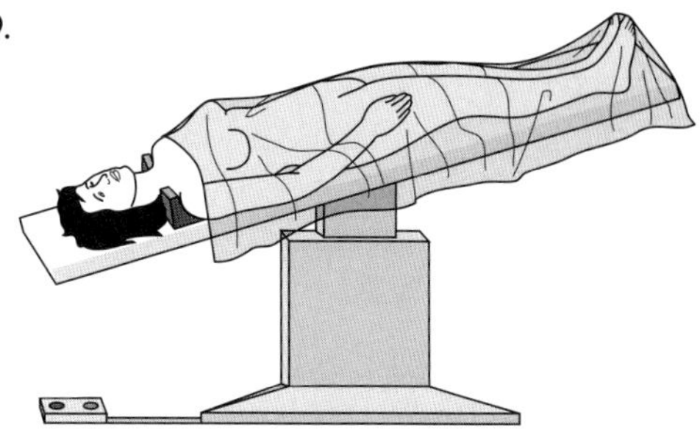

10.
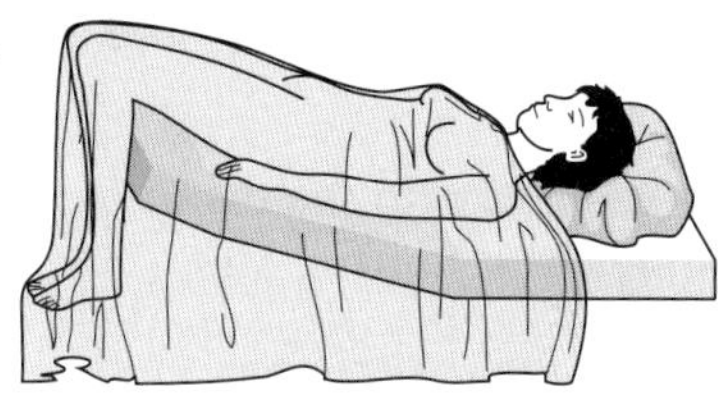

11.
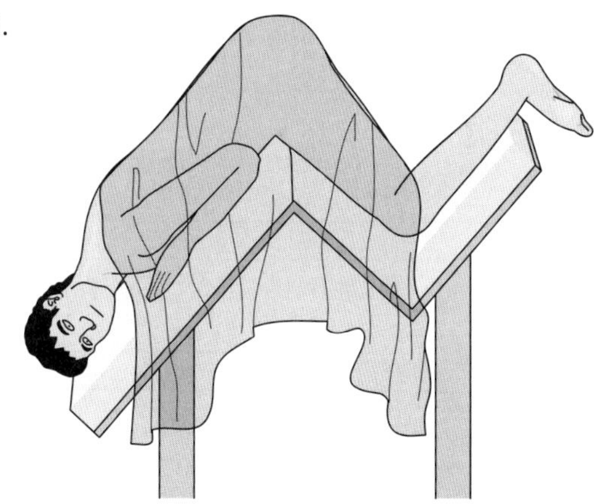

1. ________________________________________
2. ________________________________________
3. ________________________________________
4. ________________________________________
5. ________________________________________
6. ________________________________________
7. ________________________________________
8. ________________________________________
9. ________________________________________
10. ________________________________________
11. ________________________________________

# Chapter Application

## Case Studies with Critical Thinking Questions

### Scenario 1

Kelly escorts Mrs. Leonard into the exam room for her yearly Pap test and pelvic exam. Kelly didn't have time to clean the room before escorting Mrs. Leonard to the back office, so she asks her to have a seat on the stool while she tidies the room. She disposes the used gown and table paper and sets up all the supplies. She then asks Mrs. Leonard to disrobe and prepares her for the exam.

1. What was Kelly's first *big* mistake? ________________________________________.

2. What should Mrs. Leonard have been instructed to do before disrobing? ________________________________________.

3. Should equipment and supplies be set up in the presence of the patient? ________________________________________.

### Scenario 2

Mr. Johnson is being seen in the office for a sigmoidoscopy. The medical assistant gives Mr. Johnson disrobing instructions and leaves the room for a few minutes. When she returns, she places Mr. Johnson in the knee-chest position, and he complains about how uncomfortable it is for him. The medical assistant assures the patient that it will be only a few more minutes before the provider is ready.

1. When should the patient have been placed into the position for the exam? ________________________________________.

2. What should the medical assistant have done to make the patient more comfortable? ________________________________________.

3. What is an alternative position that can be used for this procedure? ________________________________________.

Chapter

# 5

# The Physical Exam, Specialty Exams, and Procedures

## OBJECTIVES

In this chapter, you will learn the following:

### KB KNOWLEDGE BASE

1. Spell and define, using the glossary at the back of the text, all the Words to Know in this chapter.
2. Discuss the reasons a complete physical examination is performed.
3. Explain the role of the medical assistant in the examination process.
4. Discuss patient education as it relates to breast and testicular self-examination and why physical examinations are performed.
5. Name the six examination techniques used by physicians and give examples of each.
6. Discuss the physical examination format for providers and the body systems that are examined.
7. Discuss the examination and specialty procedures routinely performed on patients. (Refer to Table 40–1.)
8. Explain why irrigation of the ear is performed.
9. Describe the audiometric assessment procedures used to assess hearing acuity.
10. Explain why irrigation of the eye is performed.
11. Identify three vision screening tests and explain what they determine.
12. Describe a spirometry test and state the purpose of it.
13. Explain what a peak flow meter measures and why its use may be indicated.
14. Describe pulse oximetry testing and why it is performed.
15. Explain what a flexible sigmoidoscopy can help diagnose.

### S SKILLS

1. Prepare a patient for and assist with a routine physical exam.
2. Perform ear irrigation.
3. Perform eye irrigation.
4. Measure distant vision acuity with a Snellen chart.
5. Measure near vision acuity with a Jaeger chart.
6. Determine color vision acuity using Ishihara plates.
7. Perform spirometry testing.
8. Perform peak flow measuring.
9. Perform pulse oximetry testing.
10. Assist with a flexible sigmoidoscopy procedure.

### B BEHAVIOR

1. Apply critical thinking skills in performing patient assessment and care.
2. Use language and verbal skills that enable patients' understanding.
3. Demonstrate respect for diversity in approaching patients and families.
4. Demonstrate awareness of the territorial boundaries of the person with whom communicating.

## WORDS TO KNOW

acuity
audiometer
auscultation
bimanual
bruit
cerumen
coordination
decibel
digital rectal exam (DRE)
duration
enema
evacuant
fecal
flexible sigmoidoscope
funduscopy
gait
guaiac test paper
heartburn
heart murmur
hernia
inspection
irrigate
Ishihara
Jaeger chart
lavage
laxative
lumen
manipulation
mucosa
obturator
occluder
occult
palpation
peak flow
percussion
peripheral
physical
pitch
polyps
proctoscope
pulse oximetry
resonance
scribe
Snellen chart
spirometer
symmetry
tonometry
turgor
vertex
visceral
vital capacity

## THE COMPLETE PHYSICAL EXAMINATION

The primary reason for performing a complete physical examination (CPE) is to determine the general state of health and well-being of the patient. The CPE can be performed for various reasons, such as an insurance examination before issuing a policy, as a requirement with a patient's employment, as a request by a patient, or to assess a patient's state of health. The exam will cover all major organs and systems of the body. The provider's findings enable him or her to establish an opinion about the patient's condition and establish either a tentative or definitive diagnosis when there are abnormal signs and symptoms. Often, laboratory tests or diagnostic procedures are ordered to provide additional information upon which to base the diagnosis. After all data is obtained, the diagnosis is defined and the treatment plan, if indicated, can be established.

### The Medical Assistant's Role

As you read in Chapter 39, the medical assistant has many responsibilities in preparing for examinations, including setting up the room and supplies as well as preparing the patient for the exam. During the CPE, you will position the patient, hand examination instruments and supplies to the provider, and provide comfort to the patient as needed. Assisting with the CPE, the general physical exam, history and physical (H and P), physical exam (PE), or just plain **physical** (as it is often termed) is not difficult but is complex in that it is a *set* of procedures. You might also assist with the exam or scribe the findings per the provider.

In many facilities, the medical assistant accompanies the provider in the examination room and records the findings. The term **scribe** is given to the medical assistant who writes what the provider dictates during the exam. To perform this duty well, it is important to have sound knowledge in medical terminology, anatomy, and physiology in addition to good spelling and writing skills. Because the provider bases the diagnosis on these findings, accuracy is vital. Many providers prefer to write their own findings on the progress notes or preprinted physical forms in an outlined order of their choice (see Figure 40–1). Other providers prefer to dictate the findings of an examination into a recorder for transcription later by the medical assistant or medical transcriptionist. With the use of EHR becoming more common, the provider enters findings directly into the software as the examination is conducted (Figure 40–2).

There is no one set format for the examination as long as the provider is consistent, thorough, and complete with each patient. Some providers use the review of systems and physical examination portion of a history and physical examination form (Figure 40–3). In your career as a medical assistant, you might work with providers who may be quite different in their systematic approach to patient examination.

# Physical Exam

PLACE PATIENT LABEL HERE

Patient ID #______________________ DATE OF EXAM ___ /___ /___

❑ New Pt. Well-Woman Exam ❑ New Pt. Problem ❑ Est. Pt. Well-Woman Exam ❑ Est. Pt. Problem

**NAME**

**AGE** **DOB** **LMP**

**Current MEDS**

**Current BCM**

**ALLERGIES**

**PFSH of** ___/___/___ **Reviewed** ❑ No changes ❑ Updated

**STI RISKS:** Change in partner since last exam? ❑ Yes ❑ No

Are both pt and partner mutually monogamous? ❑ Yes ❑ No

Current partner's STI status: ❑ HSV ❑ HBV ❑ HCV ❑ Unknown

Partners: ❑ Men ❑ Women ❑ Both

❑ Vaginal ❑ Oral ❑ Anal Sex

With partner_________ wks / mos / yrs

**EDUCATION [if oral, if written]**

- ❑ Contraceptive options
- ❑ Method education
- ❑ Exam/lab findings discussed
- ❑ Breast health
- ❑ Problem education
- ❑ UTI / Cystitis
- ❑ Anemia / Iron / Diet
- ❑ Cholesterol management
- ❑ Infertility
- ❑ Menopause
- ❑ HT / ET
- ❑ Parental involvement
- ❑ Medications prescribed
- ________________
- ❑ Initial PT education
- ❑ Assessment / Plan discussed
- ❑ STI / HIV education / Safer sex
- ❑ Vaginitis / Vaginal infection
- ❑ Partner treatment
- ❑ Stop smoking
- ❑ Weight control / Diet / Exercise
- ❑ Options × 3 (Pregnancy)
- ❑ Preconception / Folic Acid
- ❑ Osteoporosis / Calcium
- ❑ EC offered
- ❑ Abstinence
- ❑ HPV vaccine
- ❑ Other ________________

**PATIENT INFORMATION (PI) PROVIDED**

**PIICs**

- ❑ The Pill
- ❑ The Ring
- ❑ The Patch
- ❑ Special Considerations
- ❑ HOPE
- ❑ DMPA
- ❑ EC
- ❑ POPs
- ❑ IUC
- ❑ IUC with Special Conditions
- ❑ IUC Use Beyond Recommendations
- ❑ Misoprostol for GYN Procedures
- ❑ Barriers
- ❑ Implants
- ❑ STI TX without an Exam
- ❑ Treatment of Genital Warts
- ❑ Treatment of Bartholin's Duct

**Cyst or Abscess**

- ❑ PID
- ❑ Endometrial Biopsy
- ❑ Services Related to the Menopause

**PIs**

- ❑ Herbal Medicine
- ❑ Instructions for use of the Ring
- ❑ Instructions for use of the Patch
- ❑ Pregnancy with an IUC in Place
- ❑ Condoms and Female Condoms
- ❑ Sepermicide for Birth Control
- ❑ Directions for Chlamydia

**PIs Provided in:**

- ❑ English
- ❑ Other:____________

**Treatment of Sex Partners**

- ❑ UTI
- ❑ Pregnancy Testing, Evaluation & Options Services

**S: Reason for Visit / Chief Complaint / History of Present illness**

**VITAL SIGNS**

❑ BP_________ ❑ Weight__________ ❑ Height __________ ❑ Temp _________

**O; Examination / Physical Findings**

| **SYSTEM** | **WNL** | **OTHER** |
|---|---|---|
| GENERAL | ❑ No acute distress, grossly WNL | |
| EYES | ❑ Grossly WNL | |
| ENMT | ❑ Grossly WNL | |
| CV | ❑ RRR ❑ Murmurs | |
| RESP | ❑ Clear to auscultation, equal breath sounds | |
| GI | ❑ Abdomen soft / non-tender, no masses<br>❑ Liver / spleen non-palpable<br>❑ Rectal exam (req. ≥ age 50) no masses / blood | |
| GU | ❑ Breasts w/no masses/discharge/tenderness<br>❑ No urethral discharge ❑ No CVAT<br>❑ Vulva, no lesions, skin intact w/no discoloration<br>❑ Vagina, normal color, no unusual discharge, no Bartholin enlargement / tenderness<br>❑ Cervix, no lesions, no contact bleeding<br>❑ Uterus, NS / NT / mobile / no CMT<br>❑ AF ❑ AV ❑ RF ❑ RV<br>❑ Adnexa, non-tender w/no masses | |
| MUSC. | ❑ Back w/no curvature ❑ Extremities full ROM | |
| SKIN | ❑ Intact w/no lesions<br>❑ Piercing ❑ Tattoo If yes, where ? _____ | |
| ENDO | ❑ Thyroid NS / NT / equal bilateral | |
| LYMPH | ❑ No lymphadenopathy neck / axilla / groin | |

**LAB TESTS DONE**

❑ Hct ___________

❑ Urine Dip (circle): Glucose Protein Nitrites Leukocytes

❑ Pregnancy Test Pos Neg ❑ Slide Pap ❑ Liquid Based Pap ❑ HSV ❑ GC ❑ CT

❑ HPV ❑ Other: ___________

❑ Wet Mount: KOH Saline WNL + Clue/+ Whiff pH____ +Hyphae +Trich WBC _____hpf

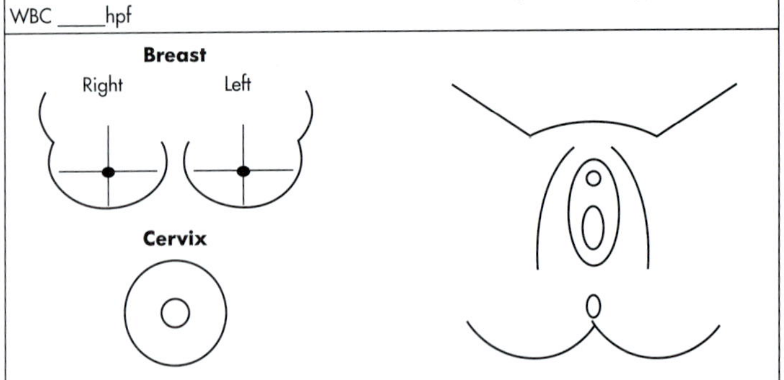


**Figure 40–1:** Example of a preprinted general physical exam form. *Delmar/Cengage Learning.*

# Physical Exam

PLACE PATIENT LABEL HERE

**ASSESSMENT**

**PLAN**

Referral provided for ______________________ Referral to ______________________
❑ Explained nature and implication of abnormal findings.
❑ Explained consequences of not receiving additional care.
❑ Explained management option and referral.
❑ Explained responsibility to obtain follow-up care.

Patient demonstrated understanding of education / findings / plan by
❑ Asking appropriate questions / returning
❑ Interpreter / Language Line. Provided by (name/relationship) ____________
❑ Other____________

**PRESCRIPTION**

❑ DMPA 150 mg IM/Sq q 12 weeks × 5 ❑ Given today
❑ OCs________ Sig: 1 qd × 1 yr # ______ today ______
❑ NuvaRing PV × 3 wks; out for 1 wk. × 1 yr # ______ today
❑ Ortho Evra 1 patch/wk × 3, none for 1 wk. × 1 yr # ______ today
Start: ❑ Sunday p next menses ❑ Day ____ ❑ Today ❑ Continue
❑ IUD ❑ ParaGard ❑ Mirena Date inserted: _________
❑ Implanon Date inserted _________
❑ Condoms #______ requested by client for ❑ contraception/BUM ❑ STD prevention
❑ Other____________

❑ OK for emergency pack of pills if needed
❑ Advanced Rx EC × 1 year ____ today ❑ EC now: ____

INTERVIEWER ______________________ CLINICIAN ______________________

DATE ______________________

**Figure 40–1:** *(continued)*

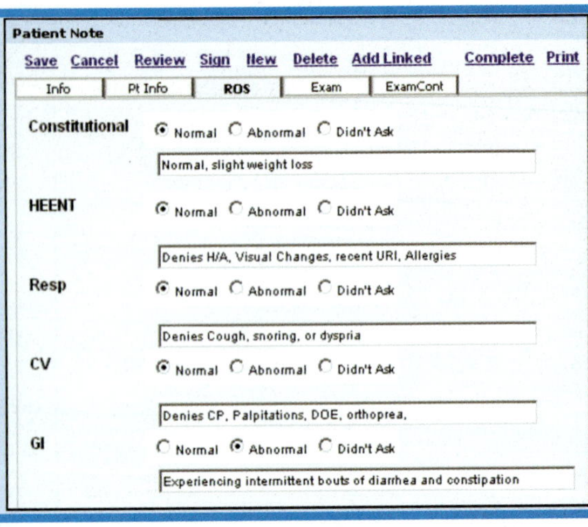

Patient Note

Save Cancel Review Sign New Delete Add Linked Complete Print

Info | Pt Info | ROS | Exam | ExamCont

Constitutional ◉ Normal ○ Abnormal ○ Didn't Ask
Normal, slight weight loss

HEENT ◉ Normal ○ Abnormal ○ Didn't Ask
Denies H/A, Visual Changes, recent URI, Allergies

Resp ◉ Normal ○ Abnormal ○ Didn't Ask
Denies Cough, snoring, or dyspria

CV ◉ Normal ○ Abnormal ○ Didn't Ask
Denies CP, Palpitations, DOE, orthoprea,

GI ○ Normal ◉ Abnormal ○ Didn't Ask
Experiencing intermittent bouts of diarrhea and constipation

**Figure 40–2:** Part of a physical exam screen in an EHR. *Courtesy of TriMed Technologies, Corp.*

## EXAMINATION TECHNIQUES

Providers are skilled in a variety of techniques used to evaluate patients in the examination process. You are expected to have a basic knowledge of these six techniques used to evaluate patients during physical examinations. Each technique provides specific information regarding the condition of the patient's body.

1. **Inspection** is evaluation by the use of sight. This is usually the initial part of the exam, when the provider looks at the patient to observe the skin's color and condition (rashes and discoloration), the general appearance (grooming, apparent state of health, posture), the level of anxiety, and **gait**. Awareness of person, place, and time as well as any visible injuries or deformities are noted.

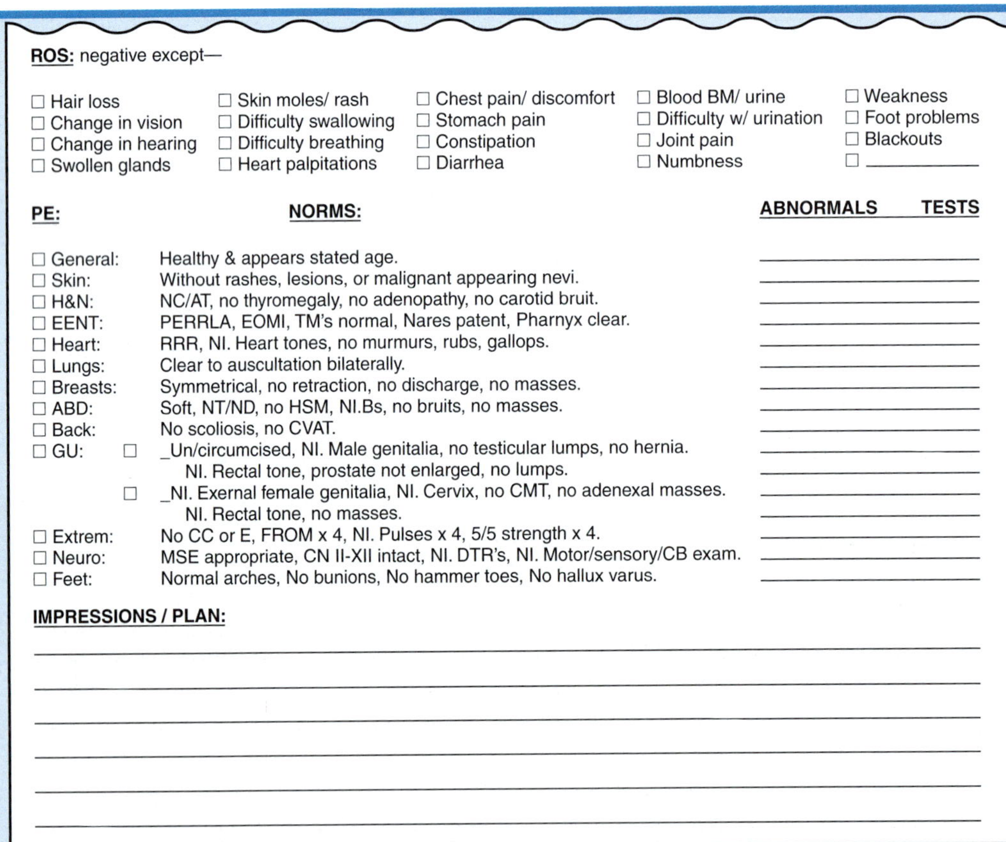

**ROS:** negative except—

☐ Hair loss ☐ Change in vision ☐ Change in hearing ☐ Swollen glands
☐ Skin moles/ rash ☐ Difficulty swallowing ☐ Difficulty breathing ☐ Heart palpitations
☐ Chest pain/ discomfort ☐ Stomach pain ☐ Constipation ☐ Diarrhea
☐ Blood BM/ urine ☐ Difficulty w/ urination ☐ Joint pain ☐ Numbness
☐ Weakness ☐ Foot problems ☐ Blackouts ☐ ______

| PE: | NORMS: | ABNORMALS | TESTS |
|---|---|---|---|
| ☐ General: | Healthy & appears stated age. | | |
| ☐ Skin: | Without rashes, lesions, or malignant appearing nevi. | | |
| ☐ H&N: | NC/AT, no thyromegaly, no adenopathy, no carotid bruit. | | |
| ☐ EENT: | PERRLA, EOMI, TM's normal, Nares patent, Pharnyx clear. | | |
| ☐ Heart: | RRR, Nl. Heart tones, no murmurs, rubs, gallops. | | |
| ☐ Lungs: | Clear to auscultation bilaterally. | | |
| ☐ Breasts: | Symmetrical, no retraction, no discharge, no masses. | | |
| ☐ ABD: | Soft, NT/ND, no HSM, Nl.Bs, no bruits, no masses. | | |
| ☐ Back: | No scoliosis, no CVAT. | | |
| ☐ GU: | ☐ _Un/circumcised, Nl. Male genitalia, no testicular lumps, no hernia. Nl. Rectal tone, prostate not enlarged, no lumps. | | |
| | ☐ _Nl. Exernal female genitalia, Nl. Cervix, no CMT, no adenexal masses. Nl. Rectal tone, no masses. | | |
| ☐ Extrem: | No CC or E, FROM x 4, Nl. Pulses x 4, 5/5 strength x 4. | | |
| ☐ Neuro: | MSE appropriate, CN II-XII intact, Nl. DTR's, Nl. Motor/sensory/CB exam. | | |
| ☐ Feet: | Normal arches, No bunions, No hammer toes, No hallux varus. | | |

**IMPRESSIONS / PLAN:**

**Figure 40–3:** Review of systems and physical examination portion of an H and P form. *Delmar/Cengage Learning.*

2. **Palpation** is evaluation using the sense of touch. The body can be felt using one hand, two hands (**bimanual** as in vaginal and rectal examinations), or one finger only (digitally as in **digital rectal examination [DRE]**). Examination of the breasts is done with the flat surfaces of the fingers of both hands. Palpation can determine skin temperature, size and shape of organs, the position and presence of abnormal structures, and the degree of abdominal rigidity and aortic pulsations.
3. **Percussion** is a means of producing sounds by tapping various parts of the body. The provider listens to the sounds to determine the size, density, and location of underlying **visceral** organs. **Pitch**, quality, **duration**, and **resonance** are terms used by providers when referring to percussion. Direct

percussion is termed *immediate* and is done by striking the finger against the patient's body. The type of percussion most often used is *indirect* or *mediate*. With indirect percussion, the examiner's finger is placed on the area and struck with a finger of the other hand.

4. **Auscultation** is listening to sounds made by the patient's body. Indirect or mediate auscultation is done with the stethoscope to amplify sounds that arise from the lungs, heart, and visceral organs. Sounds heard by this method of examination include **bruits**, murmurs, rales, rhythms, and bowel sounds. Direct or immediate auscultation is done by placing the ear directly over the bare surface area. Auscultation skill is acquired with experience. The provider must be able to determine normal from abnormal sounds. Some, such as the heart valve sounds, last only a fraction of a second and demand concentrated listening.
5. Mensuration, as you learned in Chapter 38, means measurement. In this part of the examination, the patient's chest and extremities are measured and recorded. Usually, a standard flexible tape measure is used. Mensuration includes all the following measurements: height, weight, head, chest, and other parts of the body as appropriate; temperature; pulse; respirations; and blood pressure. All measurements should be recorded in centimeters, inches, or feet; and pounds or kilograms; being consistent is especially necessary in keeping track of the pediatric patient's growth and development or in assessment and evaluation of any patient's change in readings that may contribute to a diagnosis.
6. **Manipulation** is the passive movement of a joint to determine the range of extension and flexion. This evaluation is especially important when patients have had joint injuries or have arthritis. Orthopedic providers evaluate range of motion following surgical procedures such as knee and hip replacements. Insurance companies and state industrial commissions may request evaluation to determine continuation of coverage following trauma injuries and industrial accidents.

## PHYSICAL EXAMINATION FORMAT

In reviewing the medical examination form in Figure 40–3, notice that the section immediately following "Review of Systems" has the areas outlined for recording the findings of the complete physical examination. It is concise and requires listing only abnormal findings to conserve time and writing. Additionally, many abbreviations are used (and some may be facility-specific).

The following pages provide an explanation of each of the body areas examined to help you become familiar with what the provider does in each section of the physical examination. Even though H and P and customized physical forms vary in appearance, the contents are basically be the same. The form has small boxes to check to be sure nothing is omitted. Each exam area has conditions to be observed and a line to note any abnormalities. If an additional diagnostic test is needed, it can also be noted after the abnormal finding.

Remember that the very first part of the physical includes measurement, vital signs, and vision screening (covered later in this chapter), which you will have initially completed before the provider's examination. To make the physical examination format easier to read and understand, it is presented in a modified outline format.

1. First, the examination area is listed in the heading.
2. Next [enclosed in brackets] is the patient's position, the examination technique(s), and the equipment or supplies needed. The patient is gowned throughout the examination, positioned, and draped as explained in Chapter 39. The gown will probably be opened in the back and simply raised by you or the provider for examining the chest and abdomen. The drape will also be repositioned throughout the examination to allow inspection and examination of the patient while providing as much coverage as possible.
3. There is a brief description of how the provider may conduct this portion of the examination.
4. Within each examination area are listed characteristics the provider may be observing and, *in italics*, some applicable descriptive terms. Each provider has his or her own style and depth of examination, which may not include all the areas and characteristics mentioned. The following will help you understand the components of a complete physical examination.

### General Appearance

[Anatomical, ambulate, or sitting; inspection; no equipment or supplies, just provider observations]

The provider may ask the patient to stand in front of him in the anatomical position while he observes the patient's general appearance. A few questions may be asked to judge speech and appropriate responses. The patient is asked to walk across the room to observe the manner of walking and body movements.

- Appearance—*grooming, state of health, body stature, nourished, appears stated age*
- Awareness—*to person, place, and time; confused; distressed*
- Gait—*manner of walking: shuffle, limp, balance, evidence of stiffness or pain*
- Speech—*slurring, stutter, loss of voice, impediment*
- Hearing—*response to sound, volume of speech*
- Breath—*odors: sweet and fruity with diabetes, acetone with acidosis, oral hygiene*

## Skin

[Sitting or standing; inspection or palpation; no equipment or supplies, just provider observations]

The provider will inspect anterior and posterior skin surfaces while the patient stands in front of him or her and as he or she progresses through the examination.

- Color—*redness, bruising, birth marks, darker areas*
- Condition—*dry, flaky, soft, calloused fingers or hands, skin cracks,* **turgor** (measured by pinching back of hand and observing the length of time for return to normal; provides estimate of hydration)
- Blemishes—*moles, warts, scars, acne, rashes*
- Lumps—*palpable masses under the skin*
- Nails—*cuticles, groomed, brittle, peeling, grooved, spooning, clubbing, white lines*

## Neck

[Sitting; inspection, palpation, auscultation, or manipulation]

The provider observes the patient in a sitting position, palpating and giving instructions for movement to evaluate range of motion.

- Range of motion
- Thyroid gland for *size, nodules, and symmetry*
- Lymph nodes and parotid glands palpated,
- Observation of swallowing,
- Auscultation of carotid arteries (Figure 40–4). (Blockage of the artery causes a sound known as a *bruit.*)

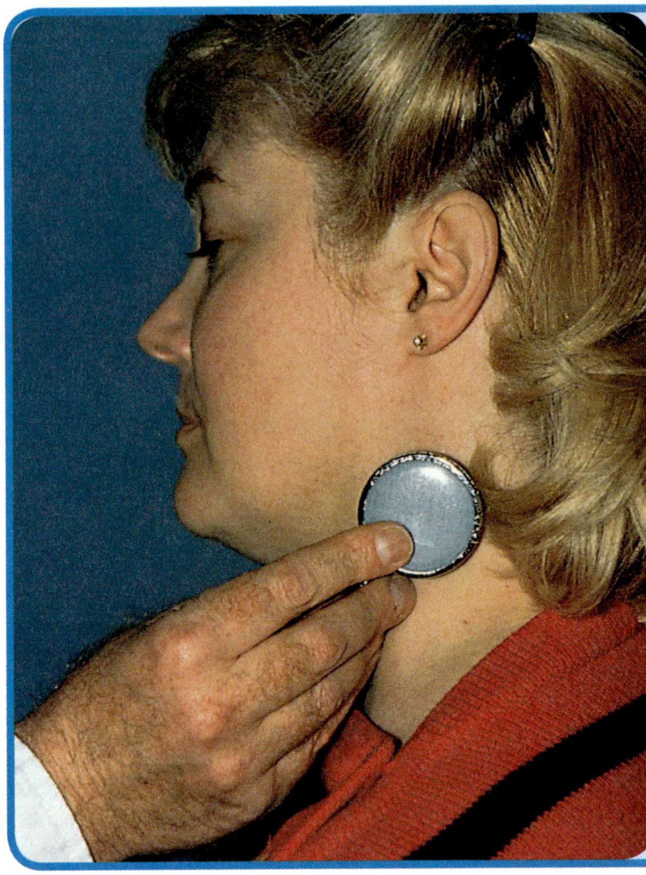

**Figure 40–4:** The physician auscultates the neck for the sounds made by blood flowing through the carotid artery. *Delmar/Cengage Learning.*

## HEENT (Head, Eyes, Ears, Nose, and Throat)

[Sitting; inspection, palpation; ophthalmoscope, otoscope, tuning fork, nasal speculum, tongue depressor, sterile gauze square]

The provider visually observes each area and uses the ophthalmoscope and otoscope to view internal structures. Eye musculature is observed by requesting patient movement. Hearing is evaluated using the tuning fork, and the nasal passages are examined with a speculum. The mouth, throat, and tongue are checked for lesions, and oral hygiene is evaluated.

- Head—**symmetry**, *nodules, hair texture and distribution, scalp*
- Face—*skin condition, presence of facial hair, facial paralysis, eye symmetry*
- Eyes—*observed for protrusion, lashes, symmetry, general condition*

  Vision—*The results of the Snellen, Jaeger, and Ishihara screening procedures previously completed following mensuration are indicated on the form.*
  Pupils (in darkened room with light source)—*These are checked for reaction to light and accommodation (LandA); if equal, it is recorded as PERRLA (pupils equal, round, and respond to light and accommodation).*
  Sclera—*color, clarity, scarring*
  Musculature—*extraocular movements (EOM) are checked for: movement up, down, right, and left while following the provider's finger.*
  **Peripheral**—*This is side vision while looking straight forward.*
  Internal structures—*Provider views these with an ophthalmoscope: retina, optic disc, blood vessels*

- Ears—*visual and otoscope inspection*

  External—*size, symmetry, lobes, structure*
  Middle—*with otoscope: external auditory canal, cerumen, drainage, tympanic membrane (should be pearly gray), scars from perforations and infection*
  Hearing—*tuning fork to test air, nerve conduction*

- Nose—*visual and nasal speculum inspection*

  Exterior—*structure: straight, curved, bulbous, color*
  Interior—*with nasal speculum and light; checks mucosa, septum, polyps*

- Throat—*inspection with light source*
- Mouth—*with light and tongue depressor, checks inside surface of cheeks and jaw alignment; with gauze to hold tongue, check under tongue and mouth floor, frenulum*

  Tongue—*surface, mobility, depress while patient says "ah" to view tonsils, posterior pharynx*
  Teeth—*oral hygiene, condition of teeth, gums, bite, dentures* (*Note:* If poor oral hygiene, provide patient education and instructional materials following examination and encourage dental visit.)

## Chest

[Sitting; inspection or palpation; no equipment or supplies, just provider observations]

The provider observes the seated patient as the chest is palpated for underlying nodes or masses. The chest structure is noted, and the movement in response to breathing is observed.

- Inspection—*for symmetry of sides, shape deformities, intercostal spaces when breathing (retract or bulge), posterior spine alignment, scapula levels*
- Palpation—*lymph nodes, nodules, tenderness* (Figure 40–5)

## Heart

[Sitting; auscultation; stethoscope]

The provider auscultates the heart from both anterior and posterior chest wall. The medical assistant and patient must maintain silence during the examination for the provider to hear the heart sounds. Abnormalities may indicate the need for further testing or a cardiologist referral.

- Rate and rhythm—*beats per minute, regularity, volume, premature contractions*
- Sounds—***heart murmurs***

## Lungs

[Sitting; auscultation or percussion; stethoscope]

The provider auscultates the lungs on posterior and anterior chest wall. Again, the medical assistant and patient must maintain silence except for the patient's making speech sounds the provider may request. Percussion may be used if fluid, excess air, or a mass is suspected within the chest cavity (Figure 40–6).

- Rate and rhythm—*breaths per minute, regularity, volume, depth*
- Sounds—*posterior auscultation (breathe with open mouth): wheeze, rales, rhonchi, crackling, bronchial constriction; percussion for lung consolidation, hyperinflation, pleural fluid*
- Capacity—*measured by the* **spirometer**; *different tests can be done: forced vital capacity involves forced inhalation followed by quick and complete exhalation to determine the capacity of lungs.* (Review the procedure for performing spirometry later in the chapter).

## Breasts

[Sitting or recumbent; inspection or palpation; no equipment or supplies, just provider observations]

The provider inspects and palpates the breasts with the patient in sitting and lying positions. The provider may provide breast self-examination instruction to the patient or defer the responsibility to the medical assistant.

- Inspection—*size, shape, symmetry, position, nipples, dimpling*

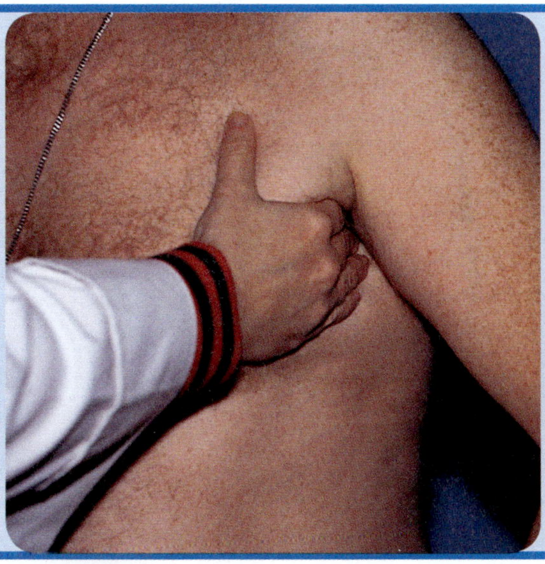

**Figure 40–5:** Palpation of the patient's axillary region. *Delmar/Cengage Learning.*

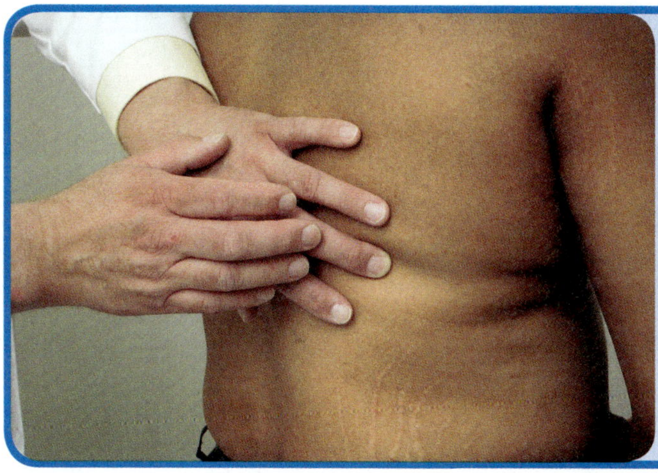

**Figure 40–6:** Using blunt percussion to examine the base of the lung. *Delmar/Cengage Learning.*

- Palpate—*lumps, nodules, tenderness, mass, in both supine and sitting position*
- Patient education—*Men can also develop breast cancer and should be examined. Instruct the female patient to perform monthly breast self-examination following her menstrual period. Provide visual educational handout. Encourage regular mammograms as appropriate for her age group.*

## PATIENT EDUCATION

### Breast Self-Examination

Breasts should be examined on a specific day every month, 7 to 10 days following the beginning of a period for women who still menstruate. Learn what your breasts feel like so you can identify a change. Normal changes of breast tissue due to hormonal fluctuations during the cycle could be mistaken for an abnormality.

1. Lie on your back with a pillow or a large folded towel under the same shoulder as the breast you're examining.
2. For the right breast, use the ends of the three middle fingers of the left hand to press the breast tissue against the chest wall to feel for lumps or thickening (Figure 40–7A). Move the fingers in a pattern: Start at the nipple and move around the breast in circles toward the chest wall or move up and down or in a wedge pattern. Use the same pattern each month. Cover the entire breast area.
3. Repeat for the left breast.
4. Stand in front of a mirror (Figure 40–7B). Look at the breasts for symmetry; observe for any area that appears to be attached or falls differently. Observe with arms at sides and with arms raised.
5. Do an extra breast exam while showering. Wet, soapy hands glide over the skin, making feeling the tissue easier.
6. Report any abnormal findings to your physician as soon as possible.

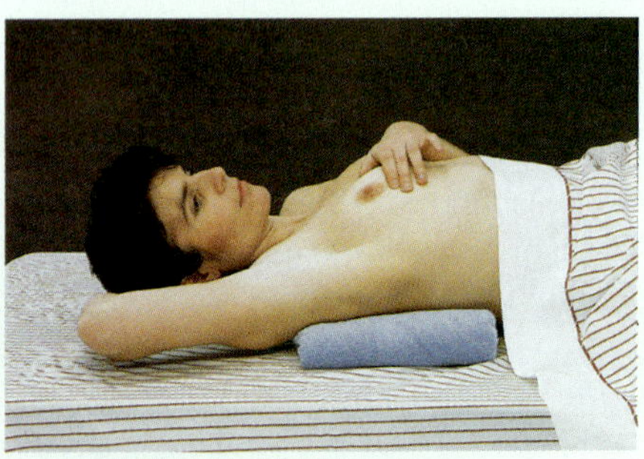

**Figure 40–7A:** Breast self-exam, lying down. *Delmar/Cengage Learning.*

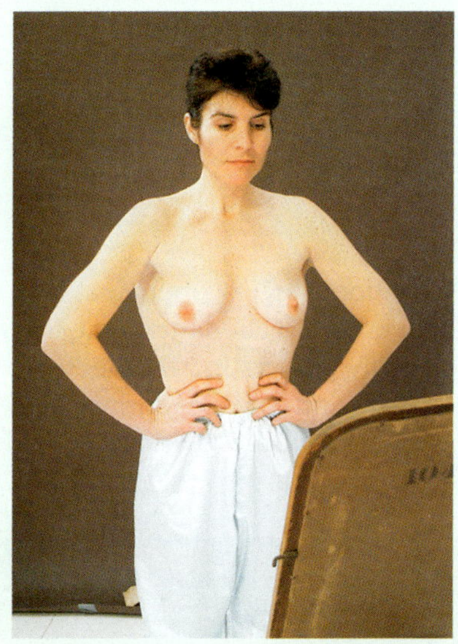

**Figure 40–7B:** Breast self-exam, in front of mirror. *Delmar/Cengage Learning.*

## Abdomen

[Supine or dorsal recumbent; auscultation, inspection, palpation, or percussion; stethoscope]

Refer to Figures 40–8A, B, and C to review the sections of the abdomen and the location of the underlying organs.

The provider stands at the side to inspect, auscultate, palpate, and percuss the abdomen with the patient in the supine and dorsal recumbent positions. A pillow under the patient's head and relaxing the abdominal muscles facilitate deep palpation of the abdominal organs. Auscultating for bowel sounds requires the medical assistant and patient to maintain silence.

- Auscultation—*(should be done first because palpation and percussion can alter bowel sounds); bowel sounds' character and frequency, bruits*
- Inspection—*symmetry, operative scars, protrusions (hernias), umbilicus*
- Palpation—*abdominal aorta pulse, masses,* ***hernias****, tenderness, organs, muscular tension*
- Percussion—*liver, spleen, and stomach size; presence of air*

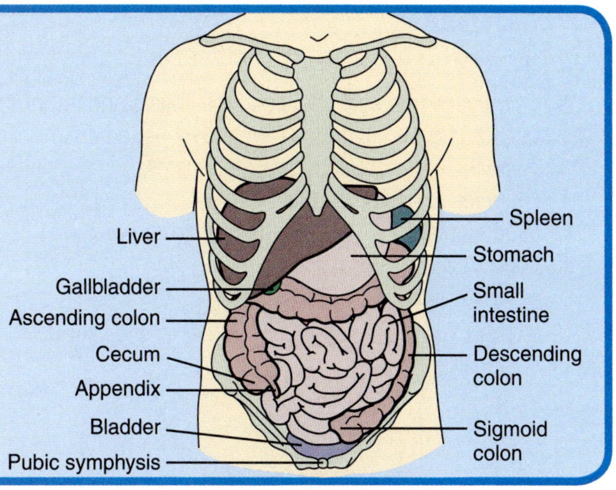


**Figure 40–8A:** Position of abdominal organs in the nine abdominal regions. *Delmar/Cengage Learning.*

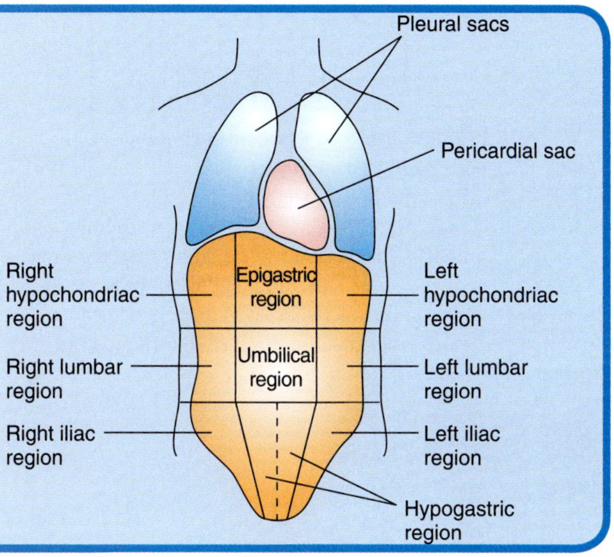


**Figure 40–8B:** Position of the nine abdominal regions. *Delmar/Cengage Learning.*

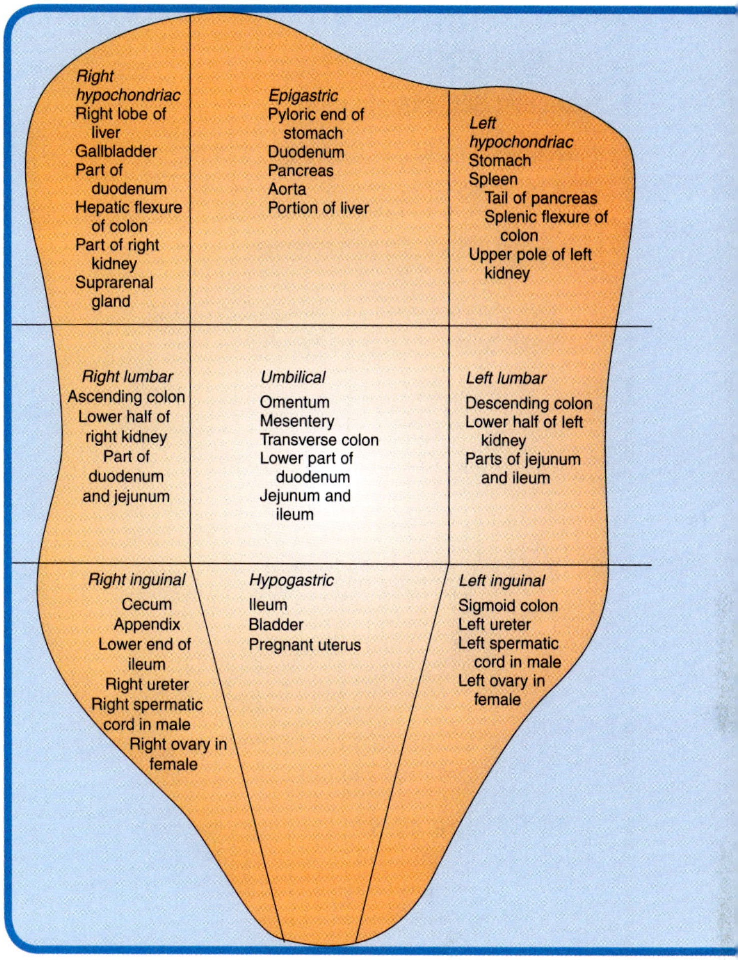


**Figure 40–8C:** The nine regions of the abdominal cavity with underlying visceral organs. *Delmar/Cengage Learning.*

## Back

[Standing; inspection, palpation, or manipulation; no equipment or supplies, just provider observations]

The provider inspects the posterior surface to observe the spine and symmetry of bony prominences. A lateral view will detect excessive anterior and posterior curvatures. The patient may be asked to twist and bend over to evaluate curvatures and flexibility.

- Spine—*straight, concave and convex curvatures, kyphosis, lordosis, scoliosis, manipulation to sides, twist, bend over, front and back, cervical manipulation and head all directions*
- Symmetry—*sides equal, pelvis and scapula even*

## Genitourinary and Rectal (Male)

[Standing; inspection or palpation; physician's senses, glove, lubricant, **guaiac test paper** (occult blood test kit), tissues]

The provider wears gloves to inspect the external genitalia of the standing male patient. When the testes are palpated, males past puberty should be instructed in testicular self-examination (TSE). Printed instructions should be provided following the examination. The patient is asked to bear down and cough while the provider checks for hernias in the scrotum and inguinal ring. The patient is then instructed to turn around and bend over the table. The provider inspects the anus and then inserts the gloved and lubricated index finger into the anal canal to evaluate sphincter tone and internal hemorrhoids. The prostate is palpated through the anterior wall of the rectum. A test for **occult** blood is taken from a small amount of stool on the withdrawn index finger placed on the guaiac test paper. Tissues are used to remove the excess lubricant.

- Pubis—*lesions, infestation, distribution of hair*
- Penis—*lesions, scars, deformity, discharge, circumcision, urinary meatus*

## PATIENT EDUCATION

### Testicular Self-Examination

It is recommended that men begin routine testicular self-examination at about 15 years of age. The testes should be carefully palpated after a warm shower or bath when the scrotal skin is relaxed.

1. Manually examine each testis. It is normal for one testis to be larger than the other.
2. Gently roll the testes between the fingers and thumbs of both hands (Figures 40–9A and B). Become familiar with the structure and feel of the testes.
3. Feel for lumps or nodules.
4. See Figure 40–9C to identify the structures.
5. Report any abnormal findings to your physician as soon as possible.

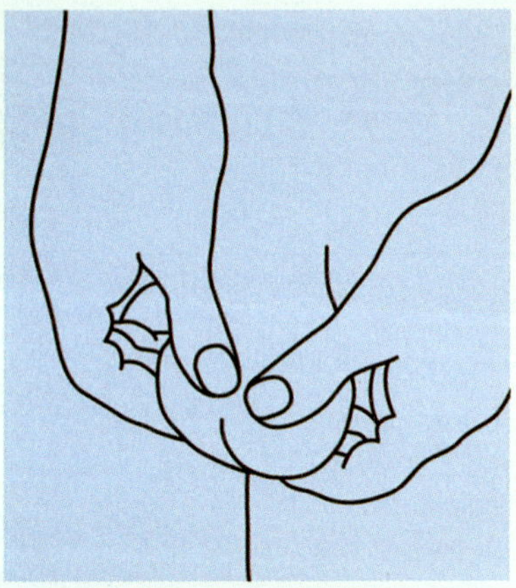

**Figure 40–9A:** Testicular self-exam. Stand in front of the mirror. Look for swelling on the skin of the scrotum. *Delmar/Cengage Learning.*

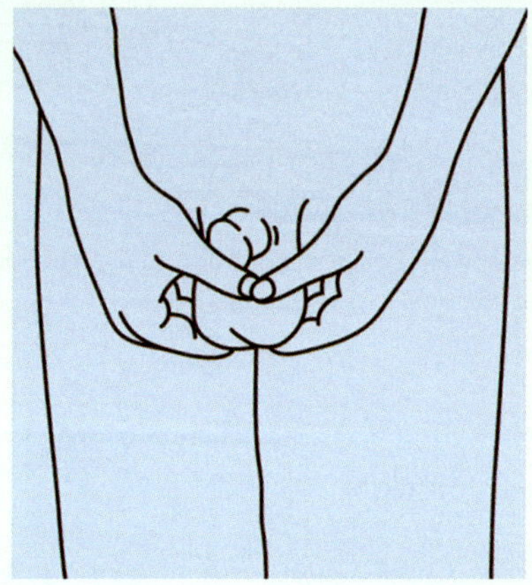

**Figure 40–9B:** Examine each testicle with both hands. Position your index and middle fingers under the testicle with the thumbs on top. Gently roll the testicle between your thumbs and fingers. (Having one testicle larger than the other is normal.) Men should be advised to be examined by a physician as soon as possible if there are any abnormal findings, such as lumps or nodules, when doing TSE. *Delmar/Cengage Learning.*

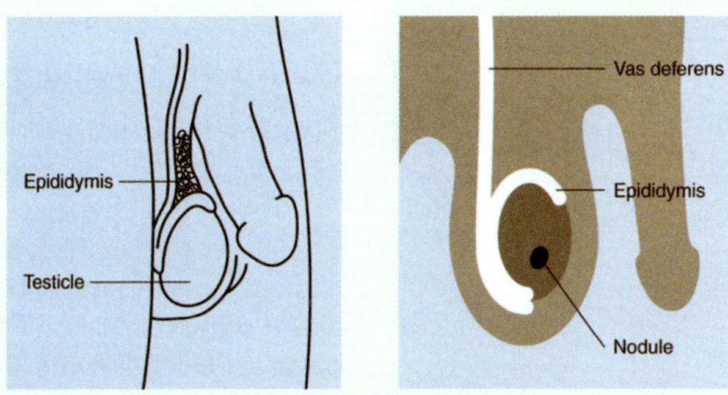


**Figure 40–9C:** Illustration of testicular structures. *Delmar/Cengage Learning.*

- Scrotum—*symmetry, swelling, varicosities, fluid, masses, presence of hernia*
- Anus—*hemorrhoids, lesions, fissures, prolapse, sphincter tone*
- Prostate—*size, tenderness, nodules*

**Genitourinary and Rectal (Female)**

[Lithotomy; inspection or palpation; gloves, lubricant, vaginal speculum, examination stool, exam lamp, guaiac paper (occult blood test kit), tissues]

The medical assistant assists the patient into the lithotomy position. The provider puts on gloves or is assisted into gloves by the medical assistant. The provider usually sits on a stool at the foot of the table, with the light coming over his or her shoulder. First the perineal and anal areas are inspected. Then the speculum, which the medical assistant has warmed in running water, has lubricant applied and is inserted into the vagina to view internal structures. A bimanual examination follows. The provider inserts two fingers of the well-lubricated gloved hand into the vagina and examines internal structures by deep palpation with the other hand, and then the index finger is inserted into the anus to examine the anal and rectal area. A test for occult blood is taken from a small amount of stool on the withdrawn index finger placed on the guaiac test paper. Tissues are used to remove the excess lubricant. Additional tissues are offered to remove any residual lubricant. For information on gynecological exams and collecting a Pap test, refer to Chapter 41.

- Pubis—*lesions, infestation, distribution of hair*
- Labia—*edema, redness, cysts, masses, varicosities*
- Vaginal orifice—*hymen, inflammation, bleeding, discharge, lesions*
- Vagina—*discharge, redness, lesions, mass, cervix*

Bimanual examination by palpation:

- Uterus—*size, masses, symmetry, tenderness, position*
- Ovaries—*size, masses, symmetry, tenderness*
- Anus—*Inspection for hemorrhoids, lesions, fissures, prolapse; palpation: sphincter tone, internal hemorrhoids, masses*

## Extremities

[Recumbent; mensuration and manipulation; tape measure]

The provider sometimes measures different parts of the body; however, the lower extremities are probably the most frequently measured, especially if the patient complains of back problems. It is very common to find one leg slightly longer than the other, but when the difference is too great, the pelvis and back are out of alignment, and muscles, therefore, might react with spasms.

- Leg—*Medial surface is measured bilaterally from the anterior superior iliac spine to the bony prominence of the tibia at the ankle; legs and ankles are assessed for edema.*
- Feet—*Arches, toes, and toenails are examined, and feet are checked for deformities and bunions.*

All extremity joints are observed for range of motion (refer to Chapter 56) by the provider either requesting the patient to move extremities or by passively flexing, extending, and rotating the arms and legs to evaluate the shoulders, hips, elbows, knees, wrists, and ankles. This can be combined with evaluating muscle strength.

## Muscle Strength

Muscle strength is sometimes observed by asking the patient to perform a set of movements that the provider counteracts with resistance. Figure 40–10 shows some examples.

- Fingers—The patient is asked to spread his or her fingers (abduction); then the provider tries to force them together to measures ulnar nerve function.
- Grip—The patient is asked to squeeze the index and middle finger of the provider as the provider tries to remove them to evaluate forearm muscles and condition of the hands.
- Elbow—The patient pushes and pulls against the provider's resistance to check flexion and extension strength of the arms.
- Hip—Flexion of the hip is evaluated by having the patient try to raise his or her leg while the provider pushes down on the thigh.
- Knee—Flexion of the knee is evaluated by having the patient flex the leg with the foot on the table and maintaining the position as the provider tries to straighten the leg.
- Knee—Extension of the knee is evaluated by having the patient try to straighten the leg while the provider holds the leg flexed and exerts pressure at the ankle.
- Ankle—The patient pushes or pulls against the provider's hand to evaluate the plantar flexion and dorsiflexion.

## Reflexes

[Sitting or supine; percussion; percussion hammer]

The provider systematically evaluates *involuntary* reflex action at several locations on the body with the patient in a sitting or lying position. The patient is instructed to relax the muscle. The provider positions the extremity so that the muscle is mildly stretched. Then the partially stretched tendon is tapped sharply to stimulate the sensory nerve endings in the muscle to cause a reaction (Figure 40–11). These tests evaluate the condition of the sensory nerve, the *automatic* synapse in the spinal cord, the motor nerve, and the innervated muscle. The biceps, triceps, patellar, Achilles, and plantar reflexes are checked. The plantar reaction is stimulated by stroking the plantar surface with the handle of the hammer or an object such as a key. Note on the physical exam form in Figure 40–4 the neuro area, the examination of CN II–XII, and the motor and sensory nerves.

## Other Evaluations

In addition to the many examinations already discussed, the physician may include others such as:

1. *Romberg balance test*—Performed to detect any muscle abnormality. The patient stands with feet together and eyes open; if the balance seems all right, the examiner asks the patient to close the eyes. If there is any muscle abnormality, the patient can possibly fall. Assist by standing close enough to help prevent this from happening.

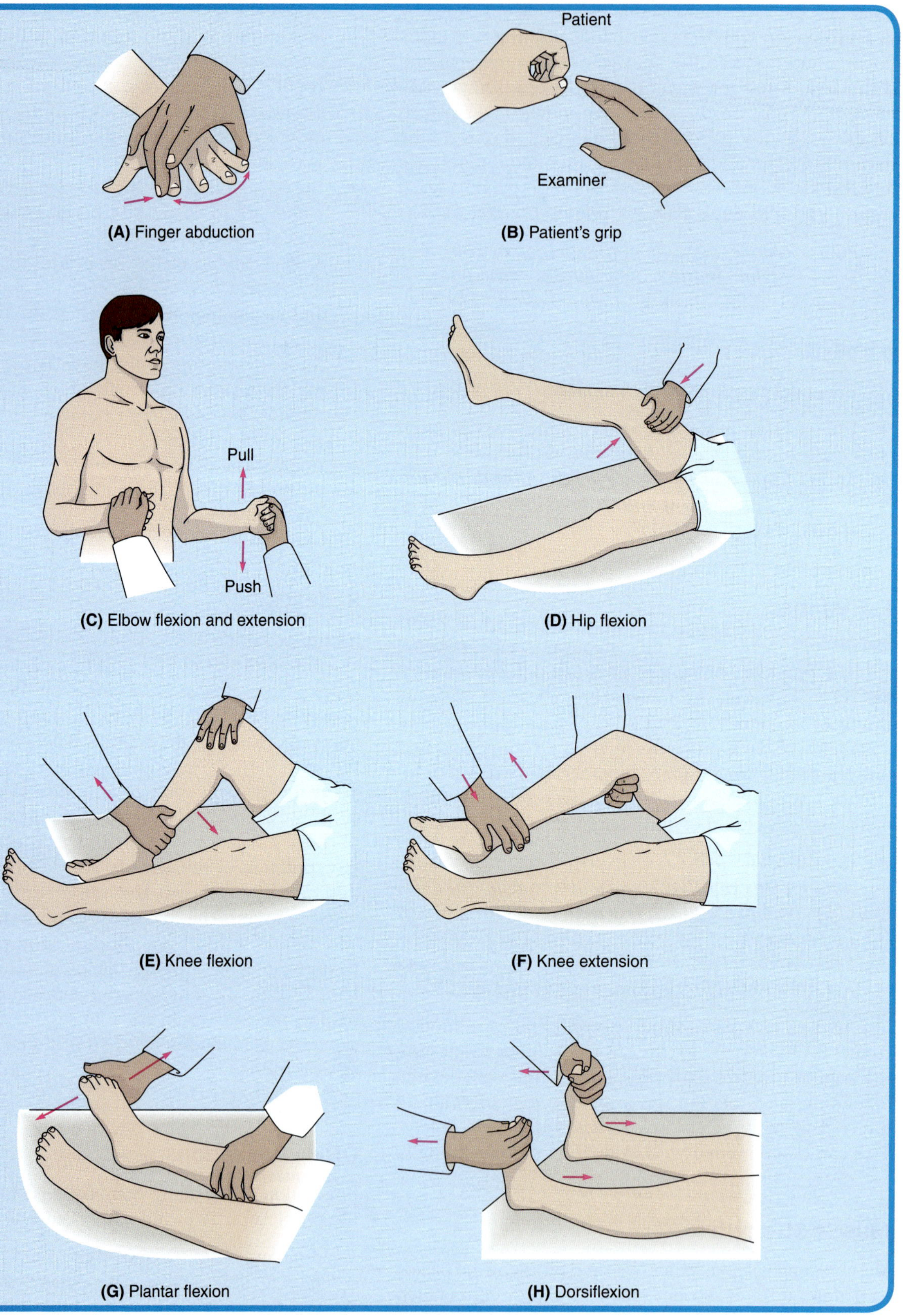


**Figure 40–10:** Testing muscle strength. *Delmar/Cengage Learning.*

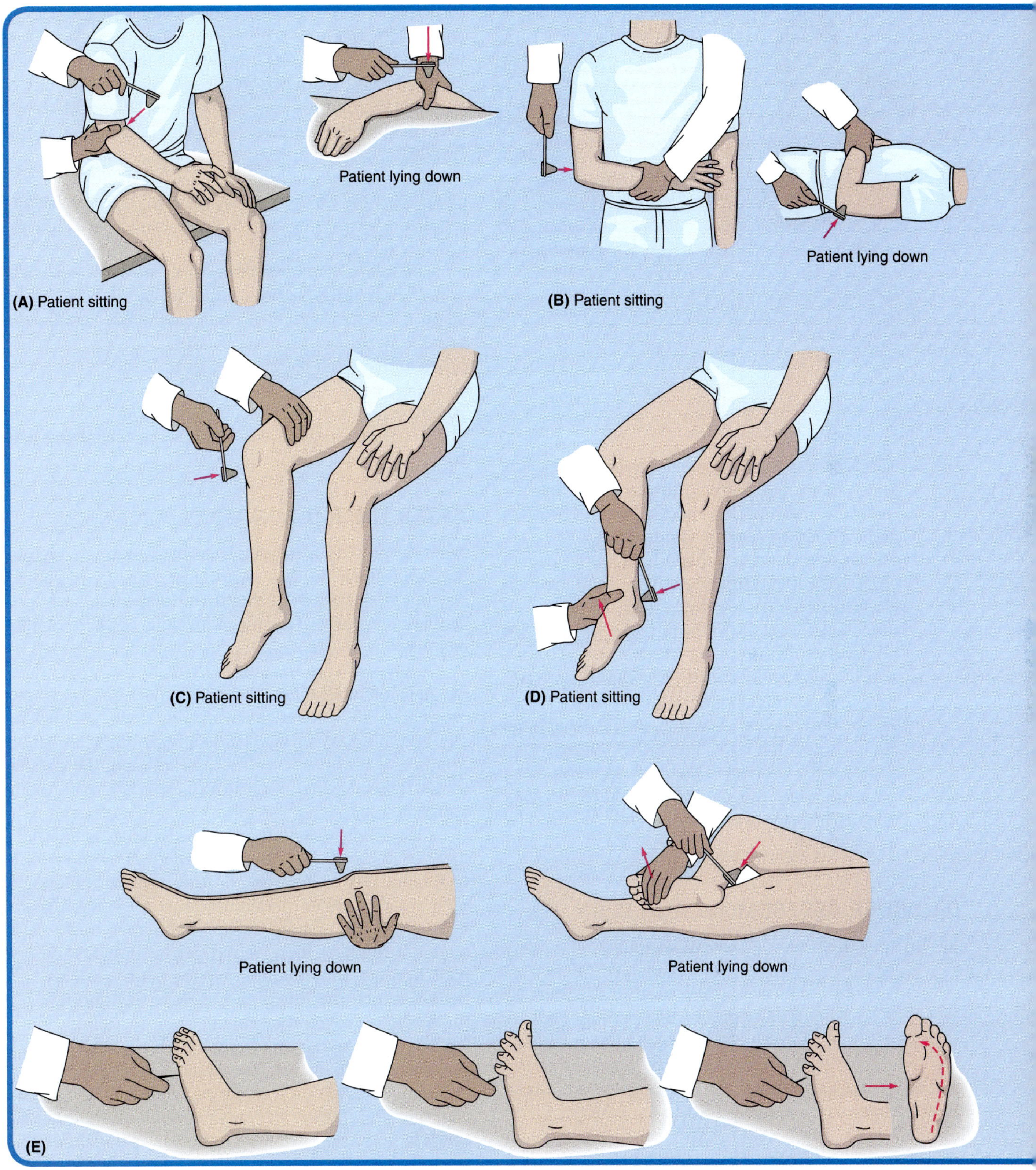


**Figure 40–11:** A percussion hammer is used to test (A) biceps, (B) triceps, (C) patellar, (D) Achilles, and (E) plantar reflexes. *Delmar/ Cengage Learning.*

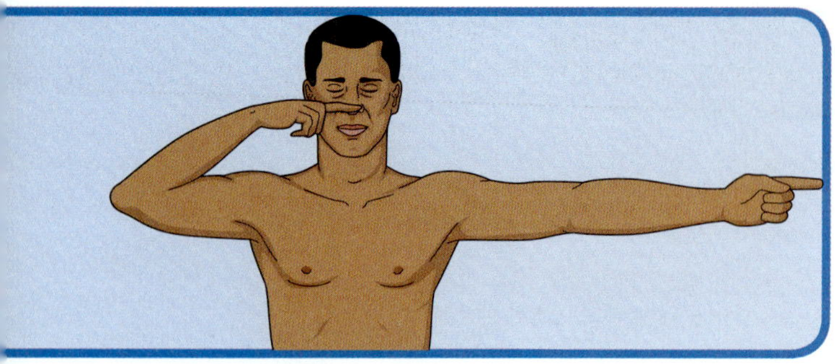

**Figure 40–12:** The provider observes patient coordination as the finger is touched to the nose to determine normal coordination. *Delmar/Cengage Learning.*

2. Other tests for **coordination**, which can include:
   a. The patient sits up, spreads the arms out wide, and touches the fingertip to the nose, first the right and then the left quickly, with eyes open and then closed (Figure 40–12).
   b. The heel-to-shin test is performed by the patient while lying in the supine position: First, the right heel traces the left leg down from the knee, and then the left heel down the right leg; this can also be done while the patient stands.
   c. Alternating motion is a test that can involve tapping the foot or clapping.
   d. The heel-to-toe test of coordination is having the patient touch the right heel to the left great toe and then the left heel to the right great toe; it can be done while the patient is standing or lying down. The patient is observed and evaluated by the examiner.

## PROVIDER ASSESSMENT AND PLAN

In documenting the physical examination, many providers use the Problem Oriented Medical Record (POMR) method, which was discussed in Chapters 13 and 37. Using this system ensures that pertinent data is recorded in logical order (SOAP) on the patient's chart with each visit to the provider. All action taken in the course of the patient's treatment generates additional information that continually adds to the patient's medical record.

The provider makes an *assessment,* or decision, about the patient's condition based on the health history, symptoms, examination findings, and any other procedures and laboratory tests thought necessary to confirm the decision. The provider may use the abbreviation R/O (rule out) to indicate that there is not yet conclusive evidence in the decision concerning a patient's condition or in confirming a diagnosis (e.g., R/O gallbladder disease—awaiting diagnostic X-ray studies).

The provider's *plan* includes *all* measures for management of the care of the patient that are listed, including diet, exercise, physical therapy, medication, surgery, and any others.

Following the completion of the physical examination, the provider provides you with the patient's chart or puts it in a confidential designated area. You should then check the chart for orders to perform any additional procedures for the patient such as ECG, lab tests, scheduling X-rays, or an appointment with a specialist. After you have finished the procedures, you should write your first initial and last name after each one, signifying that you completed the orders.

## AFTER THE EXAMINATION

After the provider has completed the physical examination, you might need to perform or assist in additional screening tests. Some of the testing, screening, and procedures are covered in the remaining sections of this chapter.

Always be sure to help the patient down from the examination table. Often after sitting there for some time, especially if the patient has been lying down, the patient can become dizzy or lightheaded, and a fall is possible. You can also offer the courtesy of assisting the patient to get dressed when appropriate, especially with older adults.

Answer any questions about the follow-up appointment or further studies. Let the patient know how long to expect to wait for reports from the lab, radiology, or other diagnostic procedures. It is a common practice to give the patient an appointment 7 to 10 days after the physical for a report of the findings; others mail a report. Still others phone the patient or have the patient phone the office at a specific day and time. If this is the case, tell the patient when to call and with whom to speak when phoning for the report. Whatever the policy is where you are employed, realize that the patient is usually very concerned about what the physician will find. Letting patients know about their health status as soon as possible in a professional manner will be appreciated.

Procedure 40–1 provides step-by-step instruction for assisting with a general physical examination.

## PROCEDURE 40–1 Prepare a Patient for and Assist with a Routine Physical Examination

**PURPOSE:** To have the patient, the room, and the examination equipment prepared for the physician to complete a physical examination as you assist with the process as needed

**EQUIPMENT:** Gown, drape, stethoscope, ophthalmoscope, otoscope, tongue depressors, sterile gauze squares, tuning fork, nasal speculum, tape measure, percussion hammer, vaginal speculum, guaiac test kit, disposable gloves, lubricant, tissues, towel, Mayo tray, examination stool, exam lamp, regular and biohazardous waste container, patient chart or EMR, and a pen

S **SKILL:** Prepare a patient for and assist with a routine physical exam.

| Procedure Steps | Detailed Instructions and/or *Rationales* |
|---|---|
| 1. Prepare the examination room as in Procedure 39–1. | |
| 2. Review the patient's chart for completed history and the physical examination form. | Have a pen ready if you are to scribe for the physician. |
| 3. Wash hands. | |
| 4. Prepare the examination equipment on the Mayo tray in order of use and cover with a towel. | Place the Mayo tray in a convenient location in the room. |
| 5. Pull out the step from the table. Place a gown and drape on the table. | |
| B 6. Identify the patient, introduce yourself, check the chart, and explain the procedure to the patient, ***using language the patient can understand.*** | *Ensures that you have the correct patient. Ask the patient to follow you to the room. Using appropriate language ensures that the patient understands the examination process.* |
| 7. Measure and record vital signs, height, and weight. | If the physical follows the in-person interview and history, the mensuration would have been completed and recorded. |
| 8. Instruct the patient to go to the bathroom to empty the bladder. | Provide a labeled specimen bottle for a urine sample to be tested later. |
| 9. Instruct the patient to remove clothing and place it on a chair, to put on the gown with the opening in back, to sit at the end of the table, and to cover the legs with the drape. | Evaluate ability to undress and to get onto the table unassisted. Assist the patient as needed, especially the elderly, weak, or disabled. Do not leave disoriented, weak, dizzy, or ill patients alone. Request temporary family assistance if you must leave the room. |
| 10. Ensure that the patient is ready and notify the provider. | |
| 11. Assist the provider as needed with the examination. Position and drape the patient, adjust lights, and hand equipment as appropriate for each body system. | • **General appearance and skin inspection—**When instructed, remove the drape, help the patient from the table for inspecting posterior surface and gait evaluation and assist to sit again.<br>• **Neck—**Stand by.<br>• **HEENT—**If provider requests, turn off lights for pupil and ophthalmoscope evaluation. (If physician desires, hand ophthalmoscope, then otoscope, nasal speculum, tongue blade, gauze squares, and tuning fork.) |

*(continues)*

*(continued)*

| Procedure Steps | Detailed Instructions and/or *Rationales* |
|---|---|
| | • **Chest—**Might need to raise gown<br>• **Heart—**Ensure silence. Might need to raise the gown. Note whether ECG is requested.<br>• **Lungs—**Ensure silence. Might need to raise the gown. Note whether vital capacity is requested.<br>• **Breasts—**Raise gown for sitting exam and then assist the patient to lie back. Expose the breasts and cover with the drape.<br>• **Abdomen—**Raise gown to the breasts and then cover with the drape. Stand away from the side of the table.<br>• **Back—**Provider's preference; may be done while the patient is standing for general inspection. If not, assist the patient to sit and then stand in front of the provider.<br>• **Extremities—**Position the patient in supine position and cover with the drape. Hand tape measure.<br>• **Reflexes—**Position patient in sitting position (most common). Hand percussion hammer.<br>• **Muscle strength—**Begin with sitting patient *and t*hen assist to supine and drape.<br>• **Genitourinary and rectal (female)—**assist the patient into lithotomy position and drape. Assist the provider to glove and then adjust lamp. Warm the speculum; hand when ready. Apply lubricant to a gloved finger. Prepare the guaiac paper. |
| 12. When the exam is completed, allow the patient to relax a moment and then help to sitting position. | |
| 13. Provide tissues to remove excess lubricant and instruct the patient to dress. | |
| 14. Take specimens from the room to the laboratory for testing. | |
| 15. Return to the room, provide patient instructions, and see the patient out. | • Determine whether the patient has any questions.<br>• Provide instructions and schedule any additional procedures requested by the physician.<br>• Provide information for receiving the examination results. |
| 16. Properly clean the room and prepare it for the next patient. | • Put on gloves to wrap up the table paper and dispose of used supplies in appropriate waste containers.<br>• Disinfect table tops, exam lamp, and examination table.<br>• Remove and discard gloves in the appropriate waste container; wash hands. |

| Procedure Steps | Detailed Instructions and/or *Rationales* |
|---|---|
| | • Replace used supplies and cover the table and pillow with clean paper. |
| 17. Give the room a visual check for completeness. | |

**Charting Example**

| | |
|---|---|
| 2-14-XX<br>11:30 am | Patient here for a complete physical today. Refer to physical form for findings.<br>T. EDWARDS, CMA(AAMA) |

## Patient Follow-up

Patients might ask how often they need to have a physical. Some providers recommend annual physicals for their patients, others every two to three years unless a specific or chronic medical problem exists. *The physical exam schedule in Table 40–1 is meant to serve as a guide. The medical needs of patients will vary, as will physicians' recommendations. You will need to check with the provider who employs you because office policies can vary.*

**TABLE 40–1 Physical Examination Frequency**

| Procedure/Screening | Age |
|---|---|
| Hearing | Annually 65 years+, or as necessitated by symptoms |
| Vision | Annually 65 years+, or as necessitated by symptoms<br>Tonometry or funduscopy at 40, then every 4 years |
| Urinalysis | Annually 65 years+, or as necessitated by symptoms |
| Skin for melanoma | Begin at 40, then annually |
| Fecal occult blood test | Begin at 50, then annually |
| Males: Digital rectal exam (DRE) and Prostate Specific Antigen (PSA) | Begin at 50, then annually |
| Sigmoidoscopy (flexible fiber-optic) | Begin at 50, then annually |
| Colonoscopy | Starting at age 50, every 10 years or as directed by provider |
| Pulmonary function tests | As needed for high-risk patients (COPD and smokers) |
| Total blood cholesterol | At age 20, start screening every 5 years or as directed by provider. |
| Thyroid testing | As needed for symptoms; baseline for females at menopause, then every 2 years |
| H and P | 20–39, every 3 years; then annually after 40 |
| Height and weight | Annually 13–65+, then as directed by provider |
| Blood pressure | Annually 13–65+, then as directed by provider if higher than 140/90 |
| Males: testicular self-exam | Monthly (13–65+ as needed for symptoms) or as directed by provider |
| Females: mammogram | Baseline at 40, every 1–2 years, then annually at 50 |
| Breast self-exam | Monthly self performed, 18–39, at least every 3 years; 40+, annually (by provider) |
| Pap test and pelvic exam | Begin no later than age 21. At least every 1–3 years for sexually active women |

## EYE AND EAR EXAMINATIONS

In assisting with eye and ear examinations, you may be expected to hand instruments to the provider as needed. Assembling the instruments in the order of use will be most helpful. You will be responsible for making sure that the instruments are clean and in working order.

Most often, wall-mounted otoscope and ophthalmoscope instruments with electrically powered light sources are used in the medical office (Figure 40–13). Otoscopes and ophthalmoscopes should be checked to be sure the light bulbs are providing strong enough light and changed periodically. If these instruments are the handheld portable type, the batteries must also be changed or charged periodically (Figure 40–17A and B). Cleaning of the scopes after patient use is performed by wiping them down with a gauze pad and disinfectant or disinfectant wipe as discussed in Chapter 39.

You might also be responsible for providing education and assurance to the patient and recording the procedure performed along with documenting the results in the patient's chart or EHR.

### Ear Examinations

Most physicians use a disposable plastic ear speculum to prevent disease transmission. If non-disposable specula are used, they must be sanitized after every use with a mild detergent and sterilized so they can be reused safely to examine another patient. (Refer to Chapter 36 for infection control techniques.) If the patient has an infected ear that has a discharge containing blood, a disposable ear speculum is preferred and protective gloves must be worn.

Sometimes it is difficult for the provider to inspect the patient's ear due to a buildup of **cerumen** (earwax) in the ear. Patients sometimes try to remove it by using a cotton-tipped swab, but this often pushes it farther into the ear canal, where it becomes lodged and hardens. This buildup can become very uncomfortable and eventually impair hearing. The ear may require **irrigation** (also known as **lavage**) to remove the excessive wax. The provider will determine whether the ear needs to be irrigated and direct the medical assistant to perform the procedure. Occasionally, it is necessary to instill a softening solution in the ear to soften ear wax before an irrigation procedure can be performed. Refer to Chapter 52 for the procedure for ear medication instillation.

Patients should have impacted cerumen removed to avoid further discomfort or possible injury to the ear. Many offices have adopted Waterpik® or electronic ear irrigators for this purpose because of the gentle flow produced and convenience for irrigation procedures. A bulb, metal, or plastic syringe may also be used to perform the ear irrigation procedure.

After irrigation procedures are performed, even with gentle care, many patients feel a little dizziness. Be sure that patients are completely stable before permitting them to leave. After the ear wax is removed, the provider will be able to visualize the ear canal to determine whether infection or other conditions are occurring. Perform irrigations of the ear following the steps in Procedure 40–2.

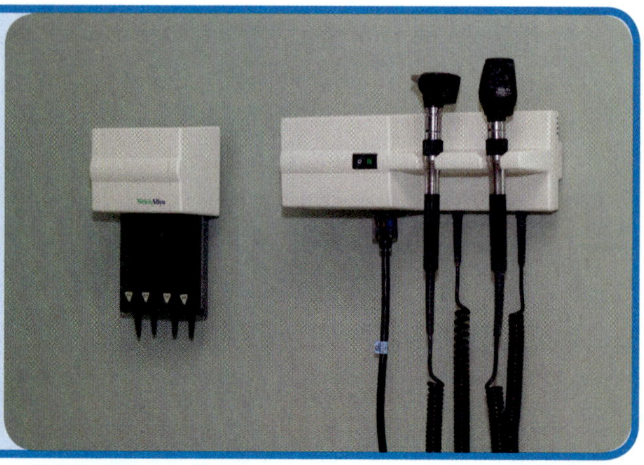

**Figure 40–13:** Wall-mounted set of scopes. *Delmar/Cengage Learning.*

#### PATIENT EDUCATION

1. Advise patients not to put anything into their ears to avoid damaging the tympanic membrane. Cerumen is produced to protect and moisten the membrane of the ear canal. Many people feel that they must completely remove this daily with a swab, which often results in it being packed down into the ear canal, where it hardens. Impacted cerumen must be removed by a health care professional.
2. Instruct patients that ear drops and other ear medications should be used only with the advice of their provider. Earache, pain, or discharge should be reported to and examined by the provider as soon as possible.
3. Discuss the possibility of permanent hearing loss with patients who work around extremely loud noise or who listen to audio systems, radios, or TVs with the volume up high. Suggest to these patients to wear protective ear coverings or ear plugs and turn down the volume on audio systems to avoid nerve damage.
4. Urge patients to have regular hearing tests to detect loss of hearing or other related problems. It is recommended this to be done annually, unless otherwise instructed by the provider, if there is a noticeable difference or problem with hearing. If there is a history of ear infections, the patient should have periodic hearing tests.

## PROCEDURE 40–2 Irrigate the Ear

**PURPOSE:** To irrigate the ear canal to remove foreign objects, impacted cerumen, or drainage

**EQUIPMENT:** Gloves, small basin, ordered lukewarm irrigation solution, towel, ear basin, syringe, gauze squares, otoscope, ear speculum, tissues, patient chart or EMR, and a pen

S **SKILL:** Perform ear irrigation.

| Procedure Steps | Detailed Instructions and/or *Rationales* |
|---|---|
| 1. Wash hands. Prepare the solution as ordered and assemble the necessary items for the procedure. | The solution is usually between 99°F and 100°F for patient comfort. |
| B 2. Identify the patient, introduce yourself, and explain the procedure, ***using language the patient can understand.*** | This *ensures* that *you are performing the procedure on the correct patient.* |
| 3. Assist the patient onto the examination table or to a chair. | |
| 4. Put on gloves. | |
| 5. View the affected ear with an otoscope to see where cerumen or the foreign object is located so that the flow of solution can be directed properly. | The flow should be directed upward and to one side. To use the otoscope, place one hand gently against the patient's head, and grasp the auricle with your thumb and index finger, pulling up and back for adults and older children and down and back for infants up to 36 months. Avoid using too much pressure as you insert the speculum into the ear canal. |
| 6. Ask the patient to turn his or her head to the affected side and toward the back. Place a towel over the patient's shoulder to protect his or her clothing. | For pediatric patients, ask a parent to hold the child on his or her lap and assist you during the procedure. |
| 7. Position the ear basin under the ear for the patient to hold to catch the solution. | |
| 8. Use a gauze square to wipe away any particles from the outer ear before proceeding. | |
| 9. Fill the syringe with the ordered solution. | |
| 10. With one hand, gently pull the auricle up and back for an adult (or down and back for an infant or small child) (Figure 40–14A–B). With the other hand, place the tip of the syringe into the canal and aim the flow of solution upward so the entire ear canal will be irrigated.<br>11. Use gauze squares to wipe the excess solution from the outside of the patient's ear. | *Pulling the auricle straightens the ear canal.* DO NOT direct the flow of the solution straight into the ear or use force, or the result will be quite painful for the patient and may damage the tympanic membrane. |
| 12. Give the patient several gauze squares or tissues and have the patient tilt his or her head to the side to allow drainage of excess solution from the canal. | All material must be removed to inspect the ear canal and tympanic membrane adequately. Patients sometimes feel a little dizzy following this procedure. Allow the patient time to gain balance; assist the patient from the examination table or call the provider to examine. |
| 13. Inspect the ear canal with an otoscope to determine whether the desired results have been obtained. Repeat irrigation if necessary. | |

*(continues)*

*(continued)*

| Procedure Steps | Detailed Instructions and/or *Rationales* |
|---|---|
| 14. Record the procedure on the patient's chart. | Include which ear was irrigated, the solution used, the results of the procedure, and any other important observations. |
| 15. Wash equipment and return it to the proper storage area. | |
| 16. Remove gloves and wash hands. | |

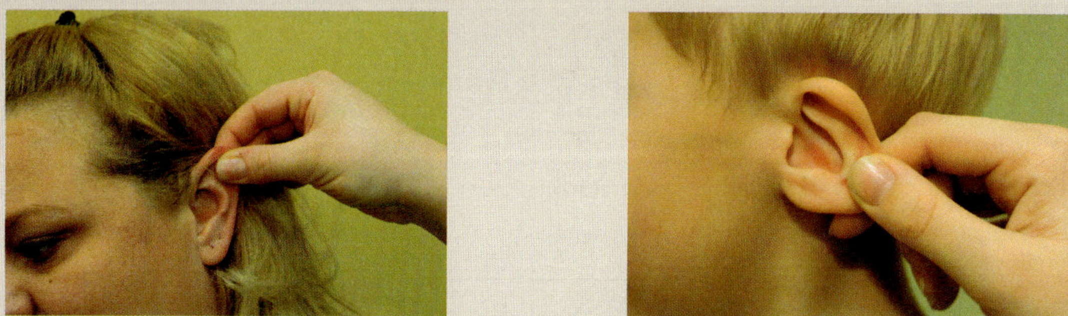

**Figure 40–14:** (A) Positioning the ear up and back for an adult. (B) Positioning the ear down and back for a child. *Delmar/Cengage Learning.*

### Charting Example

| | |
|---|---|
| 5-20-XX<br>11:30 am | Irrigated pt's right ear with water @ 100°F, per Dr. Long; returned three pieces of cerumen (1.25 cm each). Eardrum is shiny with a pearl-gray color. T. Edwards, CMA(AAMA) |

## Auditory Acuity

The function of the ear is to enable sound to be perceived. If this process is impaired, hearing loss results. Diseases or conditions of the ear, if not treated, can cause damage to nerves and tissues, which can result in mild to profound deafness.

Sometimes an auditory problem may be as simple as the patient having impacted cerumen, and after irrigation, the person's hearing returns to normal. Other times, further measures are necessary. One of your most important duties is relaying important information observed to the provider about patients. Often, it is a family member who makes the appointment for a patient with an obvious hearing problem. You can watch for any behaviors as you have contact with the patient or when you talk to him or her over the phone.

Common behaviors of patients that indicate the loss of hearing ability are:

- Frequently asking to repeat what was said during conversation.
- Talking in an inappropriately loud voice.
- Not responding when spoken to if out of sight range.
- Not pronouncing words well.
- Responding only when you speak very loudly.

Certain complaints can suggest hearing loss or auditory nerve damage. When patients disclose any of the following symptoms, you should bring it to the attention of the provider for further assessment:

- Ringing in the ears
- Decreased hearing in one ear (or both), sometimes caused by impacted cerumen
- Infection or injury to the ear
- Bleeding or discharge from the ear(s)
- Any unusual noise or feeling inside the ears

These signs and any others that patients tell you should be documented in the chart during in-person screening. Further examination by the provider is necessary to determine the extent of the problem and its treatment.

**CLINICAL PEARL**

Some patients might try to hide hearing loss if they perceive it to be embarrassing or are afraid they might have to wear a hearing aid or undergo surgery. A patient may try to compensate for the hearing loss by:

- Learning to read lips
- Turning the best ear toward the sound source
- Pretending that he or she heard
- Increasingly turning up the volume on audio equipment
- Standing very close during conversation
- Sometimes withdrawing

If family members of the patient relate this information to you, advise the person to have the patient schedule a time to have a provider examine the ears and have a hearing test. Note the information on the patient's chart and bring it to the provider's attention. The provider will discuss the problem with the patient during the scheduled appointment.

## Hearing Assessment

Providers use several audiometric assessment procedures to determine the cause of the patient's hearing loss, some of which are a part of the complete or routine physical examination.

An **audiometer** is an instrument that measures one's hearing; it determines the hearing thresholds of pure tones of frequencies that are normally audible by an individual. Tone frequency refers to the sound vibrations per second; tone intensity refers to the loudness. Some also measure bone and air conduction. The threshold of hearing is the point at which a sound can barely be heard. Figure 40–15 illustrates the **decibels** of common environmental noise levels. The audiometer is cleaned after patient use by wiping the unit down with disinfectant wipes or a disinfectant cleaner and gauze squares.

Audiometric devices are powered by either batteries or electricity. The devices should be checked periodically for proper performance and accuracy. If the batteries need to be changed or if a wire is frayed, it should be taken care of before being used with patients, not only for their safety but to make sure that it works efficiently. Several types of audiometers are available for use in determining hearing acuity. Many are still used that require the operator to turn a dial manually to emit the various frequencies for the patient to hear during the test. Companies that manufacture audiometers offer in-service demonstrations to make sure their equipment is used properly. Operational manuals should be kept with the instrument for handy reference.

The procedure for most audiometers is basically the same. The patient is instructed to place the earphones (marked red for the right ear and blue for the left ear) over the ears. The medical assistant tells the patient how the earphones are to be placed and how to work the

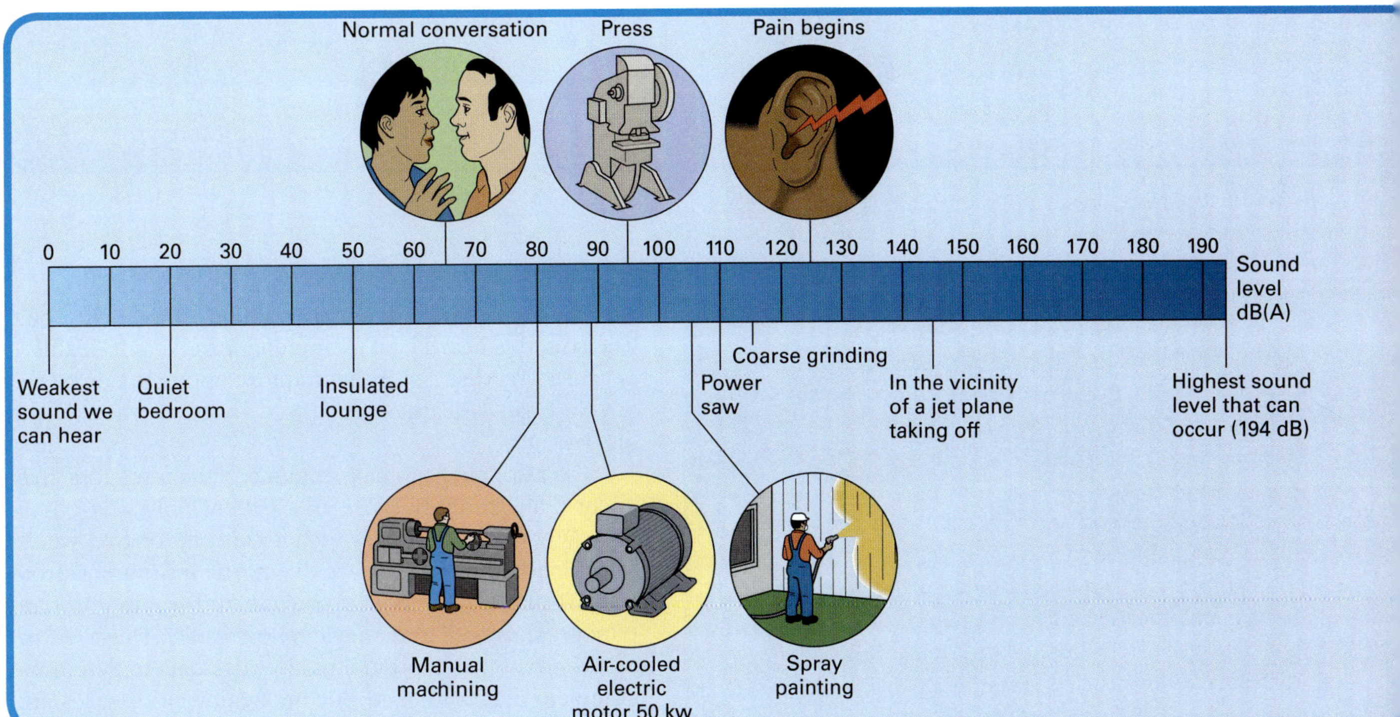


**Figure 40–15:** Noise levels associated with selected environments and machinery. *Delmar/Cengage Learning.*

control signal. The printer records the results of the hearing test or, if not an automatic machine, you might need to fill out the form manually with the patient's responses. The printout is called an audiogram and is filed in the patient's chart after the provider reads the results of the test and makes an evaluation.

During the procedure, the machine tests one ear at a time. In the ear that is being tested, the machine provides a series of tones. The sound is automatically blocked in the ear that is not being tested. The patient listens and signals (either by raising a finger or by using a handheld control) as the various sounds are heard. The tones range in frequencies from very low to very high with a varied level of decibel intensity. After the right ear has been tested, the machine switches automatically to test the left ear. Report any complaints the patient may have and any unusual behavior before or during the hearing test to the provider and in the patient's chart, along with the results of the test, and place your initials indicating that you have completed the test.

Tympanometry is a procedure that determines the ability of the middle ear to transmit sound waves and is commonly performed on children to diagnose middle ear infections. A probe is inserted into the ear canal to measure the air pressure of the ear canal in relation to the air pressure found in the middle ear.

During the physical examination, the provider will use a tuning fork to test the patient's hearing. A two-pronged metal tuning fork is used, its frequency varying with the size of the instrument. The common tests done are the Rinne and the Weber (Figure 40–16A–C).

In the Rinne test, the examiner strikes the fork and then holds the shank (stem) against the patient's mastoid bone until the patient no longer hears the sound; this is performed to assess nerve or conduction deafness (Figure 40–16A). The prongs of the tuning fork are then placed about 1 inch from the auditory meatus (opening to the ear) and then next to it (Figure 40–16B). In a normal ear, the sound is heard about twice as long by air conduction as by bone conduction. If hearing by bone conduction is greater, the result is spoken of as a negative Rinne.

In the Weber test, the vibrating tuning fork is held against the **vertex** (crown of the head) or against the skull or forehead in the midline (Figure 40–16C). The sound is heard best by the unaffected ear if deafness is caused by disease of the auditory apparatus or by the affected ear if deafness is caused by obstruction of the air passages.

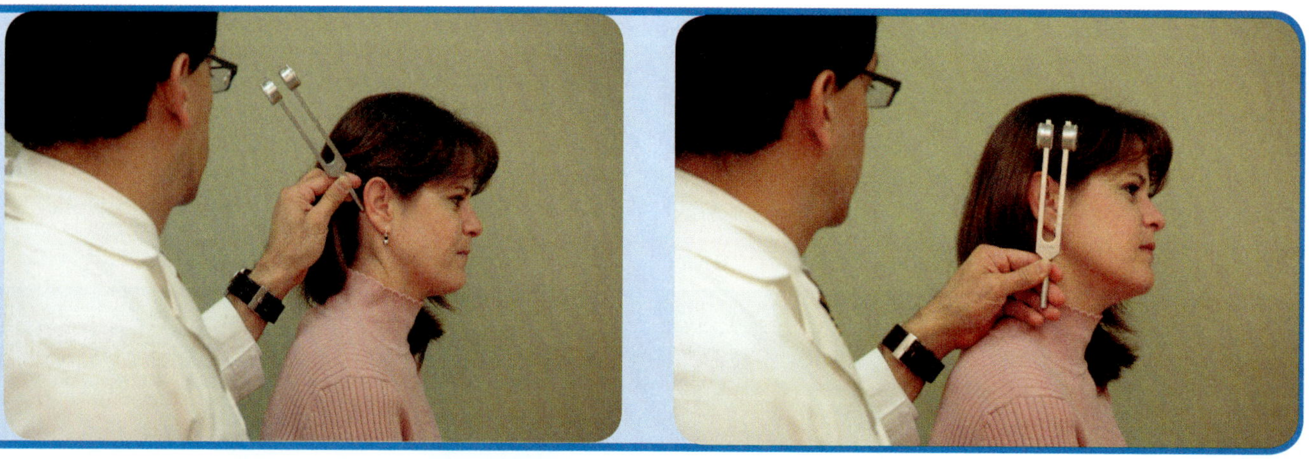

**Figure 40–16A and B:** Rinne test. *Delmar/Cengage Learning.*

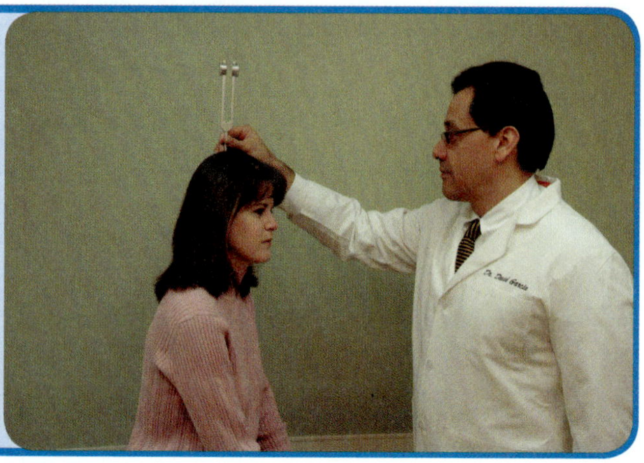

**Figure 40–16C:** Weber test. *Delmar/Cengage Learning.*

Occasionally, a small amount of hearing loss may occur temporarily because of a patient's physical condition. When this occurs, a recheck in one or two weeks may be advisable. There are diagnostic instruments from various manufacturers that provide audiogram and tympanogram as well as acoustic reflex results. These instruments are useful in providing objective data to determine complete diagnoses and documentation of diseases and disorders of the ear as well as evaluation of follow-up treatment.

## Eye Examinations

For examinations of the eye, the provider uses an ophthalmoscope, an instrument used to examine the internal structures of the eye. Visual examinations can be performed if a patient has an eye infection or injury or needs additional screening to check vision acuity or color vision. Often, the screenings are performed prior to the provider's examination so the results can be discussed during the physical exam. The provider will advise you to do this, depending upon his or her preference.

Occasionally, the eye may need to be irrigated if there is inflammation, secretions in the eye due to infection, a chemical contamination, or a foreign particle in the eye. Your role may be to perform the irrigation. Eyes that have come in contact with a chemical are usually flushed with plain water using an eyewash station, whereas other flushing may be performed with a rubber bulb syringe or Waterpik. For these types of irrigations, a sterile saline solution is used.

Patients should be instructed to lie on their side with their face turned to the side of the eye being irrigated. A basin will be placed under the eye to catch the solution. A water-absorbent pad may also be placed under the patient. The eye should be flushed from the inner canthus or corner of the eye to the outer canthus to prevent any debris being removed from reentering the eye. Procedure 40–3 lists the steps on how to perform eye irrigation.

### PATIENT EDUCATION

1. While performing procedures involving the eye, the medical assistant may want to remind patients to use eye protection when indicated, such as the use of safety glasses or goggles when working with tools that could cause particles of material to fly into the eye and cause injury.
2. Remind patients to wear protective sunglasses when out in direct sunlight for extended periods.
3. Remind patients to have routine eye examinations, especially when the family medical history includes glaucoma, cataracts, or diabetes. **Tonometry** and **funduscopy** are recommended every four years for patients past 40 years old.
4. Explain to patients that over-the-counter eye drops should be used carefully and only as directed because extended use can cause tissue damage. Used only when necessary and with the advice of the provider.
5. Advise patients not to rub their eyes because further irritation and possibly tissue damage could result. Itching, burning, or watering eyes can be signs of infection. Rubbing the eyes can transmit the infection to others.
6. In the event of a chemical splash in the eye, patients should flush the eye with clear, room temperature water for 20 minutes (nonstop) and seek medical attention immediately.

## PROCEDURE 40–3 Irrigate the Eye

**PURPOSE:** To irrigate the patient's eye(s) to soothe tissues, relieve inflammation, and remove foreign objects and discharge

**EQUIPMENT:** Gloves, small basin of lukewarm irrigation solution, towel, emesis basin, irrigation syringe or bottle of solution, gauze squares, patient chart or EMR, and a pen

S **SKILL:** Perform eye irrigation.

| | Procedure Steps | Detailed Instructions and/or *Rationales* |
|---|---|---|
| | 1. Wash hands. Assemble the items needed for the procedure; prepare lukewarm solution. | |
| B | 2. Identify the patient, introduce yourself, and explain the procedure, ***using language that the patient can understand.*** | *Ensures that you are performing the procedure on the correct patient.* |
| B | 3. ***Ask the patient which position would be more comfortable, sitting or lying down.*** Drape the patient with a towel to protect clothing. | Assist onto the examination table if desired. |

*(continues)*

*(continued)*

| Procedure Steps | Detailed Instructions and/or *Rationales* |
|---|---|
| 4. Put on gloves. | |
| 5. Ask patient to tilt his or her head back and to the side. Place the emesis basin against the head. Instruct patient to hold the basin to catch the solution during irrigation (Figure 40–17). | Placing several tissues, gauze squares, or a towel between the face and the basin will help prevent the patient from getting wet during the procedure. You might have to hold the basin yourself. |
| 6. Gently wipe eye with gauze square from the inner to outer canthus to remove any particles before proceeding with irrigation. | |
| 7. Fill syringe with ordered solution. | |
| 8. Hold the affected eye open with the thumb and index finger and slowly release the solution over the eye gently and steadily. | This must be done from inner canthus to outer canthus *to prevent any solution from entering the other eye, which may not be affected, and for ease of catching solution.* |
| 9. When irrigation is completed, use gauze squares or tissues to blot the area dry. | |
| 10. Record the procedure in the patient's chart. | Record the type of solution that was used, which eye was irrigated, results, and any other important information you may have observed while performing the procedure. |
| 11. Wash the items and return them to the proper storage area. | |
| 12. Remove gloves and wash hands. | Deposit gloves in an appropriate container based upon the conditions under which irrigation was performed. |

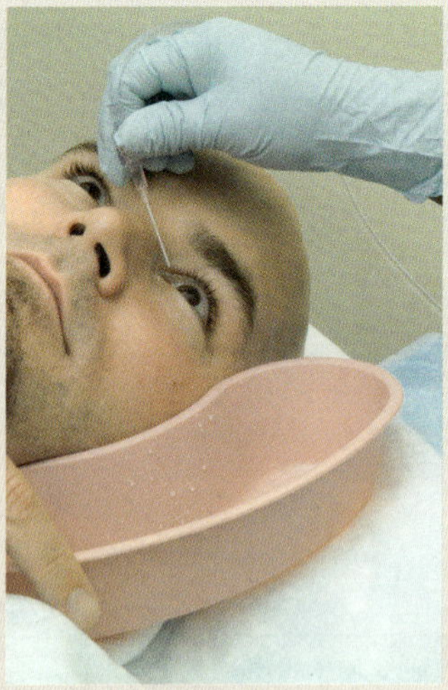

**Figure 40–17:** Irrigating the eye. *Delmar/Cengage Learning.*

## Charting Example

| | |
|---|---|
| 3-30-XX<br>11:30 am | Right eye irrigated w/ $H_2O$ to remove sand, per Dr. White; tolerated well. Pt. states, "eyes less scratchy."<br>T. EDWARDS, CMA(AAMA) |

## Visual Acuity

Measuring visual **acuity** is a diagnostic screening procedure most often done by the medical assistant on the patient's initial visit, prior to the physical examination. It should be performed in a well-lighted area with no interruptions. Observation of the patient for any conditions or behaviors that may indicate visual disturbances is an essential part of the overall examination.

The following are examples of what to look for when performing visual acuity tests:

- Tilting the head to the side or forward
- Blinking or watering of the eyes
- Frowning or puckering of the face
- Closing of one eye when testing both eyes
- Any sign of straining to see

The most common screening device for *distance* vision is a **Snellen chart**, which shows at what distance the chart can be read by the patient. The regular chart has letters arranged in rows from largest to smallest. Those who might have difficulty with reading or are non-English speakers should be tested with the chart or cards of the letter *E* arranged in different directions. The patients are directed to use their hand, particularly the three middle fingers to show the direction the E is facing. Figure 40–18 shows two Snellen vision screening charts, which are made to standard specifications. These charts are hung on the wall with a mark 20 feet away to show where the patient should stand or sit to read the chart. The chart should be at the patient's eye level. The patient covers one eye with an **occluder** so each eye may be tested individually.

Distance visual acuity is written as a fraction. The numerator is the number of feet, or the distance from the chart; the denominator is the numbered line the patient can read. If one's distant visual acuity results are 20/100, it means that the person stood 20 feet from the chart and read the line that should be read at 100 feet. One who has 20/10 acuity can see at 20 feet what should be seen at a distance of 10 feet. A finding of 20/20 is average. Patients should be screened with and without their corrective lenses and the results recorded as such on their charts. Note that if visual acuity is 20/200 or less in the better eye with corrective lenses, the patient is considered legally blind.

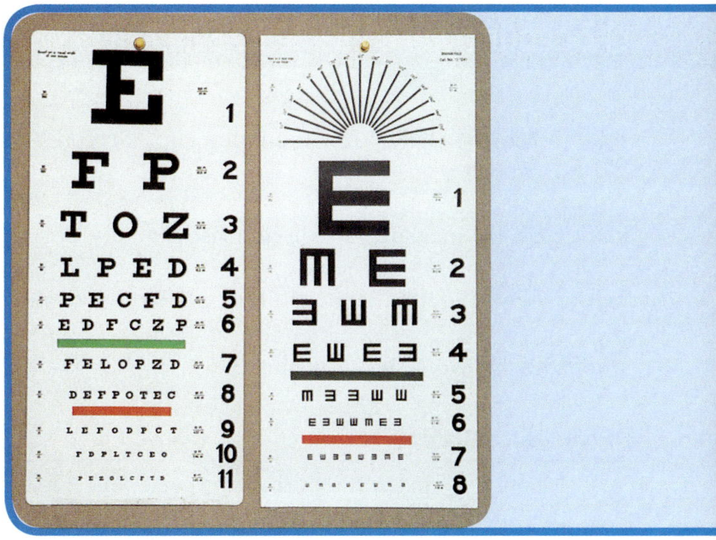


**Figure 40–18:** Snellen visual acuity screening charts. *Delmar/Cengage Learning.*

Common complaints that can indicate vision problems are listed in Table 40–2. These complaints pertain to both children and adults. Perform Procedure 40–4 to measure distance vision.

**TABLE 40–2 Possible Indications of Visual Disturbance**

| During Activities That Require Reading | Conditions | Behaviors | Complaints |
|---|---|---|---|
| 1. Exhibits difficulty with near or distance vision | 1. Redness of the eye(s) or eyelid(s) | 1. Looks cross-eyed | 1. Blurriness of vision |
| 2. Avoids reading, writing, and related activities | 2. Sties or crusting or swelling of eyelid(s) | 2. Rubbing eyes frequently | 2. Nausea |
| | 3. Poor eye coordination | 3. Confuses letters (e.g., *a* and *c*, *f* and *t*, *m* and *n*) | 3. Headaches often |
| | 4. Watering or discharge | 4. Turns head or leans forward to see better | 4. Dizziness |
| | 5. Accident or injury to the eye | 5. Blinks continually | 5. Eyes sensitive to light |
| | | 6. Irritable at attempting close work | 6. Feels like something in the eye(s) |

## PROCEDURE 40–4 Screen Visual Acuity with a Snellen Chart

**MEDIA LINK:** View the video clip, "Screen Visual Acuity," on the Premium Website.

**PURPOSE:** To measure the distant visual acuity of a patient

**EQUIPMENT:** Snellen chart, pointer, ocular eye occluder, patient chart or EMR, and a pen

**S SKILL:** Measure distant vision acuity with a Snellen chart.

| Procedure Steps | Detailed Instructions and/or *Rationales* |
|---|---|
| **B** 1. Identify the patient, introduce yourself, and explain the procedure, ***using language that the patient can understand.*** | *Ensures* that *you are performing the procedure on the correct patient.* The patient is to read each line from the chart as you point to it with a pointer. Tell the patient to keep both eyes open when covering one eye. This prevents squinting and blurring. |
| 2. Ask the patient to read the chart with both eyes (OU) first, standing 20 feet from the chart. | The chart should be at the patient's eye level. Follow office policy in giving the test. Asking patients to read only certain lines of the chart may be less time consuming (e.g., "Begin at line 6."). |
| 3. To test acuity of the right eye, have the patient cover the left eye with an occluder. | If patient wears corrective lenses, the procedure should be performed first wearing lenses and then without and recorded as such. |
| 4. Record the smallest line the patient can read without making a mistake. | Some physicians allow up to two errors on the smallest line read. Record any observations of individual accommodations made to read chart, such as squinting or turning the head. |
| 5. Have the patient cover his or her right eye and test acuity of the left, following the same procedure. | |
| 6. Record the number of the smallest line the patient can read. | |

### Charting Example

| | |
|---|---|
| 2-14-XX<br>11:30 am | Snellen findings: Vision screening per Dr. White, right eye 25/30, left eye 20/40, no squinting observed.<br>T. EDWARDS, CMA(AAMA) |

The **Jaeger chart** is a common method of screening for **near** vision acuity. The screening procedure should be conducted in a well-lighted room without interruptions. The patient should be tested with and without wearing corrective lenses, and each eye is tested separately for a complete assessment to be made by the provider. The chart used for this procedure is a card held by the patient between 14 and 16 inches from the eye (measure with a yardstick, a meterstick, or a tape measure for accuracy). This is the distance at which one with normal vision is able to read printed material (a magazine) or work on something that requires close attention (sewing). The Jaeger screening test consists of reading material that has ascending sizes of type ranging from 0.37 mm to 2.5 mm (Figure 40–19). The test contains excerpts from a manuscript sectioned into short paragraphs, none of which are the same. Observe the patient for any difficulty (e.g., holding the

**No. 1.**
.37M

In the second century of the Christian era, the empire of Rome comprehended the fairest part of the earth, and the most civilized portion of mankind. The frontiers of that extensive monarchy were guarded by ancient renown and disciplined valor. The gentle but powerful influence of laws and manners had gradually cemented the union of the provinces. Their peaceful inhabitants enjoyed and abused the advantages of wealth.

**No. 2.**
.50M

fourscore years, the public administration was conducted by the virtue and abilities of Nerva, Trajan, Hadrian, and the two Antonines. It is the design of this, and of the two succeeding chapters, to describe the prosperous condition of their empire; and afterwards, from the death of Marcus Antoninus, to deduce the most important circumstances of its decline and fall; a revolution which will ever be remembered, and is still felt by

**No. 3.**
.62M

the nations of the earth. The principal conquests of the Romans were achieved under the republic; and the emperors, for the most part, were satisfied with preserving those dominions which had been acquired by the policy of the senate, the active emulations of the consuls, and the martial enthusiasm of the people. The seven first centuries were filled with a rapid succession of triumphs; but it was

**No. 4.**
.75M

reserved for Augustus to relinquish the ambitious design of subduing the whole earth, and to introduce a spirit of moderation into the public councils. Inclined to peace by his temper and situation, it was very easy for him to discover that Rome, in her present exalted situation, had much less to hope than to fear from the chance of arms; and that, in the prosecution of

**No. 5.**
1.00M

the undertaking became every day more difficult, the event more doubtful, and the possession more precarious, and less beneficial. The experience of Augustus added weight to these salutary reflections, and effectually convinced him that, by the prudent vigor of

**No. 6.**
1.25M

his counsels, it would be easy to secure every concession which the safety or the dignity of Rome might require from the most formidable barbarians. Instead of exposing his person or his legions to the arrows of the Parthinians, he obtained, by an honor-

**No. 7.**
1.50M

able treaty, the restitution of the standards and prisoners which had been taken in the defeat of Crassus. His generals, in the early part of his reign, attempted the reduction of Ethiopia and Arabia Felix. They marched near a thou-

**No. 8.**
1.75M

sand miles to the south of the tropic; but the heat of the climate soon repelled the invaders, and protected the unwarlike natives of those sequestered regions

**No. 9.**
2.00M

The northern countries of Europe scarcely deserved the expense and labor of conquest. The forests and morasses of Germany were

**No. 10.**
2.25M

filled with a hardy race of barbarians who despised life when it was separated from freedom; and though, on the first

**No. 11.**
2.50M

attack, they seemed to yield to the weight of the Roman power, they soon, by a signal

**Figure 40–19:** Example of a Jaeger chart. *Delmar/Cengage Learning.*

chart right in front of the face, squinting, or blinking) while trying to read the card. You then record the section number that the patient can read easily. Refer to Procedure 40–5.

Electronic devices that screen both near and distance visual acuity are also available. Some products are capable of fully automating the screening process and generating a final results report.

## PROCEDURE 40–5 Screen Visual Acuity with the Jaeger System

**PURPOSE:** To determine near distance visual acuity of a patient by using the Jaeger system

**EQUIPMENT:** Jaeger near vision acuity chart, patient chart or EMR, and a pen

S **SKILL:** Measure near vision acuity with a Jaeger chart.

| Procedure Steps | Detailed Instructions and/or *Rationales* |
|---|---|
| B 1. Identify the patient, introduce yourself, and explain the procedure, ***using language that the patient can understand.*** | *Ensures that you are performing the procedure on the correct patient.* |
| 2. Have the patient sit up straight but comfortably in a well-lighted area. | |

*(continues)*

*(continued)*

| Procedure Steps | Detailed Instructions and/or *Rationales* |
|---|---|
| 3. Hand the Jaeger chart to the patient to hold, between 14 inches and 16 inches from the eyes. | Figure 40–20 shows proper positioning of the card. |
| 4. Instruct the patient to read (out loud to you) the various paragraphs of the card with both eyes open, first without wearing corrective lenses and then with. | Each eye should be tested individually having the person cover the left eye first while reading the card and then the right. Observe carefully for any difficulty the patient has in reading any of the lines on the card. Listen also to any remarks made by the patient and note them on the chart. |
| 5. Record the results and problems, if any, on the patient's chart to assist the provider in determining the visual acuity of the patient. | The smallest line of print that the patient can read should be recorded and initialed. |
| 6. Thank the patient for cooperation and answer any questions. | |
| 7. Return the Jaeger chart to proper storage. | |

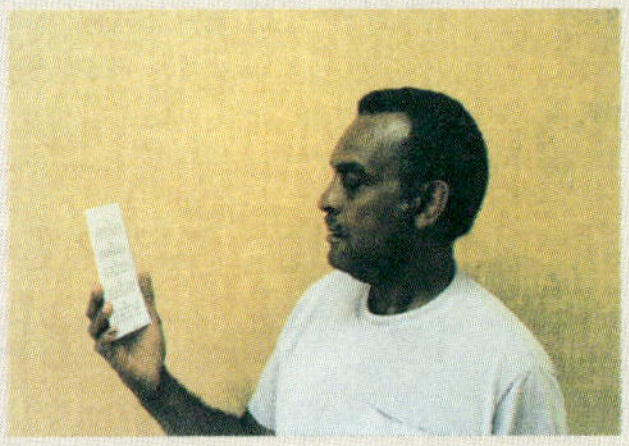

**Figure 40–20:** Proper distance for near visual acuity screening. *Delmar/Cengage Learning.*

### Charting Example

| | |
|---|---|
| 8-17-XX 11:30 am | Screened vision w/Jaeger per Dr. White; read No 3 (62M) both eyes w/corrective lenses; No 11 (2.5) right eye (squinting); No 10 (2.2) left eye. T. EDWARDS, CMA(AAMA) |

*Color vision* acuity means that one can accurately recognize colors. The inability to perceive colors of the spectrum distinctly is commonly termed *color blindness* or the technically correct and preferred term, *color deficient*. This is caused by changes that happen in the pigments of the cones in the retina of the eyes as they react to red, green, and blue light wavelengths.

There are two primary types of color deficiency: daltonism and achromatic vision. Daltonism, which is the most common, is a hereditary visual disorder in which the person cannot tell the difference between red and green. Achromatic vision is total color blindness (the person cannot recognize any color at all) and is very rare. These people see everything in white, gray, and black. The probable cause for this condition is defective cones in the retina or complete absence of them.

Several other conditions involve one's inability or weakness in distinguishing certain colors. In deuteranopia, a person has trouble telling any difference between varying shades of green and of bluish reds and neutral shades. Protanopia is partial color blindness. These people have trouble with the perception of reds, and sometimes yellows and greens are confused. This condition is often referred to as red blindness. Tritanopia, which is the rarest, means that the person cannot distinguish blue color.

Although electronic devices are available for screening color vision, the most common method for screening patients for defects in distinguishing color vision acuity is with an **Ishihara** color plates book. A sample of the series of multicolored charts in the test book is shown in Figure 40–21. In these pictures of the color plates, a person with normal color vision acuity can see a pink-red number 8 against a blue-green background and a blue-green number 5 against a pink-red background.

Patients may be asked to trace the patterns of color with a cotton swab as you observe them. Instruct the patients not to use their fingers for the tracing because the oil on their skin can discolor the plates. There are letters

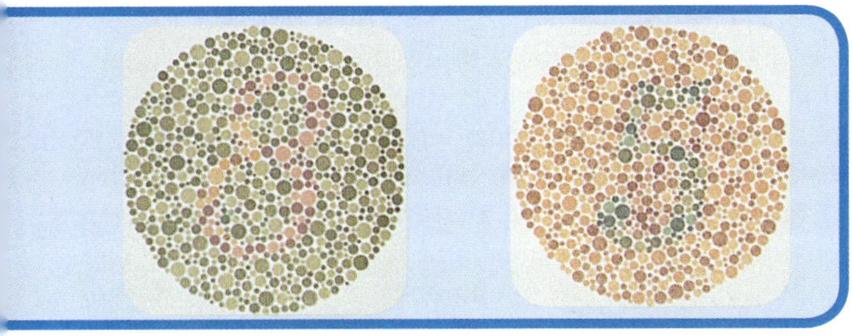

**Figure 40–21:** Sample of Ishihara color plates. *Delmar/Cengage Learning.*

and numbers (and curved lines and shapes for nonreaders) that are one color within another. When administering this procedure, make sure that the room is well-lit, preferably with natural daylight (not direct sunlight), so that the patient is able to follow your instructions without straining to see. Whatever method of color vision assessment is used where you are employed, it is vital for you to be accurate in reporting the results. You need to have your own eyes tested first to determine whether they have normal color vision before administering the test to patients. Perform Procedure 40–6 to measure color vision acuity.

Patients with thyroid conditions should be routinely screened for color vision acuity during scheduled visits. The procedure should include testing with both eyes first and then each eye separately to see whether there is any difference in the perception of color in either eye. The eye not used should be covered with an occluder and not held shut. Grave's disease patients especially need frequent assessment of their color vision acuity changes. The color vision test results may lead to earlier diagnosis and treatment of Grave's ophthalmopathy.

## PROCEDURE 40–6 Determine Color Vision Acuity by the Ishihara Method

**MEDIA LINK:** View the video, "Color Vision Acuity," for this chapter on the Premium Website.

**PURPOSE:** To determine color vision acuity of a patient by using the Ishihara method

**EQUIPMENT:** Ishihara book, proper lighting, occluder, patient chart or EMR, and a pen

S **SKILL:** Determine color vision acuity by using Ishihara plates.

| Procedure Steps | Detailed Instructions and/or *Rationales* |
|---|---|
| 1. Obtain the chart from the back of the book. | Before administering this screening test, you should be tested. |
| B 2. Identify the patient, introduce yourself, and explain the procedure, ***using language that the patient can understand.*** | *Ensures that you are performing the procedure on the correct patient.* |
| 3. Ask the patient first to read the plates with both eyes. | If the patient wears corrective lenses, perform the testing with the patient wearing them and be sure to document it in the patient's chart. |
| 4. Have the patient cover the left eye to test the right eye and then cover the right to test the left. | Make sure to note any difficulty or complaint of the patient during the screening process. |
| 5. Compare answers given with those on chart. Record those frames the patient misses and write down what the patient reports so that the degree of color deficiency may be determined by the provider. | |
| 6. Document results in the patient's chart. | |

### Charting Example

| | |
|---|---|
| 9-24-XX<br>11:30 am | Color vision screening per Dr. White; Ishihara color plates—accurately read.<br>T. EDWARDS, CMA(AAMA) |

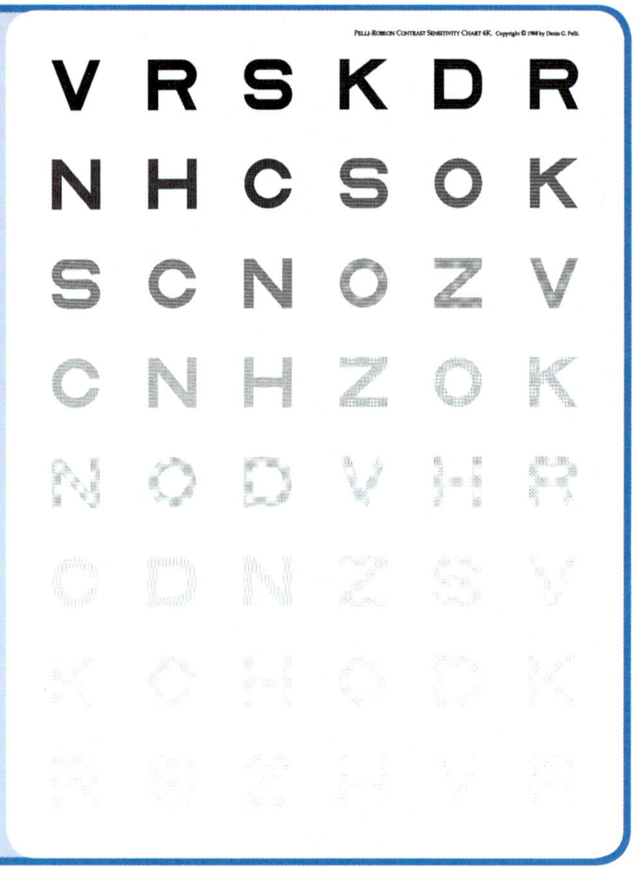


**Figure 40–22:** Pelli–Robson contrast sensitivity chart. *Courtesy of Dr. Denis Pelli, NYU.*

## Contrast Sensitivity Screening

The Pelli–Robson *contrast sensitivity* chart measures contrast sensitivity by determining the faintest contrast an observer can see (Figure 40–22). Clinical evidence shows that contrast sensitivity is affected by all the major eye diseases—diabetic retinopathy, macular degeneration, glaucoma, and cataract. Therefore, measuring contrast sensitivity provides a sensitive screening test for eye disease to provide earlier diagnosis and treatment.

Another contrast sensitivity screening method is the CSV-1000, developed by Vectorvision. All patients can be tested with this method, but it is especially useful in screening small children, internationals, and people who are illiterate. This test has a series of four groups of circles. In these rows of circles, some are solid gray in color and some have vertical lines. The patient is instructed to look at the first group and tell which circles have lines within them. The last correctly identified circle in each group is charted on a graph. The results of this test are interpreted by the provider.

## RESPIRATORY EXAMINATIONS

When the patient arrives for his or her visit, recall that one of the first procedures performed is the monitoring of his or her vital signs, including the respiratory rate. (Refer to Chapter 38.) The provider will recheck the patient's breathing during the physical examination to determine whether there are any abnormalities that warrant additional testing. Many patients have risk factors or infections that would encourage further diagnostic testing to be performed, such as smoking, environmental exposures, and infections such as bronchitis, influenza, or pneumonia. A variety of testing may be incorporated into their exam, depending on the patient's symptoms.

### Vital Capacity Tests

**Vital capacity** is defined as the greatest volume of air that can be expelled during a complete, slow, unforced expiration following a maximum inspiration. Vital capacity should equal inspiratory capacity plus expiratory reserve. Vital capacity is usually reported in both absolute values and statistically derived values based on the age, sex, and height of the patient. The statistical value is reported as a percentage.

The spirometer is an instrument that tests the capacity of the lungs. Many providers prefer to use the handheld spirometer, which comes with vital capacity charts. Vital capacity testing is performed to evaluate patients who are suspected of having pulmonary insufficiency. Vital capacity testing aids in the diagnosis and degree of functional or obstructive abnormalities. It also helps the provider find the cause of dyspnea and evaluate the effectiveness of medication and therapy.

**PATIENT EDUCATION**

When scheduling patients for vital capacity tests, it is important to advise them to eat lightly and not to smoke for at least six hours before the appointment. Patients should refrain from routine treatment, and medication should not be taken until after the test is completed.

In preparing to perform this diagnostic procedure, instruct the patient regarding the necessary steps and demonstrate the use of the spirometer. Routine procedures, such as height, weight, and vital signs, should have already been taken and recorded in the patient's chart. Showing the patient how to hold the instrument and what is expected will yield a more accurate test result. Disposable mouthpieces are used to prevent disease transmission. Most spirometers are computerized and have a printout of the results within minutes of administering the test. Type in the patient's name, age, height, race, gender, account number, and any other information, if applicable, before you start the test.

Figure 40–23 pictures a medical assistant coaching a patient through the procedure. A clip is placed on the patient's nose to force the expired air out of the lungs directly into the mouthpiece (make sure patient's mouth is sealed around the mouthpiece) and into the spirometer. Instruct the patient to stand up straight and to take in a slow deep breath. Coach the patient to expel all the air from the lungs quickly until it is not possible to exhale any more, within approximately 15 seconds. Give the patient several practice runs before beginning the official test because it is an awkward procedure for most people. Follow each of the expirations with a few seconds of resting for the patient. Watch for signs of stress, dizziness, coughing, or other problems the patient might have during the test. Generally, three to five expirations are tested. The results are analyzed by the computerized instrument, and the diagnostic data are printed for evaluation by the provider. Test results below 80 percent are usually considered abnormal. This spirometry reading is placed in the patient's chart, along with a notation of any symptoms or problems the patient might have had during the test and your initials. Spirometry tests should not be performed when the patient has been diagnosed with angina, acute coronary insufficiency, or recent myocardial infarction. Allow the patient to sit and relax to wait for consultation with the provider. Instruct the patient to resume medication and therapy routine as directed by the provider. Procedure 40–7 provides step-by-step instruction.

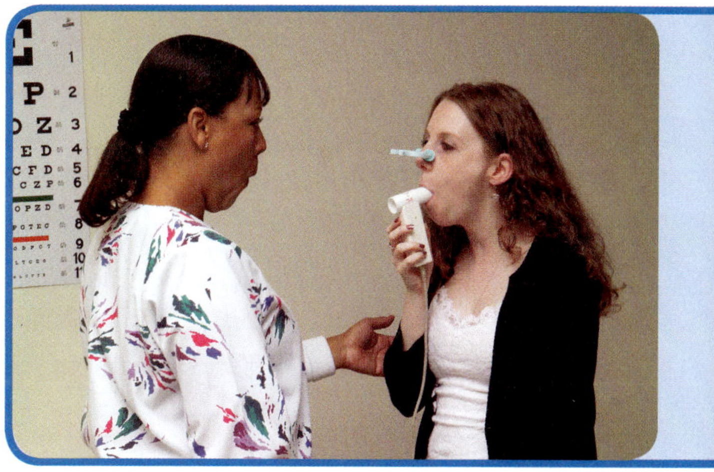

**Figure 40–23:** The medical assistant coaches the patient during the spirometry test. *Delmar/Cengage Learning.*

## PROCEDURE 40–7 Perform Spirometry Testing

**PURPOSE:** Evaluate patients suspected of having pulmonary insufficiency

**EQUIPMENT:** Spirometer and disposable mouthpieces, patient chart or EMR, and a pen

S **SKILL:** Perform spirometry testing.

| Procedure Steps | Detailed Instructions and/or *Rationales* |
|---|---|
| 1. Obtain the spirometer machine, assemble the necessary equipment and supplies; wash hands. | |
| B 2. Identify the patient, introduce yourself, and explain the procedure and equipment, ***using language the patient will understand.*** | *Ensures that you are performing the procedure on the correct patient.* Let the patient become familiar with the equipment by having the patient breathe into the machine. |
| B 3. ***Be sure the patient is in a comfortable position and any restrictive clothing (such as a tie or collar) is loosened before initiating the procedure.*** | |
| 4. Instruct the patient to sit or stand as straight as possible and not bend at the waist while blowing into the disposable mouthpiece. | |

*(continues)*

*(continued)*

| Procedure Steps | Detailed Instructions and/or *Rationales* |
|---|---|
| 5. Instruct the patient to make a tight seal around the mouthpiece with the lips. | |
| 6. After telling the patient to take deep breaths in (inhalation), coach the patient to breathe all the air out of the lungs until unable to exhale any longer, usually about 15 seconds. | |
| 7. Allow the patient to have a practice run before performing the actual test. | |
| 8. Support the patient during the test and have the patient keep blowing into the mouthpiece until told to stop. | Watch for signs of stress, dizziness, coughing, or other problems during the test. |
| 9. Document the procedure in the patient's chart and place the results in the chart for the provider's review. | |

**Charting Example**

| | |
|---|---|
| 3-30-XX<br>11:30 am | Spirometry testing performed per Dr. White. Patient tolerated well.<br>T. EDWARDS, CMA(AAMA) |

## Peak Flow Testing

**Peak flow** testing measures a patient's ability to exhale. A peak flow meter is a monitoring device that measures the peak expiratory flow rate, that is, the highest speed at which one can forcibly blow air from the lungs after taking in as deep a breath as possible (Figure 40–24). Peak flow testing may be used if a patient had an inconclusive or normal spirometry test but is still presenting with asthma symptoms. It can also be performed to monitor the effectiveness of medications or to determine whether another form of treatment should be tried. Daily peak flow readings can help detect subtle changes in lung function, sometimes even before the patient is aware of them. Patients can benefit from a peak flow meter in several ways: to recognize that asthma may be occurring at night, to improve perception of asthma, to identify factors that worsen asthma and to predict worsening of asthma. Peak flow measurements can change over time, depending on the patient's current medical condition, age, weight, and the time of day it is taken. Procedure 40–8 provides complete steps on how to perform a peak flow measurement on a patient.

Although the predicted "normal" peak flow is determined by height, age, and sex, it is preferable to gauge asthma control by comparing daily peak flow readings with the patient's personal best reading. This is defined as the highest measurement the patient can achieve in the middle of a good day, after using any prescribed inhaled bronchodilators. The patient might need to use a peak flow meter for one or two weeks to arrive at the personal best number. After a personal best peak flow has been established, every effort must be made to maintain values within 80 percent of this number. If the reading falls between 50 percent and 70 percent, the patient will usually need to take a quick action inhaler; if it falls below 50 percent, the patient must seek emergency care. Providers will have guidelines they want their patients to follow.

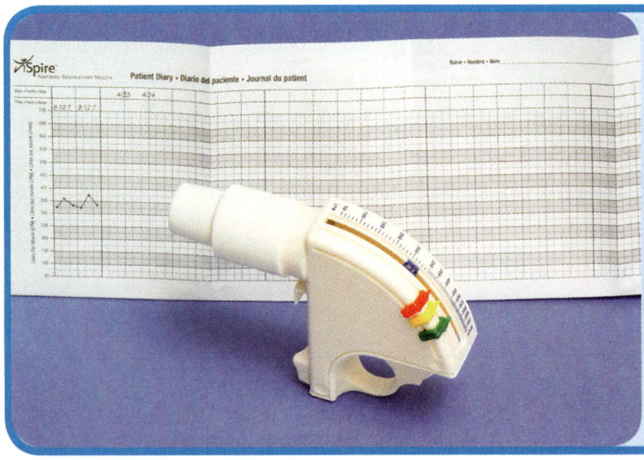


**FIGURE 40–24:** Peak flow meter with patient diary. *Delmar/Cengage Learning.*

## PROCEDURE 40–8 Perform Peak Flow Testing

**MEDIA LINK:** View the animation, "Peak Flow Testing," for this chapter on the Premium Website.

**PURPOSE:** Correctly instruct the patient to measure his or her peak expiratory flow rate

**EQUIPMENT:** Peak flow meter, mouth piece, medical order, waste container, patient chart or EMR, and a pen

S **SKILL:** Instruct the patient to measure his or her peak expiratory flow rate.

| Procedure Steps | Detailed Instructions and/or *Rationales* |
|---|---|
| 1. Assemble equipment and supplies; wash hands. | |
| B 2. Identify the patient, introduce yourself, and explain the procedure and equipment, ***using language the patient will understand.*** | *Ensures* that *you are performing the procedure on the correct patient.* |
| B 3. ***Be sure the patient is in a comfortable position, and any restrictive clothing (such as a tie or collar) is loosened before initiating the procedure.*** | Help the patient to a standing position (if needed). |
| 4. Set the indicator to the bottom (lowest number) of the scale. | |
| 5. Instruct the patient to take in a deep breath, place the meter to mouth, close lips around the mouthpiece, and blow as hard as he or she can. | |
| 6. Write down the number the patient achieved. | |
| 7. Repeat steps 5, 6, and 7 two more times. | |
| 8. Instruct the patient to do a peak flow 2–3 times a day. | Instruct the patient to take readings in the AM, PM, and when he or she is short of breath. |
| 9. Explain to the patient how to establish his or her "Personal Best"; explain the "Three Zone" system and how to record results in his or her peak flow diary. | |
| 10. Dispose of mouthpiece in the waste container. | |
| 11. Document. | |

### Charting Example

| | |
|---|---|
| 3-30-XX 11:30 am | Patient instructed on how to measure peak expiratory flow, using a peak flow meter, how to obtain personal best, and how to monitor the three zones with their results. T. EDWARDS, CMA(AAMA) |

## Pulse Oximetry

As discussed in Chapter 38, **pulse oximetry** is a simple, noninvasive test that measures the patient's pulse rate and oxygen saturation (SAT) level in the blood. Many cardiopulmonary conditions could warrant the provider seeking a patient's oxygen saturation level. Common cardiac and pulmonary conditions include heart attacks, congestive heart failure (CHF) and coronary artery disease (CAD), asthma, pneumonia, and respiratory syncytial virus (RSV), a common but serious respiratory virus often seen in infants and children.

Many oximeter models are available; common ones are small, handheld devices with a monitor and a sensor that is clipped onto the patient's finger (Figure 40–25). The sensor has an infrared light in it that transmits through the patient's tissues to a photo detector on the opposite side of the clip. The device measures the amount of light that is absorbed by the hemoglobin, which is then displayed as a percentage on the monitor. Additional attachments can be used in the event of poor circulation, calloused fingers, nail polish, or if the patient is an infant or small child. The attachment can be wrapped around the toe, earlobe, or bridge of the nose and is held in place similar to a bandage. A normal pulse oximeter reading is 95 percent or higher. Refer to Procedure 40–9 for instructions on how to perform a pulse oximeter test.

You may be instructed to schedule patients for further pulmonary function studies to be performed by a pulmonary and thoracic specialist. More sophisticated equipment may be necessary to evaluate a patient's condition.

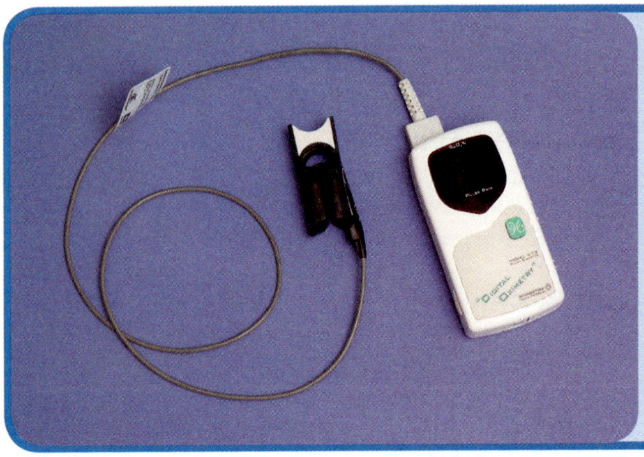

**Figure 40–25:** Pulse oximeter. *Delmar/Cengage Learning.*

## PROCEDURE 40–9 Perform Pulse Oximetry Testing

**PURPOSE:** To measure a patient's oxygen level in the blood

**EQUIPMENT:** Pulse oximeter, alcohol wipes, nail polish remover if needed, patient chart or EHR, and a pen

**SKILL:** Perform pulse oximetry testing.

| Procedure Steps | Detailed Instructions and/or *Rationales* |
|---|---|
| 1. Wash hands and assemble equipment. | |
| 2. Identify the patient, introduce yourself, and explain the procedure and equipment, ***using language the patient will understand.*** | *Ensures that you are performing the procedure on the correct patient.* |
| 3. Select a site for the sensor. | The finger is commonly used. If the patient has poor circulation, use another site such as the bridge of the nose, earlobe, or forehead (you need a special sensor for this). |
| 4. Clean the site with alcohol. Remove nail polish if needed. Wash with soap and water. | |
| 5. Apply sensor, read results. | |
| 6. Note the results (including pulse) according to the manufacturer's instructions. (Take reading after 10 seconds.) | |
| 7. ***Apply critical thinking skills in performing patient assessment and care, notifying provider immediately of abnormal results.*** Abnormal results are less than 95%. | |
| 8. Document procedure, site of application, (sensor applied to left index finger), and results. | |

### Charting Example

| | |
|---|---|
| 3-30-XX<br>11:30 am | Pulse oximetry sensor applied to L index finger per Dr. White. P 70 SpO2 99%.<br>T. EDWARDS, CMA(AAMA) |

## PROCTOLOGIC EXAMINATIONS

In the diagnosis of hemorrhoids, fissures, and ulcerations, the provider usually begins investigative procedures by examining the anus and the interior of the rectum with a **proctoscope**. The proctoscope permits viewing of the anal canal and lower rectal area when sigmoidoscopy is not necessary; for example, the provider may view the intestinal **mucosa** following a normal bowel movement. Figure 40–26 shows a tray setup for a basic rectal exam.

Some of the instruments used in these procedures are shown in Figure 40–27A through C. The rectal speculum (A) allows viewing of the anal canal and rectum, the biopsy forceps (B) permit removing a tissue sample for examination, and the snare (C) is used to detach polyps or other pendulous growths from the mucosa to be examined. All instruments and items that come in contact with a body cavity must be free from microorganisms. The medical assistant is generally responsible for this task. Some instruments can be disinfected and then autoclaved. Delicate instruments and those with plastic or rubber parts will require processing in a germicidal solution. (Refer to Chapter 36.)

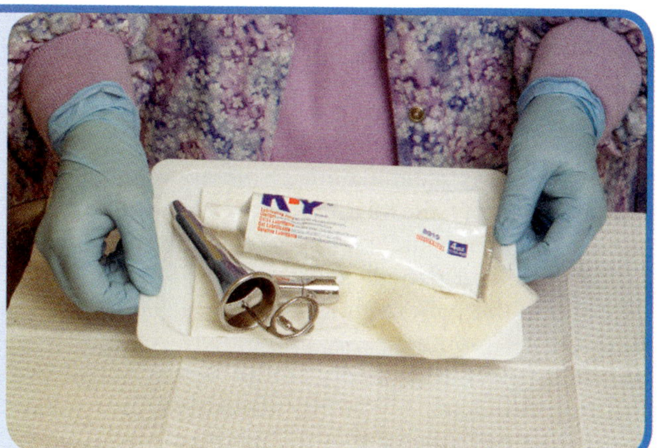

**Figure 40–26:** Tray setup for a rectal exam. *Delmar/Cengage Learning.*

Proper positioning of patients during the exam is important for both the provider's viewing of the rectum and sigmoid colon and for the patient's comfort. Proctology tables (refer to Figure 39–9) are designed especially for this procedure. They provide support of the patient's chest and head with the arm resting against the headboard as the table is tilted to the knee-chest position. Those who cannot tolerate this position are assisted into a Sims' position for the exam. You should ask about the provider's preference in patient position because there are variations.

### Patient Instructions and Preparation

Patients may be instructed to eat a light diet containing plenty of clear liquids and avoiding dairy products for 24 hours before the exam and to have a plain cleansing **enema** the morning of, or two hours before, the exam. Other providers may wish patients to use **laxatives** the day before and an enema the night before and the morning of the exam.

Some exams require the use of **evacuants** by the patient before the exam; if this is the case, instructions should be made clear to the patient before the appointment is scheduled. Helping him or her choose a convenient appointment time and explaining the reasons for the preparations they must undergo will usually be appreciated.

For the patient's convenience, make sure that you use an examination room that is close to the restroom if an enema is administered. The enema is a simple procedure, one that patients can do at home when advised by the provider. Your patience and understanding are needed here because most patients are embarrassed to have this done.

Occasionally, even when the patient follows the list of instructions, the enema solution is not retained long enough for it to work. Encourage the patient to hold the contents of the enema longer and perhaps explain that the longer the contents are held, the more successful

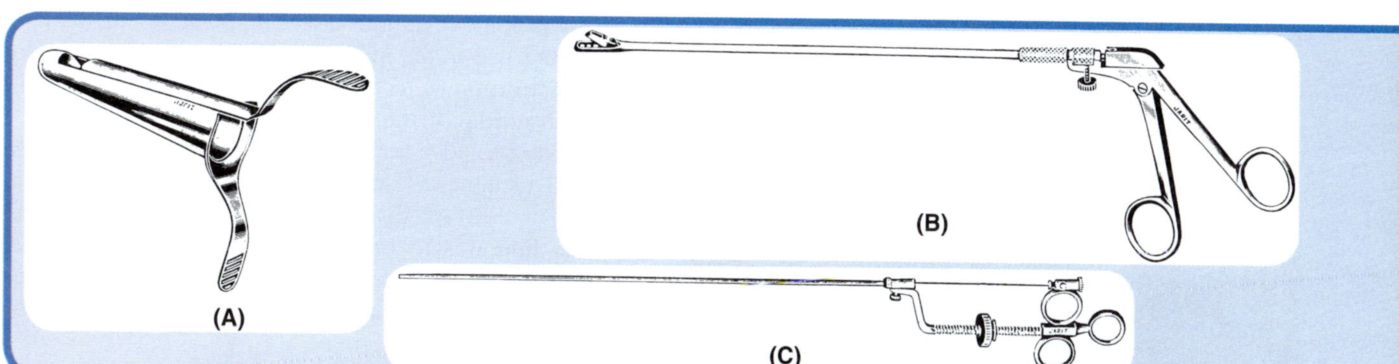


**Figure 40–27A–C:** Instruments used in proctological procedures: (A) rectal speculum, (B) biopsy forceps, and (C) rectal snare. *Courtesy of JARIT Surgical Instruments.*

the results will be. Often, encouraging deep breathing and placing a couple of tissues over the anal opening and applying gentle pressure will aid in retaining the fluid. Otherwise, it may have to be repeated or the exam rescheduled.

## Sigmoidoscopy

Sigmoidoscopy is a diagnostic examination of the interior of the sigmoid colon. It is a useful aid in the diagnosis of cancer of the colon, ulcerations, **polyps**, tumors, bleeding, and other lower intestinal disorders. The sigmoidoscope is an instrument with a light source and a magnifying lens, which permits viewing the mucous membranes of the sigmoid colon. Many providers use a **flexible sigmoidoscope** (Figure 40–28), although metal and plastic (disposable) scopes are still occasionally used. The flexible sigmoidoscope can be inserted much farther into the colon with less discomfort. This instrument makes it possible to view more of the interior of the colon.

When using the metal or plastic type, an **obturator** (a tool with a solid, rounded end) is inserted into the sigmoidoscope. The tip of the obturator and scope are lubricated and carefully inserted into the rectum and sigmoid. Then the obturator is removed so that the S shape of the colon can be seen. Patients find this an uncomfortable and unpleasant procedure.

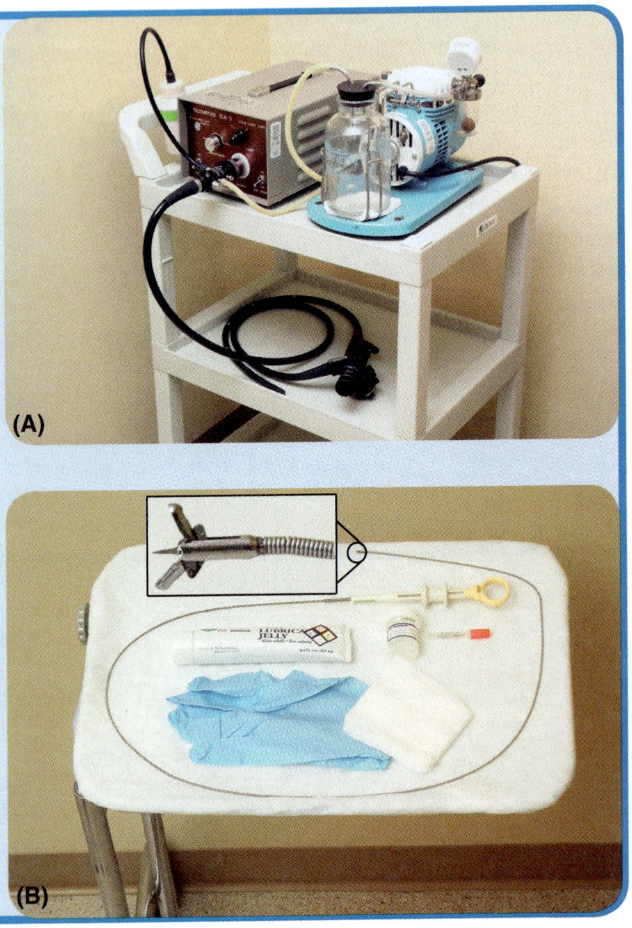


**Figure 40–28A–B:** Setup for sigmoidoscopy with flexible sigmoidoscope. *Delmar/Cengage Learning.*

### PATIENT EDUCATION

The medical assistant often instructs the patient in how to prepare for the sigmoidoscopy and explains how the test is performed. For successful examination, proper preparation is essential. In addition to having the patient restrict dairy products, raw fruits and vegetables, and grains and cereals from his or her diet, encourage the patient to drink plenty of clear liquids and eat lightly the day before the scheduled appointment for the sigmoid colon exam.

Manufactured preps are used to clean the colon and, usually, an enema should be self-administered at home approximately two hours before the exam. Providers may vary the instructions according to the patient's condition, so it is best to ask before proceeding with instructions. If patients are not completely informed about preparations and the exam is attempted with unsatisfactory results, it will have to be repeated. It is best to give patients both oral and written instructions.

As with any examination of the abdomen, ask the patient to empty the bladder and evacuate the bowel before the procedure begins to make the exam easier for both the patient and the provider. During the procedure, the patient should be instructed to breathe through the mouth deeply and slowly relax abdominal muscles to reduce discomfort. Patients may feel the urge to defecate during any colon examination because of the stretching of the intestinal wall from the instrument passing through and air being introduced with it. The procedure should last only a minute or two, especially if patients have followed preparation instructions.

Air is sometimes introduced into the colon (by the examiner's use of the inflation bulb attached to the rigid scope with tubing) to distend the wall of the colon for easier insertion of the **lumen** of the scope. The flexible scope provides for inflation by instilling air through a length of attached small tubing. It is controlled by a switch on the box that also controls the light source. Patients find this to be uncomfortable and sometimes painful. The provider may need to use a suction pump to remove mucus, blood, or **fecal** material that is obstructing the view of the colon.

When the patient has been prepared and the examiner is ready to begin the exam, you hand the necessary instruments and supplies to the provider as needed and provide support to the patient. During the sigmoidoscopy, the provider might want to take a biopsy of questionable tissue from the sigmoid colon to aid in confirming the diagnosis. A biopsy lab request form must be completed and accompany any tissue sent to the lab. Containers for biopsy specimens have a preservative solution to preserve the tissue until the analysis is done.

Remember to advise patients to report any problems, such as bleeding, discharge, swelling, or any other unusual discomfort, following any proctologic procedure.

The examinations discussed in this chapter are by no means the only ones performed in medical offices and clinics. You will learn many others as you gain experience and knowledge in assisting.

## PATIENT EDUCATION

When patients come in for rectal or sigmoidoscopy examinations, here are a few informative topics you might discuss with them:

1. Laxatives and enemas should be used only at the direction of the provider.
2. Constipation may be avoided or relieved by including fresh fruits and vegetables and cereals and grains in the diet, drinking plenty of liquids (water), and getting regular exercise.
3. If patients have any of the following symptoms persistently, consulting the provider is strongly advised because it could mean that a disease or an abnormal condition is present: **heartburn** or indigestion; nausea, vomiting, or both; constipation or diarrhea; excessive gas or bloating; or feces that is tarry (black) or other than a normal brown color.
4. Inform patients over age 40 that they should routinely test their stool for blood every two years for detection of cancer of the colon or more often if advised by the provider. Patients over age 50 should test annually.

## PROCEDURE 40–10 Assist with a Flexible Sigmoidoscopy

**PURPOSE:** To assist in examination of the sigmoid colon

**EQUIPMENT:** Gloves; water-soluble lubricant; gauze squares; flexible sigmoidoscope; long cotton-tipped swabs; drape sheet (fenestrated optional); suction machine (container with room temperature water); tissues; if ordered by physician: biopsy forceps, specimen container for transport to lab; lab request form; patient chart or EMR; and a pen

S **SKILL:** Assist with a flexible sigmoidoscopy procedure.

| | Procedure Steps | Detailed Instructions and/or *Rationales* |
|---|---|---|
| B | 1. Identify patient, introduce yourself, and explain the procedure, ***using language that the patient understands.*** | *Ensures that you are performing the procedure on the correct patient.* Ask the patient to empty the bladder and bowel. |
| | 2. Assemble all needed items on a Mayo tray near the end of the examination table. | If a biopsy is scheduled, complete the lab request form and label the specimen container. |
| | 3. Plug in cord of light source to make sure it works properly; then turn it off. | *If left on, it will be uncomfortably warm for the patient and can cause a burn.* |
| B | 4. ***Instruct the patient to disrobe from the waist down and let you know when he or she is ready. Assist the patient to sit at the end of the table and cover him or her with the drape sheet for privacy.*** | |
| | 5. Wash hands and put on gloves. | |

*(continues)*

*(continued)*

| Procedure Steps | Detailed Instructions and/or *Rationales* |
|---|---|
| 6. Just before the provider is ready to begin the exam, assist the patient into a knee-chest or Sims' position, whichever the provider prefers. | Many providers have an examining table that permits the patient to kneel on a pad and then be placed in a proctological position to facilitate the procedure. |
| 7. Assist the provider by applying about two tablespoons of lubricant on gauze square for the tip of the gloved fingers. | The provider makes a digital examination of the anus and rectum prior to insertion of the endoscope. |
| 8. As the provider finishes the digital exam, plug the sigmoidoscope into the light source. Secure the air-inflation tubing and have it ready to hand to the provider; activate the switches for air inflation and light. | |
| 9. As the provider inserts the sigmoidoscope, be ready to hand items as needed. | Have the suction machine plugged in and suction tip secured. *Often, fecal material or unexpelled enema fluid is present and must be removed before adequate viewing can be accomplished.* |
| 10. Be prepared to rinse the suction tip in water if it becomes clogged. | Flexible scopes aspirate through the attached tubing when suction is activated. |
| 11. If biopsy is indicated, hand biopsy forceps to the provider and have a specimen container open so the provider can place tissue in it. Place the cap on the container securely. | |
| 12. Use tissues to clean lubricant and waste from the patient's anal area and discard it into the waste container. | |
| 13. Place a small pad or dressing over the anal area in case of light bleeding. | |
| 14. Assist the patient to resting prone position (or return table to starting position). | |
| B 15. ***Assist the patient to a sitting position, allowing time for balance to return before helping him or her down from the table. Instruct the patient to dress.*** | |
| 16. Wear gloves to clean the exam table and instruments. The scope and suction tip should be cleaned with detergent and water and placed in a disinfectant to be sterilized. | Follow the manufacturer's instructions for cleaning, disinfecting, and sterilization. |
| 17. Remove gloves and wash hands. | |
| 18. Attach a label and the completed requisition form to the specimen container. Place the specimen container in the area for laboratory pickup. | |
| 19. Restock the room and return the instruments to storage. | |
| 20. Document the procedure on the patient's chart. | |

## Charting Example

| | |
|---|---|
| 4/19/XX 11:30 am | Flexible sigmoidoscopy exam tolerated well by patient; biopsy of lesion on anterior wall at 10 inches. Pad placed over anal area in case of light bleeding. Specimen sent to lab. Follow-up when results received. T. EDWARDS, CMA(AAMA) |

## CHAPTER SUMMARY

- The primary reason for performing a complete physical examination (CPE) is to determine the general state of health and well-being of the patient. The CPE can be performed for various reasons such as an insurance examination before issuing a policy, as a requirement with a patient's employment, as a request by a patient, or to assess a patient's state of health.
- Your role in the physical examination process in addition to preparing the room is to provide assistance and instruction to the patient, assist the provider by anticipating the provider's needs during the exam, handing him or her instruments, positioning and draping the patient, and performing as a scribe if needed.
- You may be expected to provide patient education on a variety of topics. When you know about the pamphlets and other resources available in your office, you can talk with the patient and indicate that you will supply the material after the exam if the provider concurs with the necessity of it.
- The provider uses six examination methods while performing a physical examination. They are inspection, palpation, percussion, auscultation, mensuration, and manipulation.
- The physical examination is performed by the provider. Within each examination area are characteristics the provider may be observing and some applicable descriptive terms. Providers have their own style and depth of examination, which may not include all the areas and characteristics mentioned. You must be aware of the various examination components and the significance of each.
- Patients may ask how often they need to have a physical or a checkup, as they call it. You may use Table 40–1 as a guide in giving advice to adult patients about examination and specialty procedures routinely performed on patients.
- Sometimes it is difficult for the provider to inspect the patient's ear due to a buildup of cerumen (earwax) in the ear. This buildup can become very uncomfortable and eventually impair hearing. The ear may require irrigation (also known as lavage) to remove the excessive wax.
- Providers use several audiometric assessment procedures to determine the cause of the patient's hearing loss: Audiometry is a procedure that measures one's hearing; tympanometry is a procedure that determines the ability of the middle ear to transmit sound waves and is commonly performed on children to diagnose middle ear infections; and a two-pronged metal tuning fork, its frequency varying with the size of the instrument, tests nerve or conduction deafness.
- Occasionally, the eye might need to be irrigated if there is inflammation, secretions in the eye due to infection, a chemical contamination, or a foreign particle in the eye.
- Measuring visual acuity is a diagnostic screening procedure most often done by the medical assistant. Common vision screening tests include the Snellen chart, which measures *distance* vision; the Jaeger system, which screens for *near* vision acuity; and the Ishihara color plates book, which screens patients for defects in distinguishing *color vision* acuity.
- The spirometer is an instrument that tests the capacity of the lungs. Vital capacity testing aids in the diagnosis and degree of functional or obstructive abnormalities. It also helps the provider find the cause of dyspnea and evaluate the effectiveness of medication and therapy.
- Peak flow testing measures a patient's ability to exhale. A peak flow meter is a monitoring device that measures your peak expiratory flow rate, the highest speed that you can forcibly blow air from your lungs after taking in as deep a breath as possible. Peak flow testing can be used if a patient had an inconclusive or normal spirometry test or to monitor the effectiveness of medications.
- Pulse oximetry is a noninvasive test that measures the patient's pulse rate and oxygen saturation (SAT) in the blood. It is a simple test that is performed in many clinical facilities to determine a patient's oxygen status.
- Flexible sigmoidoscopy is a diagnostic examination of the interior of the sigmoid colon. It is a useful aid in the diagnosis of ulcerations, polyps, tumors, bleeding, cancer of the colon, and other lower intestinal disorders.

## STUDY TOOLS

| | |
|---|---|
| **Workbook** | Activities for Chapter 40 |
| **Premium Website** MEDIA LINK | View these **Media Links** for Chapter 40:<br>• Screen Visual Acuity<br>• Screen Color Vision Acuity<br>• Peak Flow Testing |

| StudyWARE | Activities and Quizzes on the **StudyWARE™ Software** for Chapter 40 |
|---|---|
| | Complete the following **Competency Challenge 2.0** activities:<br>• Tuesday, 11:00 AM, Prepare and Assist with Procedures, Treatments, and Minor Office Surgeries<br>• Wednesday, 1:00 PM, Perform Respiratory Testing<br>• Thursday, 3:00 PM, Provide Patient Instructions |
| | **Audio Library** of medical terms |
| | Online access to the **Critical Thinking Challenge 2.0** |
| **CourseMate** | Activities and Quizzes for Chapter 40 |
| **WebTutor** | Activities and Quizzes for Chapter 40 |

## CHECK YOUR KNOWLEDGE

1. The following examination technique uses a means of producing sounds by tapping various parts of the body.
   a. Inspection
   b. Palpation
   c. Percussion
   d. Manipulation
2. Which examination technique must be used to detect sounds, including bruits, murmurs, rales, rhythms, and bowel sounds?
   a. Auscultation
   b. Inspection
   c. Mensuration
   d. Percussion
3. The Rinne and Weber tests are performed by using the following piece of equipment.
   a. Ophthalmoscope
   b. Otoscope
   c. Audiometer
   d. Tuning fork
4. The breast examination is best done on the ________ days following the menstrual cycle of menstruating women.
   a. 21–28
   b. 7–10
   c. 5–10
   d. 7–14
5. At what age should men begin a routine testicular self-examination?
   a. 12
   b. 15
   c. 16
   d. 18
6. What is the name of the chart used most commonly for screening distance vision?
   a. Jaeger
   b. Snellen
   c. Ishihara
   d. Pelli-Robson
7. Which of the following devices are used to measure the capacity of the lungs?
   a. Spirometer
   b. Peak flow
   c. Tuning fork
   d. Both a and b
8. In the diagnosis of ulcerations, polyps, tumors, bleeding, cancer of the colon, and other lower intestinal disorders, the examination of the interior of the sigmoid colon can be done using a:
   a. proctoscope.
   b. rectal speculum.
   c. rectal snare.
   d. sigmoidoscope.

## WEB LINKS

Centers for Disease Control and Prevention: www.cdc.gov/nip

Hearing Loss Web: www.hearinglossweb.com

## RESOURCES

Estes, M. E. Z. (2010). *Health Assessment & Physical Examination* (3rd ed.). Clifton Park, NY: Delmar Cengage Learning.

Heller, M., and Veach, L. (2009). *Clinical Medical Assisting: A Professional, Field Smart Approach to the Workplace*. Clifton Park, NY: Delmar, Cengage Learning.

Lindh, W., Pooler, M., Tamparo, C., and Dahl, B. (2010). *Delmar's Comprehensive Medical Assisting Administrative and Clinical Competencies* (4th ed.). Clifton Park, NY: Delmar Cengage Learning.

Venes, D. (ed.). (2009). *Taber's Cyclopedic Medical Dictionary* (21st ed.). Philadelphia: F. A. Davis.

CHAPTER 5

# The Physical Exam, Specialty Exams, and Procedures

## Words to Know Challenge

**Spelling: Each line contains three spellings of a word. Underline the correctly spelled word.**

| | | |
|---|---|---|
| 1. auscultation | auscutatuion | asscultation |
| 2. menipulation | manipulation | maniputation |
| 3. bimanual | bymanual | bimanule |
| 4. bruet | bruit | brute |
| 5. gate | gait | gaite |
| 6. hurnia | hernea | hernia |
| 7. laxative | laxetive | laxitive |
| 8. luman | luemen | lumen |
| 9. mucosa | mucousa | mycousa |
| 10. obtruator | obturator | abturator |
| 11. evakuant | evacuent | evacuant |
| 12. occluder | ocluder | aucluder |

**Matching: Match the term in column I to its definition in column II.**

| | COLUMN I | COLUMN II |
|---|---|---|
| ____ | 1. audiometer | A. means "to wash out" |
| ____ | 2. acuity | B. unit for measuring volume of sound |
| ____ | 3. cerumen | C. medical term for earwax |
| ____ | 4. decibel | D. another word for lavage |
| ____ | 5. irrigate | E. clarity/sharpness of perception |
| ____ | 6. lavage | F. instrument that measures hearing |
| ____ | 7. Snellen Chart | G. a screening tool for near vision acuity |

(continues)

| | | |
|---|---|---|
| ____ | 8. Jaeger Chart | H. a screening tool for distant visual acuity |
| ____ | 9. scribe | I. test for occult blood in stool |
| ____ | 10. guaiac test paper | J. documents provider's dictation during an exam |
| ____ | 11. enema | K. part of preparation for sigmoidoscopy |

MODULE 5

# Working in the Patient Electronic Medical Record

## OBJECTIVES

In this module, you will:

1. Use the appointment schedule on the EHR side of the program, indicating patients have been admitted to an exam room.
2. Create new patient notes in an electronic patient record.
3. Enter patient history information into the patient record.
4. Enter vital signs information into the patient record.
5. Record Review of Systems (ROS) information from a patient questionnaire for provider review.
6. Record past history, family history, social history in the patient record for provider review.

## TASK 5-1: ADMITTING PATIENTS USING THE EHR SCHEDULE

Today is October 16, 2008.

You are working with Dr. Venus today as a clinical medical assistant. Perry Marshall, a patient of Dr. Venus, arrives for his annual exam. He completes an ROS form while in the waiting area, and the administrative medical assistant confirms that there are no registration updates at this time. Once Perry has been brought into the exam room, you will change his appointment status to Admitted.

1. Log in to e-Medsys®.

2. Using the steps learned in Module 4, indicate on the appointment schedule that Perry has Arrived and Registered.

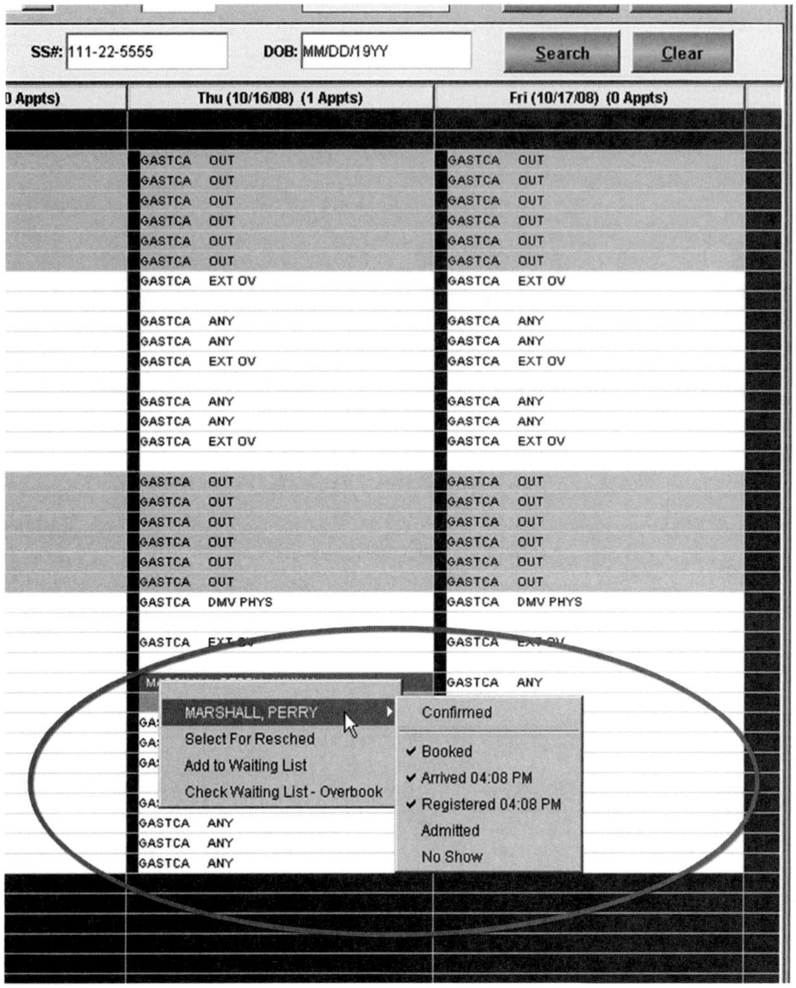


Reprinted with permission of TriMed Technologies, Corp.

3. At the top of the screen, click on EHR, and then click on EHR Home Page from the drop-down box.

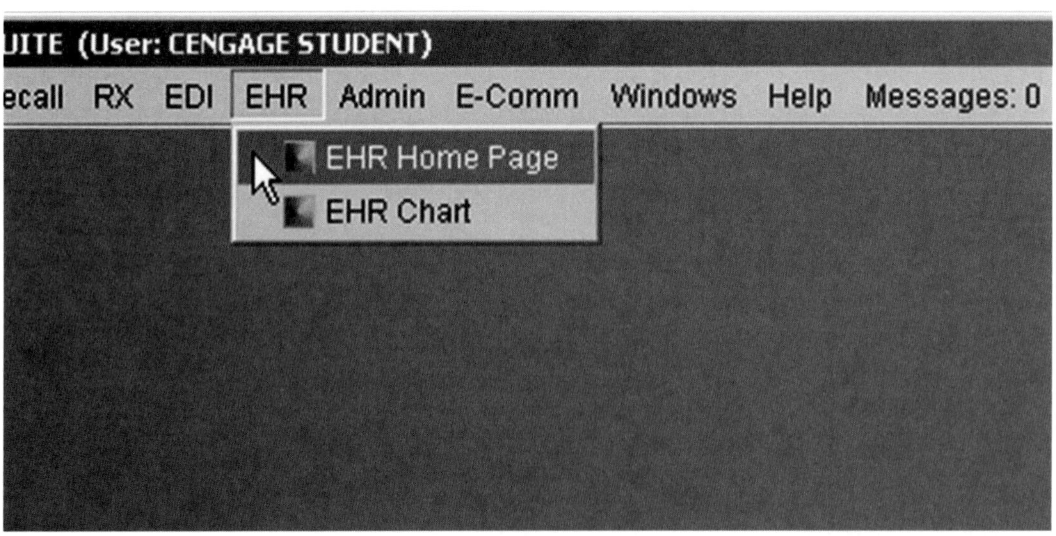


Reprinted with permission of TriMed Technologies, Corp.

4. This opens the EHR page in a new window.

5. Now, you will open Dr. Venus's schedule—in the EHR side of the program
   - On the right side of the screen, select Dr. Venus from the list of providers.
   - Type in 10/16/2008 and press the TAB button on your keyboard to find the correct date.
   - Below the calendar, be sure the radio buttons next to Cal and Daily are selected (this indicates that you want to view the Calendar for only today's date).

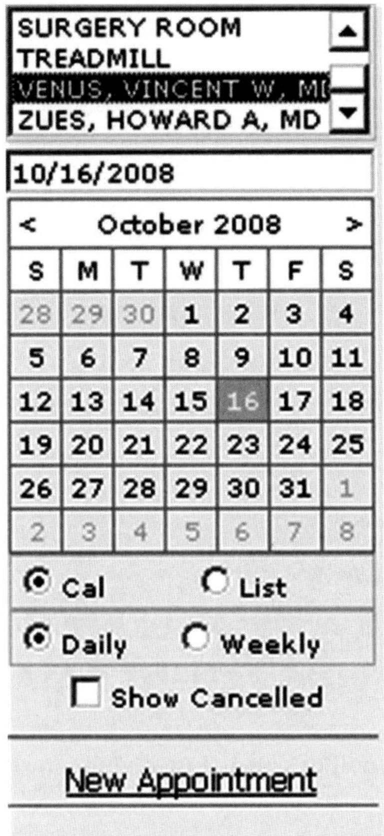


Reprinted with permission of TriMed Technologies, Corp.

6. Dr. Venus's schedule appears in the center of the page. You will see Perry Marshall's appointment on the schedule.

7. Now, right click on Perry Marshall's name on the schedule.
8. Roll your mouse over Status ▶ and then click on Admitted. This provides a timestamp for when the patient was admitted to an exam room.

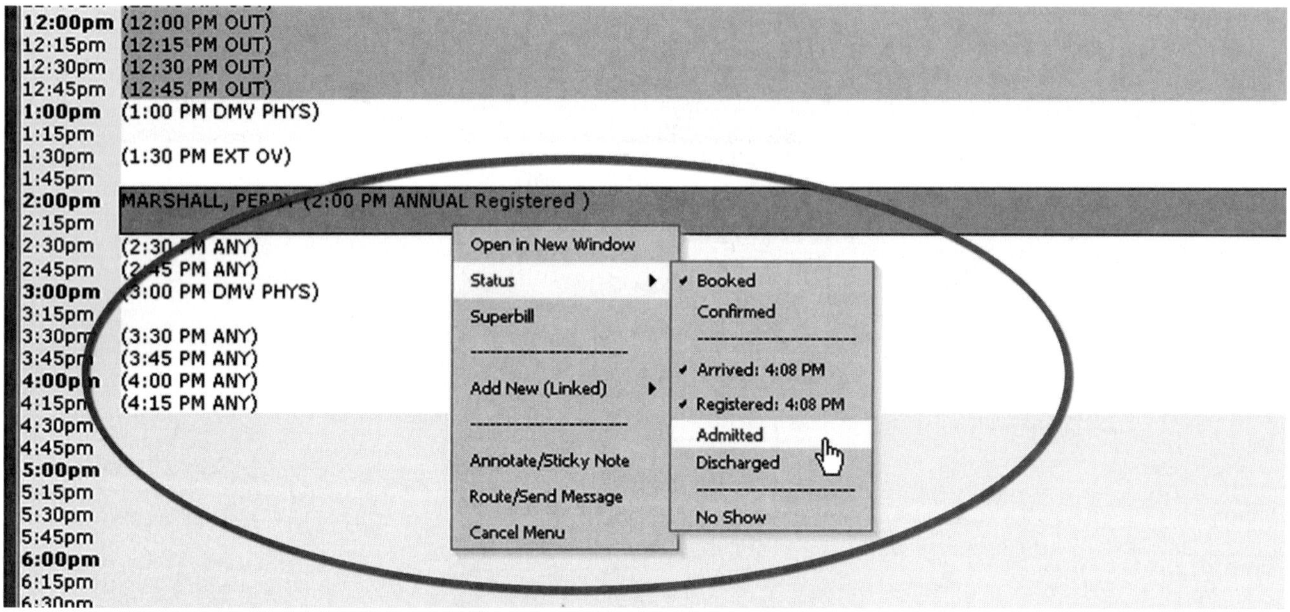


Reprinted with permission of TriMed Technologies, Corp.

## TASK 5-2: LINKING A NEW ANNUAL EXAM NOTE TO A PATIENT APPOINTMENT AND ENTERING PATIENT DATA

Now that you have indicated Perry Marshall has been admitted to an exam room, you will create a new patient note in his patient record.

1. While still on Dr. Venus's schedule, right click on Perry Marshall's name again.
2. This time, select Add New (Linked) ▶ and then click on Patient Note from the menu.

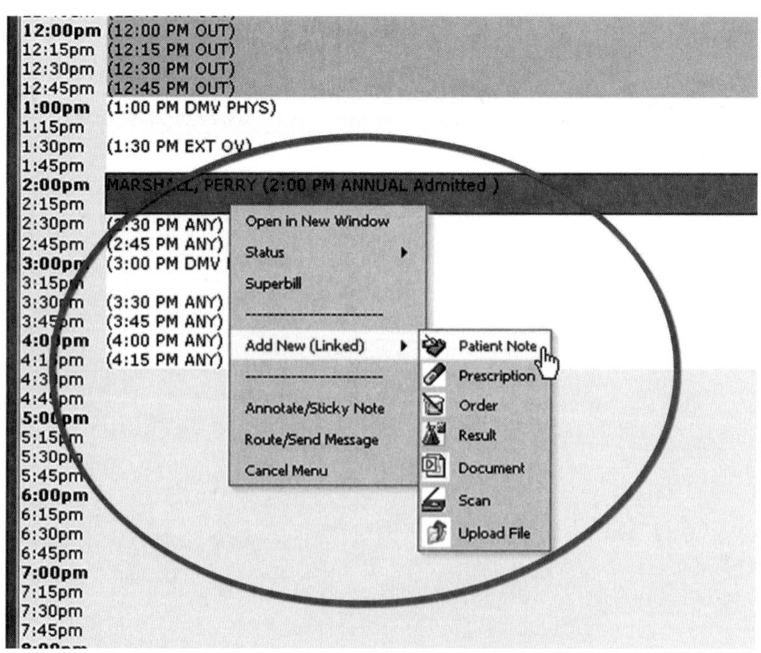


Reprinted with permission of TriMed Technologies, Corp.

3. Now you are in the patient's individual chart, and a New Note has opened on the bottom right side of the screen. You can click on the Box on the right side of the screen above the envelope icon (as shown in the following screen shot) to enlarge the New Note while you are working in it.

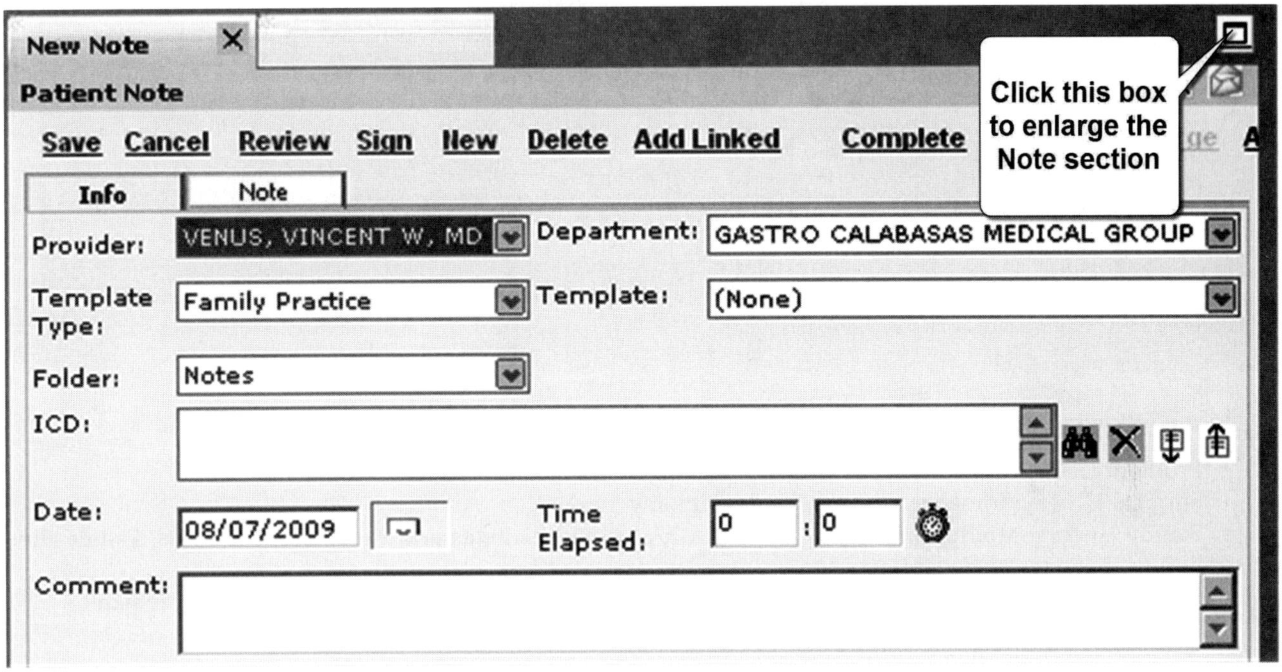


Reprinted with permission of TriMed Technologies, Corp.

4. In the Template field, use the drop-down to select Routine Exam Male. In the date field, enter 10/16/2008. (In a medical office setting, the date would be autopopulated based on today's date.)

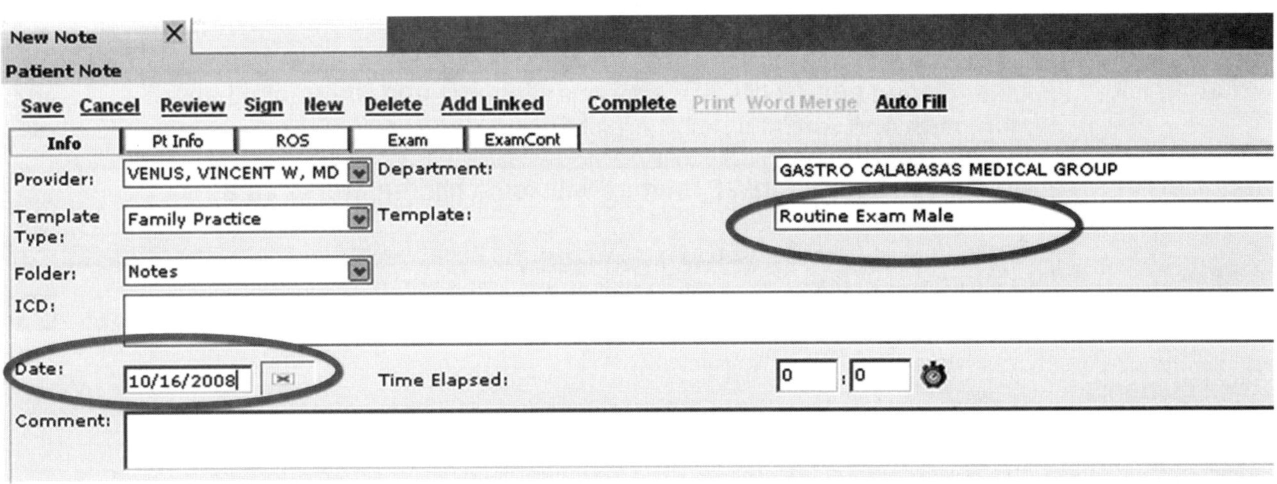


Reprinted with permission of TriMed Technologies, Corp.

5. Click Save.
6. Select the Pt Info tab.
7. Change the Date of Visit to 10/16/2008.

8. Click on the plus sign (+) next to Chief Complaint. This action will bring up a script, which lets you add additional drop-down items to the chief complaint list. Type in Annual Physical Exam and then click OK.

Reprinted with permission of TriMed Technologies, Corp.

9. In the following fields PMH (patient medical history), enter the following:
   - Problem List: Arthritis; hypertension
   - Surgical History: Cholecystectomy; appendectomy
   - Family History: Mother died at age 70 of CAD, also had diabetes and rheumatoid arthritis; Father alive and well at age 74; no siblings
   - Social History: Nonsmoker, social drinker, married with four children, works as a longshoreman

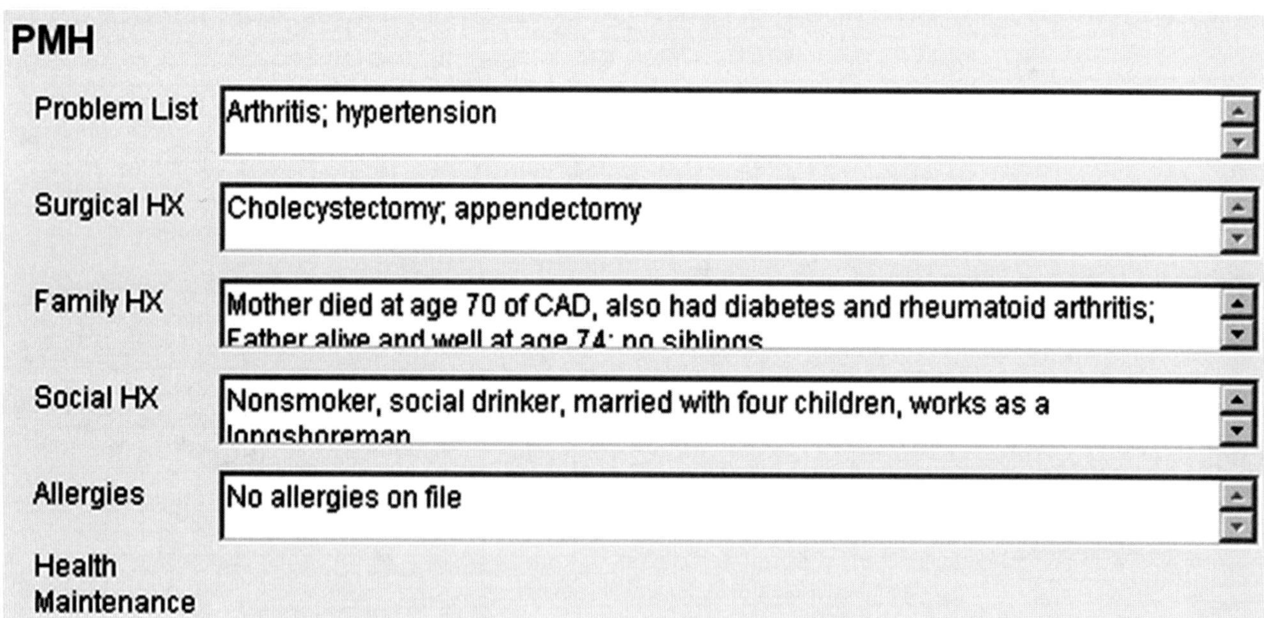


Reprinted with permission of TriMed Technologies, Corp.

10. Leave the rest of the screen for the provider to fill out. Click Save when you are finished.

# TASK 5-3: ENTERING ROS INFORMATION FROM PATIENT QUESTIONNAIRE

Recall that in the waiting area, Perry completed a Patient Questionnaire to update the provider on his state of health. The medical assistant will enter the information into the patient's chart. All of this information will be reviewed with the patient and signed by Dr. Venus.

1. Still in the Perry Marshall's new Note, select the ROS tab. Note that the default settings are "normal," which helps save time when working in the chart. The person documenting needs to enter only remarkable or abnormal items.
2. In the first entry, Constitutional, keep the radio button set to normal, but in the free text section beneath, type Normal, slight weight loss.

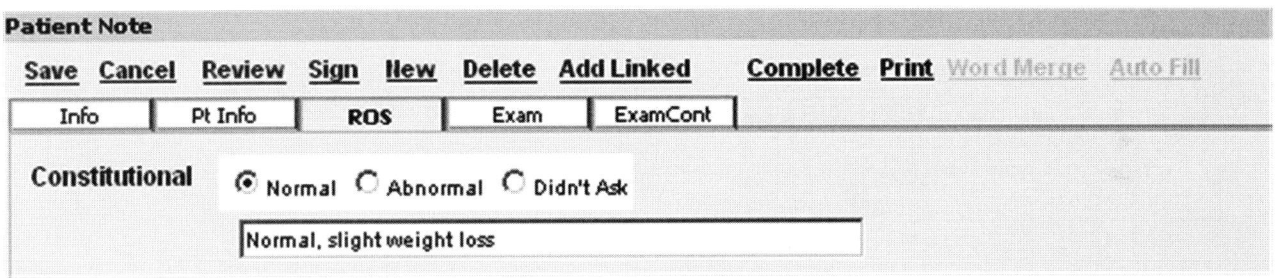


Reprinted with permission of TriMed Technologies, Corp.

3. Now enter the following information for the MS (musculoskeletal), GI (gastrointestinal), and GV (genitourinary) systems:
   - GI: Abnormal; Experiencing intermittent bouts of diarrhea and constipation
   - GV: Abnormal; Frequent urination during the night
   - MS: Abnormal; Joint pain in fingers and elbows

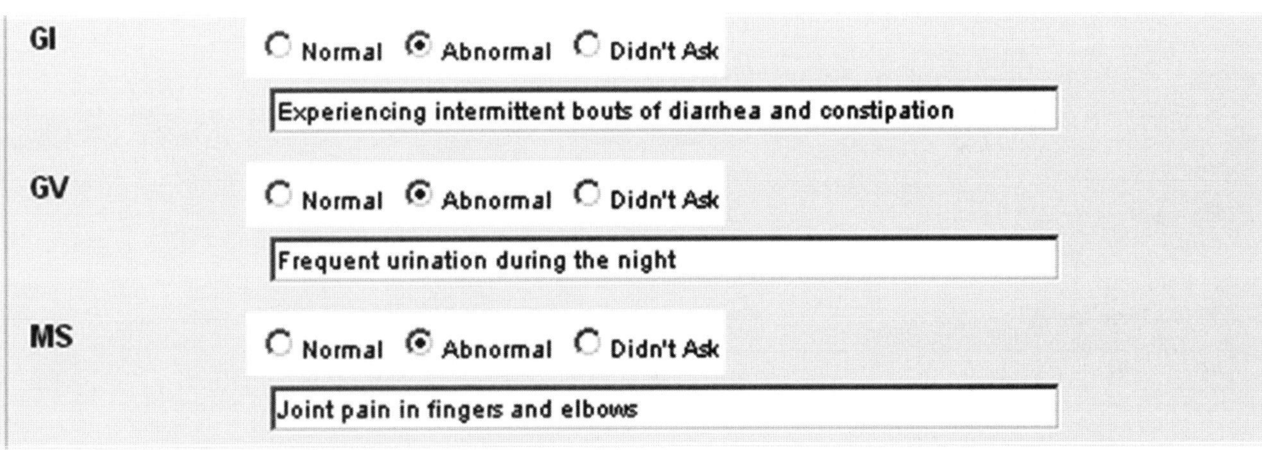


Reprinted with permission of TriMed Technologies, Corp.

4. Click Save when you are finished.

# TASK 5-4: ENTERING PATIENT VITAL SIGNS ON A PATIENT NOTE

After taking the patient's vital signs, enter them into the new Note.

1. Still in Perry Marshall's chart, select the Exam tab.
2. Enter the following information in the appropriate fields:
    - Height: 73 inches
    - Weight: 210 pounds
    - Blood Pressure (sitting): 120/65
    - Pulse: 67
    - Respiration: 17
    - Temperature: 98.6°F

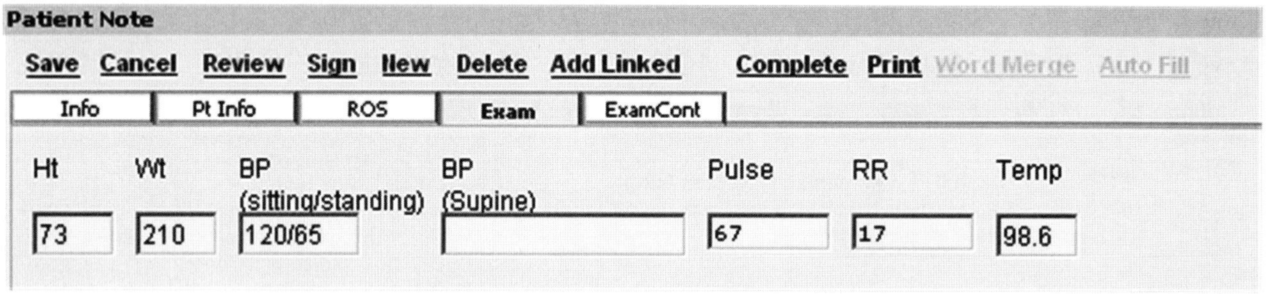


Reprinted with permission of TriMed Technologies, Corp.

3. Click Save when you are finished. The provider will complete the rest of this page during the exam.
4. Now click the Print button, and select PDF Form. Print to your local printer, and label the printout as Task 5-4.
5. When you are done, minimize the right side of the screen by clicking on the same Box on the right of the screen, above the envelope icon.
6. Then, click the X on the Routine Exam tab.

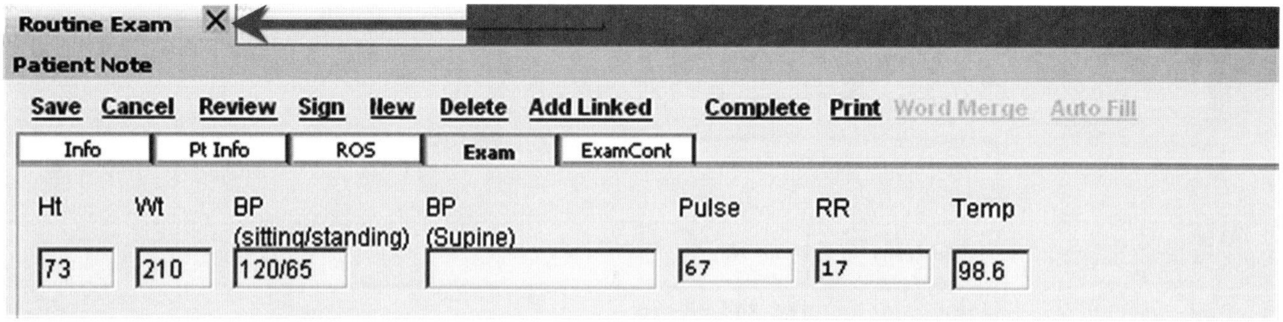


Reprinted with permission of TriMed Technologies, Corp.

# TASK 5-5: NAVIGATING THE PATIENT CHART USING TREE VIEW

This exercise is designed to familiarize you with the navigation of individual patient charts. You should still be in Perry Marshall's chart.

1. So far, you have learned how to enter information in one area of the chart (creating a new Note). On the lower left side of the screen, you should see a group of vertical tabs. This is your "left navigation" bar.

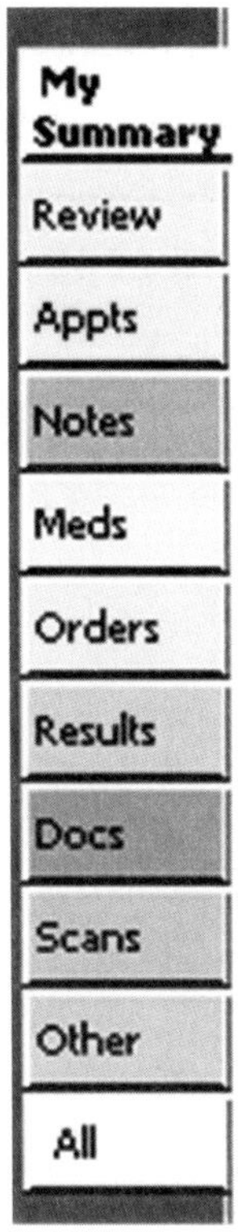


Reprinted with permission of TriMed Technologies, Corp.

2. Click on Appts. This will show all of the appointments that have been scheduled for Perry at the medical office. Make sure the box next to "Tree" is selected (the next step gives more explanation on Tree View). Make sure the box next to "Appts: Inc. Canc" is *not* selected. This suppresses appointments that were cancelled.

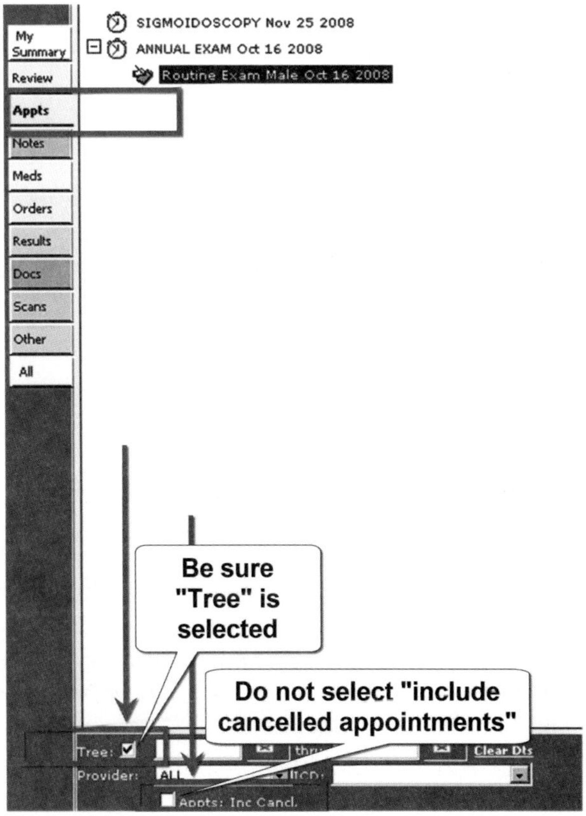


Reprinted with permission of TriMed Technologies, Corp.

3. Tree View shows items as they are connected with one another. So, on your screen, you should see that Perry Marshall has two appointments (one on November 25, and one on October 16). The October 16 appointment has a patient Note associated with it. The Tree View will continue to build when additional items are added to the patient's chart during each appointment.

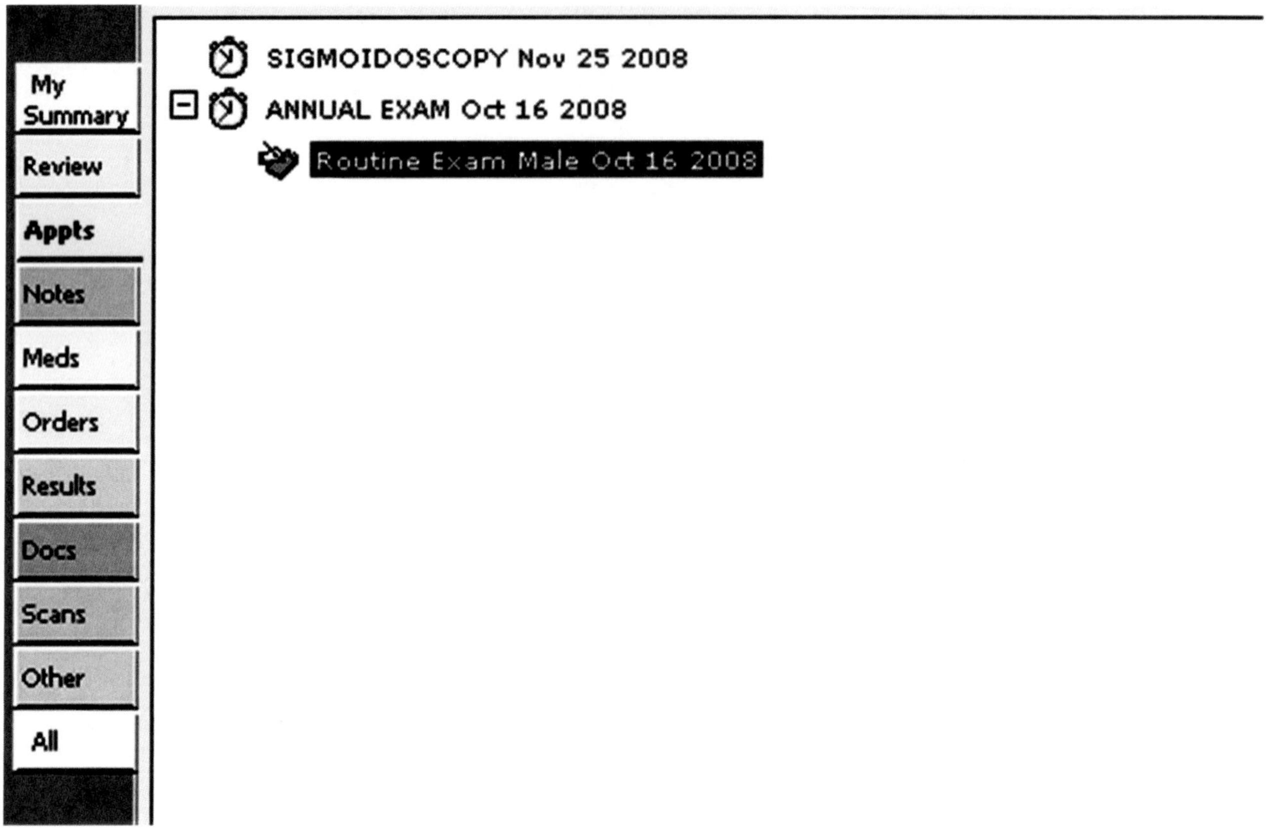


Reprinted with permission of TriMed Technologies, Corp.

4. Click on the Home button at the top of the screen to return to the EHR schedule.

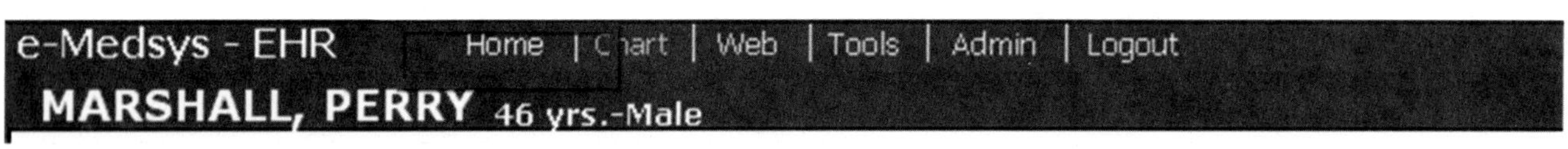


Reprinted with permission of TriMed Technologies, Corp.

# PUTTING IT ALL TOGETHER

## TASK 5-6: LINKING A NEW ANNUAL EXAM NOTE TO A PATIENT APPOINTMENT

Without using step-by-step instructions as given in the previous tasks, this task requires you to (1) receive the patient (indicating Arrived on the schedule), (2) update patient information (indicating Registered on the schedule), (3) admit the patient using the EHR schedule, (4) link a new Note to the patient's appointment, and (5) enter information and vital signs in the new Note.

Garfield Poindexter arrives for his appointment on November 18, 2008. Using the following information, enter data in his chart prior to being seen for his annual exam with Dr. Zues. Upon check-in, Mr. Poindexter indicates that he has a new work phone number, (310) 558-2893 x112, and he now has a cell phone number, (779) 438-3388. He has also advised you that his emergency contact is Gayle Rafferty with a contact number of (779) 438-2397.

When you have finished entering the information in the patient's record, print your work and label it Task 5-6.

| | |
|---|---|
| Chief Complaint | Annual Physical Exam (*hint:* this is now in the drop-down list) |
| Also here to discuss: | Sore shoulder for past two weeks, palpitations |
| Surgical History | Arthroscopic surgery on left knee |
| Family History | Mother alive and well; Father deceased one year ago at age 60 by massive heart attack; older brother with history of chronic asthma; younger brother healthy |
| Social History | Single, nonsmoker, social drinker, no illicit drug use, drinks five to eight cups of coffee per day |
| Constitutional | Healthy appearing, no significant weight fluctuations |
| Musculoskeletal | Pain in left shoulder, left ankle gives out sometimes |
| Neurological | Headaches (several per week) |
| Gastrointestinal | Frequent nausea without vomiting |
| Height | 75 inches |
| Weight | 237 pounds |
| Blood Pressure | 118/70 (sitting) |
| Pulse | 70 |
| Respiration | 19 |
| Temperature | 99.1 |

## TASK 5-7: LINKING A NEW MULTISYSTEM EXAM NOTE TO A PATIENT APPOINTMENT AND ENTERING VITAL SIGNS

Today is October 23, 2008.

You are working with Dr. Appolo today. Delores Bartel is a patient of Dr. Appolo and is being seen today for a cough that has lingered for over a week. The patient does not have registration updates today.

1. Log in to e-Medsys®.
2. Using the steps learned in Module 4, indicate on the appointment schedule that the patient has arrived and is registered.
3. Click on EHR from the top menu, and then select EHR Home Page from the drop-down box. This opens the EHR Home Page in a new window.
4. Open Dr. Appolo's schedule on the EHR schedule, and navigate to today's date.
5. Find Delores's appointment, and indicate that she has been Admitted.

6. Using the EHR schedule, right click on the patient's appointment, and link a new Note to the appointment.

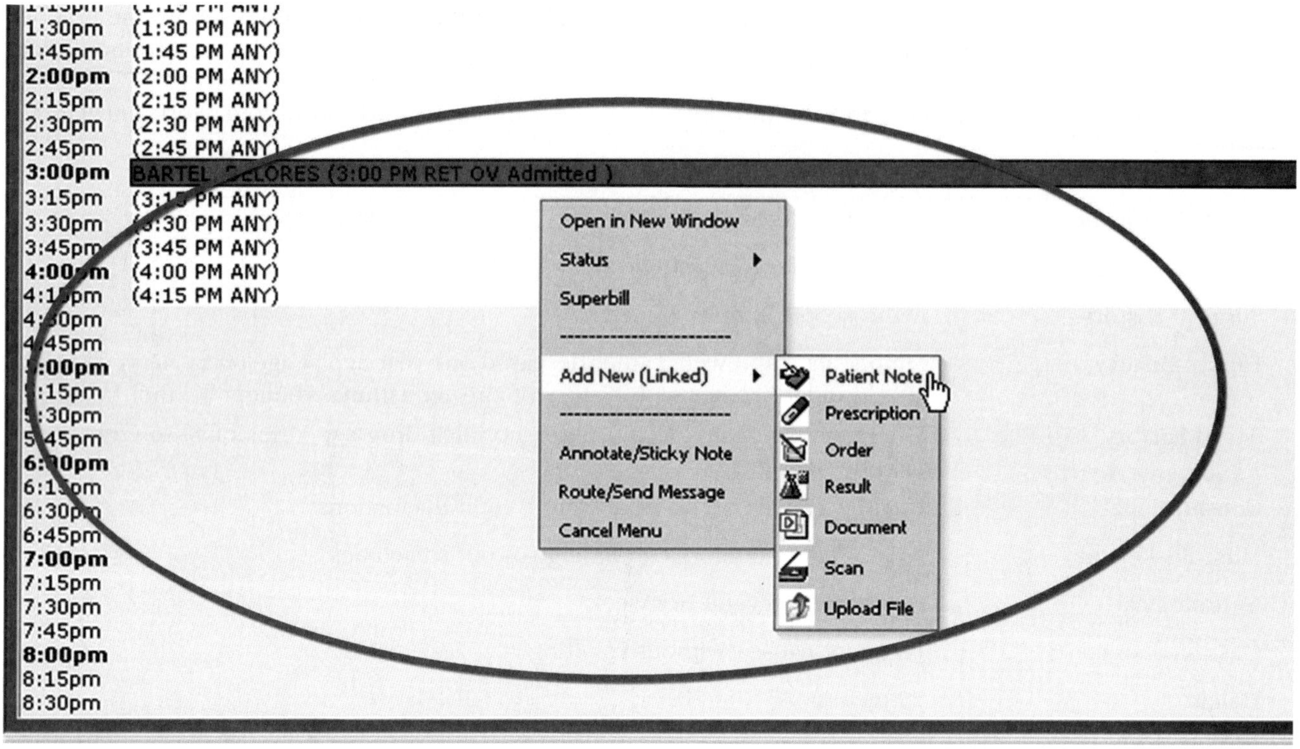

Reprinted with permission of TriMed Technologies, Corp.

7. Now the patient's individual chart appears on the screen, and the lower right side of the screen has a New Note. (Recall that you can enlarge the New Note while you are working in it.) In the Template field, use the drop-down to select MultisystemE&M1. Change the Date to 10/23/2008. Click Save.

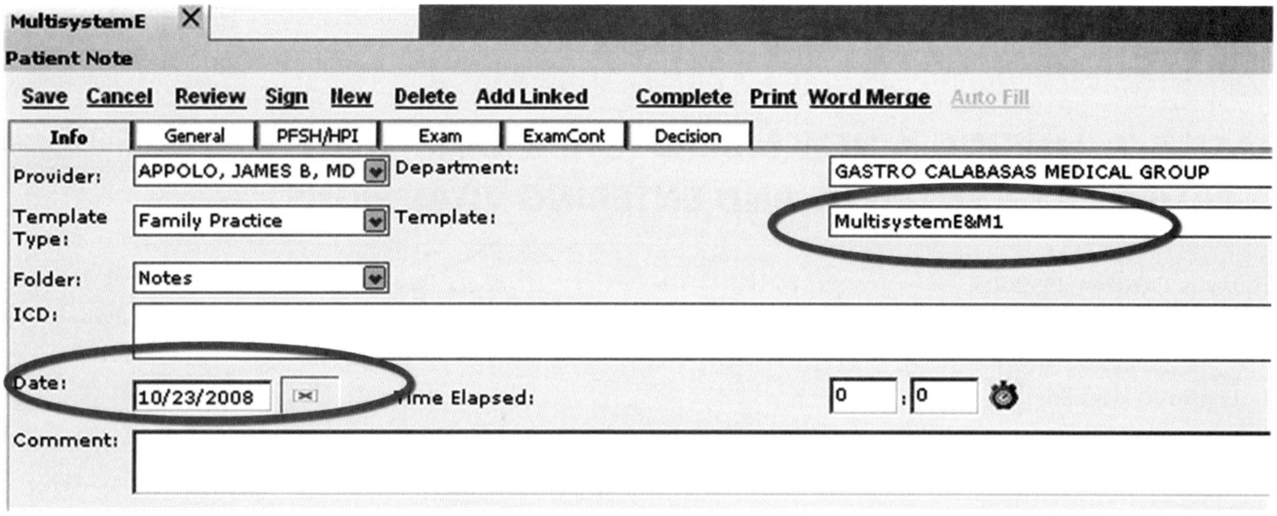

Reprinted with permission of TriMed Technologies, Corp.

8. Now, click on the General tab. Enter the following information:

- Height: 66 inches
- Weight: 148 pounds
- Blood Pressure: 117/67 (sitting)
- Pulse: 66
- Respiration: 25 (rapid and shallow)
- Temperature: 102°F
- General appearance: Ashen, lethargic
- CC: Has had a lingering cough for over a week

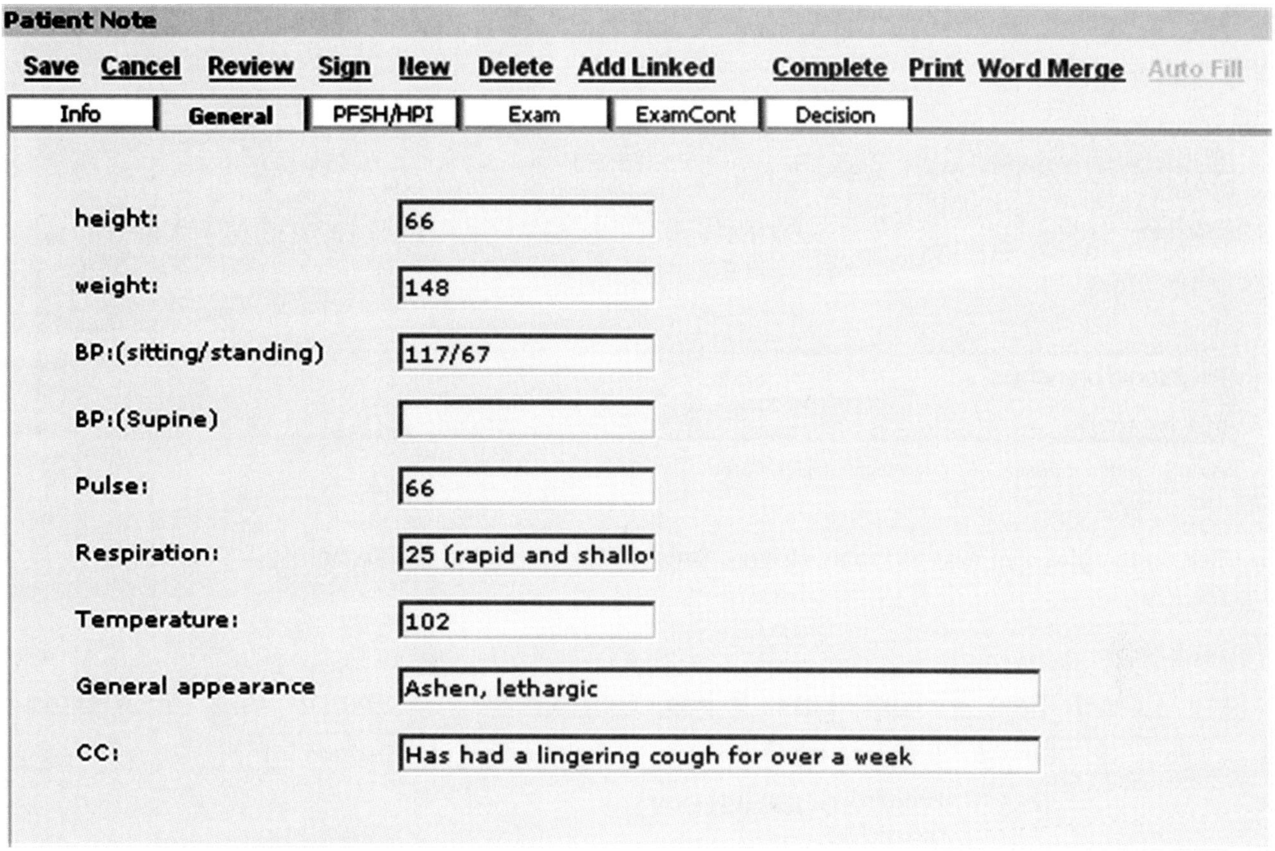


Reprinted with permission of TriMed Technologies, Corp.

9. When you are finished entering this information, click Save.

## TASK 5-8: ENTERING PATIENT, FAMILY, AND SOCIAL HISTORY (PFSH) ON A PATIENT NOTE

1. Still in the same note, click on the PFSH/HPI tab.
2. Click on the box with the three dots next to the Social History field and select "smokes" and "drinks." (Clicking anywhere outside of the drop-down box will return you to the PFSH screen.)

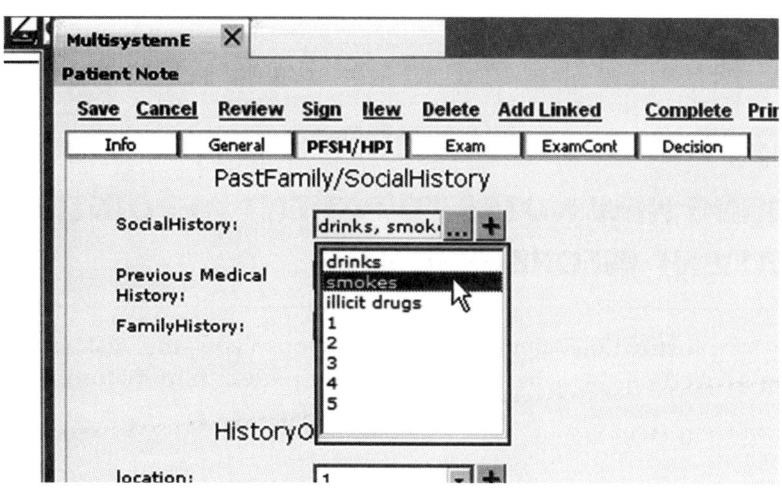


Reprinted with permission of TriMed Technologies, Corp.

3. Click on the plus sign next to Previous Medical History.
4. Enter Chronic bronchitis in the pop-up box and click OK.

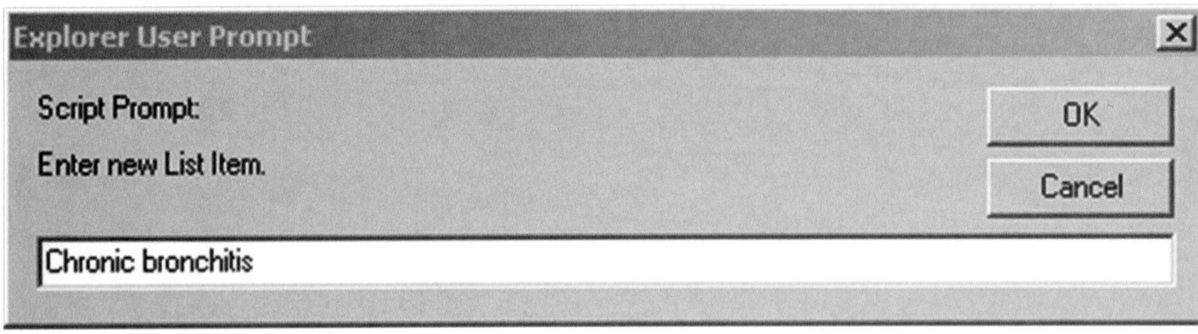


Reprinted with permission of TriMed Technologies, Corp.

5. Click on the plus sign next to Family History. Enter COPD in the pop-up box and click OK.

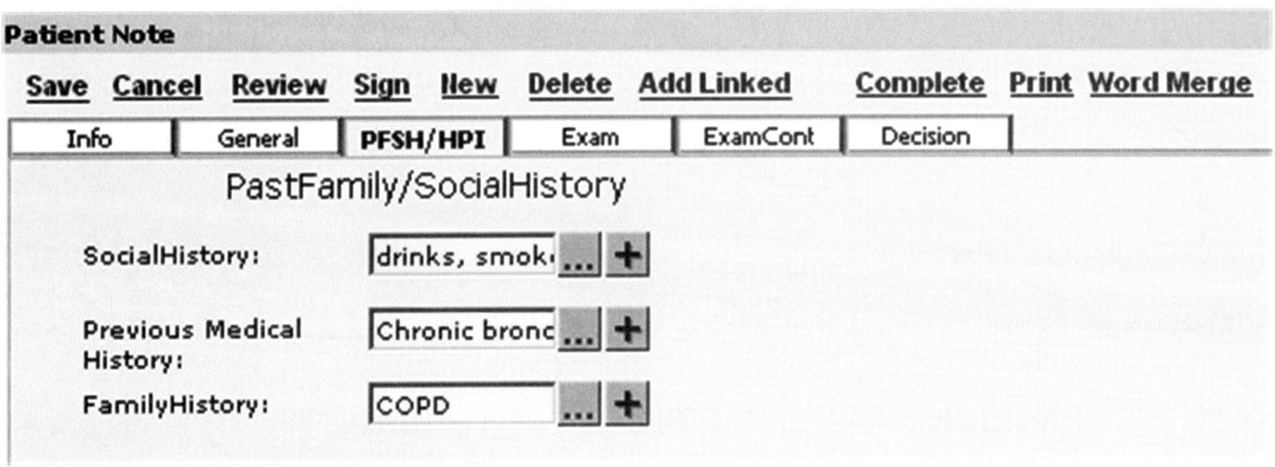


Reprinted with permission of TriMed Technologies, Corp.

6. Click Save when you have finished. The provider will complete the rest of this page during the exam.
7. Now click the Print button, and select PDF Form. Print to your local printer, and label the printout as Task 5-8.
8. When you are done, minimize the right side of the screen.
9. Then, click the X on the MultisystemE tab.

# PUTTING IT ALL TOGETHER

## TASK 5-9: LINKING NEW NOTES TO PATIENT APPOINTMENTS AND RECORDING PATIENT INFORMATION

Without using step-by-step instructions as given in the previous tasks, this task requires you to (1) receive the patient (indicating Arrived on the schedule), (2) update patient information if appropriate (indicating

Registered on the schedule), (3) admit the patient using the EHR schedule, (4) link a new Note to the patient's appointment, and (5) enter information and vital signs in the new Note.

1. Bruce Sawtelle arrives for his appointment on November 14, 2008. He has no updates to his registration information. Using the following information, create a multisystem exam template note for Bruce Sawtelle, who is being seen by Dr. Appolo for gastroenteritis. When you have finished entering the information in the patient's record, print your work and label it Task 5-9A.

| | |
|---|---|
| Height | 69 inches |
| Weight | 186 pounds |
| Blood Pressure | 120/72 (sitting) |
| Pulse | 67 |
| Respirations | 16 |
| Temperature | 100.4°F |
| General Appearance | Slightly flushed, guarded |
| Social History | Married with two children, both healthy; nonsmoker, drinks two bottles of beer per day during the week and about one six-pack per day on weekends, sometimes accompanied by hard liquor |
| Previous Medical History | Chronic asthma |
| Family History | Mother alive—hypertension, diabetes, and ulcerative colitis; Father alive—prostate Ca, and hypercholesterolemia; younger sister healthy with no chronic conditions |

2. Cory Haines arrives for his appointment on November 17, 2008. He has no updates to his registration information. Using the following information, create a new multisystem exam template for Cory Haines who is being seen by Dr. Zues for a tick bite on his lower leg. When you have finished entering the information in the patient's record, print your work and label it Task 5-9B.

| | |
|---|---|
| Height | 72 inches |
| Weight | 198 pounds |
| Blood Pressure | 117/67 (sitting) |
| Pulse | 65 |
| Respirations | 17 |
| Temperature | 98.6°F |
| General Appearance | Healthy, in no acute distress |
| Social History | Single, nonsmoker, social drinker. Physically active, involved in hiking and working out at the gym. Employed as a surgical technician |
| Previous Medical History | Fractured tibia—right leg |
| Family History | Mother alive and healthy; Father alive and healthy; younger sister and two brothers all healthy with no chronic conditions |

3. Julie McMurrey arrives for her appointment on October 7, 2008, to discuss her recent unexplained weight loss with Dr. Venus. Using the information in the following table, enter data in her chart prior to being seen for her annual exam with Dr. Venus. Additionally, when she checks into the office, she says she and her husband have moved to a new address: 439 Crandall Wood Drive, Simi Valley, CA 93065. All other information remains the same. She would like to add her husband, Brian Austin, as her emergency contact. His cell phone number is 805-312-6765. When you have finished entering the information in the patient's record, print your work and label it Task 5-7C.

| | |
|---|---|
| Height | 67 inches |
| Weight | 106 pounds |
| Blood Pressure | 117/68 (sitting) |
| Pulse | 68 |
| Respiration | 18 |
| Temperature | 98.4°F |
| General Appearance | Healthy appearing |
| Social History | Married, three children all alive and healthy, nonsmoker, nondrinker, works in healthcare as an RN, no illicit drug use |
| Previous Medical History | T&A; appendectomy |
| Family History | Mother, uterine Ca at 55 TAH performed, hypertension; Father, chronic bronchitis due to smoking, hypertension, hypercholesterolemia; two sisters, both alive and healthy |

MODULE 7

# Recording Therapeutic Injections and Immunizations

**OBJECTIVES**

In this module, you will:

1. Document administration of therapeutic injections ordered by the provider and administered by the medical assistant.
2. Complete a superbill for the administration of therapeutic injections.

## TASK 7-1: DOCUMENTING ADMINISTRATION OF A THERAPEUTIC INJECTION FOR JODIE MILLER

Today is October 28, 2008.

Jodie Miller is a patient of Dr. Zues and is coming in today at 10 a.m. for an injection for her rheumatoid arthritis (714.0). She is seeing only the MA today; there will be no physician visit. Dr. Zues has ordered 3 mg of Celestone to be administered to the patient.

1. Log in to e-Medsys®.
2. Using the steps learned in Module 4, indicate on the appointment schedule that the patient has Arrived and Registered. (The patient has no registration updates.)
3. Then, open the EHR Home Page, and using the steps learned in Module 5, indicate on the EHR schedule that the patient has been Admitted.
4. Double click on Jodie's appointment on the EHR schedule to bring up Jodie's chart.

5. In Jodie's chart, on the left side of the screen, right click on today's appointment.

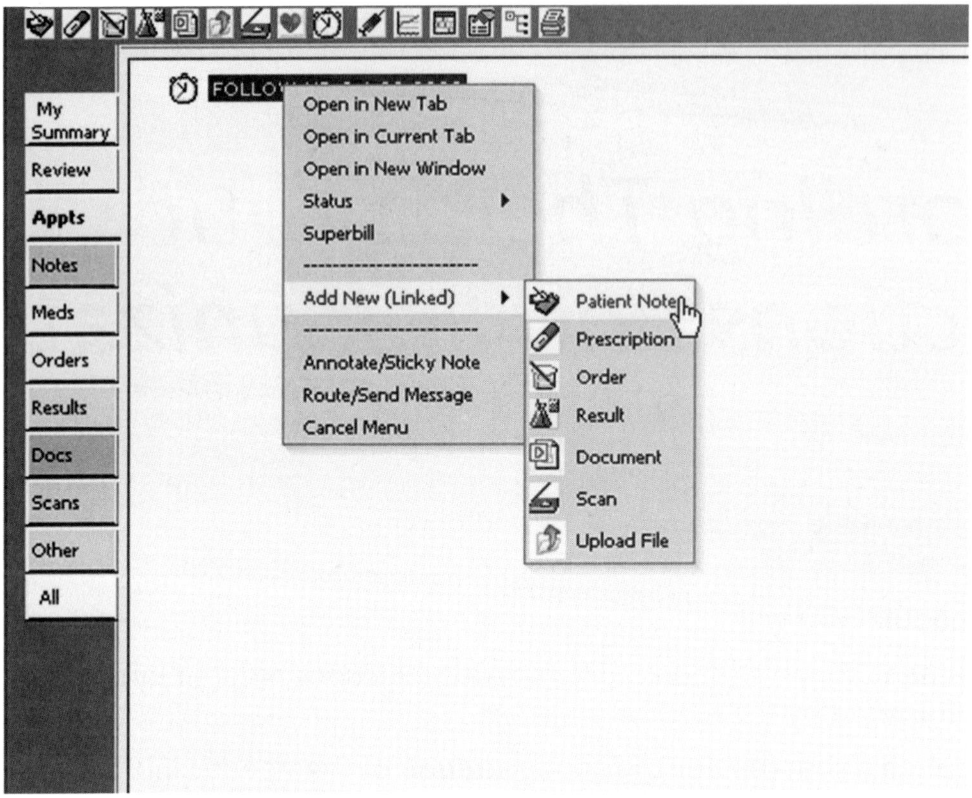


Reprinted with permission of TriMed Technologies, Corp.

6. Select Add New (Linked) ▶ and then Patient Note. The new Note appears on the right side of the screen. You may enlarge the note if you prefer.
7. The Provider, Department, Template Type, and Folder are autopopulated. Be sure that in the Template field None is selected.
8. In the ICD field, click on the binoculars to search for rheumatoid arthritis.
9. With the radio button next to Search selected, type rheu and press Enter on your keyboard. Now the ICD field is populated with the correct code, 714.0.
10. Enter the date of administration, 10/28/2008.
11. In the Comments section, type "3 mg of Celestone administered by *<insert your name and credentials>*, per Dr. Zues."
12. Check your work with the following screen shot and then click Save.

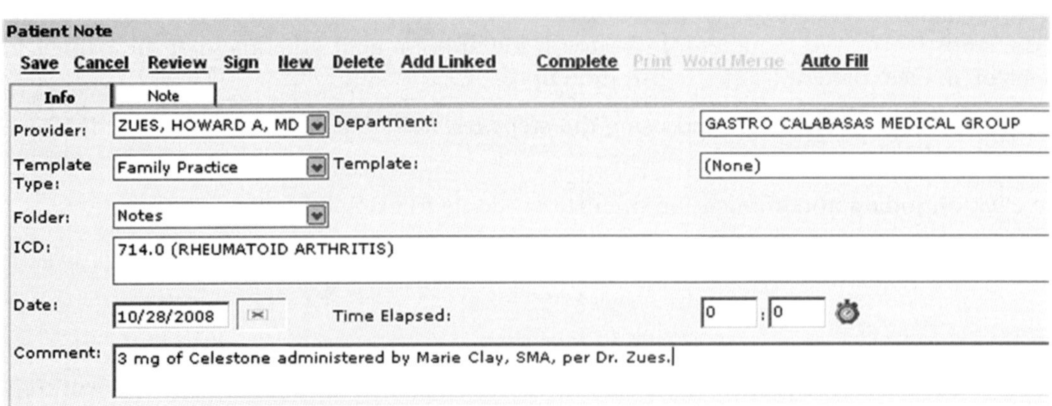


Reprinted with permission of TriMed Technologies, Corp.

13. When you are certain that the information documented is accurate, you will sign off on this note. Click Sign.
14. A new window opens. *Your sign off password is your user Login* (the one that you logged into e-Medsys® with; for example, "user15"). Enter your user Login and click Save.

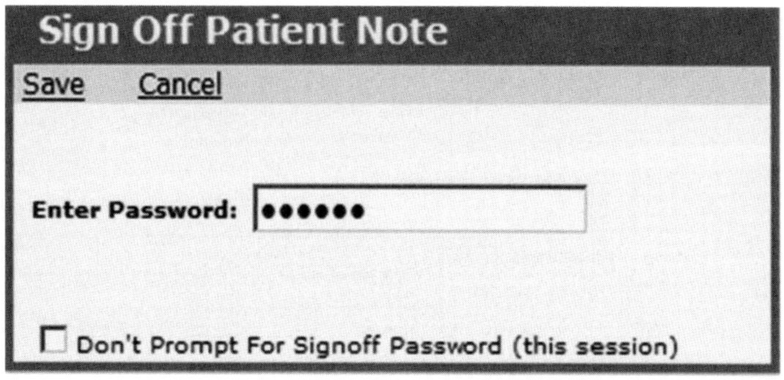


Reprinted with permission of TriMed Technologies, Corp.

15. Now the information that you entered appears grayed out on the screen. This information is part of the patient's permanent record and cannot be further modified.

> **Note:** You must complete this Task and sign off on the note in order to continue to Task 7-2.

## TASK 7-2: COMPLETING A SUPERBILL FOR JODIE MILLER

Complete a superbill indicating the diagnosis of rheumatoid arthritis (714.0), the administration of the drug (90782), and the supply of Celestone (J0702).

1. Still in Jodie Miller's chart, on the left side of the screen, left click on the 10/28/2008 FOLLOW UP appointment, highlighting it.

Reprinted with permission of TriMed Technologies, Corp.

2. When you do this, the right side of the screen brings up more information regarding the appointment. From the right-hand corner of this screen, select the Superbill tab.

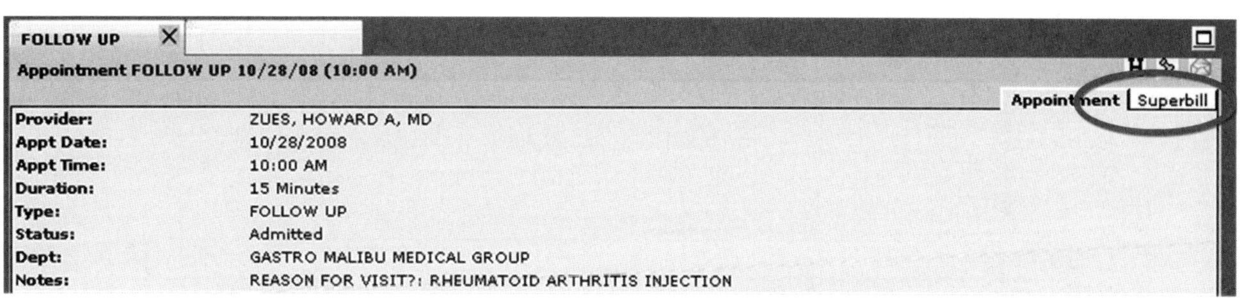


Reprinted with permission of TriMed Technologies, Corp.

3. The electronic superbill appears. Click on the corner box to enlarge while you are working within the superbill.

4. Make sure that Dr. Howard Zues's name appears in the Provider field. Leave the second provider field blank.
5. In the Date field, type 10/28/2008. The Insurance field is autopopulated based on the patient's insurance.

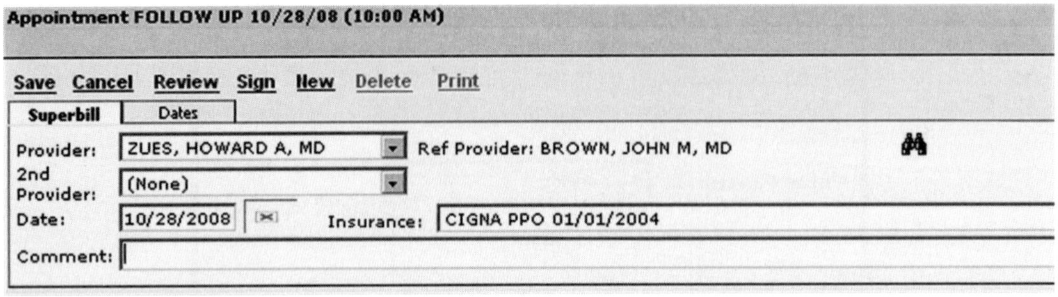


Reprinted with permission of TriMed Technologies, Corp.

6. Below the Comments section, there is a section with three tabs (Ticket, Chart, and Find). The Ticket tab is populated with some of the most common charges used in the medical office. If a charge does not appear on the Ticket tab, you can select the Find tab to look up a CPT code and add it to the superbill. Click on the Find tab.

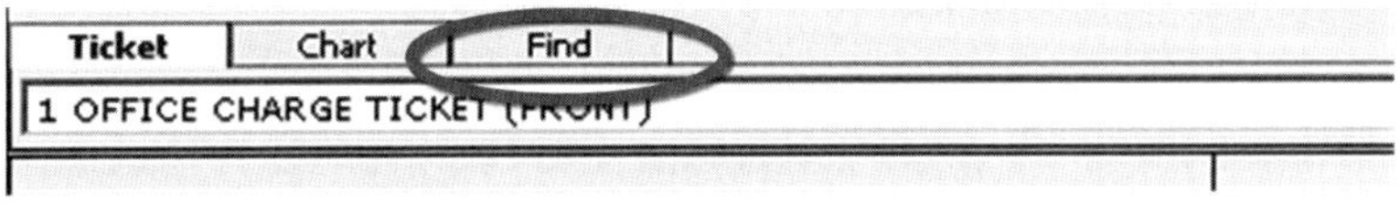


Reprinted with permission of TriMed Technologies, Corp.

7. Type 90782 (the administration of the drug) and then press Enter on your keyboard.
8. Now the procedure code appears below the search field, with a box next to it. Click on the box to select it. When you do, a row at the bottom opens that indicates your selection.

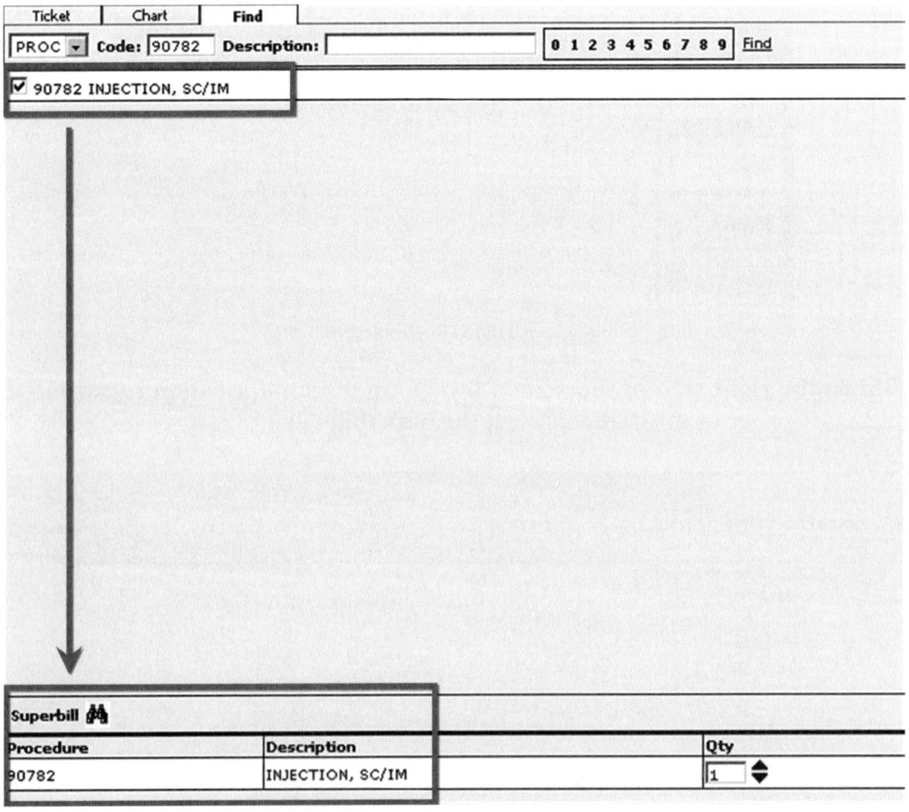


Reprinted with permission of TriMed Technologies, Corp.

9. Move your mouse into the Diag1 field. When you do, an icon of binoculars appears.

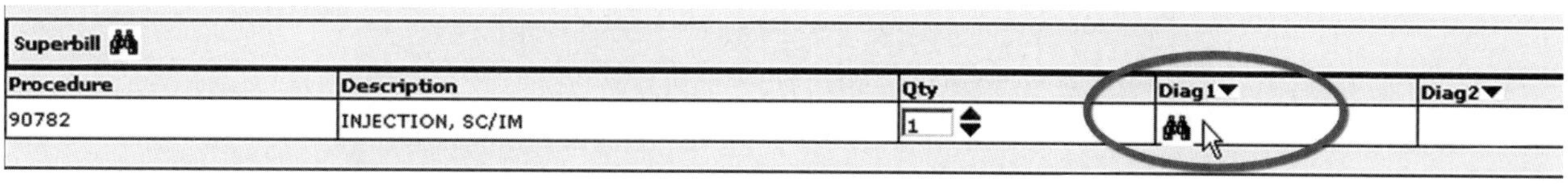


Reprinted with permission of TriMed Technologies, Corp.

10. Click on the binoculars. Now the cursor moves back up to the Code field. Type rheu in the Description field (to search for rheumatoid arthritis) and press Enter on your keyboard.
11. Now the diagnosis code appears below the search field, with a box next to it.

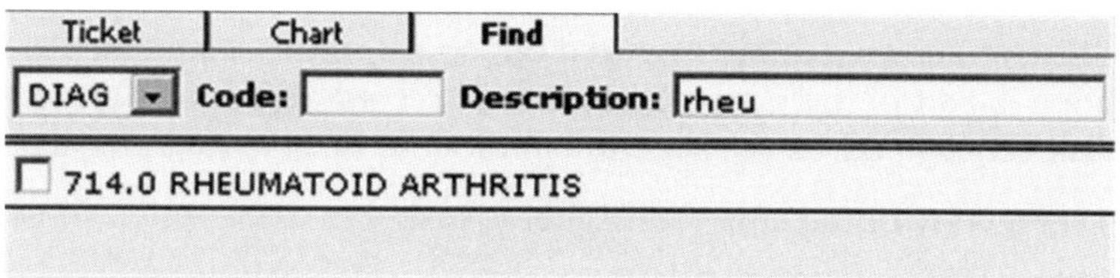


Reprinted with permission of TriMed Technologies, Corp.

12. Click on the box to select it. When you do, note that the diagnosis code now appears in the Diag1 box at the bottom.
13. Click Save. Now you are back on the Ticket tab.
14. The next CPT code is listed on the Ticket tab, so scroll down and select the box next to J0702 for the supply of Celestone. Note that when you select the box, a new row appears at the bottom.

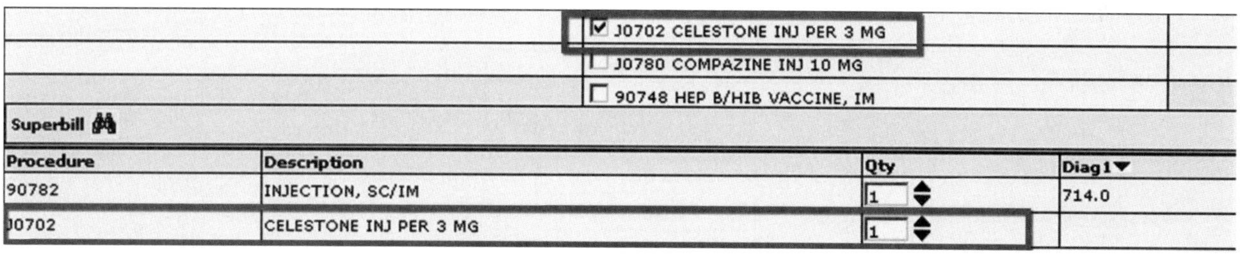


Reprinted with permission of TriMed Technologies, Corp.

15. Now, click on the triangle next to Diag1. This copies the diagnosis code that you had previously selected and enters it into the Celestone row.

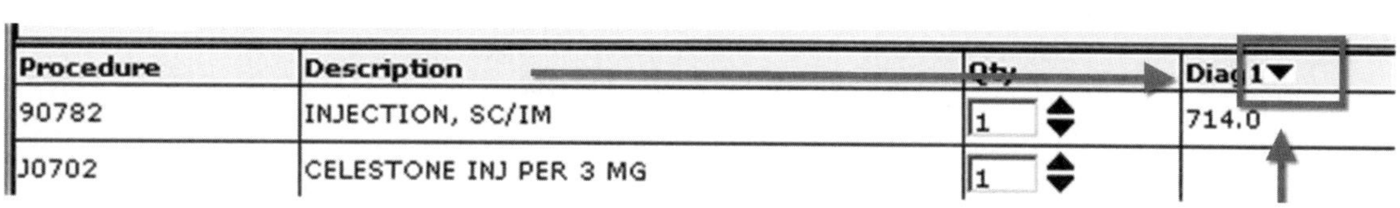


Reprinted with permission of TriMed Technologies, Corp.

16. Click Save.
17. When you are certain that the information documented is accurate, you will sign off on these charges. Click Sign.

18. A new window opens. *Your sign off password is your user Login* (the one that you logged into e-Medsys® with; for example, "user15"). Enter your user Login and click Save.

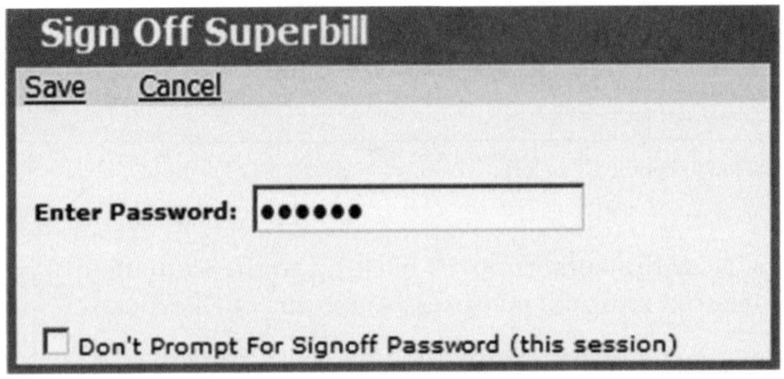


Reprinted with permission of TriMed Technologies, Corp.

19. Now the information that you entered appears grayed out on the screen, and a lock icon appears on the Superbill tab. This information is part of the patient's permanent record and cannot be further modified. *Note:* You must complete this Task and sign off on the superbill in order to be able to perform the tasks in Module 9.
20. Now click Print to print a copy of the superbill. Label it Task 7-2. Close when finished.

## Troubleshooting: Ensuring the Superbill is Signed Off

If you are unclear whether you have signed off on the superbill, follow these steps:

1. Go to the EHR schedule.
2. Find Jodie Miller's appointment on the schedule. (*Hint:* Select Dr. Zues as the provider and 10/28/2008 as the date.)
3. On the right side of the screen beneath the calendar, click on the radio button next to List.

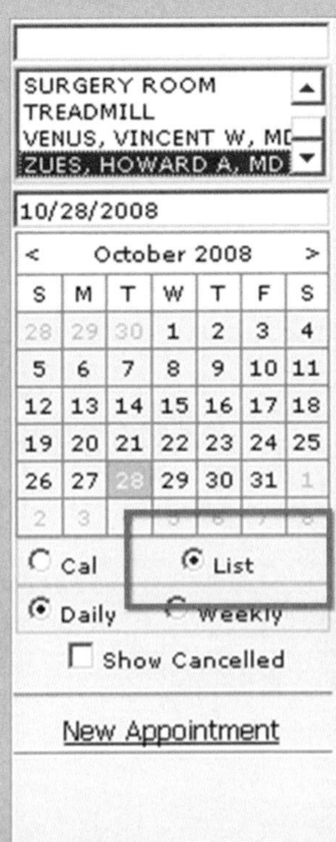


Reprinted with permission of TriMed Technologies, Corp.

4. Now, the left side of the screen brings up the schedule in List view. In this view, there is a Superbill column. In this column, the status of the superbill is indicated:
   - *Signed* means the superbill has been signed off on.
   - *Saved* means the superbill has been created, but not signed off on.
   - If there is nothing in this column, the superbill has not been created.
5. If you have followed the steps in Task 7-2, the Superbill column for Jodie Miller should indicate *Signed*.

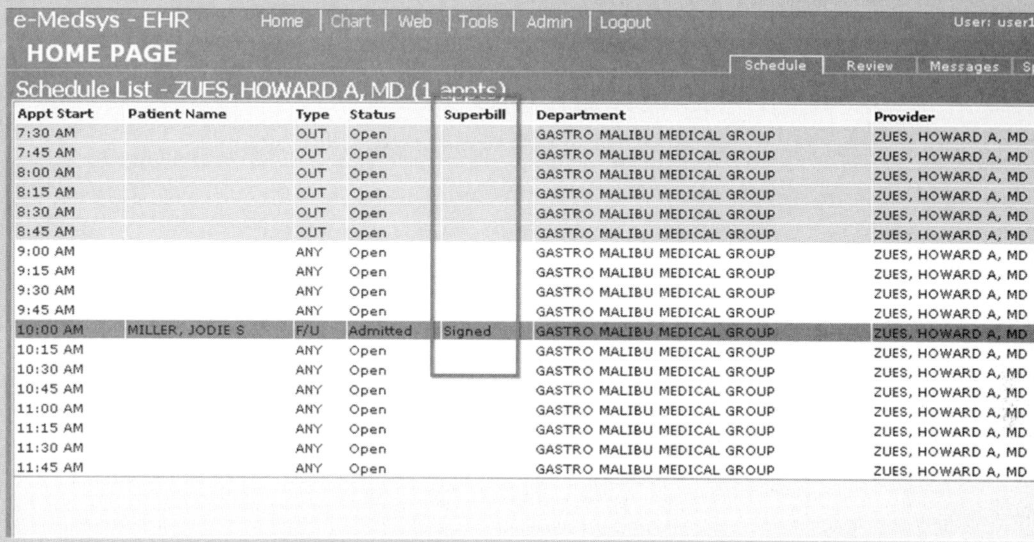

e-Medsys - EHR | Home | Chart | Web | Tools | Admin | Logout | User: user1

HOME PAGE

Schedule | Review | Messages | Sp

Schedule List - ZUES, HOWARD A, MD (1 appts)

| Appt Start | Patient Name | Type | Status | Superbill | Department | Provider |
|---|---|---|---|---|---|---|
| 7:30 AM | | OUT | Open | | GASTRO MALIBU MEDICAL GROUP | ZUES, HOWARD A, MD |
| 7:45 AM | | OUT | Open | | GASTRO MALIBU MEDICAL GROUP | ZUES, HOWARD A, MD |
| 8:00 AM | | OUT | Open | | GASTRO MALIBU MEDICAL GROUP | ZUES, HOWARD A, MD |
| 8:15 AM | | OUT | Open | | GASTRO MALIBU MEDICAL GROUP | ZUES, HOWARD A, MD |
| 8:30 AM | | OUT | Open | | GASTRO MALIBU MEDICAL GROUP | ZUES, HOWARD A, MD |
| 8:45 AM | | OUT | Open | | GASTRO MALIBU MEDICAL GROUP | ZUES, HOWARD A, MD |
| 9:00 AM | | ANY | Open | | GASTRO MALIBU MEDICAL GROUP | ZUES, HOWARD A, MD |
| 9:15 AM | | ANY | Open | | GASTRO MALIBU MEDICAL GROUP | ZUES, HOWARD A, MD |
| 9:30 AM | | ANY | Open | | GASTRO MALIBU MEDICAL GROUP | ZUES, HOWARD A, MD |
| 9:45 AM | | ANY | Open | | GASTRO MALIBU MEDICAL GROUP | ZUES, HOWARD A, MD |
| 10:00 AM | MILLER, JODIE S | F/U | Admitted | Signed | GASTRO MALIBU MEDICAL GROUP | ZUES, HOWARD A, MD |
| 10:15 AM | | ANY | Open | | GASTRO MALIBU MEDICAL GROUP | ZUES, HOWARD A, MD |
| 10:30 AM | | ANY | Open | | GASTRO MALIBU MEDICAL GROUP | ZUES, HOWARD A, MD |
| 10:45 AM | | ANY | Open | | GASTRO MALIBU MEDICAL GROUP | ZUES, HOWARD A, MD |
| 11:00 AM | | ANY | Open | | GASTRO MALIBU MEDICAL GROUP | ZUES, HOWARD A, MD |
| 11:15 AM | | ANY | Open | | GASTRO MALIBU MEDICAL GROUP | ZUES, HOWARD A, MD |
| 11:30 AM | | ANY | Open | | GASTRO MALIBU MEDICAL GROUP | ZUES, HOWARD A, MD |
| 11:45 AM | | ANY | Open | | GASTRO MALIBU MEDICAL GROUP | ZUES, HOWARD A, MD |

Reprinted with permission of TriMed Technologies, Corp.

6. If the column does not indicate *Signed*, go back into Jodie's chart. (*Hint:* Mouse over Chart on the top menu, and click on Jodie Miller from the drop-down list.) The superbill must be signed off on in order to complete Module 9.

# PUTTING IT ALL TOGETHER

## TASK 7-3: RECORDING ADMINISTRATION OF INJECTIONS AND CREATING SUPERBILLS

Without using step-by-step instructions as given in the previous tasks, this task requires you to (1) receive the patient (indicating Arrived and Registered on the schedule), (2) admit the patient using the EHR schedule, (3) create a new patient note to record the administration of injections, and (4) create and sign off on the superbill. *Note:* The superbill must be signed off on in order to complete Module 9.

1. On October 29, 2008, at 11:30 a.m., Crystal Nowell, a patient of Dr. Appolo, came in for her B-12 shot to be administered by the MA without a physician visit. Using the steps outlined in the earlier tasks and the information in the following list, document the administration of the injection and create a superbill for her. Print out the superbill and label it Task 7-3A.
   - Diagnosis: Vitamin B Deficiency
   - Diagnosis Code: 281.1
   - Administration Code: 90782
   - Substance Injected Code: J3420

2. Burt Ringer, a patient of Dr. Appolo, comes in the office for a tetanus shot on November 11, 2008, at 3 p.m. Using the steps outlined in the earlier tasks and the information in the following list, document the administration of the injection and create a superbill for him. Print out the superbill and label it Task 7-3B.

   - Diagnosis: Need for tetanus vaccination
   - Diagnosis Code: V03.7
   - Administration Code: 90782
   - Substance Administered Code: 90703

Chapter 6

# OB/GYN EXAMINATIONS

## OBJECTIVES

In this chapter, you will learn the following:

### KB KNOWLEDGE BASE

1. Spell and define, using the glossary at the back of the text, all the Words to Know in this chapter.
2. Differentiate between gynecology and obstetrics.
3. Identify five reasons the liquid-based Pap test is preferred.
4. Interpret the American Cancer Society (ACS) guidelines for frequency of Pap tests.
5. Identify four specific ACS patient preparation instructions for more accurate Pap results.
6. Stress why breast self-examination is necessary even when the provider performs an annual exam.
7. Give two reasons the medical assistant should accompany the provider when a pelvic exam is performed.
8. List the three main Pap test reporting categories.
9. Identify three processes or procedures done to confirm a diagnosis of pregnancy.
10. List five general responsibilities of the medical assistant in prenatal care.
11. Explain how to determine the estimated due date using Naegele's rule.
12. List seven assessment responsibilities of the MA before the provider performs the prenatal examination.

### S SKILLS

1. Prepare a patient for and assist with a gynecological exam and Pap test.

### B BEHAVIOR

1. Apply critical thinking skills in performing patient assessment and care.
2. Use language and verbal skills that enable patients' understanding.
3. Apply active listening skills.
4. Use appropriate body language and other nonverbal skills in communicating with patients' family and staff.
5. Demonstrate awareness of the territorial boundaries of the person with whom communicating.
6. Demonstrate recognition of the patient's level of understanding in communications.
7. Recognize and protect personal boundaries in communicating with others.
8. Explain the rationale for performance of procedure to the patient.
9. Show awareness of patients' concerns regarding their perceptions of the procedure being performed.

## WORDS TO KNOW

atypical
cervical
cytology
douche
endocervical
exfoliated
fundus
gestation
Lamaze
Naegele's rule
Papanicolaou
pregnancy
prenatal
ThinPrep
trimester
vaginitis

## GYNECOLOGICAL EXAM

In assisting with the complete physical exam (CPE, discussed in Chapter 40), the examination of the vagina and genitalia was described as part of the total exam; however, a Pap test is not necessarily done at that time. Women may schedule appointments with their general or family practitioners for a Pap test or might prefer to see a gynecologist for this type of examination. The OB/GYN (obstetrics/gynecology) practice focuses on the female reproductive system. (Refer to Chapter 35 for a complete discussion of the anatomy and physiology of this system.) Obstetrics focuses on pregnancy and childbirth, whereas the gynecology practice addresses diseases and disorders of the female reproductive system. When a patient calls a general or family practice for an appointment, be sure to make a distinction between a physical exam and a gynecological exam with a Pap test so that the appropriate amount of time is allotted and proper instructions are given. Remember that the CPE is a review of systems (ROS) of the total body, and the gynecologic exam is of the female reproductive organs only.

### PATIENT EDUCATION

Remind the patient at the time she schedules the appointment for a Pap test that she should not **douche** or engage in sexual intercourse for 48 hours before the examination. Because the specimen analysis could be misinterpreted during the menstrual flow, the patient should be advised to schedule the test about five days after her period.

## THE PAP TEST

The **Papanicolaou** (Pap) technique is a cytological screening test to detect cancer of the cervix. This method of detection was developed by an American physician, George N. Papanicolaou, in 1883. This simple smear technique used samples taken from the vagina, the cervix, and the endocervix to look for **atypical cytology**. The samples were smeared onto slides and then sprayed with a fixative or placed in an alcohol solution and sent to a lab. Studies have shown that the technique produced many inadequate specimens, sometimes requiring repeating the procedure. Up to two thirds of the false negative reports were caused by the limitations of the sampling technique and the slide preparation. Often, cells on the slide were piled up so those underneath could not be seen. Additionally, **cervical** cells were hidden by pus cells from infection, yeast cells, bacteria, and increased mucus. Therefore, precancerous cells were not visible, and the results were incorrectly reported negative. Furthermore, if the slide was not treated immediately after the smear was done, the cells dried out and became distorted, leading to possible reading errors.

In May 1996, after 50 years of conventional Pap testing, the U.S. Food and Drug Administration (FDA) approved a new, liquid-based method known by the brand names of **ThinPrep** and AutoCyte. This improved technique involves collecting the sample with a plastic **endocervical** "broom" and immediately placing it into a bottle of preservative solution (Figure 41–1). The broom is swished 10 times in the solution to remove the collected cells. The solution prevents the cells from drying out and significantly reduces the presence of mucus, bacteria, yeast, and pus cells on the slide prepared from the diluted cell samples in the solution.

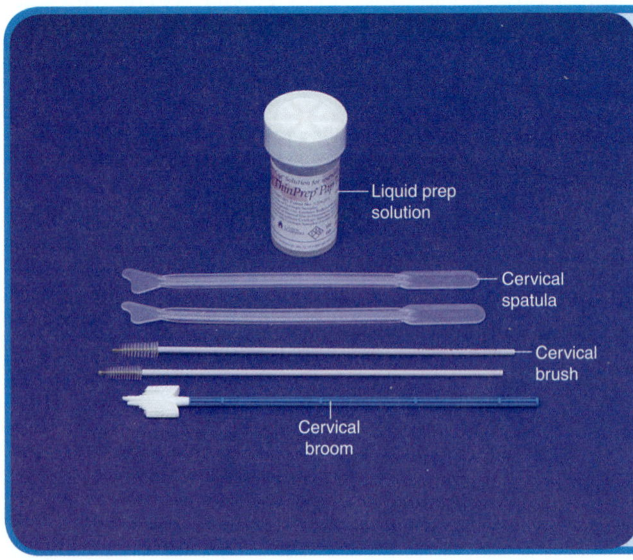


**Figure 41–1:** Liquid prep solution with cervical spatula, brush, and broom. *Delmar/Cengage Learning.*

This technique slightly improves the detection of cancers but greatly improves the detection of precancers. This method also provides the ability to do additional studies from the same sample, such as tests for the presence of HPV, chlamydia, and gonorrhea.

The AutoPap Primary Screening System has been approved by the FDA for use in screening smears before a provider or technologist analyzes them. Anything identified as abnormal would still be examined by a technologist. Additionally, these computerized instruments will retest Pap samples interpreted as normal by technologists, with the intent to detect abnormal cells that are missed by humans.

Female patients usually have the Pap test done routinely either as part of the CPE with their family doctor or by their gynecologist. Patients who have complaints of severe menstrual pain or discomfort, unusual vaginal discharge, or lower abdominal pain (or any other problems) may have a Pap smear taken during the pelvic examination to rule out gynecological problems.

The American Cancer Society recommends the following guidelines for early detection of cervical cancer:

- All women should begin screening tests about three years after they begin having vaginal intercourse but no later than 21 years old. Screening should be done every year with a regular Pap test or every two years with a liquid-based Pap test.
- At age 30, women with three normal Pap tests in a row may have a screening every two to three years with either test method. Women with risk factors such as diethylstilbestrol exposure before birth; HIV infection; or a weakened immune system due to organ transplant, chemotherapy, or chronic steroid use should continue with annual testing.
- An option for women older than 30 is screening every three years plus the HPV DNA test. Human papillomavirus (HPV) is a known risk factor for developing cervical cancer because it can cause normal cells on the cervix to become abnormal. The virus causes changes in cervical cells that can be observed from the Pap test. At least 50 percent of sexually active people will have HPV at some time in their lives, according to the Centers for Disease Control and Prevention (CDC). For more information about HPV, visit www.cdc.gov/hpv.
- Women 70 or older who have had at least three normal Pap tests in a row and no abnormal findings in the past 10 years may choose to stop cervical cancer screening. Women with the risk factors named previously should continue as long as they are in good health.
- Women who have had a total hysterectomy (cervix and uterus removed) may choose to stop screening unless surgery was performed as a treatment for precancerous cells or cervical cancer. Women who have had a hysterectomy without removal of the cervix should still follow the guidelines.

Women should be especially conscientious in scheduling Pap tests if they have a family history of uterine or cervical cancer. You should check with your provider employer for his or her preference and advise patients accordingly.

## Patient Preparation for the Pap Test

When the patient is scheduled for a Pap test, she must be given clear instructions to follow in preparation for the test. The following are recommended by the American Cancer Society for accurate results:

- Do not use tampons, birth control foams, jellies, or other vaginal creams for 48 hours before the test. (They alter the cervical and vaginal environment.)
- Do not douche for 48 hours prior to the test. (Douching could wash away **exfoliated** cancer cells and cause the test to be falsely reported as negative.)
- Do not have sexual intercourse for 48 hours before the test. (This adds extra cells and fluid to the environment, making reading more difficult.)
- Try to schedule the Pap test at least five days after the menstrual period. Avoid scheduling during the period. (Red blood cells make the test more difficult to read.)

## The Medical Assistant's Role in Gynecological Exams

Prior to bringing the patient into the examination room for the pelvic exam and Pap, the medical assistant should make the necessary preparations. As with any procedure or patient contact, wash your hands before you begin. The exam table should have a clean, protective covering. Place a gown and drape sheet on the end of the table for the patient (either cloth or disposable paper).

Prepare the Mayo tray with the instruments and supplies the provider will need to perform the pelvic exam and obtain the Pap test (Figure 41–2). Speculums can be reusable or disposable. Place the tray in a convenient location near the end of the exam table. Cover the equipment with a towel to help allay the patient's anxiety from seeing the equipment. To aid in the inspection part of the pelvic exam, an exam lamp should also be placed within reach of the examiner's stool at the end of the table. (Most lamps are expandable and attached to the wall.)

Call the patient from the reception room to prepare her for the exam. Instruct her to go to the bathroom to empty her bladder before the test. If a specimen is to be

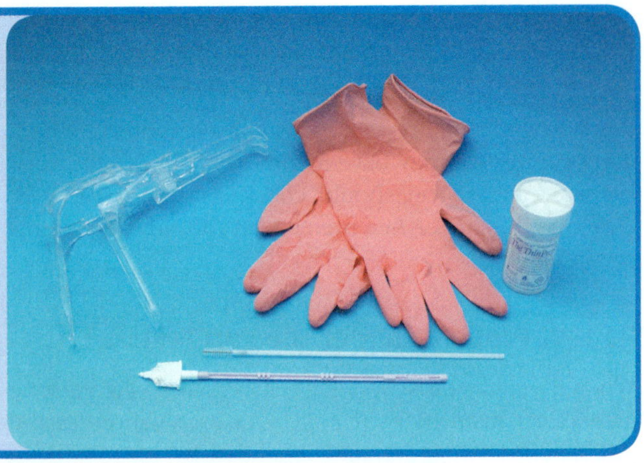

**Figure 41–2:** Equipment for a Pap smear.
*Delmar/Cengage Learning.*

obtained, instruct her in the method of collection. A pelvic examination is uncomfortable for the patient if the bladder is full, besides making the examination difficult for the provider to perform.

> **CLINICAL PEARL**
>
> Pelvic examinations that have to be delayed while the patient goes to the bathroom disrupt the schedule and should be avoided. Certainly there are exceptions; some patients may have trouble with bladder control or some other condition that requires frequent trips to the bathroom. Help these patients feel at ease because they will most likely feel embarrassed.

When the patient comes back to the examination room, try to determine her level of anxiety regarding the examination. Take time to explain the procedure, letting her know what to expect, especially if it is her first time having a pelvic exam. *Never* assume that a patient knows about a procedure. Some patients are both afraid and embarrassed to ask questions because they believe they should already know about procedures. Try to make patients feel comfortable and at ease to help them relax for the exam. Complete the cytology request form (see Figure 41–3), making sure that you ask the patient all necessary questions. Many of the questions that are asked when taking a complete GYN history will be needed for the requisition form. They should include:

- Age at onset of menstrual cycle
- Gravida (how many pregnancies the patient has had)
- Para (how many live births the patient has had)
- Abortions: How many? Were they spontaneous or elective?
- Date of last menstrual period (LMP) (you need to record the day it started)
- Regularity and duration of cycles
- Date of last Pap smear, result, and if any abnormal Pap smear results or biopsies in the past
- Contraception method used
- Hormone replacement therapy (HRT) if patient is taking any
- Date of last mammogram if had one
- Any GYN surgeries and dates
- Past and present sexual activity
- Any abnormal discharge or pain

After the patient is questioned and you fill in the required information on the requisition form, label the ThinPrep collection bottle and place it on the stand. Some requisition forms come with prenumbered stickers you can attach to specimens. This helps eliminate errors from mismatching requisitions to specimens. You can then instruct the patient to undress completely, tell her where to put her belongings, explain how to put on the exam gown with the opening in the front, and offer your assistance if needed. Allow the patient privacy for several minutes to change and then knock before entering to see whether the patient is ready.

Enter the room when the patient lets you know she is ready. Pull out the footstep at the end of the exam table and help her step up onto the exam table and sit at the end. Place the drape sheet over the top of her legs for privacy and warmth. Remember to push the footstep back in after the patient has been seated to avoid injury to you or the provider.

Alert the provider that the patient is ready to be examined. Most providers prefer the medical assistant to accompany them into the exam room, not only to assist with the procedure, but also for legal and safety reasons as discussed in Chapter 39.

Because of the importance of early detection of breast cancer, providers include the breast exam during the patient's annual appointment for the Pap test and pelvic exam. Patients should be reminded to do a breast self-examination each month following their menstrual period (see the Patient Education box in Chapter 40, page 870). Giving them a pamphlet of instructions to take with them for this procedure is recommended (Figure 41–4). Explain to the patient that the exam conducted by the provider with the annual Pap test is important but insufficient in detecting abnormal breast tissue between visits to the provider. Most women discover a lump or mass in their breasts themselves and report it to the provider. This leads to early detection and treatment, which greatly increases the survival rate.

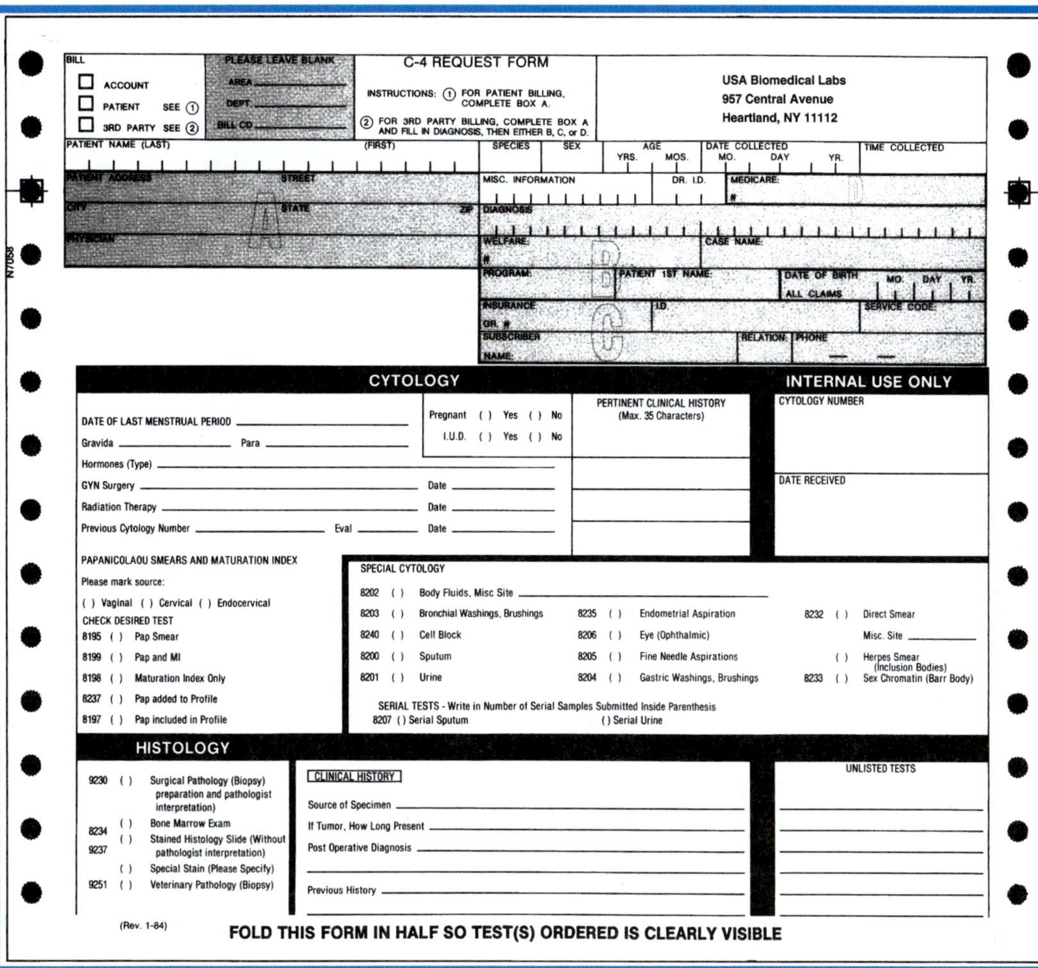

C-4 REQUEST FORM

BILL
☐ ACCOUNT
☐ PATIENT SEE ①
☐ 3RD PARTY SEE ②

PLEASE LEAVE BLANK
AREA
DEPT
BILL CO

INSTRUCTIONS: ① FOR PATIENT BILLING, COMPLETE BOX A.
② FOR 3RD PARTY BILLING, COMPLETE BOX A AND FILL IN DIAGNOSIS, THEN EITHER B, C, or D.

USA Biomedical Labs
957 Central Avenue
Heartland, NY 11112

PATIENT NAME (LAST) (FIRST) | SPECIES | SEX | AGE YRS. MOS. | DATE COLLECTED MO. DAY YR. | TIME COLLECTED

PATIENT ADDRESS | STREET | MISC. INFORMATION | DR. I.D. | MEDICARE: #

CITY | STATE | ZIP | DIAGNOSIS

PHYSICIAN

WELFARE: # | CASE NAME:

PROGRAM: | PATIENT 1ST NAME: | DATE OF BIRTH ALL CLAIMS MO. DAY YR.

INSURANCE | I.D. | SERVICE CODE:

GR. # SUBSCRIBER NAME: | RELATION | PHONE

N7/058

CYTOLOGY

DATE OF LAST MENSTRUAL PERIOD ______
Gravida ______ Para ______
Hormones (Type) ______
GYN Surgery ______ Date ______
Radiation Therapy ______ Date ______
Previous Cytology Number ______ Eval ______ Date ______

Pregnant ( ) Yes ( ) No
I.U.D. ( ) Yes ( ) No

PERTINENT CLINICAL HISTORY (Max. 35 Characters)

INTERNAL USE ONLY
CYTOLOGY NUMBER
DATE RECEIVED

PAPANICOLAOU SMEARS AND MATURATION INDEX
Please mark source:
( ) Vaginal ( ) Cervical ( ) Endocervical
CHECK DESIRED TEST
8195 ( ) Pap Smear
8199 ( ) Pap and MI
8198 ( ) Maturation Index Only
8237 ( ) Pap added to Profile
8197 ( ) Pap included in Profile

SPECIAL CYTOLOGY
8202 ( ) Body Fluids, Misc Site ______
8203 ( ) Bronchial Washings, Brushings
8240 ( ) Cell Block
8200 ( ) Sputum
8201 ( ) Urine
8235 ( ) Endometrial Aspiration
8206 ( ) Eye (Ophthalmic)
8205 ( ) Fine Needle Aspirations
8204 ( ) Gastric Washings, Brushings
8232 ( ) Direct Smear
Misc. Site ______
( ) Herpes Smear (Inclusion Bodies)
8233 ( ) Sex Chromatin (Barr Body)

SERIAL TESTS - Write in Number of Serial Samples Submitted Inside Parenthesis
8207 ( ) Serial Sputum ( ) Serial Urine

HISTOLOGY

9230 ( ) Surgical Pathology (Biopsy) preparation and pathologist interpretation)
8234 ( ) Bone Marrow Exam
9237 ( ) Stained Histology Slide (Without pathologist interpretation)
( ) Special Stain (Please Specify)
9251 ( ) Veterinary Pathology (Biopsy)

CLINICAL HISTORY
Source of Specimen ______
If Tumor, How Long Present ______
Post Operative Diagnosis ______
Previous History ______

UNLISTED TESTS

(Rev. 1-84)

FOLD THIS FORM IN HALF SO TEST(S) ORDERED IS CLEARLY VISIBLE

**Figure 41–3:** Cytology requisition form. *Delmar/Cengage Learning.*

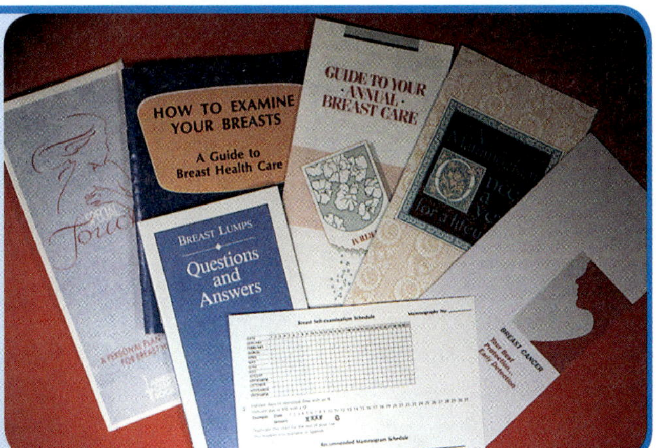


**Figure 41–4:** Breast self-examination (BSE) pamphlets and schedule. *Delmar/Cengage Learning.*

## Conducting the Examination

The provider usually listens to the heart and lungs and does a brief general check of the patient first. Then the patient's gown is lowered to the waist while the patient is still sitting up for the inspection part of the breast exam and palpation for lumps and masses. When this part is completed, you will pull the table extension out to support the patient's lower legs and feet and help the patient lie down. This assists the provider in further palpation for any abnormalities of the breast tissue. (Often, a towel is placed over the chest to provide a sense of privacy for the patient.) Next, the provider will inspect and palpate the abdominal and pelvic areas. Remind patients to breathe slowly through the mouth to help relax abdominal muscles during the exam.

The next step is for you to help the patient into the lithotomy position. Assist her in getting her feet in the stirrups, adjusting them as necessary, and place the drape sheet over her knees. Ask her to scoot down to the end of the table until the buttocks are just at the edge. Be careful in assisting patients into positions because the exam tables are usually rather narrow, and there *is* the possibility of a patient falling *off* the table. The exam lamp should be adjusted at the end of the table and the stool positioned comfortably for the provider. You will need to apply gloves as well as supply a pair for the provider to wear.

Adjust the lamp if necessary, to the provider's preference, so that the external perineal structures can be observed. When ready, hand the warmed speculum, handles first, to the provider. Some providers may want the speculum ran under warm water to facilitate insertion and comfort for the patient. After insertion (Figure 41–5), it might be necessary to adjust the light again so that the cervix can be seen clearly within the blades of the speculum.

Hand the endocervical broom or spatula to the provider if using the conventional method. The broom or spatula is inserted slightly into the cervical opening and twisted to obtain sample cells within and on the surface of the cervix (Figure 41–6A). The broom is withdrawn and immediately placed in the ThinPrep bottle (Figure 41–6B). It is swished 10 times through the solution, withdrawn to the top of the bottle, tapped a couple times to knock off any remaining solution and cells, and discarded on the Mayo stand. The labeled bottle is promptly capped. The spatula is used to spread the cells on a glass slide which is then sprayed with fixative to set and placed in a protective cover.

The bimanual exam is performed following the collection of specimens (Pap smear and cultures) so that the lubricant will not interfere in the lab analysis. The examiner inserts two fingers (with a dime-size amount of water-soluble lubricant) into the vagina and palpates the pelvic area with the other hand (Figure 41–7). The provider then places one finger into the vagina and the other in the rectum simultaneously checking for any abnormalities of the pelvic organs and rectum. You should hand the doctor a clean glove and lubricant to prevent cross-contamination between the vaginal and rectal tissues for this exam. The provider might want to screen the patient for rectal bleeding at this time by providing a fecal sample obtained during the bimanual exam to a fecal occult test card as discussed in Chapter 40.

Alternately, instead of assisting, the medical assistant may be asked to write or scribe the findings of this examination while the provider conducts the exam. Regardless of your tasks, you can be a valuable assistant to both provider and patient.

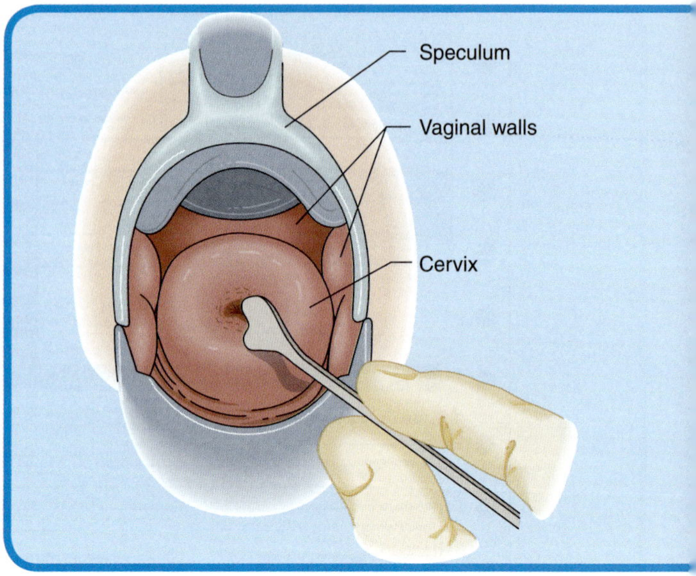


**Figure 41–6A:** The cervix is scraped with a spatula to obtain cells for a Pap test. *Delmar/Cengage Learning.*

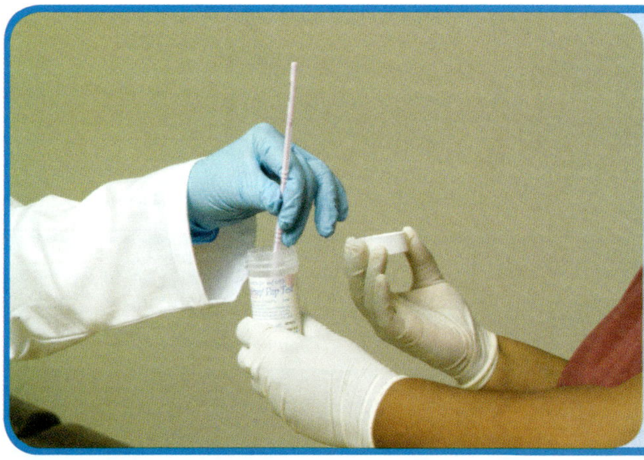

**Figure 41–6B:** The provider swishes the broom in the ThinPrep bottle. *Delmar/Cengage Learning.*

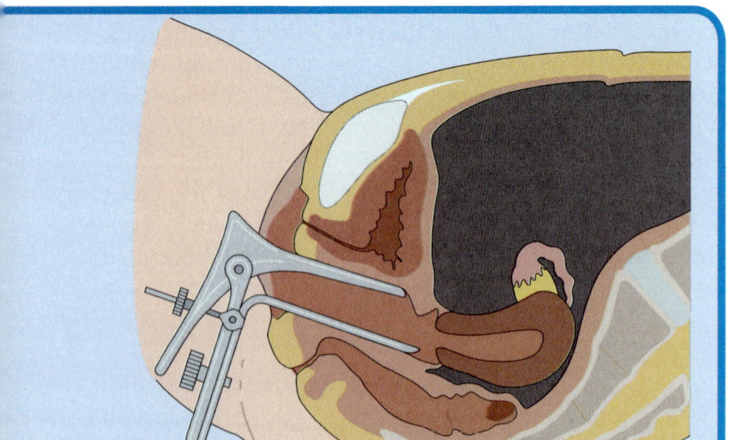

**Figure 41–5:** Lateral view of vaginal speculum in place for inspection and for obtaining specimens. *Delmar/Cengage Learning.*

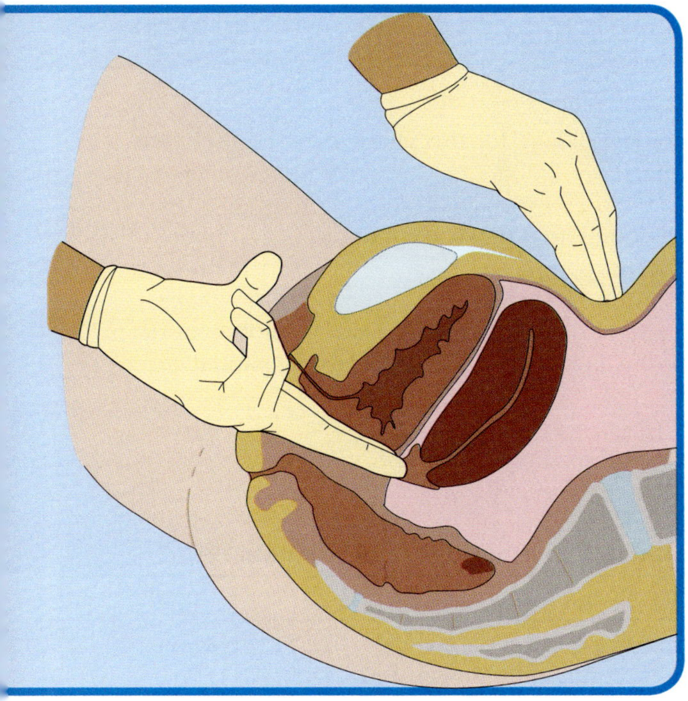

**Figure 41–7:** Bimanual pelvic exam. *Delmar/Cengage Learning.*

## After the Examination

When the exam has been completed, push the stirrups and the extension of the table in and assist the patient to sit up. After lying down for the exam, the patient may feel faint or dizzy; if she attempts to stand up too quickly, she can fall. After she has let you know that she has regained her balance, help her down from the table and offer tissues to the patient to wipe away any residual lubricant. Discard the used tissues in a waste container. Ask her to get dressed and offer assistance to the patient if needed.

Remember to advise her when to expect to receive the results of the Pap test and other reports in the mail or when she should call to find out the results. Giving these instructions will decidedly reduce unnecessary phone calls to the office. If the provider requests a return appointment for the patient, politely assist her in scheduling it or direct her to the administrative area. As time permits, you may discuss patient education topics either before or after the exam as appropriate to the age and needs of the patient.

Return to the examination room to clean up the exam area. Wear gloves to protect yourself from disease transmission. Discard all disposables in appropriate waste containers, remove gloves, and wash hands. Restock the supplies as necessary, making the room ready for the next patient to be seen. Place the labeled specimen(s) and attached requisition form in the proper area for pickup by the lab representative.

Follow the steps in Procedure 41–1 to assist the provider with a gynecological examination and a ThinPrep Pap test.

### PATIENT EDUCATION

Here are a few informative topics you might want to discuss with female patients coming in for Pap tests:

1. Explain to patients that they should *not* douche routinely because it washes away natural protective vaginal secretions that aid in the resistance of possible invading microorganisms. Douching should be done only with the provider's orders.
2. Patients who are sexually active and not in a committed, monogamous relationship should be instructed to use condoms when engaging in sexual intercourse for protection against both sexually transmitted diseases and unwanted pregnancies.
3. Educate all females to perform breast self-examination at home routinely after their menstrual period. (Refer to Chapter 40.) Pamphlets for distribution can be obtained from the American Cancer Society to help patients with the procedure.
4. Remind all female patients over age 40 to schedule a routine mammography for early detection of breast cancer.
5. Explain to female patients that any of the following symptoms could mean that infection or disease is present and that they should call for an appointment: foul vaginal odor; vaginal discharge that is other than clear; unusual bleeding; vaginal itching or soreness; or any other **vaginitis**, pain, or discomfort.
6. Advise female patients to refrain from using perfumed toilet articles such as soaps or bubble baths, vaginal sprays, tampons, toilet tissue, or feminine napkins because they may be irritating to the delicate vaginal tissues. Chronic irritation can lead to infection.

## PROCEDURE 41–1 Prepare the Patient for and Assist with a Gynecological Exam and Pap Test

**MEDIA LINK:** View the video, "Assist with a Gynecologic Exam," for this chapter on the Premium Website.

**PURPOSE:** To prepare the patient and assist the provider to complete a pelvic examination and obtain a Pap test to determine a patient's gynecological health

**EQUIPMENT:** Mayo tray, two cloth or paper towels, three pairs of disposable gloves, water-soluble lubricant, vaginal speculum, tissues, endocervical broom, ThinPrep bottle, label, laboratory requisition, patient's chart or EMR, and pen

S **SKILL:** Prepare the patient for and assist with a gynecological exam and Pap test.

| Procedure Steps | Detailed Instructions and/or *Rationales* |
|---|---|
| 1. Wash hands. | |
| 2. Prepare the room and equipment. | • Place a towel on the Mayo tray, assemble all necessary equipment, and cover.<br>• Place the requisition form on a nearby table.<br>• Place the gown and drape on the exam table. |
| 3. Call the patient from the reception room; introduce yourself and identify the patient. | *Ensures that you have the correct patient.* |
| 4. Instruct the patient to go to the bathroom to empty the bladder. | Provide instructions and a specimen container if a urine specimen is needed. |
| B 5. Explain the procedure, ***using language the patient can understand; answer any questions, making the patient feel at ease about the procedure to be performed.*** | |
| 6. Obtain the necessary information to complete the cytology requisition form. | |
| 7. Attach a label to the ThinPrep bottle and place it on the Mayo tray. | |
| B 8. Instruct the patient to remove all clothing and put on the examination gown with the opening in front. ***Leave the room to allow for privacy unless assistance is needed.*** | Show her where to put her clothing. |
| 9. When the patient is gowned, enter the room and pull out the step from the end of the table. Ask the patient sit on the table. Cover the patient's legs with the drape. Push in the table step. | Provide assistance as needed. The step is small, and the patient may step off the edge when trying to turn around to sit down. |
| B 10. Notify the provider that the patient is ready. ***If the patient is apprehensive, provide reassurance and support. Answer any questions she may have.*** | |
| 11. Accompany the provider into the room and apply critical thinking skills to provide assistance as needed. Be sure to use proper body mechanics when positioning the patient. | |

| Procedure Steps | Detailed Instructions and/or *Rationales* |
|---|---|
| 12. Position the patient in a sitting position for basic assessment and initial breast examination. Be sure to show awareness to any patient concerns regarding the procedure. | |
| 13. Assist the patient to a supine position for a continued breast exam. | Put the pillow under her head. Uncover her chest, and cover her breasts with the towel covering the Mayo tray if desired. |
| 14. When the breast exam is completed, assist the patient to cover her chest with the gown and drape and prepare for the pelvic exam. | *For modesty and patient comfort.* |
| 15. Assist the patient into a lithotomy position, helping her place her feet into the stirrups, and adjust as needed. | Push in the table extension. |
| 16. Place the drape over the patient from the chest to the feet. Push the drape down between her legs until it touches the table. Instruct the patient to slide her buttocks down to the end of the table. | *The patient's buttocks must be at the end of the table so that the vaginal speculum can be inserted without the handle hitting the table.* |
| 17. The provider will take his or her position on the exam stool at the end of the table. Remove the cover from the Mayo tray if not previously done. Hand gloves to the provider. | |
| 18. Adjust the lamp so that the light facilitates inspection of the perineal and anal areas. | |
| 19. Put on gloves and run warm water over the speculum. | |
| 20. Hand the speculum, handle first, to the provider. | |
| 21. Hand the endocervical broom, handle first, to the provider. | |
| 22. Open the labeled specimen bottle and be ready to accept the endocervical broom. | Hold the bottle securely while physician swishes the broom, or take the handle of the broom and swish thoroughly in the solution 10 times. Withdraw it from bottle, tap it against the bottle edge to dislodge any cells and excess fluid, and place it on the Mayo tray. Cap the bottle securely and place it on the Mayo tray. |
| 23. The provider will stand to perform the bimanual pelvic and rectal exam. Apply lubricant to the gloved index and middle fingers of the examining hand. | |
| 24. When the provider has finished the exam, have the patient push back up the table, help her get her feet out of the stirrups, and push the stirrups in. | |
| 25. Assist the patient to sit up. Pull out the table step. When the patient's sense of balance has returned, assist her down from the table. | |
| 26. Hand tissues to the patient to remove any residual lubricant. | |
| 27. Instruct the patient to dress. Provide assistance as needed. Remove gloves and wash hands. | |

*(continues)*

*(continued)*

| Procedure Steps | Detailed Instructions and/or *Rationales* |
|---|---|
| 28. Advise the patient when results will be available and schedule a follow-up appointment if indicated. | |
| 29. Provide any patient teaching information pamphlets that are appropriate and dismiss the patient. Record exam, Pap test, and any teaching in the chart. | |
| 30. Apply gloves; properly clean and disinfect the room and all instruments and restock supplies. | • Discard all disposable items in the appropriate waste container. Wrap up the table paper and towels and discard.<br>• If a metal speculum was used, place it in cool water, then wash, wrap, and autoclave.<br>• Disinfect table surfaces and the exam room furniture.<br>• Restock supplies. Pull down fresh table paper on the exam table. |
| 31. Place the labeled specimen bottle with the attached requisition in the lab pickup area. | |
| 32. Pull down fresh table paper on the exam table. | |
| 33. Remove gloves and wash hands. | |

### Charting Example

| | |
|---|---|
| 8/28/XX<br>2:30 PM | Annual pelvic exam and ThinPrep Pap test performed. See patient history/physical form.<br>G. Talbert, RMA(AMT) |

## Reporting Pap Test Results

The system most widely used to describe Pap test findings is the Bethesda System. It was developed in 1988 and revised in 1991 and 2001. There are three general categories:

1. Negative for intraepithelial lesion or malignancy *(Means there are no signs of cancer or precancerous changes. Other findings may be reported, such as yeast, herpes, Trichomonas, or cellular changes caused by irritation or infection.)*
2. Epithelial cell abnormalities *(Means the cells of the lining layer of the cervix show changes that might be cancer or a precancerous condition. The cells are divided into (a) atypical squamous cells, (b) low-grade squamous intraepithelial lesions (SILs), (c) high-grade SILs, and (4) squamous cell carcinoma. These findings require repeat Pap tests and other interventions such as colposcopy (examining the cervix with a magnifying lens instrument) and biopsy.*
3. Other malignant neoplasms *(Means there is likely an invasive squamous cell cancer. Additional diagnostic tests will be performed, followed by radiation, chemotherapy, or radical surgery.)*

Figure 41–8 lists and defines some terms used in the cytology reports of Pap tests.

atypical—not typical
CIN—cervical intraepithelial neoplasia
CIS—carcinoma in situ
condyloma—a lesion caused by human papillomavirus
dysplasia—precancerous lesion
epithelial—pertaining to epithelium
epithelium—cellular tissue that covers the surface of a body or that lines a body cavity
glandular—the cell making up the epithelium of a body cavity
HPV—human papillomavirus
lesion—a change in the tissue cells or a wound
malignant—a lesion that spreads out of the epithelium into underlying tissues
reactive changes—changes in cells caused by their reaction to infectious agents or a foreign body
reparative changes—changes in cells as they divide rapidly in an attempt to repair damaged tissue
SIL—squamous intraepithelial lesion (that lies within the squamous epithelium)
squamous—a type of cell that makes up the epithelium, the purpose of which is to protect underlying tissues

**Figure 41–8:** Terms and abbreviations used in cytology/Pap test reports. *Delmar/Cengage Learning.*

## OTHER GYNECOLOGICAL PROCEDURES

Other procedures can be performed to make decisions regarding the condition of the uterus and cervix. Figures 41–9A through D show gynecological instruments used in some of these procedures. The uterine sound Figure 41–9A is inserted into the uterus to explore the cavity and measure the depth. Note it is graduated in inches or centimeters. The curettes (Figure 41–9B and C) are used to scrape the lining of the uterus for a specimen and to remove growths or remnants of an abortion. The biopsy forceps (Figure 41–9D) permits taking a small piece of tissue for diagnostic examination. These instruments are most often used when performing surgical procedures.

## OBSTETRICS PATIENTS

When patients suspect that they are pregnant, their visit to the doctor is to confirm pregnancy. Usually, the patient has missed one or two menstrual periods. Because home pregnancy tests are convenient and accessible, many women have already tested their urine at home prior to coming into the office. However, even after having performed the home test, they still may not be certain of the results. The diagnosis is made by the provider only after the patient has been given a complete evaluation. This is generally done by (1) interviewing the patient and obtaining a complete **prenatal** health assessment and history; (2) doing a complete physical examination; (3) ordering laboratory tests such as urinalysis and pregnancy tests, blood tests, and cultures; and (4) performing any other diagnostic test indicated by the patient's condition.

The same principles apply in assisting with obstetrics patients as apply in assisting with the complete physical examination. Documentation of the prenatal history, vitals, and any past or current medical conditions of the patient must be complete and efficient. This enables the providers to give quality care to their patients. Refer to Chapter 35 for review of the anatomy and physiology of the reproductive system and information regarding **pregnancy**, labor, and childbirth. You need to be familiar with the terminology when discussing issues with patients.

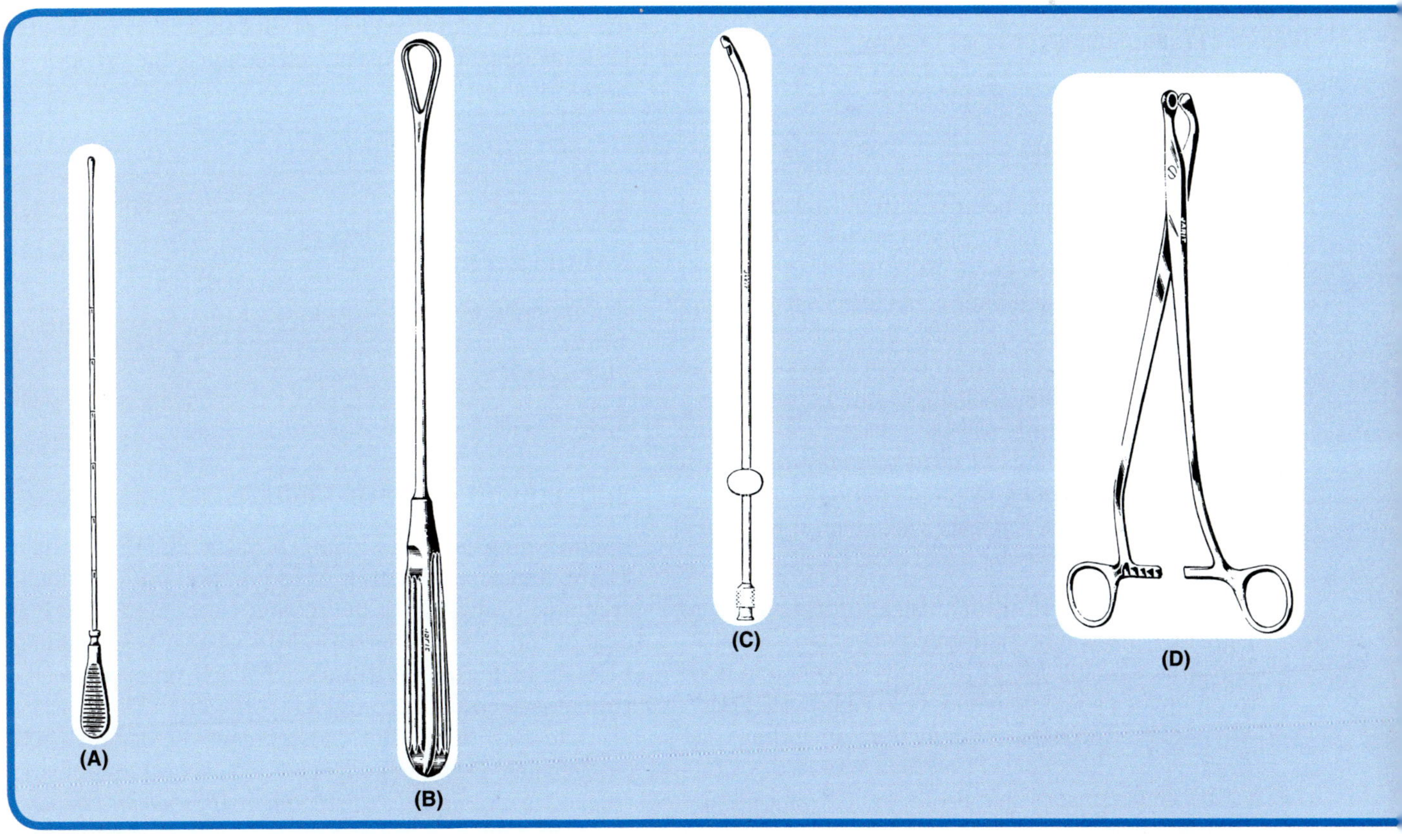


**Figure 41–9:** (A) Sims' uterine sound, can be graduated in inches or centimeters. (B) Sims' uterine curette. (C) Randall uterine curette. (D) Toms-Gaylor uterine punch. *Courtesy of JARIT Surgical Instruments.*

## The Medical Assistant's Role in Obstetrical Exams

In addition to assisting the provider with all the examinations, your role in prenatal evaluation and care of patients is to instill the importance of keeping regular appointments; encourage patients to eat a sensible, well-balanced diet; alert the doctor of any problems or concerns; and provide patient education materials with explanations. Follow your office policy regarding prenatal and childbirth classes to provide information about times and places of such programs as **Lamaze** classes.

A prenatal medical history form (Figure 41–10) and a risk assessment form (Figure 41–11) are used to assess the health status of pregnant women and is generally filled out at the patient's initial visit after the pregnancy has been confirmed. Subsequent findings during prenatal visits are recorded on the spaces provided on the bottom half of the form or on progress notes. Careful attention should be given to sections regarding (1) medications, drugs, alcohol, and smoking (consumption and use); (2) preexisting risk factors; and (3) past menstrual and obstetrical health history.

The effects on the fetus are well documented from certain medications, smoking, and alcohol as well as from illicit drug use. Risks are also associated with certain systemic disease conditions, sexually transmitted diseases, age, physical stature, and mental factors. Examine Figure 41–11 to identify risks of preterm births and poor pregnancy outcomes.

## Initial Prenatal Visit

After the pregnancy has been confirmed by means of a urine or blood test, most providers will ask you to schedule their patient to come back in for an initial or first (OB) prenatal examination. As discussed earlier, the provider will want to confirm the laboratory tests with findings obtained from a physical examination. Schedule extra time for this appointment because a complete prenatal history will be collected. A baseline of all testing and findings is used to measure against subsequent appointments.

A general guideline for what will occur at the initial examination is as follows:

- A complete medical history, using a form similar to Figure 41–10, will be performed
- A risk assessment identifying any problems related to pregnancies and deliveries (see Figure 41–11)
- A complete physical examination, including Pap smear (Procedure 41–1)
- Education regarding diet, exercise, medications, and other topics preferred by the provider
- Laboratory testing, which usually includes a prenatal profile to check the patient's blood type and RH factor; HIV, hepatitis, and VDRL screening; complete blood count to check the iron level and screen for infection; urinalysis and cultures to check for chlamydia and gonorrhea (refer to Unit 14 for descriptions on laboratory testing)
- An estimation of the date of confinement or date of delivery
- The provider's request for the patient to return in one month for the next prenatal visit

## Estimating the Date of Delivery

Probably the question of most interest to the expectant couple is when the baby will be born. This is known medically as the estimated day or date of delivery (EDD) or the estimated date of confinement (EDC). This can be determined, with a fair amount of accuracy, by using a formula known as **Naegele's rule**. The method was devised by Franz Naegele, a German obstetrician, in the early eighteenth century. The period of gestation (conception to birth) is determined by using the first day of the last menstrual period (LMP), subtracting three months, and then adding seven days plus one year.

A normal pregnancy can range from 37 to 41 weeks, so exact dates are not possible. An infant born before the 37th week is called premature, is considerably underweight, and presents challenges due to lack of development.

### EXAMPLE

**NAEGELE'S RULE**

| | |
|---|---|
| *Last menstrual period* | August 10, 2012 |
| *Minus 3 months* | May 10, 2012 |
| *Plus 7 days, 1 year* | May 17, 2013 |

## Subsequent Prenatal Visits

Routine prenatal visits to the physician's office usually follow the same format. It is very important to maintain continual evaluation of the mother's condition as well as that of the developing baby. Part of that responsibility belongs to the medical assistant. Each time before the patient is seen by the provider, you will:

- Interview the patient to determine whether any problems are being experienced and record any remarks and symptoms. (*Early treatment of problems can keep them under control and avoid later serious situations.*)

**PLEASE USE BALL POINT PEN**

NAME ____________________ SEND TOP (WHITE) COPY TO DEL. ROOM TERM ______

ADDRESS ____________________ LMP ______ LIFE ______ EDC ______

PHONE ______ RELIGION ______ NURSING ______ PEDIATRICIAN ______

AGE ______ GR ____ PARA ____ AB ______ ANESTHESIA ______

BLOOD TYPE ______ RH ____ SEROLOGY ______ REFERRING M.D. ______

HUSB. BL. TYPE ______ RH ____ GENOTYPE ______ PRENATAL PREPARATION ______

HUSBAND IN DELIVERY ROOM? ______

______ RUBELLA TITER ______

MENSTRUAL CYCLE ______

PAP SMEAR ______ G.C. CULTURE ______

| PP AR SE T G. | | DATE | WHERE CONFINED | WEEKS GESTATION | LENGTH OF LABOR | INFANT WT. | COMPLICATIONS |
|---|---|---|---|---|---|---|---|
| | 1 | | | | | | |
| | 2 | | | | | | |
| | 3 | | | | | | |
| | 4 | | | | | | |

HISTORY AND PHYSICAL

CHILDHOOD ______ HT. ____ NORMAL WT. ____ NORMAL B.P. ______

FAMILY ______ HEENT ______

TRAUMATIC ______ HEART & LUNGS ______

ADULT ______ BACK & BREASTS ______

BLOOD TRANSFUSIONS ______ ABDOMEN ______

ALLERGIES ______ SKIN & EXTREMITIES ______

SURGERY ______ PELVIC CAPACITY ______

COMMENTS: ______

MEDICATIONS ______

RH TITERS DATES: ______

| PERIODIC VISITS | | DATE | WEIGHT | BP | URINE | FHT | FUNDUS | PELVIC | COMMENTS |
|---|---|---|---|---|---|---|---|---|---|
| | 1 | | | | | | | | |
| | 2 | | | | | | | | |
| | 3 | | | | | | | | |
| | 4 | | | | | | | | |
| | 5 | | | | | | | | |
| | 6 | | | | | | | | |
| | 7 | | | | | | | | |
| | 8 | | | | | | | | |
| | 9 | | | | | | | | |
| | 10 | | | | | | | | |
| | 11 | | | | | | | | |
| | 12 | | | | | | | | |
| | 13 | | | | | | | | |
| | 14 | | | | | | | | |

DELIVERY ROOM - TERM SIGNATURE: M.D.

**Figure 41–10:** Prenatal health history form. *Delmar/Cengage Learning.*

- Request her first morning urine specimen, which she brought with her, or have her give you one now. (*Some complications of pregnancy can be identified by urine tests.*)
- Obtain a blood sample if needed: Some providers monitor the patient's iron level by checking the hemoglobin routinely. Also, screening tests for alpha-fetoprotein (AFP), a test to check for neural tube defects, may be performed at 15–18 weeks, and gestational diabetes, known as a glucose tolerance test, is performed during weeks 24–28 of gestation.
- Measure the patient's weight and record the findings. (*Weight reflects the mother's nutrition and the related health of the fetus. Excess as well as insufficient weight gain is undesirable. Excess gain could indicate fluid retention.*)
- Measure and record her vital signs. (*Monitoring blood pressure is extremely important. Hypertension is indicative of complications.*)

**PRENATAL RISK ASSESSMENT FORM**

Please print or type:

| Patient Name | Case Number | ADC Number | E.D.D. month / day / year |
|---|---|---|---|
| Physician Name | Physician Telephone | | |

Please check all that apply:

**AT RISK OF PRETERM BIRTH**

ABSOLUTE FACTORS *(one factor puts patient at risk)*

**OBSTETRICAL HISTORY**

- ❑ 1. PRETERM DELIVERY
- ❑ 2. DES EXPOSURE
- ❑ 3. CONE BIOPSY
- ❑ 4. SECOND TRIMESTER ABORTION
- ❑ 5. 1st TRIMESTER SPONTANEOUS ABORTIONS, more than 2

**CURRENT PREGNANCY**

- ❑ 6. UTERINE ANOMALY OR FIBROIDS
- ❑ 7. MULTIPLE GESTATION
- ❑ 8. ABDOMINAL SURGERY
- ❑ 9. CERVIX DILATED, more than 1.5 cm before 29 weeks
- ❑ 10. CERVIX EFFACED, less than 1 cm before 29 weeks
- ❑ 11. IRRITABLE UTERUS, more than 6 contractions per hr. confirmed
- ❑ 12. POLYHYDRAMNIOS
- ❑ 13. BLEEDING, if significant after 12 weeks
- ❑ 14. PYELONEPHRITIS
- ❑ 15. PRETERM LABOR
- ❑ 16. SMOKING, more than 10 cigarettes per day
- ❑ 17. PROM, confirmed

❑ YES ❑ NO At least ONE of the above conditions has been checked. Patient is at risk of preterm birth.

**AT RISK OF POOR PREGNANCY OUTCOME**

ABSOLUTE FACTORS *(one factor puts patient at risk)*

**OBSTETRICAL HISTORY**

- ❑ 18. INFANT DEATH, stillborn, neonatal, post neonatal
- ❑ 19. CONGENITAL ANOMALY, major
- ❑ 20. LOW BIRTH WEIGHT, less than 2500g.
- ❑ 21. ECLAMPSIA or severe preeclampsia
- ❑ 22. INCOMPETENT CERVIX

**CURRENT PREGNANCY**

- ❑ 23. HEART DISEASE, class III or IV
- ❑ 24. DIABETES, insulin dependent
- ❑ 25. SICKLE CELL ANEMIA or other hemoglobinopathy
- ❑ 26. MALIGNANCY or leukemia
- ❑ 27. THYROID DISEASE, confirmed
- ❑ 28. EPILEPSY or on anticonvulsant
- ❑ 29. HEPATITIS or chronic liver disease
- ❑ 30. ASTHMA, on medication
- ❑ 31. TUBERCULOSIS, active
- ❑ 32. PNEUMONIA
- ❑ 33. HYPERTENSION, on medication
- ❑ 34. DEEP VENOUS THROMBOSIS
- ❑ 35. PLACENTA PREVIA, 3rd trimester
- ❑ 36. OLIGOHYDRAMNIOS
- ❑ 37. ECLAMPSIA or preeclampsia
- ❑ 38. ALLOIMMUNIZATION associated with fetal disease
- ❑ 39. RUBELLA EXPOSURE with rising titer
- ❑ 40. POSITIVE SEROLOGY
- ❑ 41. ACTIVE HERPES or positive culture, 3rd trimester
- ❑ 42. PRIMIGRAVIDA, less than 17 years or more than 35 years
- ❑ 43. FAMILIAL GENETIC DISORDER, confirmed
- ❑ 44. PSYCHOSIS
- ❑ 45. MENTAL RETARDATION
- ❑ 46. DRUG OR ALCOHOL ABUSE
- ❑ 47. OTHER ____________________

❑ YES ❑ NO At least ONE of the above conditions has been checked. Patient is at risk of poor pregnancy outcome.

RELATIVE FACTORS *(two factors put patient at risk)*

- ❑ 48. PRIOR C-SECTION
- ❑ 49. PRENATAL CARE NON-COMPLIANCE, most recent pregnancy
- ❑ 50. GRAND MULTIPARA, more than 5 of 20 weeks or more
- ❑ 51. RECENT DELIVERY, less than 1 yr.
- ❑ 52. LATE INITIAL VISIT, after 14 weeks of pregnancy
- ❑ 53. MISSED PRENATAL APPOINTMENTS, 2 consecutive
- ❑ 54. AGE, less than 17 years or more than 35 years
- ❑ 55. Height, less than 5 ft.
- ❑ 56. OBESITY, more than 20% weight for height
- ❑ 57. UNDERWEIGHT, more than 10% weight for height
- ❑ 58. WEIGHT LOSS, continuing after 14 weeks
- ❑ 59. ANEMIA, less than 10 Hgb, or less than 30% Hct.
- ❑ 60. GONORRHEA, positive culture
- ❑ 61. DIABETES, gestational, diet controlled
- ❑ 62. CHRONIC BRONCHITIS
- ❑ 63. TRAUMA, requiring hospitalization
- ❑ 64. ILLITERACY or language barrier
- ❑ 65. DOMESTIC VIOLENCE
- ❑ 66. OTHER ____________________

❑ YES ❑ NO At least TWO of the above conditions have been checked. Patient is at risk of poor pregnancy outcome.

| Physician's Signature | Date |
|---|---|
| | |

**Figure 41–11:** Prenatal risk assessment form. *Delmar/Cengage Learning.*

- Check the chart to be sure all lab reports from tests ordered since the last visit are in the chart. Also check that any other studies or referral letters are included.
- If the provider will be performing an examination, prepare the patient by having her remove her clothes from the waist down, unless the breasts are also to be examined, and put on a gown with the opening in the front. (Providers have different preferences for how often they will do an exam; be sure to check with your provider for specifics.)
- Assist the patient onto the examination table and have her sit at the end. (Provide a drape for her lap and legs if an exam is being performed.)
- Notify the provider that the patient is ready for the examination.

After the provider reviews any returned reports and your chart notes, the patient's current general condition is discussed, and the reported problems or findings are further explored. Then it is time to proceed with the examination or additional testing if desired or needed.

- Assist the patient into supine position for the prenatal examination.
- Provide assistance to the provider as appropriate for the **trimester** (three-month period) of the patient's **gestation** (nine [ten lunar] months or 38 to 42 weeks).
- A fetoscope (special stethoscope) or a Doppler fetal pulse monitor and gel are applied to the abdomen to determine the developing fetus's heart rate.
- The provider may palpate the abdomen to evaluate fundic height as a means of estimating the duration of the pregnancy. If it is not as expected, it could be an indication of multiple fetuses, excess amniotic fluid, poor development of the fetus, or even fetal death.
- A flexible centimeter tape is used to measure the height of the **fundus** (top of the uterus) from the symphysis pubis to evaluate the growth of the fetus after approximately the third month.
- Upon completion of the examination, assist the patient to a sitting position and instruct her to dress.
- Record the appropriate information such as fundic height, fetal heart rate, procedures performed, and other pertinent patient or provider observations and remarks.
- Ultrasonography may be performed the first trimester to confirm pregnancy and later to monitor its progress (Figure 41–12). One of the most exciting times for the expectant parents is when the physician or technician locates the fetus by using ultrasound technology. The equipment is capable of displaying the image on the screen and printing out the baby's first "picture" for the proud parents to show to family and friends.

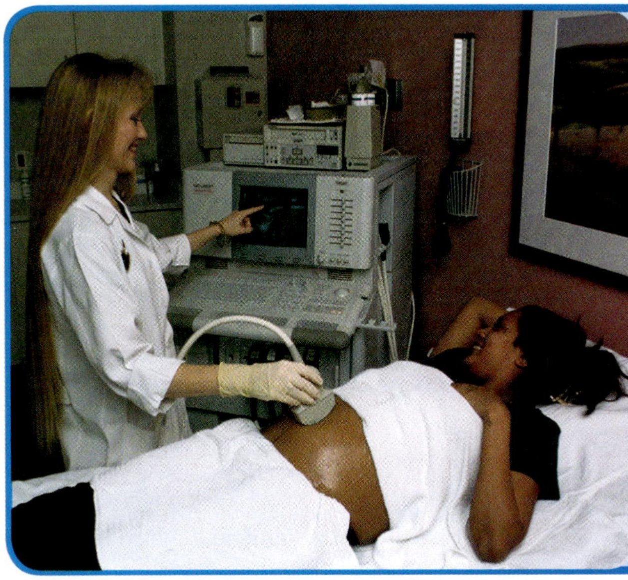

**Figure 41–12:** An ultrasound being performed.
*Delmar/Cengage Learning.*

### PATIENT EDUCATION

It is very important for prenatal patients to receive regular, systematic evaluation. You must stress the importance of keeping scheduled appointments so the mother and baby can be monitored closely.

## Patient Care

After the provider has completed the examination and talked with the patient, offer to answer any questions the patient might have. Encourage the patient to make her next appointment before leaving the facility. Figure 41–13 illustrates the frequency of office visits for a normal pregnancy. Persons experiencing difficulties or at high risk require more frequent evaluation. Give support and assistance by reminding her to call if she has any questions or problems.

The medical assistant should return to the exam room to clean up the area. Wear gloves to protect yourself from disease transmission. Discard all disposables in appropriate waste containers, remove gloves and dispose of them properly, and wash hands. Restock supplies as necessary, making the exam room ready for the next patient. Place any specimens in the area for pickup by the lab representative.

**GENERAL SCHEDULE FOR PRENATAL OR OBSTETRICAL APPOINTMENTS**

**FIRST AND SECOND TRIMESTER:**
Monthly or every four weeks through the 28th week.

**THIRD TRIMESTER:**
Every two weeks in the 30th–36th weeks. Every week in the 36th+ week up to delivery.

**Figure 41–13:** Prenatal appointment schedule.
*Delmar/Cengage Learning.*

**CLINICAL PEARL**

Especially in an OB/GYN practice, the possibility exists of patients who might be bleeding or who have an infection that can be transmitted by body fluids and therefore could be a threat to others.

To be of further assistance to both provider and patient, you might want to check all patients' charts to make sure that findings are documented in a neat and legible manner and signed by the provider. Remember, records are legal documents and may be requested at any time by insurance providers to verify the diagnosis and coding, leading to more efficient and expedient payment.

## CHAPTER SUMMARY

- Obstetrics focuses on pregnancy and childbirth, whereas the gynecology practice addresses diseases and disorders of the female reproductive system.
- The ThinPrep Pap test technique slightly improves the detection of cancers but greatly improves the detection of precancers. This method also enables additional studies from the same sample, such as tests for the presence of HPV, chlamydia, and gonorrhea.
- The ACS recommends that all women should begin Pap screening tests about three years after they begin having vaginal intercourse but no later than 21 years old. Screening should be done every year with a regular Pap test or every two years with a liquid-based Pap test. At age 30, women with three normal Pap tests in a row may have a screening every two to three years with either test method. Women with risk should continue with annual testing or follow provider's recommendations.
- The ACS has recommendations in place for women to follow to assist in making their Pap results more accurate.
- Breast self-exams need to be performed by the patient monthly. Although the breast exam conducted by the provider with the annual Pap test is important, it is insufficient in detecting abnormal breast tissue between visits to the provider. Most women discover a lump or mass in their breasts themselves and report it to the provider. This leads to early detection and treatment, which greatly increases the survival rate.
- Most providers prefer the medical assistant (or nurse) to accompany them into the exam room, not only to assist with the procedure, but also to verify their behavior in case of patient accusations.
- Three main reporting categories for Pap smears are: negative for intraepithelial lesion or malignancy; epithelial cell abnormalities; and other malignant neoplasms.
- To confirm pregnancy, the diagnosis is made only after the patient has been given a complete evaluation by (1) interviewing the patient and obtaining a complete prenatal health assessment and history; (2) doing a complete physical examination; (3) ordering laboratory tests, such as urinalysis and pregnancy tests, blood tests, and cultures; and (4) performing any other diagnostic test indicated by the patient's condition.
- In addition to assisting the provider with all the examinations, your role in prenatal evaluation and care of patients is to instill the importance of keeping regular appointments; encourage patients to eat a sensible, well-balanced diet; alert the doctor of any problems or concerns; and provide patient education materials with explanations.
- Naegele's rule is determined by using the first day of the last menstrual period (LMP), subtracting three months, and then adding seven days plus one year.
- Your role in assessing the patient prior to her prenatal appointment can include: interviewing the patient to determine whether any problems are being experienced; requesting lab and urine specimens; measuring the patient's weight and recording the findings; measuring and recording her vital signs; checking the chart to be sure all lab reports from tests ordered since the last visit are in the chart; preparing the patient if the provider will be doing an examination; and notifying the provider that the patient is ready for the examination.

## STUDY TOOLS

| | |
|---|---|
| **Workbook** | Activities for Chapter 41 |
| **Premium Website** | |
| **MEDIA LINK** | View this **Media Link** for Chapter 41:<br>• Assist with a Gynecologic Exam |

| StudyWARE | Activities and Quizzes on the **StudyWARE™ Software** for Chapter 41 |
|---|---|
| | **Audio Library** of medical terms |
| | Online access to the **Critical Thinking Challenge 2.0** |
| **CourseMate** | Activities and Quizzes for Chapter 41 |
| **WebTutor** | Activities and Quizzes for Chapter 41 |

## CHECK YOUR KNOWLEDGE

1. Over what age is it recommended that women start routine yearly mammograms?
   a. 21
   b. 30
   c. 40
   d. 50
2. All women should begin screening tests about three years after they begin having vaginal intercourse but no later than ______ years old.
   a. 16
   b. 21
   c. 18
   d. 40
3. The system most widely used to describe Pap test findings is the Bethesda System, which reports the test results by using _______ general categories:
   a. three
   b. two
   c. four
   d. six
4. Which of the following gynecological instruments are inserted into the uterus to explore the cavity and measure the depth of the uterus?
   a. Sims' uterine curette
   b. Randall uterine curette
   c. Toms-Gaylor uterine punch
   d. Sims' uterine sound
5. During the 24th to 28th week of gestation, the following blood test is obtained from the mother:
   a. Alpha-fetoprotein (AFP)
   b. Glucose tolerance test
   c. HIV
   d. Hepatitis
6. Using Naegele's rule, the period of gestation (conception to birth) is determined by using the:
   a. first day of the last menstrual period (LMP), subtracting three months, and then adding seven days plus one year.
   b. last day of the last menstrual period (LMP), subtracting three months, and then adding seven days plus one year.
   c. first day of the last menstrual period (LMP), subtracting nine months, and then adding seven days plus one year.
   d. last day of the last menstrual period (LMP), subtracting three months, and then adding seven days plus one year.

## WEB LINKS

American Cancer Society: www.cancer.org

## RESOURCES

Estes, M. E. Z. (2010). *Health Assessment & Physical Examination* (3rd ed.). Clifton Park, NY: Delmar Cengage Learning.

Heller, M., and Veach, L. (2009). *Clinical Medical Assisting: A Professional, Field Smart Approach to the Workplace*. Clifton Park, NY: Delmar, Cengage Learning.

Lindh, W., Pooler, M., Tamparo, C., and Dahl, B. (2010). *Delmar's Comprehensive Medical Assisting Administrative and Clinical Competencies* (4th ed.). Clifton Park, NY: Delmar Cengage Learning.

Venes, D., (ed.). (2009). *Taber's Cyclopedic Medical Dictionary* (21st ed.). Philadelphia: F. A. Davis.

CHAPTER **6**

# OB/GYN Examinations

## Words to Know Challenge

**Spelling: Each line contains three spellings of a word. Underline the correctly spelled word.**

| | | |
|---|---|---|
| 1. cervical | servical | cervacal |
| 2. fundas | fundes | fundus |
| 3. gestation | jestation | guestation |
| 4. Lamazae | Lamaze | Lemaze |
| 5. trymester | triemister | trimester |

**Matching: Match the term in column I to its definition in column II.**

| | COLUMN I | COLUMN II |
|---|---|---|
| ____ | 1. Atypical | A. Fetus in the uterus |
| ____ | 2. Cytology | B. Not the usual |
| ____ | 3. Douche | C. Before birth |
| ____ | 4. Endocervical | D. Cells shedding |
| ____ | 5. Exfoliated | E. Method to estimate expected date of delivery |
| ____ | 6. Naegele's rule | F. Doctor who developed cervical cancer test |
| ____ | 7. Papanicolaou | G. Within the cervix |
| ____ | 8. Pregnancy | H. Cleansing the vagina |
| ____ | 9. Prenatal | I. Inflammation of the vagina |
| ____ | 10. Vaginitis | J. Study of cells |

# Chapter 7 Pediatric Examinations

## OBJECTIVES

In this chapter, you will learn the following:

### KB KNOWLEDGE BASE

1. Spell and define, using the glossary at the back of the text, all the Words to Know in this chapter.
2. Interpret from the AAP's Recommendations for Preventive Pediatric Health Care chart for frequency and types of recommended screenings and procedures for pediatric patients.
3. Explain the Early and Periodic Screening, Diagnostic, and Treatment (EPSDT) program.
4. Identify and discuss developmental stages of life.
5. Identify gross motor activities that are appropriate for 6-month-, 1-year-, and 18-month-old children using childhood growth and development tables.
6. Explain how to plot height and weight measurements on a National Center for Health Statistics growth chart.
7. Explain the difference between a well-child and sick-child visit.
8. List five responsibilities of the medical assistant when assisting with pediatric examinations.
9. Explain the difference between neglect and abuse, citing five examples of each.
10. Identify immunizations given to 2- and 12-month-old children according to the Childhood and Adolescent Immunization Schedule.
11. Identify two charts used to perform pediatric vision acuity and explain how each is used.

### S SKILLS

1. Measure length, weight, and head and chest circumference measurements of an infant and child.
2. Plot pediatric patients' measurements on a growth chart.
3. Perform pediatric vision acuity screening.

### B BEHAVIOR

1. Apply critical thinking skills in performing patient assessment and care.
2. Explain the rationale for performance of procedure to the patient.
3. Show awareness of patients' concerns regarding their perceptions of the procedure being performed.

## WORDS TO KNOW

Apgar
attachment
bonding
caregiver
child abuse
child neglect
chronologic
circumference
development
failure to thrive (FTT)
immunization
intercede
lethargic
listlessness
malnutrition
pediatric
percentile
preventive
vaccination information statement (VIS)

## PEDIATRICS

**Pediatrics** is a specialty of medicine that cares for children from birth until essentially adulthood. The initial pediatrician's examination will often be done in the hospital a few hours after birth, but the state of health of the newborn actually began many months before with the prenatal care of the mother. Some practices limit care at 16 years of age, whereas others may continue until patients reach 18 years of age or high school graduation.

Almost immediately after birth, the infant is evaluated by the **Apgar** scoring system, which is an indication of the newborn's well-being (described in Chapter 35). This score, from 0–10, determines the infant's first individual experience with medical care. A score of 10 is considered the best possible condition; a score below 4 requires immediate intervention and continued evaluation.

With many hospital discharges occurring between 24 and 48 hours after birth, infants begin their journey through the pediatrician's office at approximately one to two weeks of age. At this visit, the height and weight are measured, diet and eating concerns discussed, and any lab tests such as PKU and bilirubin screenings or other procedures deemed necessary are performed. By 2 months, infants return for another examination and evaluation and begin the **immunization** schedule.

After that, infants continue to be examined at 2- to 3-month intervals throughout the first 18 months, and immunizations should be completed. Children continue to be examined on a yearly basis to monitor their development toward maturity. The American Academy of Pediatrics (AAP) has established Recommendations for Preventive Pediatric Health Care, a chart that outlines the types and frequency of examinations to provide **preventive** care for normally developing, healthy children. Go to the AAP's Website at www.aap.org and search for "Recommendations for Preventive Pediatric Health Care" to view and download the most up-to-date, comprehensive chart. If health or development problems occur, a more frequent schedule will be necessary.

Another program that requires regular health maintenance exams and careful documentation of examination findings is the Early and Periodic Screening, Diagnosis, and Treatment (EPSDT) program, Medicaid's comprehensive and preventive child health program. This is for eligible Medicaid patients who are between birth and 21 years of age. This program requires regular routine health maintenance checkups to detect and treat medical problems before they become serious or beyond treatment stages. The parent or primary **caregiver** must accompany the child at each visit.

The program includes the following screening services:

- Comprehensive health and developmental history (assessment of both physical and mental health development)
- Comprehensive unclothed physical exam
- Appropriate immunizations
- Laboratory tests
- Lead toxicity screening
- Health education
- Vision services
- Dental services
- Hearing services
- Other necessary health care (states must provide other necessary health care, diagnosis services, treatment, and other measures to correct problems discovered by the aforementioned screening services.)

## PEDIATRIC GROWTH AND DEVELOPMENT

Pediatric patients are examined much more frequently than adults and must be monitored carefully because of their rapid growth and **development**, especially in the first year. Growth refers to the changes in height and weight that can be measured as the infant begins to mature. Development refers to an infant's ability to control his or her body and use verbal and mental skills. These areas of assessment, as well as the apparent intellectual and social development of the developing child, are closely observed and compared with acceptable national standards. This comparison determines whether the child is at the appropriate level of development as compared to the **chronologic** age. Children will vary in individual development, but when characteristics are beyond acceptable levels, intervention will be initiated to identify the reason.

A great deal of physical, mental, and social development occurs within a relatively short period of 2 years. The ability to sit, stand, and walk; hold and use toys and utensils; and progress from babbling sounds to words all unfold over that time period. Children develop their own personality and exhibit a degree of independence (Figure 42–1). Table 42–1 highlights growth and development during infancy and toddlerhood. The table shows the age at which the average child should be able to perform the activities listed.

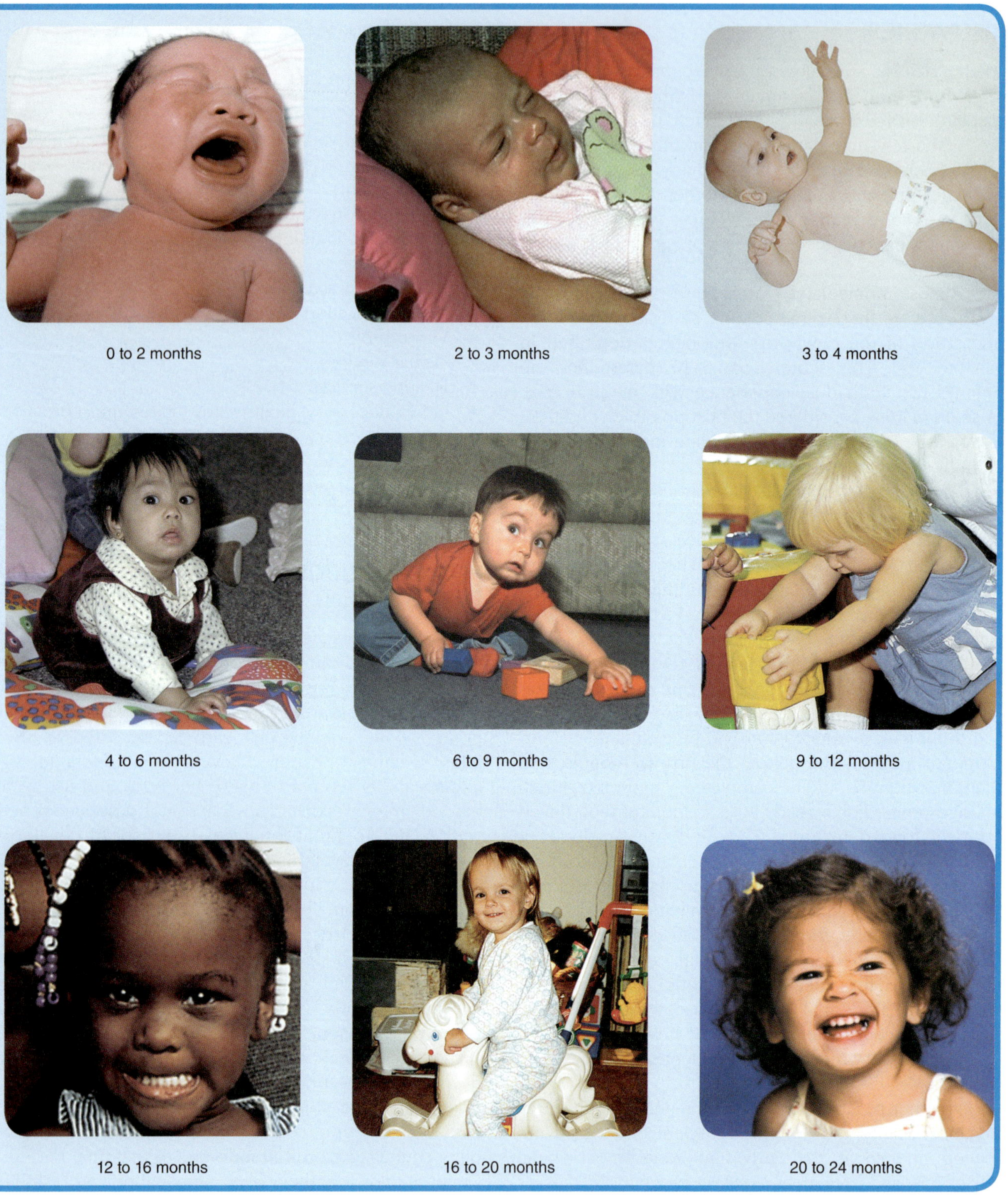


**Figure 42–1:** Growth and development stages of infants and toddlers. *Delmar/Cengage Learning.*

**TABLE 42–1 Growth and Development from Newborn to 30 Months**

| Age | Gross Motor | Fine Motor | Language | Sensory |
|---|---|---|---|---|
| Birth to 1 month | • Assumes tonic neck posture<br>• When prone, lifts and turns head | • Holds hands in fist<br>• Draws arms and legs to body | • Cries | • Comforts with holding and touch<br>• Looks at faces<br>• Follows objects when in line of vision<br>• Alert to high-pitched voices<br>• Smiles |
| 2 to 4 months | • Can raise head and shoulders when prone to 45–90 degrees; supports self on forearms<br>• Rolls from back to side | • Hands mostly open<br>• Looks at and plays with fingers<br>• Grasps and tries to reach objects | • Vocalizes when talked to; coos, babbles<br>• Laughs aloud<br>• Squeals | • Smiles<br>• Follows objects 180 degrees<br>• Turns head when hears voices or sounds |
| 4 to 6 months | • Turns from stomach to back and then back to stomach<br>• When pulled to sitting, almost no head lag<br>• By 6 months, can sit on floor with hands forward for support | • Can hold feet and put in mouth<br>• Can hold bottle<br>• Can grasp rattle and other small objects<br>• Puts objects in mouth | • Squeals | • Watches a falling object<br>• Responds to sounds |
| 6 to 8 months | • Puts full weight on legs when held in standing position<br>• Can sit without support<br>• Bounces when held in a standing position | • Transfers objects from one hand to the other<br>• Can feed self a cookie<br>• Can bang two objects together | • Babbles vowel-like sounds, "ooh" or "aah"<br>• Imitation of speech sounds ("mama," "dada") begins<br>• Laughs aloud | • Responds by looking and smiling<br>• Recognizes own name |
| 8 to 10 months | • Crawls on all fours or uses arms to pull body along floor<br>• Can pull self to sitting<br>• Can pull self to standing | • Beginning to use thumb-finger grasp<br>• Dominant hand use<br>• Has good hand-mouth coordination | • Responds to verbal commands<br>• May say one word in addition to "mama" and "dada" | • Recognizes sounds |

*(continues)*

**TABLE 42–1** *(Continued)*

| Age | Gross Motor | Fine Motor | Language | Sensory |
|---|---|---|---|---|
| 10 to 12 months | • Can sit down from standing<br>• Walks around room holding onto objects<br>• Can stand alone | • Picks up and drops objects<br>• Can put small objects into toys or containers through holes<br>• Turns many pages in a book at one time<br>• Picks up small objects | • Understands "no" and other simple commands<br>• Learns one or two other words<br>• Imitates speech sounds<br>• Speaks gibberish | • Follows fast-moving objects<br>• Indicates wants<br>• Likes to play imitative games such as patty cake and peek-a-boo |
| 12 to 15 months | • Can walk alone well<br>• Can crawl up stairs | • Can feed self with cup and spoon<br>• Puts raisins into a bottle<br>• May hold crayon or pencil and scribble<br>• Builds a tower of two cubes | • Says four to six words | • Binocular vision developed |
| 18 months | • Runs, falling often<br>• Can jump in place<br>• Can walk up stairs holding on<br>• Plays with push and pull toys | • Can build a tower of three to four cubes<br>• Can use a spoon | • Says 10 or more words<br>• Points to objects or body parts when asked | • Visual acuity 20/40 |
| 24 months | • Can walk up and down stairs<br>• Can kick a ball<br>• Can ride a tricycle | • Can draw a circle<br>• Tries to dress self | • Talks a lot<br>• Approximately 300-word vocabulary<br>• Understands commands<br>• Knows first name, refers to self<br>• Verbalizes toilet needs | |
| 30 months | • Throws a ball<br>• Jumps with both feet<br>• Can stand on one foot for a few minutes | • Can build a tower of eight blocks<br>• Can use crayons<br>• Learning to use scissors | • Knows first and last name<br>• Knows the name of one color<br>• Can sing<br>• Expresses needs<br>• Uses pronouns appropriately | |

## PEDIATRIC MEASUREMENTS

Precise measurements of the pediatric patient are essential for monitoring the growth and development of the child. In addition to monitoring normal physical development, the provider may use growth patterns and developments to assist in diagnosing diseases. Routine measurements that are obtained at every well-child visit include height or recumbent length, weight, and **circumference** of the head and chest.

## Measuring Height

Measuring the height of a baby from infancy to 36 months by recumbent length is recommended as the most accurate method of measurement. The baby should be placed on a pediatric scale with built-in height measurement apparatus or on an infant height measurement chart board with the placement of the baby's head at the headboard. If necessary, someone holds the head in position while you stretch the legs out straight. (Infants tend to flex their legs.) You then slide the footboard up to the infants' heels and measure from the vertex of the head to the heel of the baby. Refer to Figure 42–2 and Procedure 42–1 regarding how to place the baby on the exam table for measuring the recumbent length.

It is also possible to measure the recumbent length of an infant without a measuring scale or chart. Place the infant lying on an examination surface that is covered with paper and make a mark on the paper at the top of the infant's head. (Enlist the parent or another medical assistant to help position the infant.) With the parent holding the infant in position, straighten out one leg and mark on the paper at the bottom of the heel. Ask the parent to pick up the infant. Using a flexible tape or ruled measuring device, measure the distance between your two markings on the paper to obtain the recumbent length of the infant. Whether you are using a table that has a headboard, a measuring scale, or a portable measuring chart (shown in Figure 42–2), follow the directions for that particular device in your facility.

When the child reaches 3 years of age (36 months), he or she generally is old enough to cooperate, and you can begin to measure the height and weight on a regular balance beam scale, following the same procedure as an adult patient (refer to Procedure 38–1). The child's shoes should be removed and the measuring bar placed on the top (vertex) of the child's head to get an accurate measurement (Figure 42–3). The child must stand still in the center of the platform until the height measurement is obtained. To reduce the amount of time the child is in place on the platform of the scales, look at the chart and see what the measurement was at the last exam so that you can have an idea where the measurement will be.

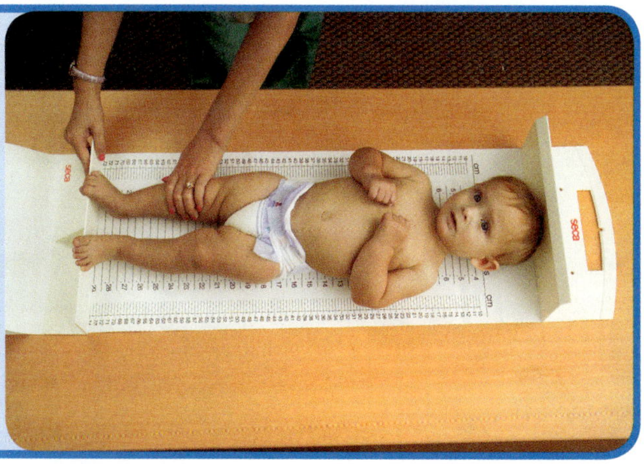

**Figure 42–2:** Measuring recumbent length of an infant, measuring from the vertex of the child's head to the heel. *Delmar/Cengage Learning.*

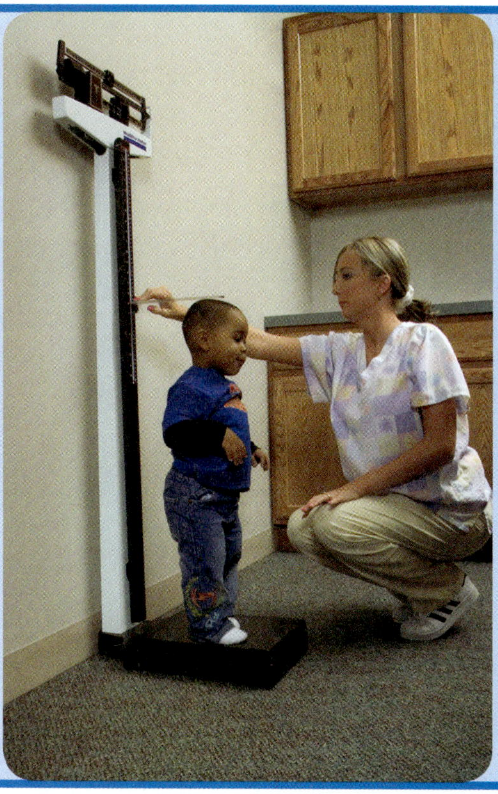

**Figure 42–3:** Measuring the child's height on a regular balance beam scale, placing the measuring bar at the vertex of the patient's head. *Delmar/Cengage Learning.*

## Weighing the Pediatric Patient

It is customary to weigh infants unclothed for greater accuracy. Remember, a wet diaper can weigh several ounces, which would lead to an inaccurate measurement of the infant's true weight. Because you cannot control an infant's elimination, a disposable, waterproof pad should be placed on the scale, and a dry diaper can be placed over the genital area in case urination occurs. It is possible to adjust the weight to accommodate for the pad and diaper if the infant's weight is of great concern. Simply place it on the scale and adjust the balance weight to zero *before* the infant is placed on the scale. If an infant gains or loses weight too quickly, it could be a signal of a disease or disorder and should be brought to the provider's attention. It is also important to ask the

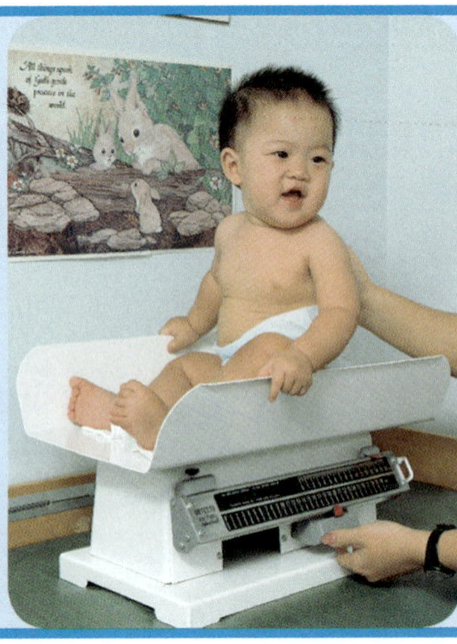

**Figure 42–4:** A baby weighed in sitting position; place your hand close to the child for safety. *Delmar/Cengage Learning.*

caregiver about the feeding schedule and appetite of the infant or child.

In some offices and clinics, the pediatric scale is kept on a stainless steel cart and simply wheeled to the patient's room. In a family or general practice office, the facility may have a pediatric room where all infants and children are examined. In a pediatric office, every patient room may have an infant scale, or the scale may be kept in a specific location where all infants and children are examined. Figures 42–4 and 42–5 show the proper positioning of the baby on the scales. Follow Procedure 42–1 to weigh an infant or baby up to 36 months or 38 pounds.

As the infant grows into the toddler stage and on to a preschooler and passes the weight limit of the infant scale, the weight can be measured on the regular balance beam scale used for older children and adults. (Refer to Procedure 38–1.) Often, the provider asks for the weight to be taken with the child unclothed except for the underwear. This is a good time for you to provide a gown for the patient, as mentioned earlier, for while he or she waits for the provider. Remember that children have feelings and may be embarrassed without their clothes.

## Head Circumference

The head circumference is measured by placing a flexible tape measure around the infant's or child's head. You want the tape measure to go around the back part of the skull that protrudes out the farthest and around in front on the forehead. It is often necessary to ask for assistance in keeping the child from pulling on the tape while you are measuring the head. Place the tape under the head if the patient is lying down, about an inch above the ears, and around to the forehead. To get an accurate measurement, you should take the measurement more than once. This measurement should be performed and recorded routinely at each office visit until the child is 36 months of age. This is important for

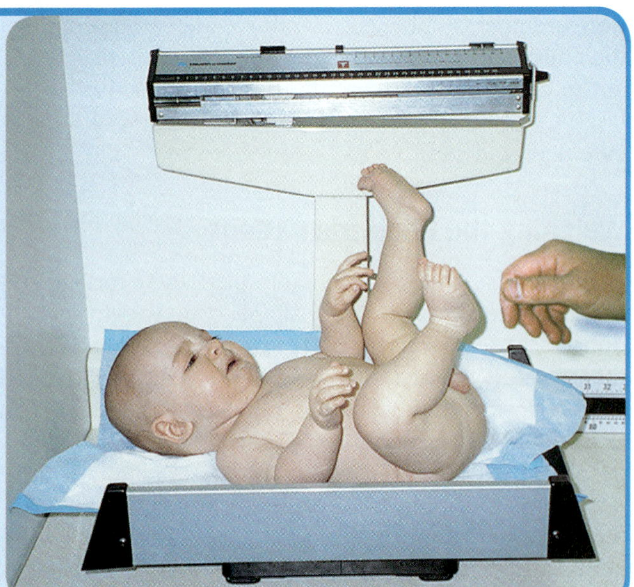

**Figure 42–5:** Infants too young to sit are weighed lying down; place your hand close to the child for safety. *Delmar/Cengage Learning.*

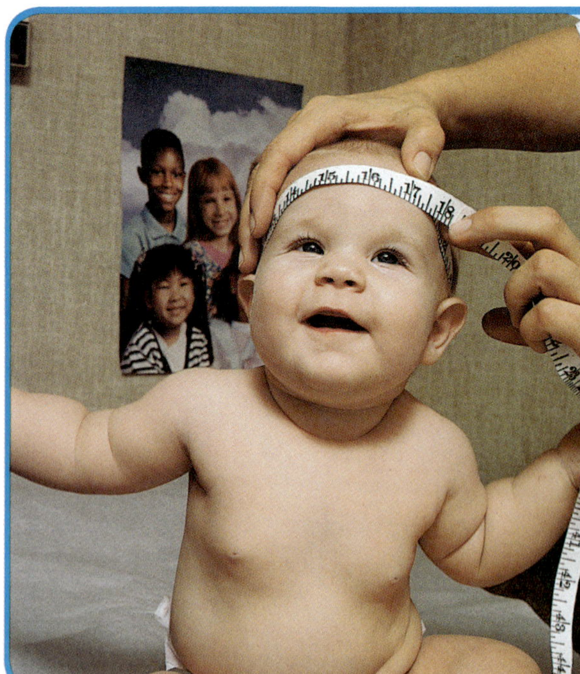

**Figure 42–6:** Measuring the head circumference of an infant. *Delmar/Cengage Learning.*

alerting the provider of abnormal development. Refer to Figure 42–6 to see the correct placement of the measuring tape. Procedure 42–1 will help you perform this measurement.

## Chest Circumference

The chest circumference is measured by placing the flexible measuring tape around the child's chest just above the nipples (Figure 42–7). Often, it is difficult to keep the baby from moving. As said before, ask for assistance from the caregiver or another medical assistant. Place the measuring tape under the child and bring it around the baby's back to the chest to meet the zero mark. This measurement is not required on the growth graph but should be recorded on the chart. Refer to Procedure 42–1 for measuring an infant's chest circumference.

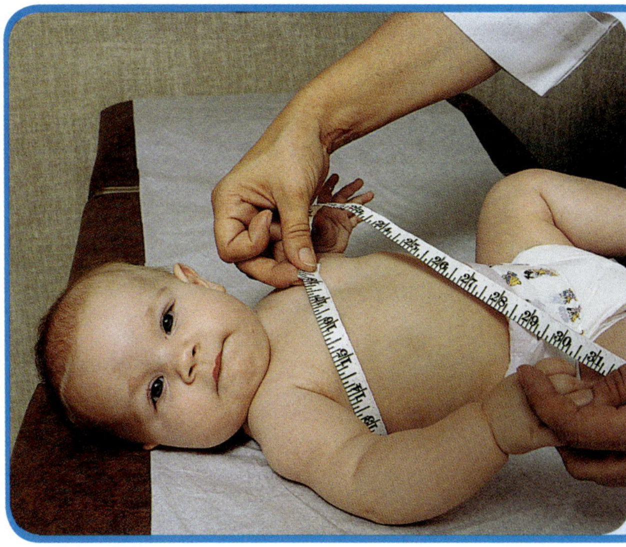

**Figure 42–7:** Measuring the chest circumference of an infant. *Delmar/Cengage Learning.*

## PROCEDURE 42–1 Measure Length, Weight, and Head and Chest Circumference of an Infant or Child

**PURPOSE:** To obtain an accurate measurement of an infant or child's length, weight, and head and chest circumference

**EQUIPMENT:** Exam table with table paper, portable measurement chart board, measuring tape, patient's chart with growth chart or EMR; parents' record booklet, pediatric scale, and pen

S **SKILL:** Measure length, weight, and head and chest circumference of an infant or child

| Procedure Steps | Detailed Instructions and/or *Rationales* |
|---|---|
| **Measure Weight** | |
| B 1. Introduce yourself, identify the patient, and explain the procedure to the parent or caregiver, ***using language that the parent or caregiver will understand.*** Wash hands. | |
| 2. Ask the parent to undress the infant or child, including diaper. | *This alleviates the infant's apprehension and conserves your time.* |
| 3. Place both weights to the left of the scale to check the balance. | |
| 4. Place a water absorbent pad on the scale; reset scale to zero if necessary. | *To avoid disease transmission and decrease shock from the cold metal for the infant. This will decrease the chance that the infant will move because of being uncomfortable or afraid.* |

*(continues)*

*(continued)*

| Procedure Steps | Detailed Instructions and/or *Rationales* |
|---|---|
| B 5. Gently place the infant on his or her back on the scale; ***place your hand slightly above the child to ensure safety.*** | The age of the baby may determine how the child is placed on the scales. Small infants will be easier to weigh lying down; those who can sit up on their own will most likely be more cooperative sitting on the scales. In either case, the safety of the baby is primary. |
| 6. Place the bottom weight to the highest measurement that will not cause the balance bar to drop to the bottom edge. | |
| 7. Slowly move upper weight until the balance bar rests in the center of the indicator. Read the infant's weight while he or she is lying still. | |
| 8. Return both weights to their resting position to the extreme left. | |
| 9. Gently remove infant and assist parent to apply diaper. | |
| 10. Discard the used absorbent pad. | |
| **Measuring Length** | |
| B 1. Explain the procedure to the parent or caregiver, ***using language that the parent or caregiver will understand.*** | |
| 2. Gently place infant on his or her back on the portable measurement chart board with the top of the infant's head flush to the top of the board. Keep the legs straight and slide the footboard up so it is flush with the infant's heels. | There can be discrepancies with measurement of newborns because they are so used to the fetal position that it is difficult to straighten the legs. |
| 3. Gently remove the infant. Measure the distance the between the headboard and the footboard. Read the length in inches to the nearest ¼, ½, or ¾ inch. | |
| **Measuring Head Circumference** | |
| B 1. Explain the procedure to the parent or caregiver, ***using language that the parent or caregiver will understand.*** | |
| 2. Place measuring tape snug around the forehead at the widest part. | Pull the tape snugly to compress any hair. |
| 3. Read measurement to the nearest ¼, ½, or ¾ inch. | |
| **Measuring Chest Circumference** | |
| B 1. Explain the procedure to the parent or caregiver, ***using language that the parent or caregiver will understand.*** | |

| Procedure Steps | Detailed Instructions and/or *Rationales* |
|---|---|
| 2. Use one thumb to hold the tape measure at the zero mark against the infant's chest at the midsternal area and around the nipples. | The infant or child may lie down on the examination table or be held by a parent or guardian for the procedure. Children of 2 or 3 years and older may sit or stand on their own if they will cooperate and remain still for the procedure. Accurate measurement cannot be achieved if the child is crying. The measurement should be taken when the child is breathing normally, not with forced inspiration or expiration. |
| 3. Read measurement to the nearest ¼, ½, or ¾ or inch. | |
| 4. Document the measurements in the patient's medical record and growth chart. | No chest measurements are included on the growth chart. The next section, and Procedure 42–2, details the steps in plotting measurements on growth charts. |

**Charting Example**

| | |
|---|---|
| 5-12-XX<br>11:30 am | Wt. 16 lbs 9 oz, Ht. 26 in., head circumference 16 ¼ inches., Chest circumference 64 cm.<br>G. Jenks, CMA(AAMA) |

## GROWTH CHARTS

All babies grow at different rates. The growth and development of the child is recorded in the patient's chart, in the caregiver's record booklet (if he or she has one), and on growth charts from the National Center for Health Statistics (NCHS), a division within the Centers for Disease Control and Prevention (CDC). These charts can be downloaded from the CDC's Website at www.cdc.gov/growthcharts and allow providers to see at a glance the child's growth and development pattern. The growth chart shows the normal growth of infants and children up to 20 years of age. The provider can then compare the child's measurements in relation to the **percentile**, that of other children the same age. (This percentile is to the far right of the graph; see Figure 42–8A.) The percentiles are calculated by plotting the child's measurements on the graph paper and locating the percentile it falls into by following the line it is plotted on to the outside of the paper where the percentiles are listed. The curved-line section closest to the top of the page, is where the height, length, and stature are recorded. The curved-line section below that is for plotting the weight of children. If the percentile of the height and weight of the child combined is wanted, the back section of the chart contains an area in which you draw an imaginary line from the child's weight to the height and plot it. You can then follow the line up the curved graph to the percentile on the right. If the measurements of a baby or child fall above or below the normal height or weight areas and the family history does not warrant it, further examination and diagnostic testing is usually scheduled.

If using an EMR system for documentation, the growth chart will display the height and weight information that you enter into the system through either the physical examination and vitals section or onto the growth chart itself, depending on the system. The record will then show the data points of the infant or child in comparison to other infants and children of that same age. The EHR provides a screen shot of this graphical data for the provider to use to monitor the child's physical development as is done with the paper chart documentation.

The growth charts become a permanent record of the child's development and are to be filed in the patient's chart. At each subsequent visit, the child's growth should be recorded. These growth graphs aid in the diagnosis of growth abnormalities, nutritional disorders, and diseases of children from birth to 20 years of age. Of course, hereditary factors also influence growth patterns, hence the importance of having a complete family health history in the medical record.

Refer to Figures 42–8A through D to see the growth graphs for boys and girls. Two graphs record growth patterns of infant males and females from birth to 36 months, and two record growth patterns record growth patterns of boys and girls from 2 to 20 years of age.

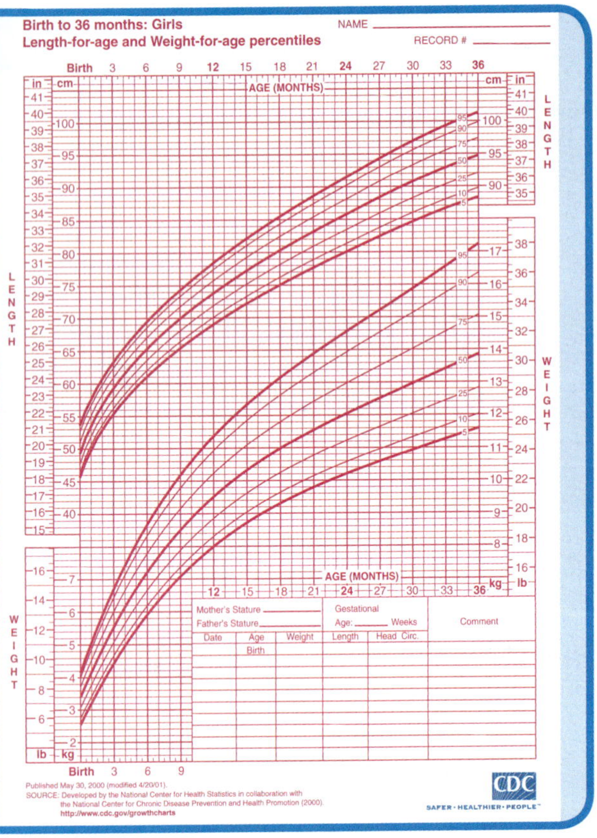


**Figure 42–8A:** Growth graph for height and weight, girls 0–36 months. *Courtesy of the Centers for Disease Control and Prevention.*

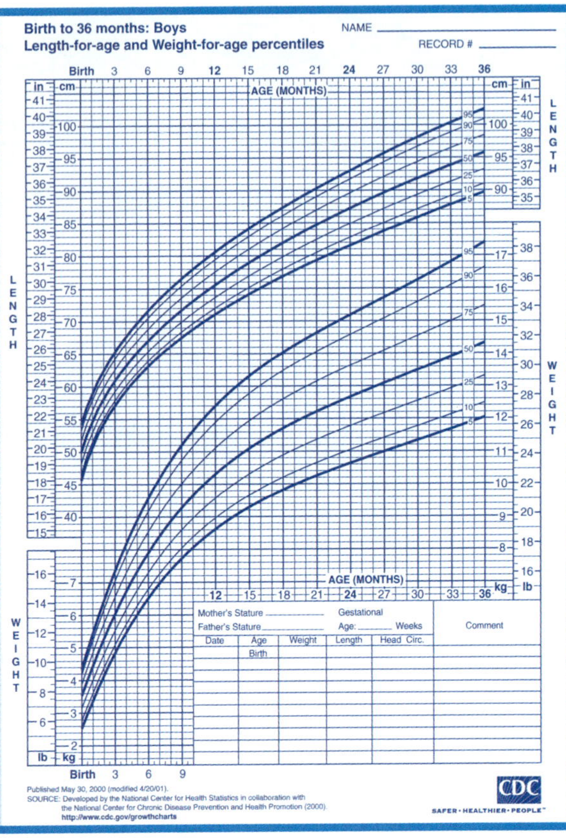


**Figure 42–8B:** Growth graph for height and weight, boys 0–36 months. *Courtesy of the Centers for Disease Control and Prevention.*

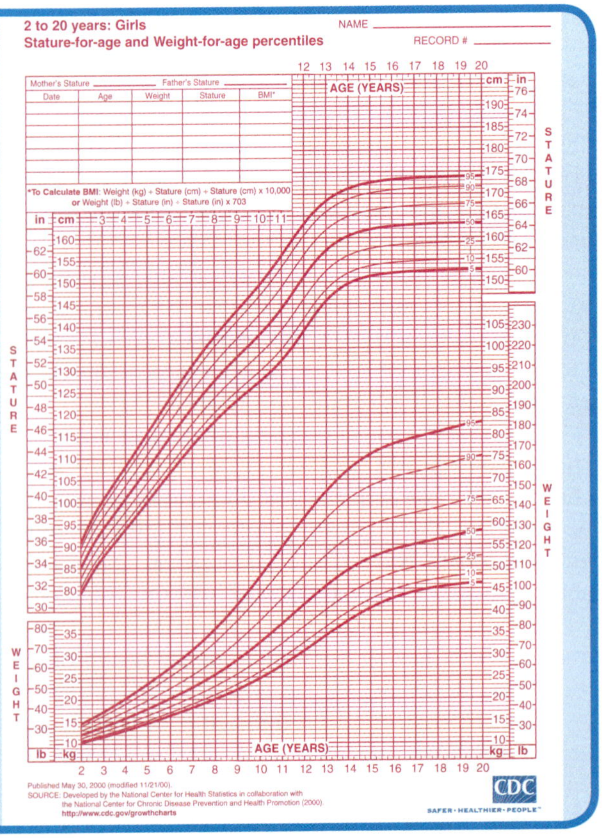


**Figure 42–8C:** Growth graph for height and weight, girls 2–20 *years. Courtesy of the Centers for Disease Control and Prevention.*

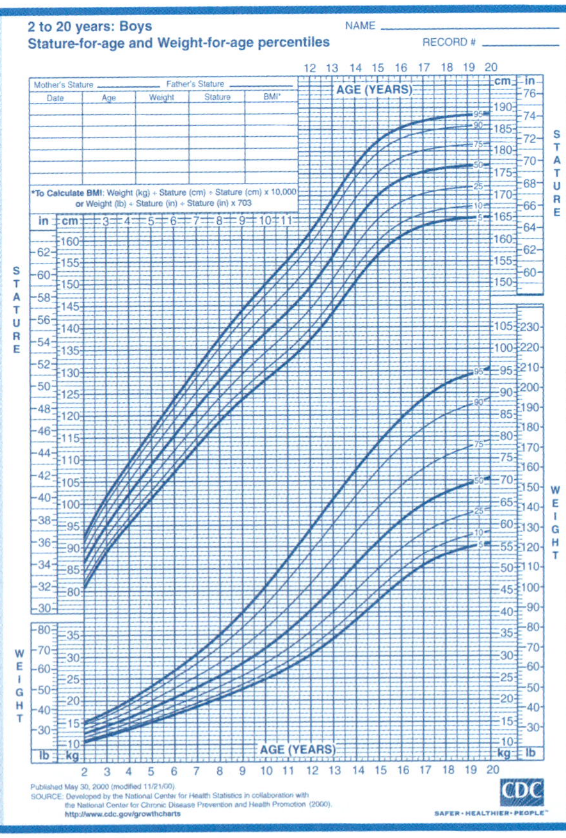


**Figure 42–8D:** Growth graph for height and weight, boys 2–20 years. *Courtesy of the Centers for Disease Control and Prevention.*

This information is printed across the top and bottom of the graph. Each of the squares across the page represents one month for the birth to 36-month graph and one year for the 2- to 20-year graph. Be sure you use the appropriate chart for the patient because the normal development and growth patterns are different for males and females. On the front of each of the graphs is a ruled section to record the date; age; length, height, and stature; and weight of the child at each appointment. The line for comments is for you to record a brief chief complaint that the caregiver (or the child, if old enough to speak) tells you. By looking at the line provided for the comments, you can see it is vital for you to print small and neatly so that it can be read easily. The complaint or problem should also be neatly recorded on the chart.

After the measurements of height, weight, and head circumference have been obtained, they are plotted on the graph where the age and the measurement intersect. To record the height measurement, simply follow the age line (vertically) to the child's length measurement (horizontally) on the left, follow the horizontal line to the point at which the two intersect, and place a dot there with your pen. For recording the weight of the infant or child, stay on the vertical (age) line and look to the right side of the graph if over 16 pounds or on the left if under. Following the horizontal line from right to left, you then place a dot at the intersection of the weight and age lines. The recumbent length of the child is recorded in inches or centimeters and the weight in either pounds or kilograms. Be consistent when measuring the child to avoid confusion.

Procedure 42–2 describes how to plot measurements on a growth chart.

## PROCEDURE 42–2 Plot Data on a Growth Chart

**PURPOSE:** To record the growth and development of a patient accurately on a growth chart

**EQUIPMENT:** Patient's chart and growth chart; pen or EHR

**S SKILL:** Plot pediatric patient's measurements on a growth chart.

| Procedure Steps | Detailed Instructions and/or *Rationales* |
|---|---|
| 1. Obtain measurement data from the patient's chart. | This should include the patient's weight, height, and head circumference. |
| 2. Locate the patient's age on the growth chart. | This runs across the top and bottom of the growth chart. |
| 3. Locate the patient's height on the growth chart. | Depending on the child's length, you will find this on the left or right margin of the chart. |
| 4. Locate the patient's weight on the growth chart. | Depending on the child's weight, you will find this on the left or right margin of the chart. |
| 5. Find where the age on the horizontal line and child's height or length on the vertical line intersect and plot the measurement by making a dot on the chart. | You can then follow the curved line that you plotted on up to the right where it ends to read the percentile. |
| 6. Do the same for the child's weight. | |
| 7. On the back side of the chart, find the graph for the head circumference. This is plotted the same way. | |
| 8. Fill in the box chart on the growth chart with the date, patient's age, weight, height, and head circumference. | This allows the provider to see the development at a glance. |
| 9. Some providers want you to connect the dots of the measurements over time with a thin line. You can also determine the child's percentile by following the line on which the measurement is plotted to the side of the paper where the percentiles are indicated. | Refer to Figure 42–9 for a sample of a completed growth chart. |

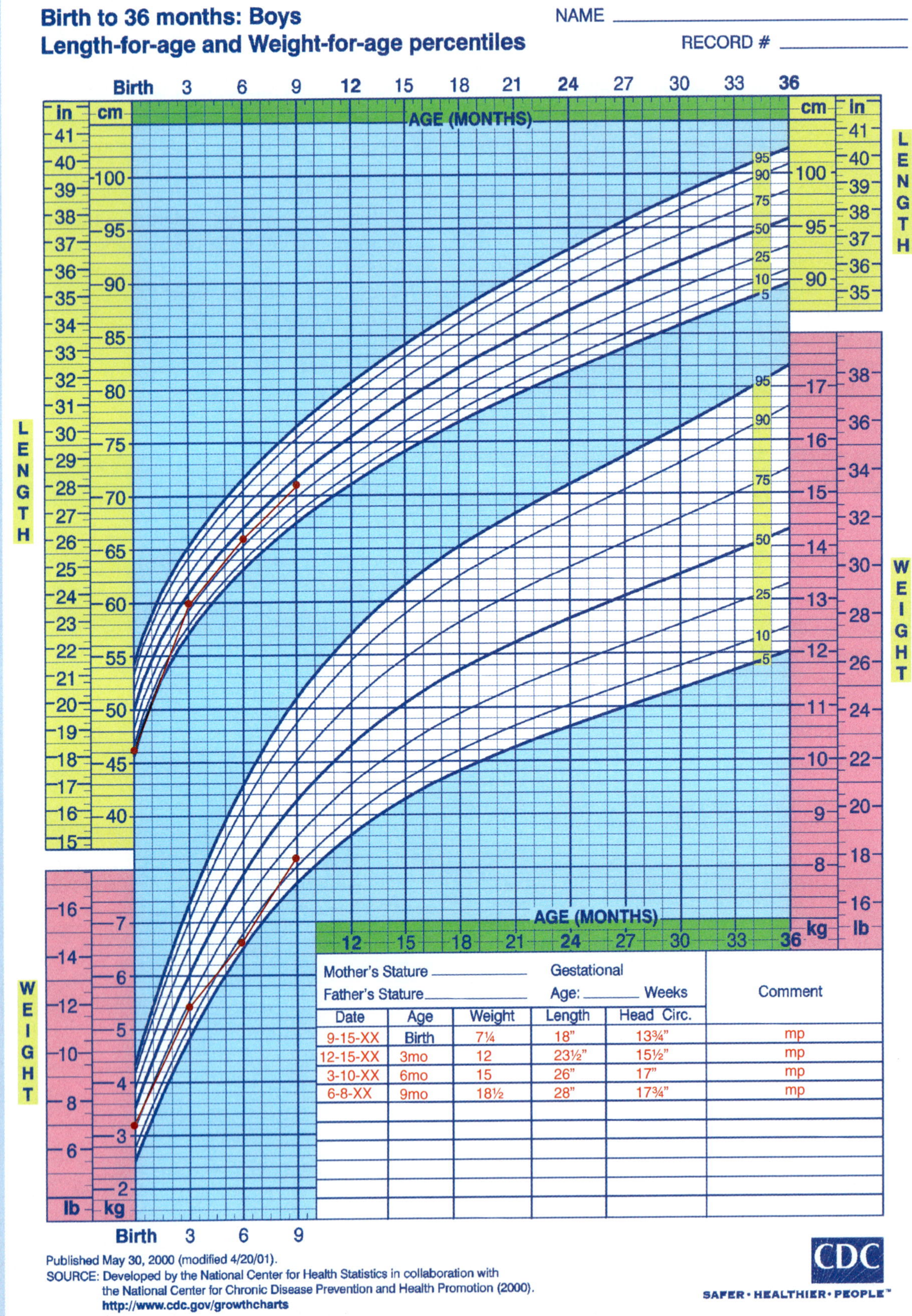


| Date | Age | Weight | Length | Head Circ. | Comment |
|---|---|---|---|---|---|
| 9-15-XX | Birth | 7¼ | 18" | 13¾" | mp |
| 12-15-XX | 3mo | 12 | 23½" | 15½" | mp |
| 3-10-XX | 6mo | 15 | 26" | 17" | mp |
| 6-8-XX | 9mo | 18½ | 28" | 17¾" | mp |

**Figure 42–9:** Completed growth chart. *Courtesy of the Centers for Disease Control and Prevention.*

### Failure to Thrive

An infant or young child who is below the third percentile on standardized growth charts is said to have a **failure to thrive (FTT)**. The cause may be from a physical problem (such as an unrepaired cleft palate or a disease condition) or associated with a poor physical and emotional environment. Normally, when a baby is born, a great deal of examining, touching, cuddling, and expressions of love are directed toward it. The infant is known to respond to this behavior, and this parent-child relationship is called **attachment** and **bonding**. When this does not occur, the baby lacks emotional support. Often, care is not provided on a consistent basis. If food is offered, the baby might be too **lethargic** to eat. Parents might lack knowledge about infant care, have anxiety about being a parent, or just be unconcerned. Parental illness, drug abuse, an unwanted or ill infant, and other factors can cause difficulty. With irregular and often absent care, the infant will show physical, emotional, and social delays in development.

When conducting the interview and performing the procedures prior to the provider's examination, the medical assistant has an opportunity to observe the parental behavior as well as the baby's condition. Some symptoms of an FTT baby are **listlessness** and avoidance of eye contact. Additionally, the infant will not seem concerned about you, a stranger, and there might be no cooing or crying. Older infants may not be interested in toys or playing. Parents may exhibit a lack of concern, not ask questions, and express negative comments about the baby. Inform the provider of any behaviors you observe that seem different to you so that awareness can be established and further examined.

## WELL-CHILD OR SICK-CHILD VISITS

When a parent calls for an appointment, it should be determined whether the visit is for a routine well-child examination or the child has symptoms of an illness. Specific well-child hours are usually set aside in each day's schedule to care for the routine examinations and procedures (as identified on the Recommendations for Preventive Pediatric Health Care chart). However, when a child is ill, most pediatricians will attempt to see the child within a few hours of a parent's call. Parents can usually phone the pediatrician's office at all hours of the day or night and someone who is on call will respond. Some practices use an answering device or service to receive parental messages and then respond to those accordingly. Practices may also set aside early office hours to see children who have become ill overnight. Check with your employer for the guidelines at your facility.

### The Pediatric Office Environment

When young patients come in to see the provider, your attitude may be the deciding factor in their cooperation during the visit. Greeting them with a smile and speaking to them on their developmental level will help gain their trust and cooperation.

**CLINICAL PEARL**

Patients of all ages are much more cooperative when they feel welcome. Some children may be fearful of health care providers or the medical office, due to prior traumatic experiences in emergency care centers because of serious illness or injury, or even because of an immunization. Some parents may even contribute to this fear by using threats of medical care and shots when disciplining children. If you take time, showing interest and patience, you can establish a rapport with the patients and help eliminate this potential problem.

The play area in the reception area helps the children feel welcome and provides a comfortable environment. A variety of safe, durable, washable, and educational toys should be provided. Toys that have many or tiny parts are not appropriate because they can be a potential choking hazard or create an unsafe walkway if left out, causing others to fall and possibly be hurt. Keeping the toys clean and contained in one area will be one of your duties.

**CLINICAL PEARL**

Often, a child will find an interesting toy while waiting to be called in to the examination room. The child's cooperation will be greater if the patient is permitted to bring the toy back to the exam room, which helps you gain compliance in performing any necessary procedures in preparation for the provider's examination. When the child is finished with the toy, ensure that it is sanitized properly before returning it to the play area for other children.

Ideally, the play area should be used only for well children who are waiting for annual physical examinations or other well visits, checkups, allergy injections, or immunizations. Every attempt should be made to provide for the separation of well and sick children in the office, including providing separate reception areas. When an ill child is brought to the office, the administrative medical assistant should be notified and accommodations made to take the sick child back into an examination or other private area immediately. At the very least, a separate area with its own toys should be set aside so that the office play area and toys are not available to the sick child.

**CLINICAL PEARL**

Children (and patients of any age) becoming sick and vomiting is a concern in any medical facility. The administrative medical assistant should keep a disposable emesis basin near the front desk for this potential situation. You should also keep a commercial preparation accessible for use in cleaning up this type of waste. Gloves, paper towels, facial tissues, and biohazardous plastic waste bags should also be easily accessible. A covered waste receptacle lined with a biohazardous plastic bag for disposal of contaminated items should be available.

There can be occasions when a parent or caregiver brings a seriously ill or injured child into the facility unannounced. You must act quickly to provide immediate care to the patient and protect others from the possible transmission of the disease.

## Medical Assistant Responsibilities

As a medical assistant, you will have certain routine responsibilities to perform with each pediatric examination. Generally, you will:

- Assist in gathering data.
- Document information.
- Perform screening tests within your skill and ability level.
- Assist the patient.
- Assist the provider.
- Provide patient education.

Some providers require all patients from age 2 to 100 years to have vital signs taken and recorded at every visit regardless of the reason for the appointment. Others feel it is necessary only periodically or when indicated by symptoms. Check with your employer for his or her preferences. Accuracy in the documentation of each of these components is essential to quality care for these young patients. You also should afford time with parents or caregivers and children to provide patient education as appropriate to the child's age and developmental stage.

When you are assisting with the examination of a child, a very important responsibility is relaying information to the provider from the parent or caregiver and from the provider to the patient and parent or caregiver. Your careful observation of the child and the parent or caregiver–child relationship could be critical information to the provider in the care and treatment of the child. Make note of any unusual observations and advise the provider before the child is seen.

## Child Neglect and Abuse

One area of awareness concerns the suspicion of **child neglect** or **child abuse**. Neglect refers to the lack of or withholding of care. Abuse refers to inflicting emotional, physical, or sexual injury. The federal Child Abuse Prevention and Treatment Act states that all threats or acts that might cause physical or mental harm to a child *must be* reported. This refers to suspicion of neglect of care as well as of abuse. Anyone, whether a teacher, neighbor, social worker, family member, or health care worker, is obligated to report neglect or abuse to the proper authorities. The law protects the person who makes the report under a confidentiality provision. It should be mentioned that although parents are responsible for their child's care, that responsibility is often given to other caregivers such as grandparents, babysitters, or boyfriends or girlfriends of the single parent. This act applies to all caregivers.

As a medical assistant, be aware of neglect and abuse symptoms, some of which are not too obvious. During your interview and performance of routine procedures, you might feel there is a possibility of inadequate care. Alert the provider of your suspicions before the examination because they must be evaluated by the provider. It is beyond your scope of practice as an MA to determine whether neglect or abuse is occurring; only the provider can make such a diagnosis and will contact the appropriate authorities. The appropriate authorities to whom the provider should make a report in your community should be identified in the office manual. Table 42–2 lists some of the more obvious examples of neglect and abuse for your information.

## Establishing Rapport

Cooperation with youngsters is generally obtained by explaining, in a calm, simple manner appropriate to their stage of development, what you and the provider are going to do and why. If you sense behavior that is not cooperative, you must ask the parent or caregiver to **intercede**. A child who is uncooperative for a necessary procedure has to be restrained safely by you and the parent or another health care worker. Doing what has to be done as quickly as possible is the best way to handle the situation.

Young children are often amused with items that are not ordinary toys during an examination, such as a plastic drinking cup or tongue depressor (with supervision, of course). Giving children non-sharp instruments

**TABLE 42–2 Symptoms of Neglect and Abuse**

| Neglect | Abuse |
|---|---|
| Excessive length of time before seeking medical attention for illness or injury | Discoloration or bruises on the back, buttocks, or any other area |
| Apparent **malnutrition** | Evidence of burns in unusual places |
| Obvious lack of dental care | Internal abdominal pain |
| Immunizations neglected or incomplete | Dislocation of joints, such as shoulder and wrist |
| Poor personal hygiene | Frequent injuries requiring medical attention |
| Inadequate clothing for season or size; unclean | An X-ray of current injury showing evidence of untreated previous fractures |
| Developmental delay | Suspicious story about the injury; difference between description by child and parent or caregiver |
| Parental comments indicating lack of concern or not wanting child | Reports by the child of sexual or physical abuse |

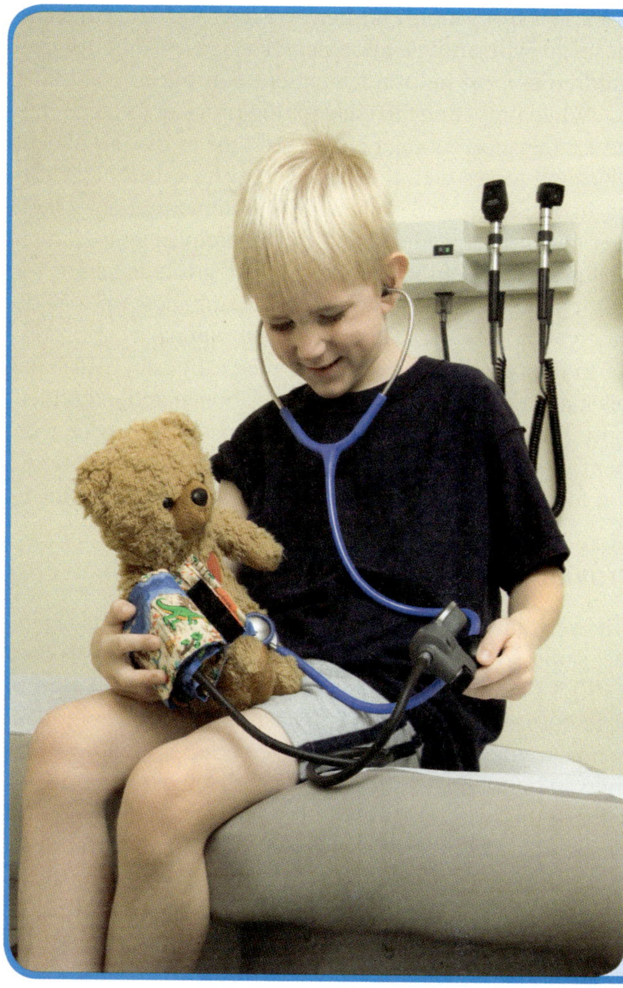

**Figure 42–10:** The child is allowed to become familiar with the blood pressure instruments the provider will use to examine him. *Delmar/Cengage Learning.*

such as a percussion hammer, stethoscope, or penlight to examine can help them overcome fear of their use by the doctor during the exam (Figure 42–10). Be sure to clean these items properly when the examination is completed.

Pediatric patients should be regarded as individuals and given the kindness and respect you give all patients. Be sure to provide a gown for them; many practices have specific gowns for pediatric patients with child-friendly prints on them. Young children are often embarrassed and chilled sitting on the examination table in their underwear, awaiting the doctor. This is an easy way to help them feel more comfortable and keep them warm, and they like the special treatment.

Another common practice to help little ones feel special is to provide them with bandages in colorful prints or cartoon characters for their minor cuts and abrasions or for injection sites following immunizations. Most health care providers in medical facilities that treat pediatric patients offer a small token reward such as stickers, balloons, or trinkets after their treatment or exam is completed. (Ask the parent or caregiver for approval first.) This gives the child positive reinforcement and helps establish and keep a good rapport between the medical team and the child.

**MEDIA LINK**

View the video, "Communicating with Pediatric Patients," for this chapter on the Premium Website.

## Examination Preparation

The initial part of the pediatric checkup and examination is the preparation of the baby or child. Remember to establish a good rapport with the child and the caregiver by being friendly and relaxed. Ask the caregiver about the child and how everything has been regarding the child's behavior and health as well as whether there are any problems or questions. Many caregivers or parents are unaware of developmental stages and what to expect from their children. Posting a chart regarding these growth and developmental stages of infants and children is most helpful for patient education.

While preparing the child for the provider to come into the examination room, it is an ideal time to discuss patient education topics with the caregiver such as the child's eating habits, sleep and daily activities, immunization schedules, toilet training, and taking and recording a temperature. This is a great help to parents and caregivers in caring for their children. Printed booklets and pamphlets on a wide variety of topics should be offered to parents as appropriate to their children's ages. Your medical facility will have this kind of information in a more elaborate and expanded form. Patient education materials for patients to take with them about specific topics, such as sleep disturbances, nutrition for toddlers, and toilet training, should be available.

### Provider Examination

The examination of a pediatric patient follows basically the same format of the comprehensive physical exam (CPE) for adults. The provider examines the patient from head to toe. Because little ones may be uncooperative at times, you should assist the provider by holding the child still until the exam is completed. Often the provider will ask the caregiver to hold the baby while listening to the heart and lungs. The provider will ask the caregiver about the baby's eating and sleeping schedule and how the development is progressing (e.g., at 2 to 3 months, is the baby playing with his or her own hands? at 6 months, is he or she crawling?). The provider also observes the parent or caregiver relationship. Part of the examination of toddlers and children is to observe their gait by placing the child across the room and observing him or her from behind as he or she walks to the caregiver.

## IMMUNIZATIONS

As part of the pediatric exam and AAP's Recommended Preventive Pediatric Health Care chart, babies and children receive their immunizations. You are required to have the proper immunizations ready for the provider to administer, or you may be asked to administer them yourself (office policies and providers differ regarding this procedure). You are required to record this information on the patient's immunization record in his or her chart and in the booklet that parents or caregivers keep.

Documentation of shot records is law, so recording them accurately is mandatory. The Immunization Action Coalition (IAC) provides excellent resources on its Website, www.immunize.org, including blank Vaccine Administration Records for Children and Teens and examples of how to document on them. Completed examples of these forms are shown in Figures 42–11A to B.

Make sure, before the immunizations are given, that you give the caregiver or parent the **vaccination information statement(s) (VIS)**, which provides detailed information about the immunization(s), including possible side effects in printed form for him or her to keep (Figure 42–12). A VIS for every immunization can be downloaded from the Centers for Disease Control and Prevention (CDC) Website at www.cdc.gov/vaccines/pubs/vis/default.htm. VISs in different languages can be found on the IAC Website at www.immunize.org.

> **CLINICAL PEARL**
>
> Go to www.immunize.org/handouts/ to search and download other educational handouts and resources from the IAC.

Allow parents or caregivers the time to read the sheets and ask questions. The parent or caregiver should sign for consent after he or she has read it or you have explained the information to him or her. Instruct the caregiver to contact the doctor immediately if a serious reaction should occur from the immunization. If the child has a fever the day of the scheduled appointment, the provider will check the child before giving any immunizations. Be sure to have the provider outline exactly what needs to be done as a routine so you will be efficient in getting pediatric patients ready for the provider to examine. Many practices post an immunization schedule near the immunizations to be used as a reference guide. The CDC releases annual Recommended Childhood and Adolescent Immunization Schedules for children in the United States. It is approved by the AAP and the American Academy of Family Physicians. Figures 42–13A and B show the schedule for the year 201X. In Chapter 53, you will learn more about immunizations and how to prepare the injections.

## VISION SCREENING

Vision and hearing screenings are also identified on the AAP Recommended Preventive Pediatric Health Care chart. On the chart, notice that for the first 36 months, vision screening is considered to be subjective or evaluated by history. At age 3, the child is old enough to identify items on a vision screening chart and can be evaluated more easily.

Unless the vision is considerably impaired, deficiencies might not be too obvious. Usually, the parent or caregiver will indicate that the child either holds books too closely to the face or rubs the eyes frequently. Other observations can include excessive blinking, looking cross-eyed, or turning and tilting the head forward to see well. The subspecialty area of pediatric ophthalmology can evaluate the vision of very small children and should be consulted if indicated. However, the routine screening can be done in general at pediatric offices by using the modified Snellen charts as discussed in Chapter 40.

(Page 1 of 2)

# Vaccine Administration Record for Children and Teens

Patient name: *Emily Jacobs*

Birthdate: *6/2/2005*

Chart number: ______

Before administering any vaccines, give copies of all pertinent Vaccine Information Statements (VISs) to the child's parent or legal representative and make sure he/she understands the risks and benefits of the vaccine(s). Always provide or update the patient's personal recor d card.

| Vaccine | Type of Vaccine[1] | Date given (mo/day/yr) | Funding Source (F,S,P)[2] | Site[3] | Vaccine | | Vaccine Information Statement (VIS) | | Vaccinator[5] (signature or initials & title) |
|---|---|---|---|---|---|---|---|---|---|
| | | | | | Lot # | Mfr. | Date on VIS[4] | Date given[4] | |
| **Hepatitis B[6]** (e.g., HepB, Hib-HepB, DTaP-HepB-IPV) Give IM.[7] | HepB | 6/2/2005 | F | RT | 0651M | MRK | 7/11/01 | 6/2/05 | JTA |
| | Pediarix | 8/2/2005 | F | RT | 635A1 | GSK | 7/11/01 | 8/2/05 | DCP |
| | Pediarix | 10/2/2005 | F | RT | 712A2 | GSK | 7/11/01 | 10/2/05 | DCP |
| | Pediarix | 12/2/2005 | F | RT | 712A2 | GSK | 7/11/01 | 12/2/05 | DLW |
| **Diphtheria, Tetanus, Pertussis[6]** (e.g., DTaP, DTaP/Hib, DTaP-HepB-IPV, DT, DTaP-IPV/Hib, Tdap, DTaP-IPV, Td) Give IM.[7] | Pediarix | 8/2/2005 | F | RT | 635A2 | GSK | 7/30/01 | 8/2/05 | DCP |
| | Pediarix | 10/2/2005 | F | RT | 712A2 | GSK | 7/30/01 | 10/2/05 | DCP |
| | Pediarix | 12/2/2005 | F | RT | 712A2 | GSK | 7/30/01 | 12/2/05 | DLW |
| | DTaP-Hib | 9/2/2006 | F | RA | P0897AA | SPI | 7/30/01 | 9/2/06 | RLV |
| | DTaP | 8/2/2010 | F | RA | 326-912 | SPI | 5/17/07 | 8/2/10 | JTA |
| | | | | | | | | | |
| | | | | | | | | | |
| ***Haemophilus influenzae type b[6]*** (e.g., Hib, Hib-HepB, DTaP-IPV/Hib, DTaP/Hib) Give IM.[7] | Hib | 8/2/2005 | F | LT | UA744AA | SPI | 12/16/98 | 8/2/05 | DCP |
| | Hib | 10/2/2005 | F | LT | UA744AA | SPI | 12/16/98 | 10/2/05 | DCP |
| | Hib | 12/2/2005 | F | LT | UA744AA | SPI | 12/16/98 | 12/2/05 | DLW |
| | DTaP-Hib | 9/2/2006 | F | RA | 7172AA | SPI | 12/16/98 | 9/2/06 | RLV |
| **Polio[6]** (e.g., IPV, DTaP-HepB-IPV, DTaP-IPV/Hib, DTaP-IPV) Give IPV SC or IM.[7] Give all others IM.[7] | Pediarix | 8/2/2005 | F | RT | 635A2 | GSK | 1/1/00 | 8/2/05 | DCP |
| | Pediarix | 10/2/2005 | F | RT | 712A2 | GSK | 1/1/00 | 10/2/05 | DCP |
| | Pediarix | 12/2/2005 | F | RT | 712A2 | GSK | 1/1/00 | 12/2/05 | DLW |
| | IPV | 8/2/2010 | F | RA | U4569-8 | SPI | 1/1/00 | 8/2/10 | DCP |
| **Pneumococcal** (e.g., PCV7, PCV13, conjugate; PPSV23, polysaccharide) Give PCV IM.[7] Give PPSV SC or IM.[7] | PCV7 | 8/2/2005 | F | LT | 489-835 | WYE | 9/30/02 | 8/2/05 | DCP |
| | PCV7 | 10/2/2005 | F | RT | 489-835 | WYE | 9/30/02 | 10/2/05 | DCP |
| | PCV7 | 12/2/2005 | F | LT | 489-835 | WYE | 9/30/02 | 12/2/05 | DLW |
| | PCV7 | 9/2/2006 | F | LA | 501-245 | WYE | 9/30/02 | 9/2/06 | RLV |
| | PCV13 | 8/2/2010 | F | LA | E44433 | PFI | 12/9/08 | 8/2/10 | DCP |
| **Rotavirus** (RV1, RV5) Give orally (po). | | | | | | | | | |
| | | | | | | | | | |
| | | | | | | | | | |

*DTaP-HepB-IPV (Pediarix)*

*DTaP-Hib (TriHIBit): 2 lot #s, 2 different VISs*

*Pediarix: 3 different VIS dates*

See page 2 to record measles-mumps-rubella, varicella, hepatitis A, meningococcal, HPV, influenza, and other vaccines (e.g., tra vel vaccines).

## How to Complete This Record

1. Record the generic abbreviation (e.g., Tdap) or the trade name for each vaccine (see table at right).
2. Record the funding source of the vaccine given as either F (federal), S (state), or P (private).
3. Record the site where vaccine was administered as either RA (right arm), LA (left arm), RT (right thigh), LT (left thigh), or IN (intranasal).
4. Record the publication date of each VIS as well as the date the VIS is given to the patient.
5. To meet the space constraints of this form and federal requirements for documentation, a healthcare setting may want to keep a reference list of vaccinators that includes their initials and titles.
6. For combination vaccines, fill in a row for each antigen in the combination.
7. IM is the abbreviation for intramuscular; SC is the abbreviation for subcutaneous.

| Abbreviation | Trade Name & Manufacturer |
|---|---|
| DTaP | Daptacel (sanofi); Infanrix (GlaxoSmithKline [GSK]); Tripedia (sanofi pasteur) |
| DT (pediatric) | Generic (sanofi pasteur) |
| DTaP-HepB-IPV | Pediarix (GSK) |
| DTaP/Hib | TriHIBit (sanofi pasteur) |
| DTaP-IPV/Hib | Pentacel (sanofi pasteur) |
| DTaP-IPV | Kinrix (GSK) |
| HepB | Engerix-B (GSK); Recombivax HB (Merck) |
| HepA-HepB | Twinrix (GSK); can be given to teens age 18 and older |
| Hib | ActHIB (sanofi pasteur); Hiberix (GSK); PedvaxHIB (Merck) |
| Hib-HepB | Comvax (Merck) |
| IPV | Ipol (sanofi pasteur) |
| PCV13 | Prevnar 13 (Pfizer) |
| PPSV23 | Pneumovax 23 (Merck) |
| RV1 | Rotarix (GSK) |
| RV5 | RotaTeq (Merck) |
| Tdap | Adacel (sanofi pasteur); Boostrix (GSK) |
| Td | Decavac (sanofi pasteur), Generic (MA Biological Labs) |

Technical content reviewed by the Centers for Disease Control and Prevention, August 2010.

www.immunize.org/catg.d/p2022.pdf • Item #P2022 (8/10)

**FIGURE 42–11A:** Vaccine Administration Records for Children and Teens, completed for a child. *Acquired from www.immunize.org/catg.d/p2022.pdf on 1/3/2010. We thank the Immunization Action Coalition.* (continues)

(Page 2 of 2)

# Vaccine Administration Record for Children and Teens

Patient name: *Emily Jacobs*

Birthdate: *6/2/2005*

Chart number: ______

Before administering any vaccines, give copies of all pertinent Vaccine Information Statements (VISs) to the child's parent or legal representative and make sure he/she understands the risks and benefits of the vaccine(s). Always provide or update the patient's personal recor d card.

| Vaccine | Type of Vaccine[1] | Date given (mo/day/yr) | Funding Source (F,S,P)[2] | Site[3] | Vaccine | | Vaccine Information Statement (VIS) | | Vaccinator[5] (signature or initials & title) |
|---|---|---|---|---|---|---|---|---|---|
| | | | | | Lot # | Mfr. | Date on VIS[4] | Date given[4] | |
| **Measles, Mumps, Rubella**[6] (e.g., MMR, MMRV) Give SC.[7] | MMRV | 6/2/2006 | P | RA | 0857M | MRK | 1/15/03 | 6/2/06 | DLW |
| | MMRV | 8/2/2010 | P | LA | 0522F | MRK | 5/21/10 | 8/2/10 | DCP |
| **Varicella**[6] (e.g., VAR, MMRV) Give SC.[7] | MMRV | 6/2/2006 | P | RA | 0857M | MRK | 12/16/98 | 6/2/06 | DLW |
| | MMRV | 8/2/2010 | P | LA | 0522F | MRK | 5/21/10 | 8/2/10 | DCP |
| **Hepatitis A** (HepA) Give IM.[7] | HepA | 6/2/2006 | P | LA | 0524L | MRK | 8/4/04 | 6/2/06 | DLW |
| | HepA | 12/2/2006 | P | LA | 0634K | MRK | 3/21/06 | 8/2/06 | MAT |
| | | | | | | | | | |
| **Meningococcal** (e.g., MCV4; MPSV4) Give MCV4 IM[7] and MPSV4 SC.[7] | | | | | | | | | |
| | | | | | | | | | |
| | | | | | | | | | |
| **Human papillomavirus** (e.g., HPV2, HPV4) Give IM.[7] | | | | | | | | | |
| | | | | | | | | | |
| | | | | | | | | | |
| **Influenza** (e.g., TIV, inactivated; LAIV, live attenuated) Give TIV IM.[7] Give LAIV IN.[7] | TIV | 12/5/2005 | F | RT | U097543 | SPI | 7/18/05 | 12/5/05 | JTA |
| | TIV | 1/5/2006 | F | RT | U097543 | SPI | 7/18/05 | 1/5/06 | DCP |
| | TIV | 10/16/2006 | F | LA | U106459 | SPI | 6/30/06 | 10/16/06 | MAT |
| | LAIV | 11/15/2007 | S | IN | 500337P | MED | 7/16/07 | 11/15/07 | ABB |
| | TIV | 10/12/2008 | S | RA | U2169MA | SPI | 7/24/08 | 10/12/08 | CAS |
| | TIV | 10/2/2009 | F | LA | 71211 | NOV | 8/11/09 | 10/2/09 | MAT |
| | TIV-H1N1 | 11/15/2009 | F | RA | UP016AA | SPI | 10/2/09 | 11/15/09 | CEL |
| | LAIV-H1N1 | 12/29/2009 | F | IN | 500756P | MED | 10/2/09 | 12/29/09 | ZAZ |
| | | | | | | | | | |
| | | | | | | | | | |
| | | | | | | | | | |
| **Other** | | | | | | | | | |
| | | | | | | | | | |

MMR-VAR (MMRV)

See page 1 to record hepatitis B, diphtheria, tetanus, pertussis, *Haemophilus influenzae* type b, polio, pneumococcal, and rotavirus vaccines.

## How to Complete this Record

1. Record the generic abbreviation (e.g., Tdap) or the trade name for each vaccine (see table at right).
2. Record the funding source of the vaccine given as either F (federal), S (state), or P (private).
3. Record the site where vaccine was administered as either RA (right arm), LA (left arm), RT (right thigh), LT (left thigh), or IN (intranasal).
4. Record the publication date of each VIS as well as the date the VIS is given to the patient.
5. To meet the space constraints of this form and federal requirements for documentation, a healthcare setting may want to keep a reference list of vaccinators that includes their initials and titles.
6. For combination vaccines, fill in a row for each antigen in the combination.
7. IM is the abbreviation for intramuscular; SC is the abbreviation for subcutaneous; IN is the abbreviation for intranasal.

| Abbreviation | Trade Name & Manufacturer |
|---|---|
| MMR | MMRII (Merck) |
| VAR | Varivax (Merck) |
| MMRV | ProQuad (Merck) |
| HepA | Havrix (GlaxoSmithKline [GSK]); Vaqta (Merck) |
| HepA-HepB | Twinrix (GSK) |
| HPV2 | Cervarix (GSK) |
| HPV4 | Gardasil (Merck) |
| LAIV (Live attenuated influenza vaccine] | FluMist (MedImmune) |
| TIV (Trivalent inactivated influenza vaccine) | Afluria (CSL Biotherapies); Agriflu (Novartis); Fluarix (GSK); FluLaval (GSK); Fluvirin (Novartis); Fluzone (sanofi) |
| MCV4 | Menactra (sanofi pasteur); Menveo (Novartis) |
| MPSV4 | Menomune (sanofi pasteur) |

Technical content reviewed by the Centers for Disease Control and Prevention, August 2010.

www.immunize.org/catg.d/p2022.pdf • Item #P2022 (8/10)

**FIGURE 42–11A:** *(continued)*

(Page 1 of 2)

# Vaccine Administration Record for Children and Teens

Patient name: *Jessica Ashley*

Birthdate: *10/15/1991*

Chart number: ______

Before administering any vaccines, give copies of all pertinent Vaccine Information Statements (VISs) to the child's parent or legal representative and make sure he/she understands the risks and benefits of the vaccine(s). Always provide or update the patient's personal recor d card.

| Vaccine | Type of Vaccine[1] | Date given (mo/day/yr) | Funding Source (F,S,P)[2] | Site[3] | Vaccine | | Vaccine Information Statement (VIS) | | Vaccinator[5] (signature or initials & title) |
|---|---|---|---|---|---|---|---|---|---|
| | | | | | Lot # | Mfr. | Date on VIS[4] | Date given[4] | |
| **Hepatitis B**[6] (e.g., HepB, Hib-HepB, DTaP-HepB-IPV) Give IM.[7] | HepB (1.0 mL) | 6/2/2004 | P | RA | 0651M | MRK | 7/11/01 | 6/2/04 | TAA |
| | HepB (1.0 mL) | 1/2/2005 | P | RA | 0651M | MRK | 7/11/01 | 1/2/05 | TAA |
| | 2-dose series of adult Recombivax given to child 12-15 yrs | | | | | | | | |
| | | | | | | | | | |
| **Diphtheria, Tetanus, Pertussis**[6] (e.g., DTaP, DTaP/Hib, DTaP-HepB-IPV, DT, DTaP-IPV/Hib, Tdap, DTaP-IPV, Td) Give IM.[7] | DTP | 12/15/1991 | P | RT | 326-912 | LED | 1/1/88 | 12/15/91 | DCP |
| | DTP | 2/15/1992 | P | RT | 326-912 | LED | 10/15/91 | 2/15/92 | DCP |
| | DTaP | 4/15/1992 | P | RT | 326-912 | LED | 3/25/92 | 4/15/92 | DLW |
| | DTaP | 4/15/1993 | P | RA | 326-912 | LED | 3/25/92 | 4/15/93 | RLV |
| | DTaP | 4/15/1996 | P | RA | 657-888 | LED | 6/10/94 | 4/15/96 | JTA |
| | Td | 10/15/2003 | P | RA | 467-854 | LED | 7/30/01 | 10/15/03 | PWS |
| | Tdap | 6/12/2010 | P | RA | AC52B023AA | GSK | 11/18/08 | 6/12/10 | DLW |
| ***Haemophilus influenzae* type b**[6] (e.g., Hib, Hib-HepB, DTaP-IPV/Hib, DTaP/Hib) Give IM.[7] | Hib | 12/15/1991 | P | LT | 1492L | MRK | 6/6/91 | 12/15/91 | DCP |
| | PedvaxHIB | 2/15/1992 | P | LT | 1492L | MRK | 6/6/91 | 2/15/92 | DCP |
| | Hib | 10/15/1992 | P | LT | 1492L | MRK | 6/6/91 | 10/15/92 | DLW |
| | | | | | | | | | |
| **Polio**[6] (e.g., IPV, DTaP-HepB-IPV, DTaP-IPV/Hib, DTaP-IPV) Give IPV SC or IM.[7] Give all others IM.[7] | OPV | 12/15/1991 | P | po | 0678A | LED | 10/15/91 | 12/15/91 | DCP |
| | OPV | 2/15/1992 | P | po | 0678A | LED | 10/15/91 | 2/15/92 | DCP |
| | OPV | 4/15/1993 | P | po | 0678A | LED | 10/15/91 | 4/15/93 | RLV |
| | OPV | 4/15/1996 | P | po | 0987A | LED | 10/15/91 | 4/15/93 | JTA |
| **Pneumococcal** (e.g., PCV7, PCV13, conjugate; PPSV23, polysaccharide) Give PCV IM.[7] Give PPSV SC or IM.[7] | | | | | | | | | |
| | | | | | | | | | |
| | | | | | | | | | |
| | | | | | | | | | |
| | | | | | | | | | |
| **Rotavirus** (RV1, RV5) Give orally (po). | | | | | | | | | |
| | | | | | | | | | |
| | | | | | | | | | |

See page 2 to record measles-mumps-rubella, varicella, hepatitis A, meningococcal, HPV, influenza, and other vaccines (e.g., tra vel vaccines).

## How to Complete This Record

1. Record the generic abbreviation (e.g., Tdap) or the trade name for each vaccine (see table at right).
2. Record the funding source of the vaccine given as either F (federal), S (state), or P (private).
3. Record the site where vaccine was administered as either RA (right arm), LA (left arm), RT (right thigh), LT (left thigh), or IN (intranasal).
4. Record the publication date of each VIS as well as the date the VIS is given to the patient.
5. To meet the space constraints of this form and federal requirements for documentation, a healthcare setting may want to keep a reference list of vaccinators that includes their initials and titles.
6. For combination vaccines, fill in a row for each antigen in the combination.
7. IM is the abbreviation for intramuscular; SC is the abbreviation for subcutaneous.

| Abbreviation | Trade Name & Manufacturer |
|---|---|
| DTaP | Daptacel (sanofi); Infanrix (GlaxoSmithKline [GSK]); Tripedia (sanofi pasteur) |
| DT (pediatric) | Generic (sanofi pasteur) |
| DTaP-HepB-IPV | Pediarix (GSK) |
| DTaP/Hib | TriHIBit (sanofi pasteur) |
| DTaP-IPV/Hib | Pentacel (sanofi pasteur) |
| DTaP-IPV | Kinrix (GSK) |
| HepB | Engerix-B (GSK); Recombivax HB (Merck) |
| HepA-HepB | Twinrix (GSK); can be given to teens age 18 and older |
| Hib | ActHIB (sanofi pasteur); Hiberix (GSK); PedvaxHIB (Merck) |
| Hib-HepB | Comvax (Merck) |
| IPV | Ipol (sanofi pasteur) |
| PCV13 | Prevnar 13 (Pfizer) |
| PPSV23 | Pneumovax 23 (Merck) |
| RV1 | Rotarix (GSK) |
| RV5 | RotaTeq (Merck) |
| Tdap | Adacel (sanofi pasteur); Boostrix (GSK) |
| Td | Decavac (sanofi pasteur), Generic (MA Biological Labs) |

Technical content reviewed by the Centers for Disease Control and Prevention, August 2010.

www.immunize.org/catg.d/p2022.pdf • Item #P2022 (8/10)

**FIGURE 42–11B:** Vaccine Administration Records for Children and Teens, completed for a teenager. *Acquired from www.immunize.org/catg.d/p2022.pdf on 1/3/2010; we thank the Immunization Action Coalition.* (*continues*)

(Page 2 of 2)

# Vaccine Administration Record for Children and Teens

Patient name: *Jessica Ashley*

Birthdate: *10/15/1991*

Chart number: ______________

Before administering any vaccines, give copies of all pertinent Vaccine Information Statements (VISs) to the child's parent or legal representative and make sure he/she understands the risks and benefits of the vaccine(s). Always provide or update the patient's personal recor d card.

| Vaccine | Type of Vaccine[1] | Date given (mo/day/yr) | Funding Source (F,S,P)[2] | Site[3] | Vaccine | | Vaccine Information Statement (VIS) | | Vaccinator[5] (signature or initials & title) |
|---|---|---|---|---|---|---|---|---|---|
| | | | | | Lot # | Mfr. | Date on VIS[4] | Date given[4] | |
| **Measles, Mumps, Rubella**[6] (e.g., MMR, MMRV) Give SC.[7] | MMR | 1/15/1993 | P | RA | 0857M | MRK | 10/15/91 | 1/15/93 | DLW |
| | MMR | 10/15/2003 | P | LA | 0946M | MRK | 1/15/03 | 10/15/03 | PWS |
| **Varicella**[6] (e.g., VAR, MMRV) Give SC.[7] | VAR | 10/15/2003 | P | LA | 0799M | MRK | 12/16/98 | 10/15/03 | PWS |
| | VAR | 10/15/2007 | P | LA | 0689M | MRK | 1/10/07 | 10/15/07 | JTA |
| **Hepatitis A** (HepA) Give IM.[7] | | | | | | | | | |
| **Meningococcal** (e.g., MCV4; MPSV4) Give MCV4 IM[7] and MPSV4 SC.[7] | MCV4 | 6/12/2010 | P | LA | 28011 | NOV | 1//28/08 | 6/12/10 | MAT |
| **Human papillomavirus** (e.g., HPV2, HPV4) Give IM.[7] | HPV2 | 12/12/2009 | P | LA | 0331Z | GSK | 2/2/07 | 12/12/09 | TAA |
| | Cervarix | 2/13/2010 | P | LA | 0331Z | GSK | 2/2/07 | 2/13/10 | PWS |
| | Garadasil | 6/12/2010 | P | LA | 0637F | MRK | 2/2/07 | 6/12/10 | DLW |
| **Influenza** (e.g., TIV, inactivated; LAIV, live attenuated) Give TIV IM.[7] Give LAIV IN.[7] | FluMist | 10/15/2007 | P | IN | 500491P | MED | 10/4/07 | 10/15/07 | MAT |
| | TIV | 10/12/2008 | P | RA | 878771P | NOV | 7/24/08 | 10/12/08 | JTA |
| | Fluzone | 10/2/2009 | P | RA | U100461 | SPI | 8/11/09 | 10/2/09 | DLW |
| | H1N1 | 12/7/2009 | P | LA | 1009224P | NOV | 10/2/09 | 12/7/09 | MAT |
| **Other** | | | | | | | | | |

*When recording the type of vaccine, use the generic abbreviation, tradename, or both. By recording the manufacturer, you will always be able to determine the brand of vaccine given.*

See page 1 to record hepatitis B, diphtheria, tetanus, pertussis, *Haemophilus influenzae* type b, polio, pneumococcal, and rotavirus vaccines.

## How to Complete this Record

1. Record the generic abbreviation (e.g., Tdap) or the trade name for each vaccine (see table at right).
2. Record the funding source of the vaccine given as either F (federal), S (state), or P (private).
3. Record the site where vaccine was administered as either RA (right arm), LA (left arm), RT (right thigh), LT (left thigh), or IN (intranasal).
4. Record the publication date of each VIS as well as the date the VIS is given to the patient.
5. To meet the space constraints of this form and federal requirements for documentation, a healthcare setting may want to keep a reference list of vaccinators that includes their initials and titles.
6. For combination vaccines, fill in a row for each antigen in the combination.
7. IM is the abbreviation for intramuscular; SC is the abbreviation for subcutaneous; IN is the abbreviation for intranasal.

| Abbreviation | Trade Name & Manufacturer |
|---|---|
| MMR | MMRII (Merck) |
| VAR | Varivax (Merck) |
| MMRV | ProQuad (Merck) |
| HepA | Havrix (GlaxoSmithKline [GSK]); Vaqta (Merck) |
| HepA-HepB | Twinrix (GSK) |
| HPV2 | Cervarix (GSK) |
| HPV4 | Gardasil (Merck) |
| LAIV (Live attenuated influenza vaccine] | FluMist (MedImmune) |
| TIV (Trivalent inactivated influenza vaccine) | Afluria (CSL Biotherapies); Agriflu (Novartis); Fluarix (GSK); FluLaval (GSK); Fluvirin (Novartis); Fluzone (sanofi) |
| MCV4 | Menactra (sanofi pasteur); Menveo (Novartis) |
| MPSV4 | Menomune (sanofi pasteur) |

Technical content reviewed by the Centers for Disease Control and Prevention, August 2010.

www.immunize.org/catg.d/p2022.pdf • Item #P2022 (8/10)

**FIGURE 42–11B:** *(continued)*

# YOUR BABY'S FIRST VACCINES

## WHAT YOU NEED TO KNOW

Babies get six vaccines between birth and 6 months of age.

These vaccines protect your baby from 8 serious diseases (see the next page).

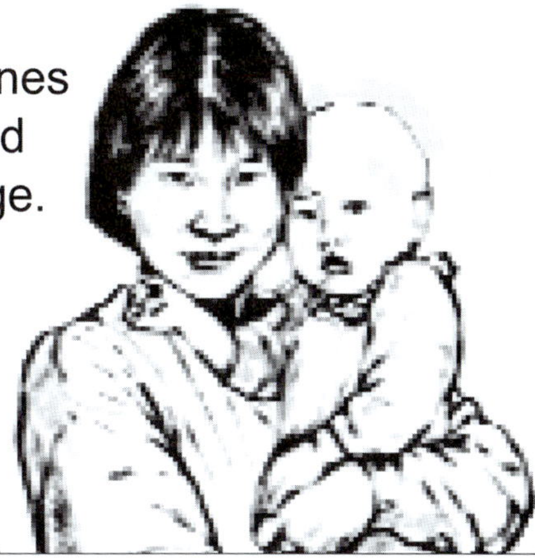

**Your baby will get vaccines today that prevent these diseases:**

☐ Hepatitis B ☐ Polio ☐ Pneumococcal Disease
☐ Diphtheria, Tetanus & Pertussis ☐ Rotavirus ☐ Hib

(Provider: Check appropriate boxes)

These vaccines may be given separately, or some might be given together in the same shot (for example, Hepatitis B and Hib can be given together, and so can DTaP, Polio, and Hepatitis B). These "combination vaccines" are as safe and effective as the individual vaccines, and mean fewer shots for your baby.

***These vaccines may all be given at the same visit. Getting several vaccines at the same time will not harm your baby.***

**This *Vaccine Information Statement* (VIS) tells you about the benefits and risks of these vaccines. It also contains information about reporting an adverse reaction, the National Vaccine Injury Compensation Program, and how to get more information about childhood diseases and vaccines.**

**Please read this VIS before your child gets his or her immunizations, and take it home with you afterward. Ask your doctor, nurse, or other healthcare provider if you have questions.**

Individual Vaccine Information Statements are also available for these vaccines.
Many Vaccine Information Statements are available in Spanish and other languages. See www.immunize.org/vis

DEPARTMENT OF HEALTH AND HUMAN SERVICES
CENTERS FOR DISEASE CONTROL AND PREVENTION

Vaccine Information Statement
(Interim)
42 U.S.C. § 300aa-26
**9/18/2008**

**FIGURE 42–12:** Example of a vaccine information statement. *Courtesy of the Centers for Disease Control and Prevention.* (*continues*)

# Vaccine Benefits: Why get vaccinated?

Your children's first vaccines protect them from **8 serious diseases,** caused by viruses and bacteria. These diseases have injured and killed many children (and adults) over the years. **Polio** paralyzed about 37,000 people and killed about 1,700 each year in the 1950s before there was a vaccine. In the 1980s, **Hib disease** was the leading cause of bacterial meningitis in children under 5 years of age. About 15,000 people a year died from **diphtheria** before there was a vaccine. Most children have had at least one rotavirus infection by their 5th birthday.

None of these diseases has completely disappeared. Without vaccination, they will come back. This has happened in other parts of the world.

## *8 Diseases Prevented by Childhood Vaccines*

### DIPHTHERIA — *Bacteria*

**You can get it from** contact with an infected person.

**Signs and symptoms** include a thick covering in the back of the throat that can make it hard to breathe.

**It can lead to** breathing problems, heart failure, and death.

### TETANUS (Lockjaw) — *Bacteria*

**You can get it from** a cut or wound. It does not spread from person to person.

**Signs and symptoms** include painful tightening of the muscles, usually all over the body.

**It can lead to** stiffness of the jaw, so the victim can't open his mouth or swallow. It leads to death in about 1 case out of 5.

### PERTUSSIS (Whooping Cough) — *Bacteria*

**You can get it from** contact with an infected person.

**Signs and symptoms** include violent coughing spells that can make it hard for an infant to eat, drink, or breathe. These spells can last for weeks.

**It can lead to** pneumonia, seizures (jerking and staring spells), brain damage, and death.

### HIB (*Haemophilus influenzae* type b) — *Bacteria*

**You can get it from** contact with an infected person.

**Signs and symptoms.** There may be no signs or symptoms in mild cases.

**It can lead to** meningitis (infection of the brain and spinal cord coverings); pneumonia; infections of the blood, joints, bones, and covering of the heart; brain damage; deafness; and death.

### HEPATITIS B — *Virus*

**You can get it from** contact with blood or body fluids of an infected person. Babies can get it at birth if the mother is infected, or through a cut or wound. Adults can get it from unprotected sex, sharing needles, or other exposures to blood.

**Signs and symptoms** include tiredness, diarrhea and vomiting, jaundice (yellow skin or eyes), and pain in muscles, joints and stomach.

**It can lead to** liver damage, liver cancer, and death.

### POLIO — *Virus*

**You can get it from** close contact with an infected person. It enters the body through the mouth.

**Signs and symptoms** can include a cold-like illness, or there may be no signs or symptoms at all.

**It can lead to** paralysis (can't move arm or leg), or death (by paralyzing breathing muscles).

### PNEUMOCOCCAL — *Bacteria*

**You can get it from** contact with an infected person.

**Signs and symptoms** include fever, chills, cough, and chest pain.

**It can lead to** meningitis (infection of the brain and spinal cord coverings), blood infections, ear infections, pneumonia, deafness, brain damage, and death.

### ROTAVIRUS — *Virus*

**You can get it from** contact with other children who are infected.

**Signs and symptoms** include severe diarrhea, vomiting and fever.

**It can lead to** dehydration, hospitalization (up to about 70,000 a year), and death.

### How Vaccines Work

***Immunity from Disease:*** When a child gets sick with one of these diseases, her immune system produces immunity, which keeps her from getting the same disease again. But getting sick is unpleasant, and can be dangerous.

***Immunity from Vaccines:*** Vaccines are made with the same bacteria or viruses that cause a disease, but they have been weakened or killed to make them safe. A child's immune system responds to a vaccine the same way it would if the child had the disease. This means he will develop immunity without having to get sick first.

**FIGURE 42–12:** *(continued)*

## Routine Childhood Vaccines

Six vaccines are recommended for children between birth and 6 months of age. They can prevent the 8 diseases described on the previous page. Children will also get at least one "booster" dose of most of these vaccines when they are older.

- **DTaP** (Diphtheria, Tetanus & Pertussis) Vaccine: 5 doses – **2 months, 4 months, 6 months, 15-18 months, 4-6 years**. Some children should not get pertussis vaccine. These children can get a vaccine called **DT**, which does not contain pertussis.
- **Hepatitis B** Vaccine: 3 doses – **Birth, 1-2 months, 6-18 months.**
- **Polio** Vaccine: 4 doses – **2 months, 4 months, 6-18 months, 4-6 years.**
- **Hib** (*Haemophilus influenzae* type b) Vaccine: 3 or 4 doses – **2 months, 4 months, 6 months, 12-15 months**. Several Hib vaccines are available. With one type, the 6-month dose is not needed.
- **Pneumococcal** Vaccine: 4 doses – **2 months, 4 months, 6 months, 12-15 months**. Older children with certain diseases may also need this vaccine.
- **Rotavirus** Vaccine: 2 or 3 doses – **2 months, 4 months, 6 months.** Rotavirus is an oral (swallowed) vaccine, not a shot. Two rotavirus vaccines are available. With one type, the 6 month dose is not needed.

## Vaccine Risks

Vaccines can cause side effects, like any other medicine. Mostly these are mild "local" reactions such as **tenderness, redness** or **swelling** where the shot is given, or a **mild fever**. They happen in up to 1 child out of 4 with most childhood vaccines. They appear soon after the shot is given and go away within a day or two.

More severe reactions can also occur, but this happens much less often. Some of these reactions are so uncommon that experts can't tell whether they are caused by vaccines or not.

Among the most serious reactions to vaccines are **severe allergic reactions** to a substance in a vaccine. These reactions happen very rarely – less than once in a million shots. They usually happen very soon after the shot is given. Doctor's office or clinic staff are trained to deal with them.

The risk of *any* vaccine causing serious harm, or death, is extremely small. Getting a disease is much more likely to harm a child than getting a vaccine.

### Other Reactions

The following conditions have been associated with routine childhood vaccines. By "associated" we mean that they appear more often in children who have been recently vaccinated than in those who have not. An association doesn't *prove* that a vaccine caused a reaction, but does mean it is probable.

### DTaP Vaccine

**Mild Problems**: Fussiness (up to 1 child in 3); tiredness or poor appetite (up to 1 child in 10); vomiting (up to 1 child in 50); swelling of the entire arm or leg for 1-7 days (up to 1 child in 30) – usually after the 4th or 5th dose.

**Moderate Problems**: Seizure (jerking or staring)(1 child in 14,000); non-stop crying for 3 hours or more (up to 1 child in 1,000); fever over 105°F (1 child in 16,000).

**Serious Problems**: Long-term seizures, coma, lowered consciousness, and permanent brain damage have been reported very rarely after DTaP vaccine. They are so rare we can't be sure they are caused by the vaccine.

### Polio Vaccine / Hepatitis B Vaccine / Hib Vaccine

These vaccines have not been associated with mild problems other than local reactions, or with moderate or serious problems.

### Pneumococcal Vaccine

**Mild Problems:** During studies of the vaccine, some children became fussy or drowsy or lost their appetite.

### Rotavirus Vaccine

**Mild Problems:** Children who get rotavirus vaccine are slightly more likely than other children to be irritable or to have mild, temporary diarrhea or vomiting. This happens within the first week after getting a dose of vaccine. Rotavirus vaccine does not appear to cause any serious side effects.

**FIGURE 42–13A:** Recommended immunization schedule 0–6 yrs. *Courtesy of the Centers for Disease Control and Prevention.*

## Precautions

**If your child is sick** on the date vaccinations are scheduled, your provider *may* want to put them off until she recovers. A child with a mild cold or a low fever can usually be vaccinated that day. But for a more serious illness, it may be better to wait.

Some children should **not get certain vaccines**. Talk with your provider if your child had a serious reaction after a previous dose of a vaccine, or has any life-threatening allergies. (These reactions and allergies are rare.)

- If your child had any of these reactions to a previous dose of DTaP:
  - A brain or nervous system disease within 7 days
  - Non-stop crying for 3 or more hours
  - A seizure or collapse
  - A fever over 105°F

  Talk to your provider before getting **DTaP Vaccine.**

- If your child has:
  - A life-threatening allergy to the antibiotics neomycin, streptomycin, or polymyxin B

  Talk to your provider before getting **Polio Vaccine.**

- If your child has:
  - A life-threatening allergy to yeast

  Talk to your provider before getting **Hepatitis B Vaccine.**

- If your child has:
  - A weakened immune system
  - Ongoing digestive problems
  - Recently gotten a blood transfusion or other blood product
  - Ever had intussusception (an uncommon type of intestinal obstruction)

  Talk to your provider before getting **Rotavirus Vaccine.**

## What if my child has a moderate or severe reaction?

### What should I look for?

Look for any unusual condition, such as a serious allergic reaction, high fever, weakness, or unusual behavior.

Serious allergic reactions are extremely rare with any vaccine. If one were to happen, it would most likely come within a few minutes to a few hours after the shot.

Signs of a serious allergic reaction can include:

- difficulty breathing
- hoarseness or wheezing
- swelling of the throat
- weakness
- dizziness
- fast heart beat
- hives
- paleness

### What should I do?

**Call** a doctor, or get the child to a doctor right away.

**Tell** your doctor what happened, the date and time it happened, and when the shot was given.

**Ask** your healthcare provider to report the reaction by filing a Vaccine Adverse Event Reporting System (VAERS) form. Or you can file this report yourself through the VAERS website at **www.vaers.hhs.gov**, or by calling **1-800-822-7967**.

*VAERS does not provide medical advice.*

### The National Vaccine Injury Compensation Program

A federal program exists to help pay for the care of anyone who has a serious reaction to a vaccine.

For information about the National Vaccine Injury Compensation Program, call **1-800-338-2382** or visit their website at **www.hrsa.gov/vaccinecompensation**.

### For More Information

Ask your healthcare provider. They can show you the vaccine package insert or suggest other sources of information.

Call your local or state health department.

Contact the Centers for Disease Control and Prevention (CDC) at **1-800-232-4636 (1-800-CDC-INFO).**

Visit CDC websites at **www.cdc.gov/vaccines** and **www.cdc.gov/ncidod/diseases/hepatitis.**

**FIGURE 42–13B:** Recommended immunization schedule 7–18 yrs. *Courtesy of the Centers for Disease Control and Prevention.*

The Snellen big E chart (Figure 42–14A) requires the child to indicate with his or her fingers which way the E is facing. The Es become smaller and less bold as the acuity gets more difficult. Results are recorded on the last line correctly identified, the same as with adults on the regular screening chart. The kindergarten version of the chart (Figure 42–14B) uses various shapes and symbols in descending size to evaluate vision. When using either of these, review the charts up close with the child to be sure they know what they are supposed to do and that they can name the symbols. This determines whether the child is actually having trouble seeing the chart or simply does not know what to call the letter or symbol you are pointing to.

Most preschoolers have a short attention span, so you might need some assistance from the parent or caregiver, who can help by restating your instructions and maintaining the child's position. He or she can also monitor the covering of one eye as you proceed through the test. Watch the child for signs of visual difficulty such as tilting the head and frowning or straining to see as he or she reads the chart. Procedure 42–3 provides instruction to screen a child's vision.

**CLINICAL PEARL**

You can make the screening fun by taking your turn first. This also helps the child to understand what he or she is to do. Remember to praise the child during the screening to encourage cooperation.

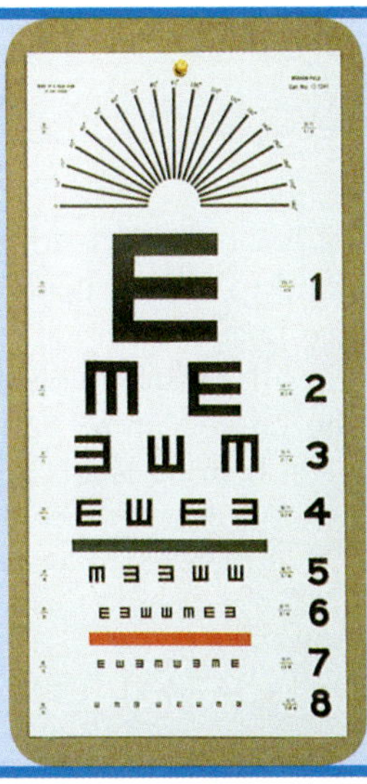

**FIGURE 42–14A:** Snellen E chart. *Delmar/Cengage Learning.*

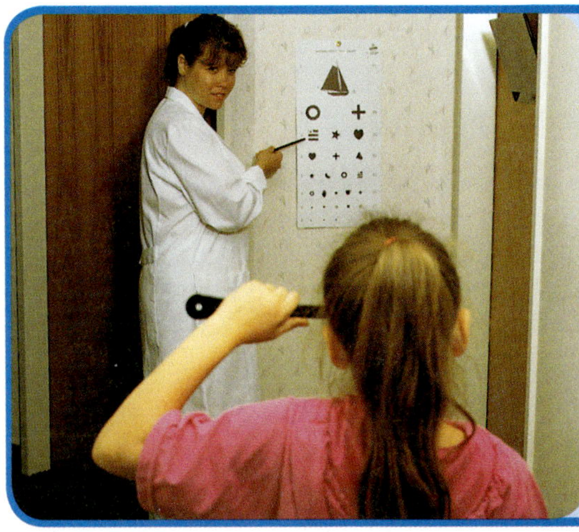

**FIGURE 42–14B:** Kindergarten chart. *Delmar/Cengage Learning.*

## PROCEDURE 42–3 Screen Pediatric Visual Acuity with a Modified Snellen Chart

**PURPOSE:** To measure distant visual acuity of a child

**EQUIPMENT:** Modified Snellen chart, pointer, eye occluder, patient's chart or EMR, and pen

**S SKILL:** Perform pediatric vision acuity screening.

| Procedure Steps | Detailed Instructions and/or *Rationales* |
|---|---|
| 1. Identify the patient and introduce yourself. | *Ensures that you are performing the procedure on the correct patient.* |
| **B** 2. Explain the procedure to the patient, ***using language that is appropriate for the patient.*** | |
| 3. Ask the patient to read the chart with both eyes at a distance of 20 feet from the chart. | |
| 4. Have the patient cover the left eye with the occluder to test the acuity of the right eye. | |

*(continues)*

*(continued)*

| Procedure Steps | Detailed Instructions and/or *Rationales* |
|---|---|
| 5. Record the smallest line the patient reads without making a mistake. | Some providers allow up to two errors on the smallest line read. |
| 6. Have the patient cover the right eye with the occluder to test the acuity of the left eye. | |
| 7. Record the smallest line read. | |

### Charting Example

| | |
|---|---|
| 4/17/XX 11:30 am | Vision screening with kindergarten screening chart per Dr. White, findings R eye 20/35, L eye 20/40; appeared to understand chart. Noticed some squinting during screening. J. Jenks, CMA(AAMA) |

## HEARING SCREENING

Hearing in infants and small children is usually observed by their reaction to surrounding sounds. Infants will respond by turning their head toward the ticking of a watch held near their ear. Older infants respond to verbal and environmental sounds. The parents or caregiver will probably be the first ones to notice a hearing deficit. The child will not respond to voice cues and will not react to surrounding noise below a certain intensity. Again, a pediatric specialist has the instruments and skills to evaluate hearing. As the child matures, an audiometer test can be given to screen hearing levels more accurately.

## CHAPTER SUMMARY

- The American Academy of Pediatrics (AAP) has established Recommendations for Preventive Pediatric Health Care, a chart that outlines the types and frequency of screening examinations and procedures. It can be downloaded from the AAP website at www.aap.org.
- Table 42–1 highlights growth and development during infancy and toddlerhood. The table shows the age at which the average child should be able to perform the activities listed.
- Pediatric growth measurements are documented on the patient's chart and on a growth chart. This chart gives the provider an ongoing quick-glance reference to the child's growth and development and is used to determine any abnormal patterns.
- Medicaid's comprehensive and preventive child health program, known as the Early and Periodic Screening, Diagnosis, and Treatment (EPSDT) program, is a program that requires regular health maintenance exams and careful documentation of examination findings for Medicaid patients who are between birth and 21 years of age.
- When a parent calls for an appointment, determine whether the visit is for a routine well-child examination or whether the child has symptoms of an illness. Specific well-child hours are usually set aside in each day's schedule.
- As a medical assistant, you have certain routine responsibilities to perform with each pediatric examination. Generally, you will assist in gathering data, document information, perform screening tests within your skill and ability level, assist the patient, assist the provider, and provide patient education.
- Child neglect refers to the lack of or withholding of care; child abuse refers to inflicting emotional, physical, or sexual injury. Examples are provided in Table 42–2.
- The CDC releases annual Recommended Childhood and Adolescent Immunization Schedules for children. You can download the latest schedule from the CDC Website at www.cdc.gov.
- To screen for visual acuity, alternate versions of the Snellen chart are used, the Snellen big E chart and the kindergarten shapes and symbols chart.

## STUDY TOOLS

| | |
|---|---|
| **Workbook** | Activities for Chapter 42 |
| **Premium Website** | |
| MEDIA LINK | View this **Media Link** for Chapter 42:<br>• Communicating with Pediatric Patients |
| StudyWARE | Activities and Quizzes on the **StudyWARE™ Software** for Chapter 42 |
| | **Audio Library** of medical terms |
| | Online access to the **Critical Thinking Challenge 2.0** |
| learninglab | Module 18: Assisting with Clinical Procedures |
| **CourseMate** | Activities and Quizzes for Chapter 42 |
| **WebTutor** | Activities and Quizzes for Chapter 42 |

## CHECK YOUR KNOWLEDGE

1. At what age will the infant begin the immunization schedule?
   a. 2 weeks
   b. 2 months
   c. 6 weeks
   d. 1 year
2. An infant or young child who is below the _________ percentile on standardized growth charts is said to be failing to thrive.
   a. third
   b. fifth
   c. seventh
   d. tenth
3. Which of the following persons are obligated to report neglect or abuse to the proper authorities?
   a. Family members
   b. Health care workers
   c. Neighbors
   d. All of the above
4. Up until what age would you record the head circumference measurement?
   a. 12 months
   b. 24 months
   c. 36 months
   d. 48 months
5. Which measurement is taken and recorded in the patient's record but not on the growth chart?
   a. Head circumference
   b. Chest circumference
   c. Height
   d. Weight
6. The kindergarten version of the Snellen chart uses:
   a. signs and symbols.
   b. the capital letter *E*.
   c. letters.
   d. numbers.
7. When using the growth chart, each month is represented by a:
   a. dot.
   b. square.
   c. line.
   d. circle.

## WEB LINKS

American Academy of Pediatrics: www.aap.org

Centers for Disease Control and Prevention: www.cdc.gov

Immunization Action Coalition: www.immunize.org

## RESOURCES


Estes, M. E. Z. (2010). *Health Assessment & Physical Examination* (3rd ed.). Clifton Park, NY: Delmar Cengage Learning.

Heller, M., and Veach, L. (2009). *Clinical Medical Assisting: A Professional, Field Smart Approach to the Workplace.* Clifton Park, NY: Delmar, Cengage Learning.

Lindh, W., Pooler, M., Tamparo, C., and Dahl, B. (2010). *Delmar's Comprehensive Medical Assisting Administrative and Clinical Competencies* (4th ed.). Clifton Park, NY: Delmar Cengage Learning.

Venes, D. (ed.). (2009). *Taber's Cyclopedic Medical Dictionary* (21st ed.). Philadelphia: F. A. Davis.

CHAPTER 7

# Pediatric Examinations

## Words to Know Challenge

**Spelling: Each line contains three spellings of a word. Underline the correctly spelled word.**

| | | |
|---|---|---|
| 1. circumfrence | circumference | circumphrence |
| 2. attachment | attachtment | atachtment |
| 3. listlessness | listlesness | lislessness |
| 4. prevantive | preventive | preventiv |
| 5. intercede | interceed | intersceed |
| 6. suscpicion | suspiscion | suspicion |
| 7. malnutrition | mallnutrition | malnutrision |
| 8. letharjic | lethargic | lethargick |

**Matching: Match the key term in column I to its definition in column II.**

| | COLUMN I | COLUMN II |
|---|---|---|
| ____ | 1. Pediatrics | A. Attachment of two persons |
| ____ | 2. Apgar | B. Inflicting emotional, physical, or sexual injury |
| ____ | 3. Child neglect | C. Lack of or withholding of care |
| ____ | 4. Child abuse | D. Advancement of abilities and knowledge |
| ____ | 5. Development | E. Scoring system used on infants after birth |
| ____ | 6. Bonding | F. Specialty medical practice that cares for infants and children |
| ____ | 7. Caregiver | G. Arrangement of events or dates in order of occurrence |
| ____ | 8. Chronologic | H. Person responsible for another's care and well-being |
| ____ | 9. Percentile | I. Lack of vigorous growth |
| ____ | 10. Failure to thrive | J. Used on a growth chart to compare a child to his or her peers. |

Chapter

# 8 Preparing for Surgery

## OBJECTIVES

In this chapter, you will learn the following:

### KB KNOWLEDGE BASE

1. Spell and define, using the glossary at the back of the text, all the Words to Know in this chapter.
2. Explain scheduling and preoperative and postoperative instructions for patients for minor office surgery.
3. Discuss the different parts of surgical instruments.
4. Describe the proper care of surgical instruments.
5. List the function of all instruments discussed in this chapter.
6. Discuss the importance of maintaining the sterile field.
7. Explain the importance of obtaining the consent form for the surgical procedure.
8. Explain the importance of proper skin preparation before an invasive procedure.
9. Differentiate between the methods of sterilization.

### S SKILLS

1. Set up a sterile tray.
2. Open packages on a sterile tray.
3. Perform hand washing for surgical asepsis.
4. Apply sterile gloves.
5. Prepare skin for a minor surgical procedure.

## WORDS TO KNOW

antiseptic
aseptic technique
contamination
fenestrated
forceps
hemostat
microbial
microorganism
needle holder
preoperative (preop)
postoperative (postop)
ratchet
retractor
scrub
serrations
speculum
strikethrough
surgical asepsis

## SCHEDULING MINOR OFFICE SURGERY

Many minor surgical procedures are now performed in the medical office, clinic, and ambulatory care center. It is usually the medical assistant's duty to schedule the surgery, educate the patient about **preoperative (preop)** and **postoperative (postop)** care, prepare the room and equipment for the surgery, and assist the physician as needed.

Many providers prefer to perform minor surgical procedures at the beginning of the day's schedule. Some might require patients to fast for a certain amount of time before the procedure. (Fasting lessens the possibility of nausea and vomiting, which some patients can experience during and following any type of surgery.)

You might be asked to schedule an appointment for a patient to have a surgical procedure as an outpatient at a large ambulatory care center or hospital. Be sure to check with the person who makes the appointment regarding the preparation for the patient. When you write the appointment date and time for the patient, make certain the patient has directions to the facility. The assistant in the hospital or surgeon's office generally phones the patient the day before the surgery to confirm the appointment.

Be sure to cover all points listed in the patient education box when scheduling a patient for a minor surgical procedure.

### PATIENT EDUCATION

When scheduling, advise patient of the:

1. Surgical procedure, by providing printed education materials.
2. Approximate length of time for procedure.
3. Appropriate clothing to wear at appointment.
4. Amount of time to fast as instructed by provider if applicable.
5. Arrangements necessary for someone to accompany the patient and drive him or her home if necessary.
6. Anticipated time off work or arranging for home care.

When patient arrives for the appointment:

1. Ascertain whether the patient has any allergies to any medications, including topical preparations, latex products, and adhesive tapes.
2. Provide written instructions regarding the surgical procedure and follow-up care.
3. Ensure that the patient has signed a surgical consent form.
4. Answer any questions concerning procedure.

Be sure the patient understands the procedure and the instructions regarding preoperative and postoperative care. Most medical facilities have printed instructions for patients. Remember that some patients you see cannot read or might not speak English. You must explain as well as you can verbally and observe the patient's reactions to your instructions. Printed instructions in other languages and the services of an interpreter should be made available to the patient. This eliminates any misunderstandings, and patients feel more at ease knowing they can refer to it. Patients should be advised of the appropriate clothing to be worn on the day of the surgery. Loose-fitting clothing, clothing easy to put on and take off, and clothing appropriate for the anatomical area of surgery should be suggested. It is a good practice to phone the patient the day prior to the appointment, not only to reassure the patient and answer any questions but to confirm the appointment.

## PREPARING THE ROOM

Prior to the scheduled surgery, get all the necessary surgical instruments and supplies ready. A routine inventory of all supplies and sterile items is vital so that a sterile tray can be set up for any surgical procedure.

### Instruments

Each instrument used in the performance of minor surgical procedures has a specific function. Many times, its function can be determined simply by a visual inspection of the instrument. Surgical instruments used in the medical office are very costly and must be carefully maintained for longevity and maximum function. Always follow manufacturer's recommendations for cleaning, sterilization, and storage of all instruments. All surgical instruments must be properly labeled and sterilized. Most of the instruments will already be sterilized (as they should be after each use). Disposable instruments are being used more frequently as a way to control the spread of infection. These instruments are designed to be used one time and then properly discarded.

#### Instrument Care and Handling

Most instruments should be cared for in the same manner. The following is a list of general rules to follow when cleaning and caring for instruments.

1. Blood, tissue, and other body fluids must not be allowed to dry on an instrument.
2. Instruments should be rinsed and then soaked in a room-temperature solution containing a detergent and a solvent immediately after each use.
3. The detergent in the soaking solution should be of a neutral pH, which will help prevent corrosion of the surfaces of the instrument.

4. The soaking solution should contain a special protein that breaks down blood and body fluids on the surface of the instrument.
5. Instruments should be placed in a plastic container for soaking to prevent damage to their points and cutting edges.
6. Separate delicate instruments from heavier ones to prevent damage.
7. Separate sharp instruments from others when cleaning and storing.
8. All surfaces and crevices must be scrubbed with a brush to remove any foreign material.
9. A careful visual inspection should be conducted during each cleaning to check for any nicks, dullness, or warping of the surfaces.
10. Damaged instruments should not be used and should be either repaired or replaced.

## Instrument Components

Each part of an instrument's structure has a specific function. Figures 49–1A through C illustrate the key components of an instrument; an explanation of their function follows.

- *Thumb handle* (Figure 49–1A): A handle similar to that of a tweezer that is squeezed between the thumb and finger.
- *Ring handle* (Figure 49–1B): Designed so that the thumb and finger can be inserted into the rings.
- *Ratchet* (Figure 49–1B): Locking mechanism designed to close in varying degrees to hold the instrument closed, used to clamp tissue and vessels.
- *Serrations* (Figure 49–1C): Little fissures engraved into the surface of the blades of hemostats and forceps designed to prevent slippage and provide a firm grip when clamping a tissue. Instruments can have serrations, cross serrations, or longitudinal serrations.
- *Teeth* (Figure 49–1C): Very sharp projections designed to hold the tissue when grasping. Teeth can be heavy or delicate, and some are classified as non-traumatic.

## Instrument Classification

Most instruments are classified according to their function as follows:

- *Cutting and dissecting*: Includes scissors, scalpels, and curettes
- *Clamping and grasping*: Includes **hemostats**, clamps, **forceps**, and **needle holders**
- *Dilating, probing, and visualizing*: Includes **retractors**, scopes, **specula**, probes, and dilators

Table 49–1 lists some common instruments along with their use.

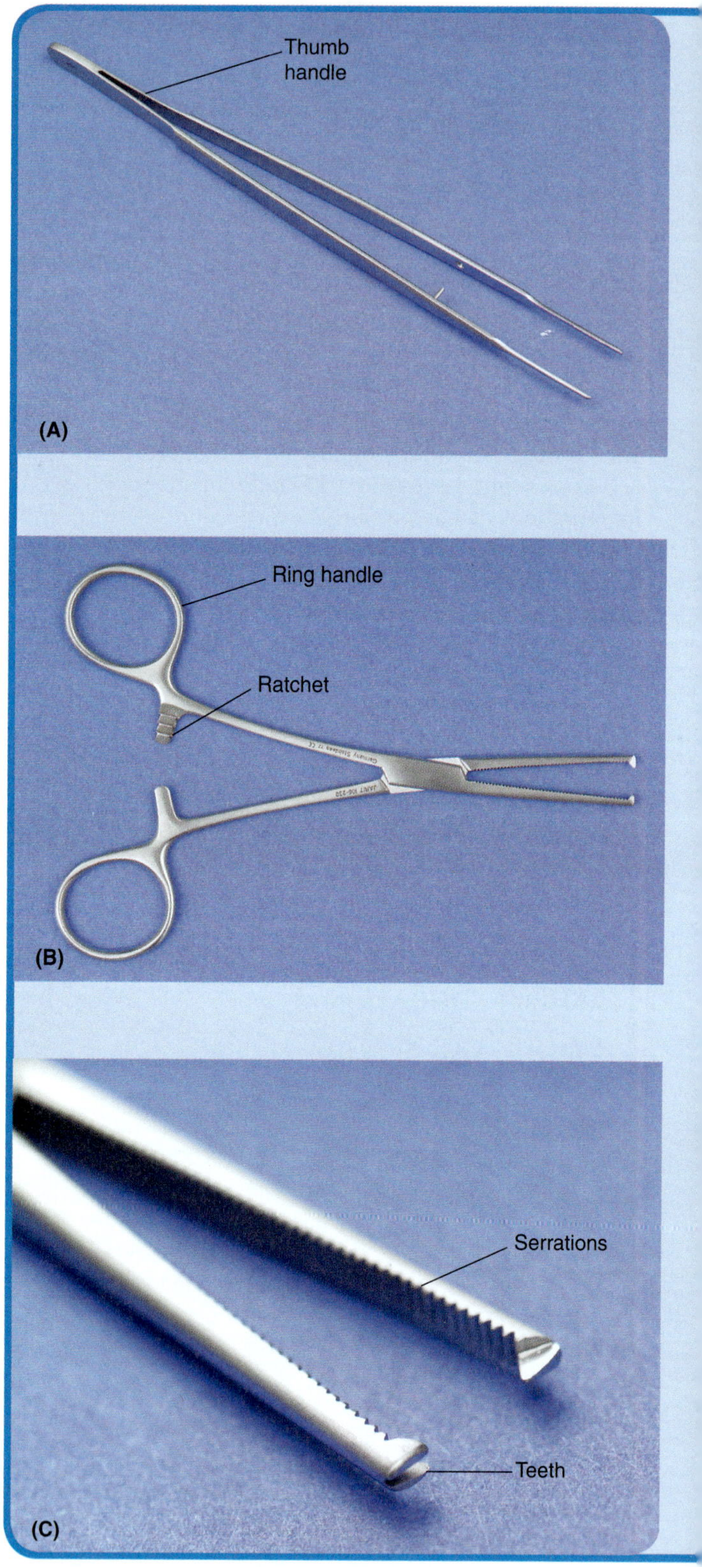


**Figure 49–1A–C:** Structural features of instruments: (A) Thumb handle. (B) Ring handle and ratchet. (C) Serrations and teeth. *Delmar/Cengage Learning.*

## TABLE 49–1 Instruments Used in Minor Office Surgical Procedures

| Figure Number | Category: Description | Use |
|---|---|---|
| | **Cutting and Dissecting** | |
| A | **Operating scissors**<br>$5\frac{1}{2}$" (14 cm), straight, sharp-blunt points | Cut tissue |
| B | **Operating scissors**<br>$5\frac{1}{2}$" (14 cm), straight, sharp-sharp points | Cut tissue |
| C | **Lister bandage scissors**<br>$7\frac{1}{4}$" (18.4 cm) | Cut dressings, tape, gauze, bandages |
| D | **Knife handle #3**<br>5" (12.7 cm), holds blades 10, 11, 12, 15 | |
| E | **Knife handle #3L**<br>$8\frac{3}{8}$" (21.3 cm), holds blades 10, 11, 12, 15 | Accepts blades; used when cutting deeper tissue |

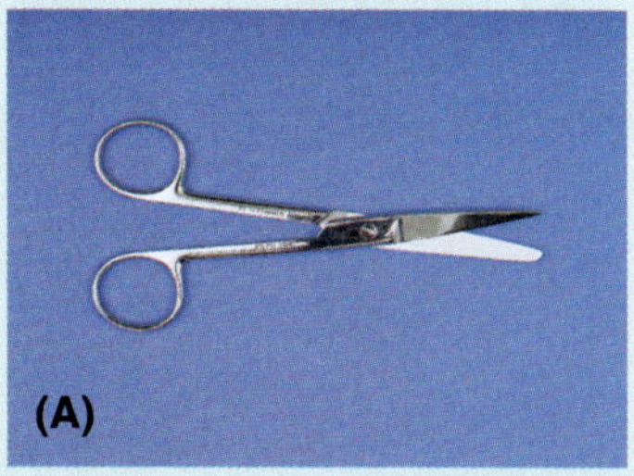
(A)

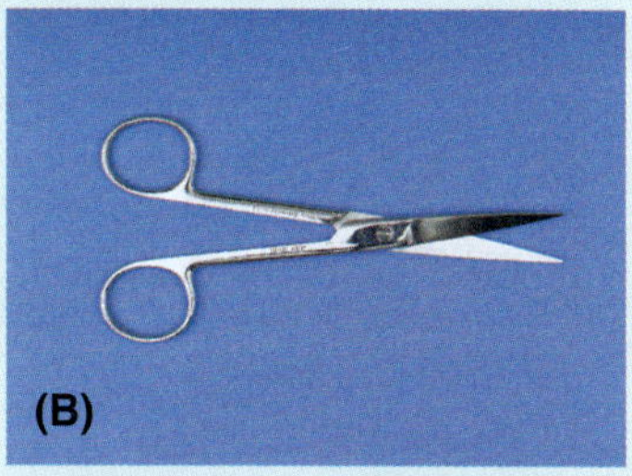
(B)

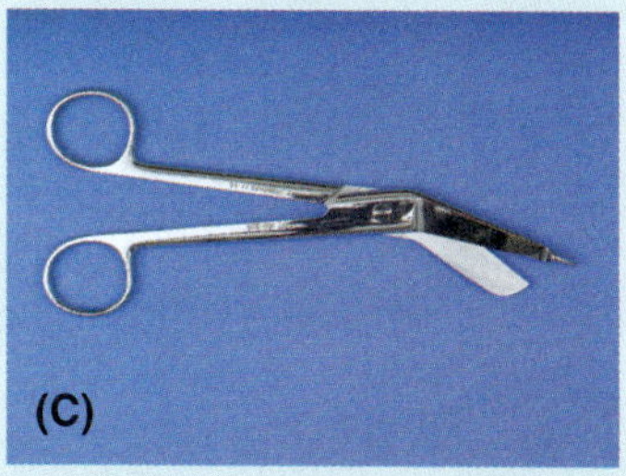
(C)

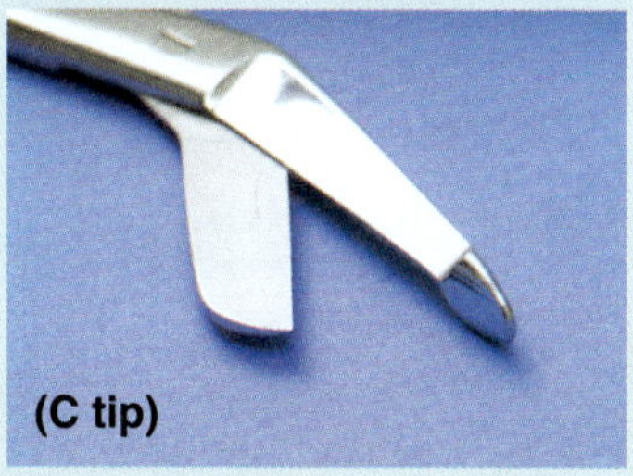
(C tip)

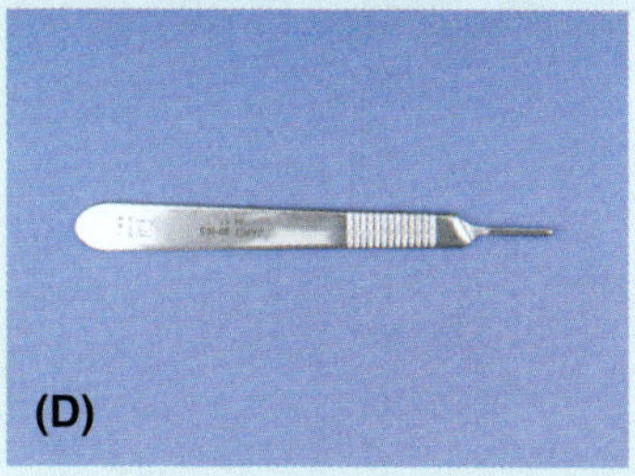
(D)

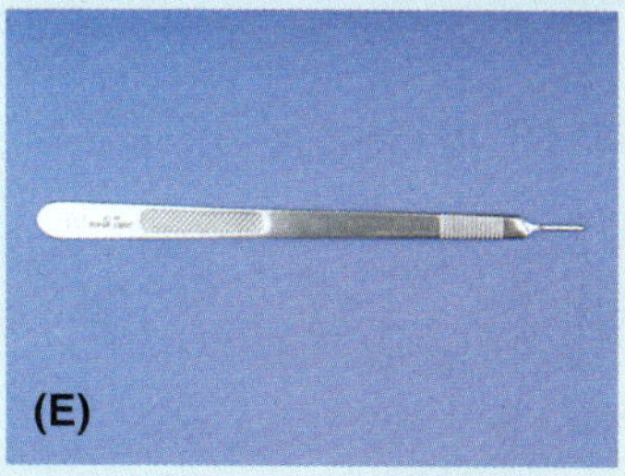
(E)

| Figure Number | Category: Description | Use |
|---|---|---|
| | **Clamping and Grasping** | |
| F | **Dressing or thumb forceps**<br>6" (15.2 cm), serrated | Pick up dressings, delicate tissue |
| G | **Adson tissue forceps**<br>$4\frac{3}{4}$" (12.1 cm), serrated | Grasp delicate tissue securely for control during dissection or suturing |
| H | **Allis tissue forceps**<br>6" (15.2 cm), 4 × 5 teeth | Grasp tissue securely for control during dissection or suturing |
| I | **Foerster sponge holding forceps**<br>$9\frac{1}{2}$" (24.1 cm), straight, serrated jaws | Pick up and hold dressings |
| J | **Hartmann mosquito hemostatic forceps**<br>$3\frac{1}{2}$" (8.9 cm), curved, serrated jaws the entire length of the tip | Grasp tissue to hold, clamp, or pull out of the way |
| K | **Kelly forceps**<br>$5\frac{1}{2}$" (14 cm), curved, partially serrated jaws | Grasp tissue to hold, clamp, or pull out of the way |
| L | **Olsen Hegar needle holder**<br>$5\frac{1}{2}$" (14 cm) | Grasp suture needle |

*(continues)*

**TABLE 49–1** *(Continued)*

| Figure Number | Category: Description | Use |
|---|---|---|
| M | **Backhaus towel forceps** | Grasp towels, dressing; hold drape towels in place (use caution—will puncture skin) |

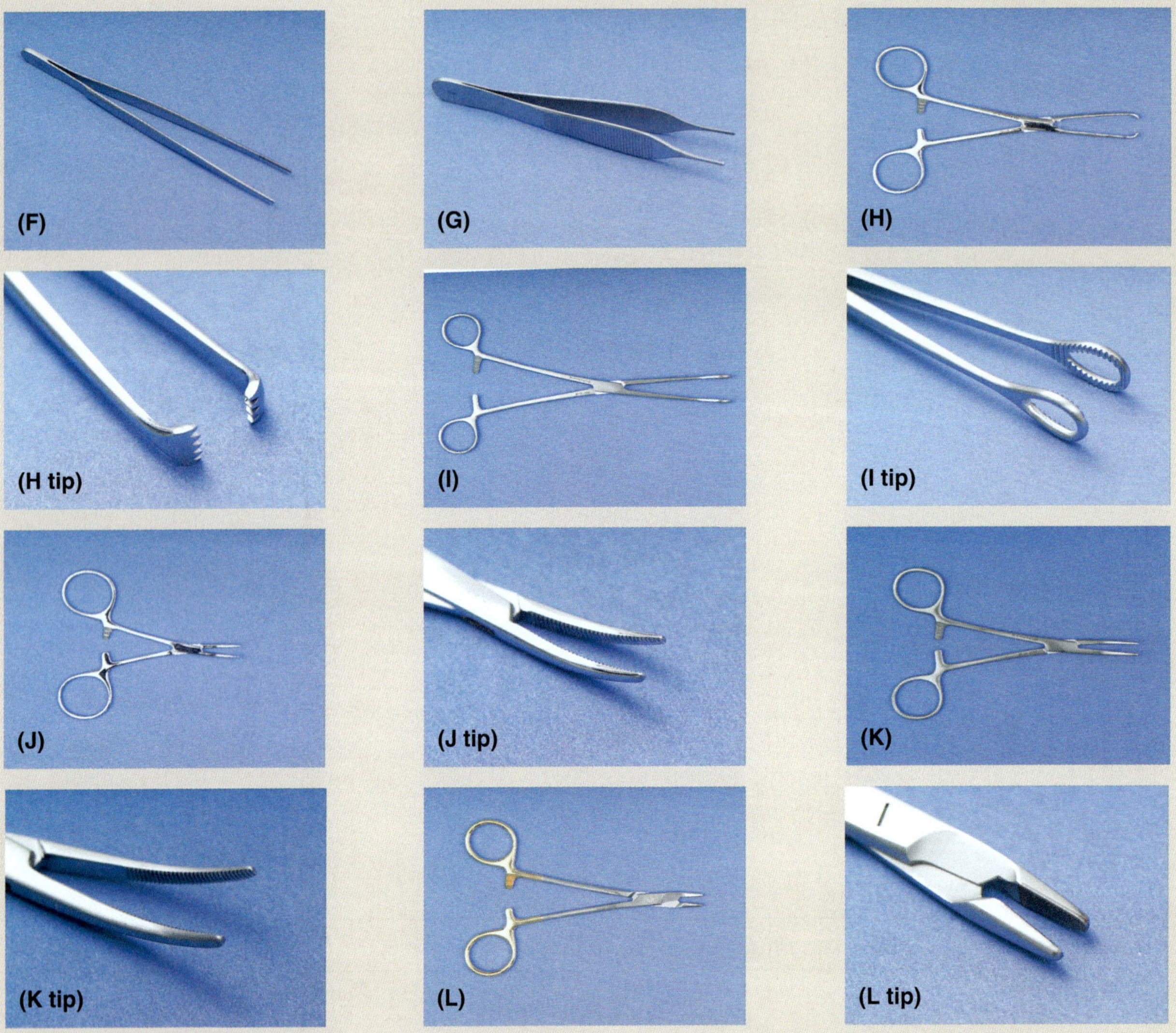


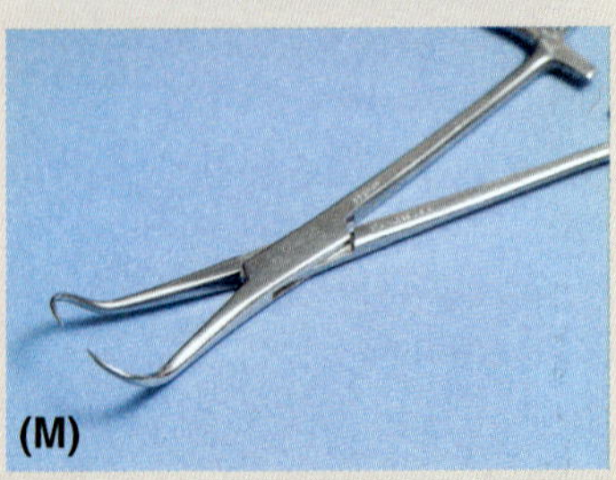


**Figure A–X:** *Courtesy of Delmar/Cengage Learning.*

| Figure Number | Category: Description | Use |
|---|---|---|
| | **Dilating, Probing, and Visualizing** | |
| N | **Senn retractor**<br>$6^1/_4$" (15.9 cm), double-ended, 3 sharp prongs, solid blade | Pull aside tissue to visualize an area better |
| O | **Ribbon retractor**<br>$1^1/_2$" (3.8 cm) wide × 13" (33 cm) long $5^1/_4$" (13.5 cm) | Pull aside tissue to visualize an area better<br>Grasp suture needle |

**TABLE 49–1** *(Continued)*

| Figure Number | Category: Description | Use |
|---|---|---|
| P | **U.S. Army retractor**<br>$^5/_8$" (1.5 cm) wide × 8-1/4" (21 cm) long | Pull aside tissue to visualize an area better |
| Q | **Deaver retractor**<br>1" (2.5 cm) wide × 13" (33 cm) long | Pull aside tissue to visualize an area better |
| R | **Richardson retractor**<br>$9^1/_2$", loop handle (1" wide × $1^1/_4$" deep) | Pull aside tissue to visualize an area better |
| S | **Flexible probe** | Explore a wound or body cavity |
| T | **Grooved director**<br>with probe tip and tongue tie | Explore a wound or body cavity |
| U | **Van Buren urethral sound**<br>Long instrument with calibrations | Measure the depth of the urethra; relieve urethral strictures |
| V | **Hegar uterine dilators**<br>Double-ended smooth rods with rounded tips | Dilate the cervix and gain access to the uterus for examination |
| W | **Grave's vaginal speculum** | Enlarge vaginal cavity (not shown) |
| X | **Vienna nasal speculum** | Enlarge nasal cavity (not shown) |

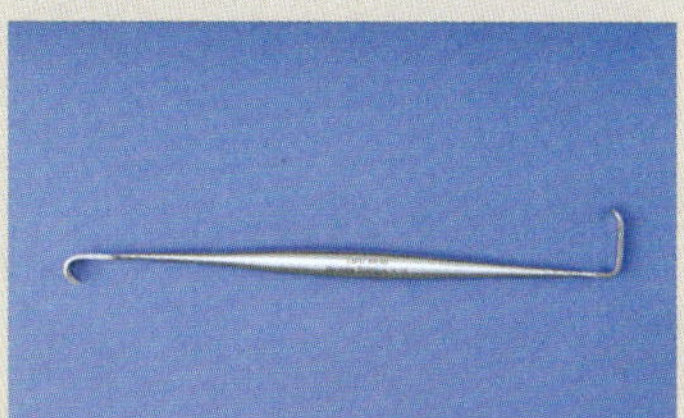
(N)

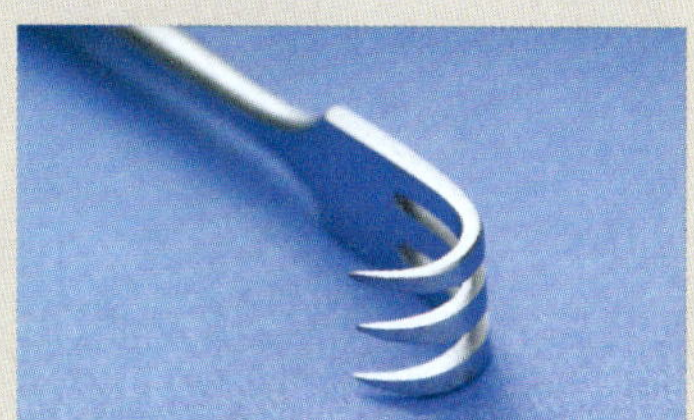
(N tip)

(O)

(P)

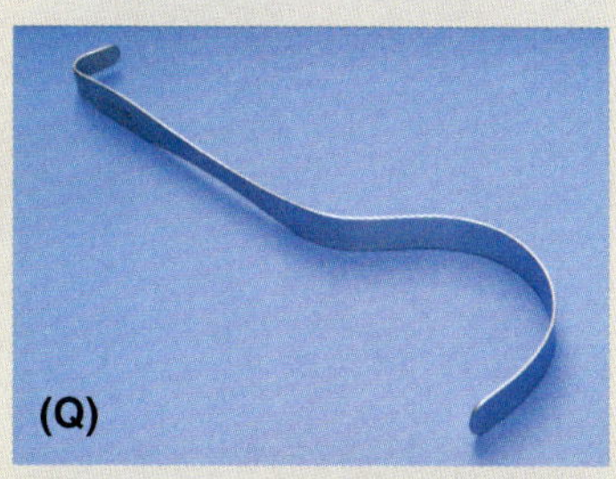
(Q)

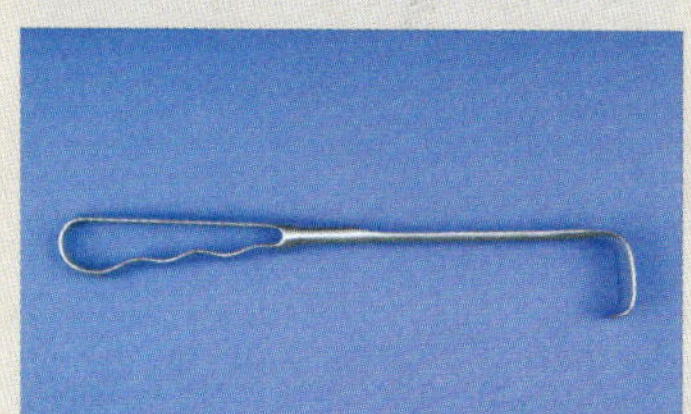
(R)

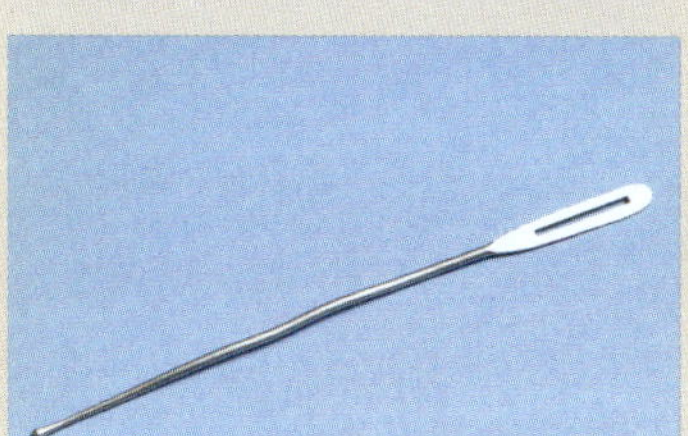
(S)

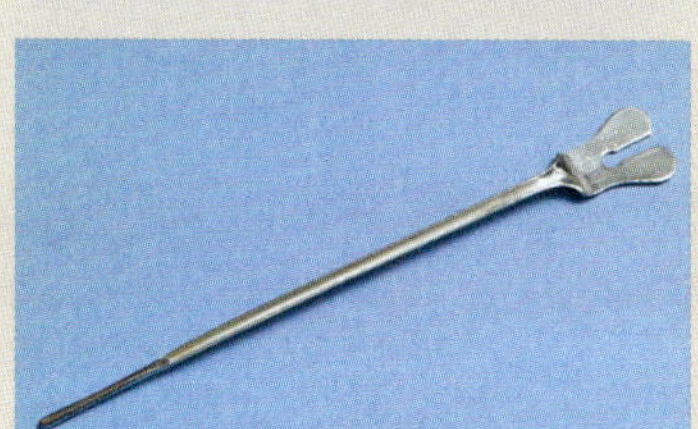
(T)

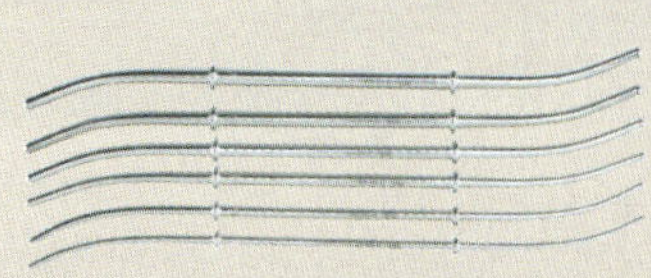
(U)

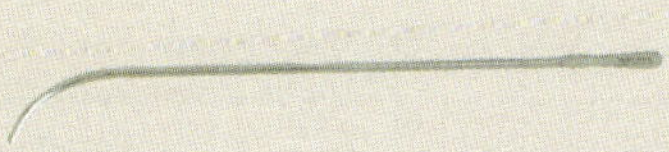
(V)

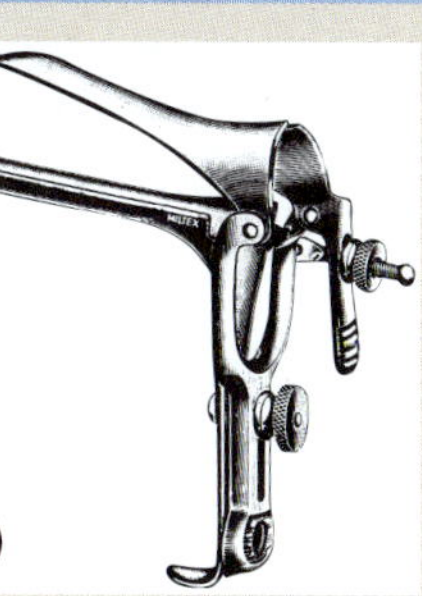
(W)

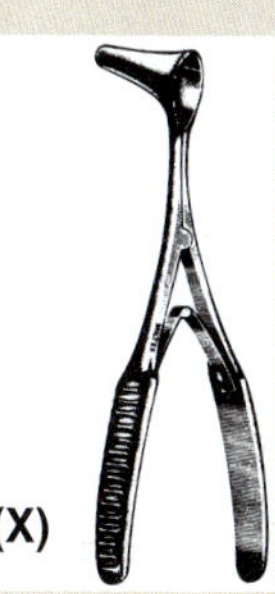
(X)

## Supplies

The basic setup for most minor surgical procedures includes the following sterile items:

- Scalpel handle and blades or disposable scalpel
- Hemostats
- Needle holder
- Needles and suture material (absorbable or nonabsorbable)
- Suture scissors
- Thumb forceps
- Probe
- Gauze squares
- Vial of **anesthetic** medication
- Needles and syringes
- Towels
- Bandages

Some of these supplies can be wrapped and sterilized together. All sterile packages must be labeled with the contents, date the package was sterilized, and the signature of the person who prepared and sterilized it. Autoclaved items remain sterile for 30 days if they have been properly processed and have been protected from moisture. Packages should be checked before use for any tears or other signs of tampering to ensure sterility.

Most items used today are disposable and come already sterile in the manufacturer's packaging. You must make sure that the package has not been torn or punctured to ensure sterility. The sterilization of the product is guaranteed only to a certain date marked on the package, and this date must be checked.

## Preparing Trays

A variety of minor surgical procedures are performed in the medical office, and each requires several instruments. Proper setup of the surgical tray is a vital part of the surgical process. The medical assistant must become familiar with the provider's preference for particular items and the way they are to be arranged for use. Until you are certain about the details of a particular procedure, you might keep a notebook handy for reference. Many offices keep a card file or computerized listing. Figure 49–2 shows an example of a specific surgical instrument tray setup and supplies commonly used in minor office procedures.

The room where the surgery will take place and the sterile tray should be set up before the patient is escorted to the area to be prepared for the procedure. Procedure 49–1 lists the steps involved in setting up a sterile tray.

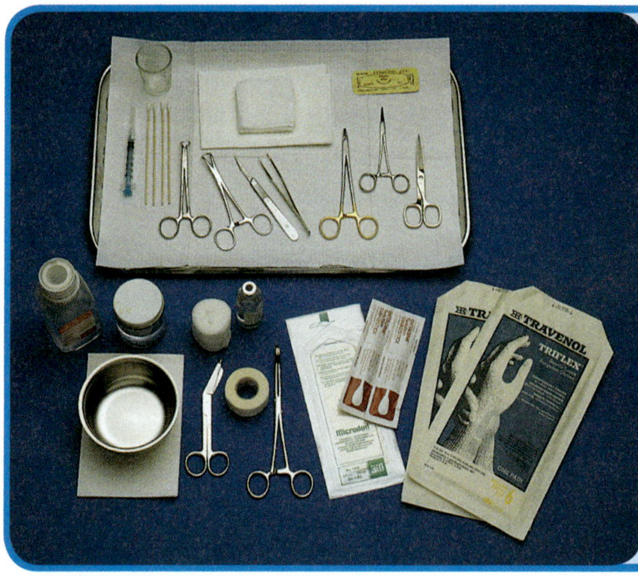


**Figure 49–2:** An example of a surgical tray setup. *Delmar/Cengage Learning.*

## PROCEDURE 49–1 Sterile Tray Setup

**PURPOSE:** Set up a sterile tray for a minor surgical procedure, according to the provider's preference

**EQUIPMENT:** Disposable sterile poly-lined drapes or sterile towels (two); Mayo instrument tray or stand positioned above the waist with stem to the right, at right angle to the counter; disposable sterile field drapes; peel-apart sterile package or autoclaved sterile package; sterile cup; container of sterile solution

**SKILL:** Set up a sterile tray.

| Procedure Steps | Detailed Instructions and/or *Rationales* |
|---|---|
| 1. Adjust the height of the Mayo tray so that the stand is at waist level (Figure 49–3A). | |

| Procedure Steps | Detailed Instructions and/or *Rationales* |
|---|---|
| 2. Clean the Mayo tray, starting from the center and working in a circular pattern (Figure 49–3B). | |
| 3. Place a sterile drape package on a clean, dry surface and open the pack, exposing the sterile drape with the corners facing you (Figure 49–3C). | *You may turn the package to position its contents properly.* |
| 4. Grasp the sterile drape by the corner and lift up enough to unfold but do not touch anything (Figure 49–3D). | *Be sure the drape does not brush up against your uniform or the counter.* |
| 5. Grasp the opposite corner, allow the drape to unfold completely, and place the drape over the Mayo tray (Figure 49–3E). Do not reach over the drape. | *Reaching over the sterile drape will contaminate it.* |

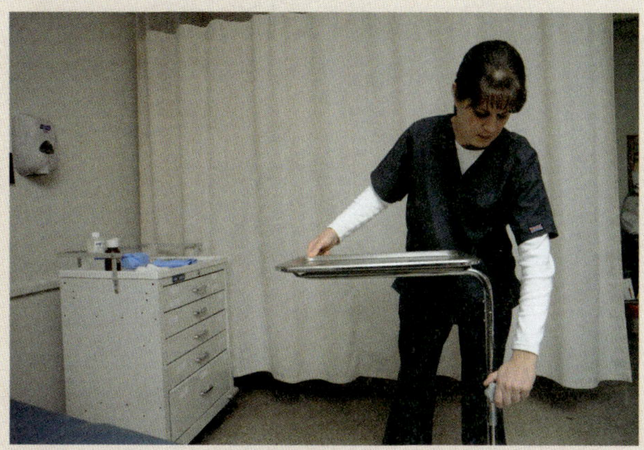

**Figure 49–3A:** Adjust the Mayo stand to the proper height. *Delmar/Cengage Learning.*

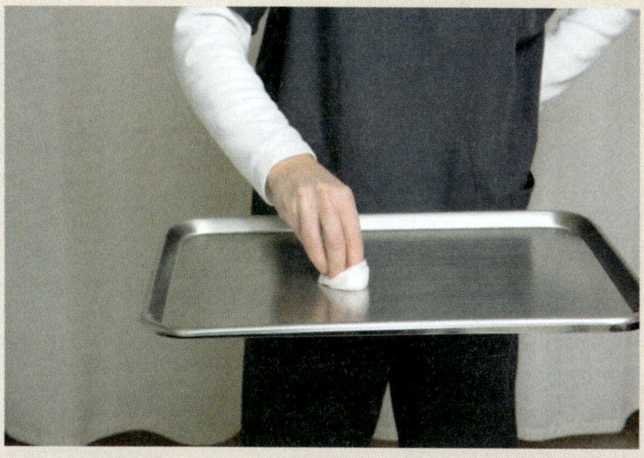

**Figure 49–3B:** Sanitize and disinfect the tray. *Delmar/Cengage Learning.*

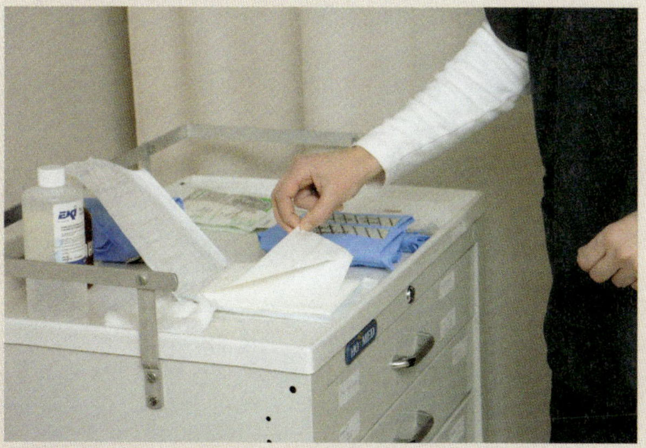

**Figure 49–3C:** Open the pack to expose the sterile drape with the corners facing toward you. *Delmar/Cengage Learning.*

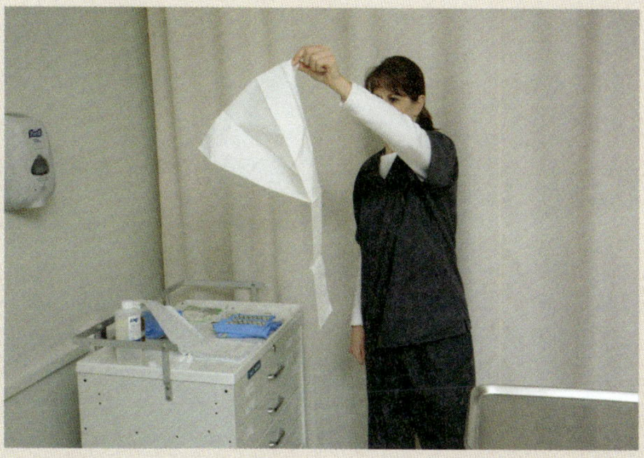

**Figure 49–3D:** Unfold the drape, without touching or reaching over it. *Delmar/Cengage Learning.*

*(continues)*

*(continued)*

| Procedure Steps | Detailed Instructions and/or *Rationales* |
|---|---|
| 6. Properly open a fanfolded (Figures 49–3F through J) or prepackaged sterile pack (Figures 49–3K and L) and allow the contents to drop onto the sterile field. | *Never reach over the sterile field because it could become contaminated.* |
| 7. After all supplies have been dropped onto the sterile field, apply sterile gloves or use sterile transfer forceps to arrange the instruments on the field according to the provider preference (Figure 49–3M). Pour any solutions as appropriate (Figure 49–3N). | |
| 8. Place a sterile drape over the field to protect it until the procedure begins (Figure 49–3O). | |

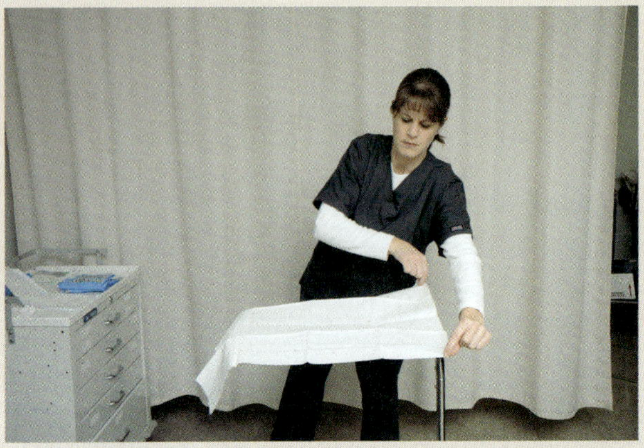

**Figure 49–3E:** Grasp the opposite corner of the unfolded drape and place the drape over the Mayo tray, without reaching over the drape. *Delmar/Cengage Learning.*

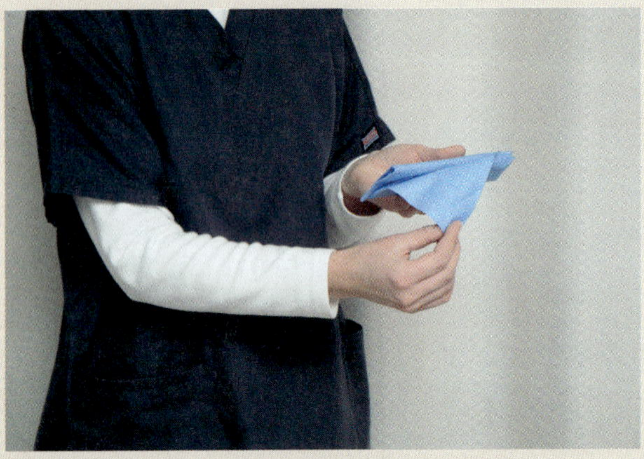

**Figure 49–3F:** To properly open a fan-folded sterile pack onto the sterile field, begin by grasping the tape on the top flap, and opening the flap away from you. *Delmar/Cengage Learning.*

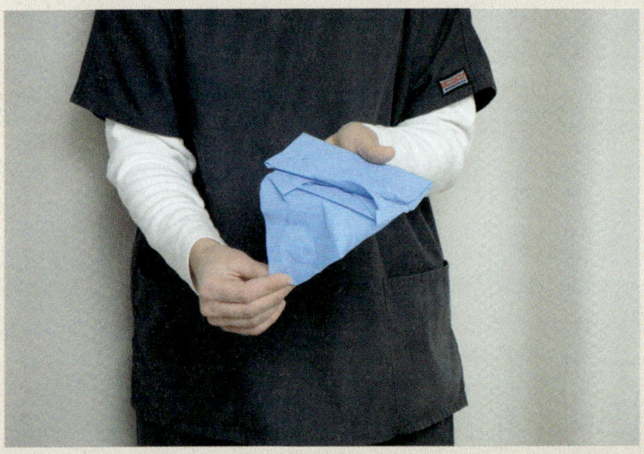

**Figure 49–3G:** Gently unroll the pack in the palm of your hand, being careful not to touch the inside of the pack. *Delmar/Cengage Learning.*

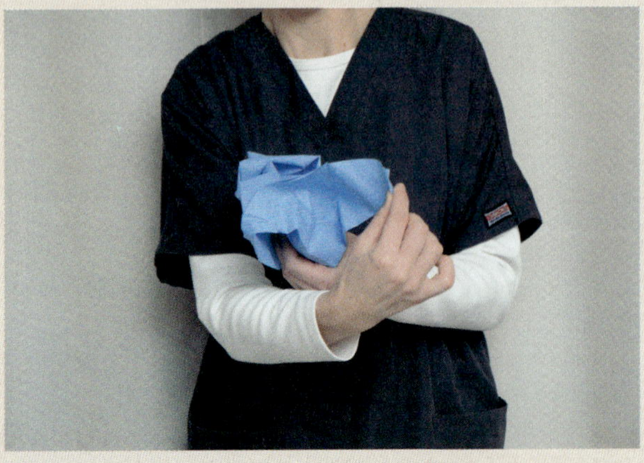

**Figure 49–3H:** Grasp the tips of the side flaps and unfold them by reaching around the side or under the pack. Do not reach over the pack. *Delmar/Cengage Learning.*

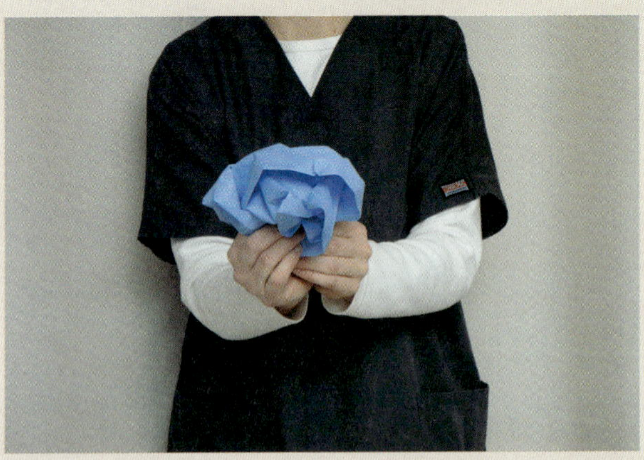

**Figure 49–3I:** Gather all the flaps together in the palm of your hand so they are back out of the way when the item is dropped onto the field. *Delmar/Cengage Learning.*

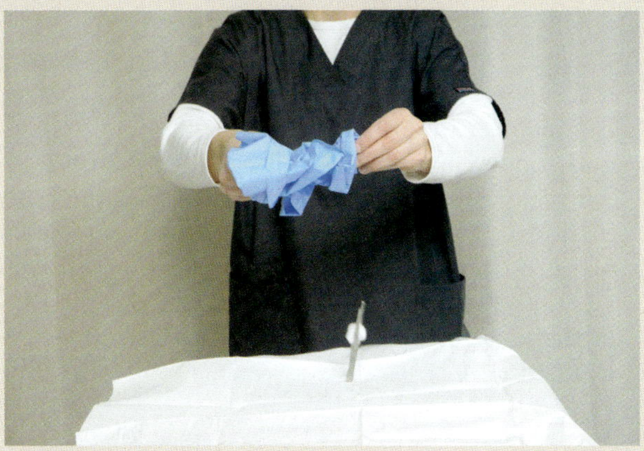

**Figure 49–3J:** Drop the instrument onto the sterile field. *Delmar/Cengage Learning.*

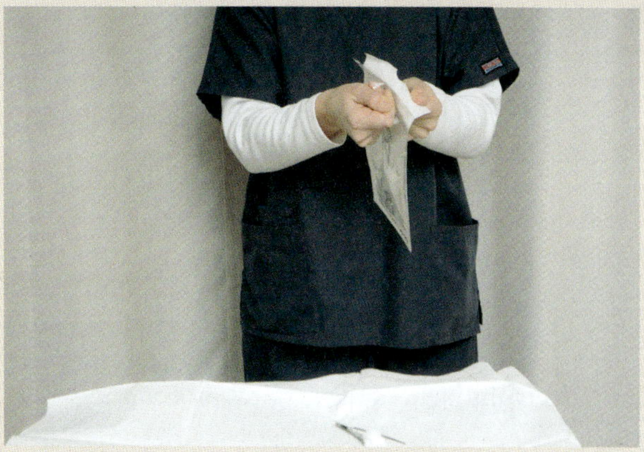

**Figure 49–3K:** To properly open a sterile peel-apart pack onto the sterile field, begin by grasping the flaps. *Delmar/Cengage Learning.*

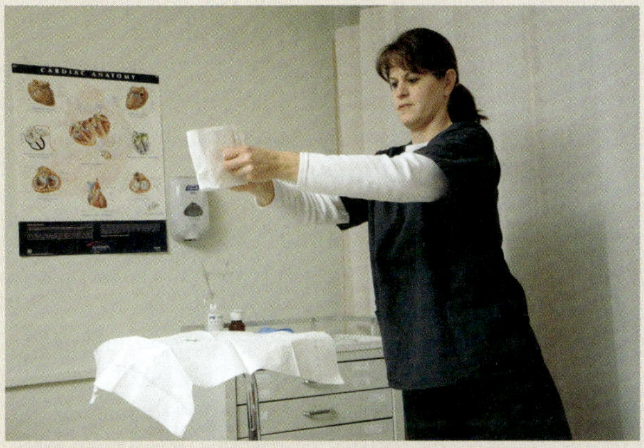


**Figure 49–3L:** Turn the pack so that the instrument will fall easily onto the sterile field when released. Drop the instrument onto the sterile field. *Delmar/Cengage Learning.*

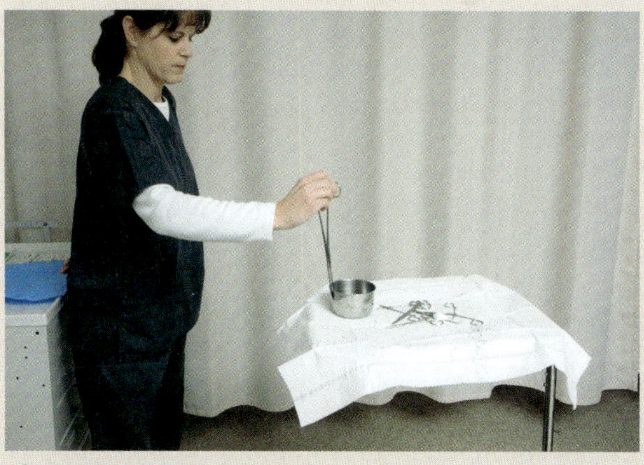

**Figure 49–3M:** Transfer forceps (or sterile gloves) may be used to arrange the instruments on the tray in the proper order. *Delmar/Cengage Learning.*

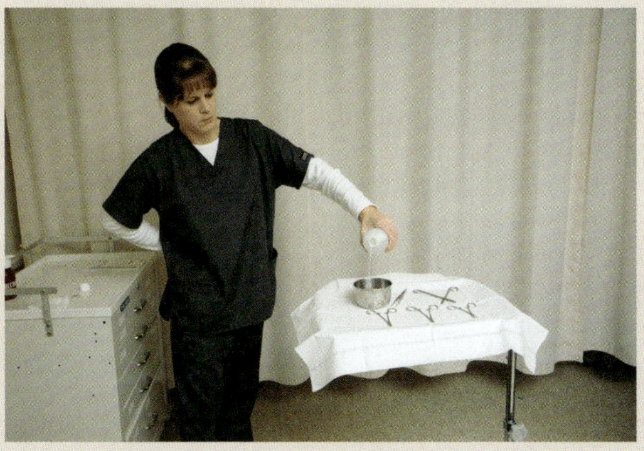

**Figure 49–3N:** Pour any solutions as appropriate. *Delmar/Cengage Learning.*

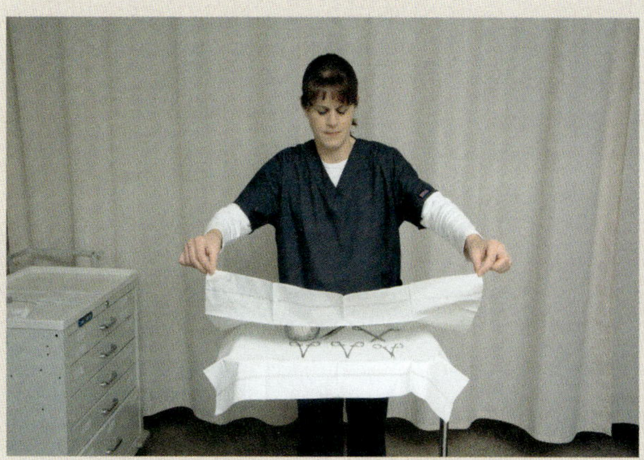

**Figure 49–3O:** Grasp another sterile drape by the corners and cover the sterile tray until the procedure begins. *Delmar/Cengage Learning.*

## SURGICAL ASEPSIS

Asepsis is defined as freedom from disease-causing agents such as microorganisms, viruses, and drug-resistant bacteria. The purpose of asepsis is to protect the patient and health care professional from disease and to stop disease from spreading. There are two types of asepsis, medical asepsis and surgical asepsis. Medical asepsis aims to reduce the number of microbes associated with diseases. **Surgical asepsis** is the total removal of all microbe-associated diseases. Even in minor surgery procedures, maintaining asepsis by aseptic technique is critical to the recovery of the surgical site and to the overall health of the patient. **Aseptic technique** is the process of maintaining sterility throughout the surgical procedure.

### Methods of Asepsis

Medical asepsis can be obtained through hand washing or cleaning agents such as antiseptics. (Refer to Chapter 36 for a complete discussion of medical asepsis.) Hand antiseptics are designed to inhibit and kill bacteria and are effective in killing many of the harmful bacteria that contribute to disease; however, hand antiseptics do not destroy all bacteria. Hand antiseptics are useful but should not take the place of proper hand washing.

Standard precautions are steps that reduce risk of infection from blood-borne pathogens. Standard precautions can be achieved by (1) treating all body fluids as if they are contaminated and (2) correctly donning personal protective equipment (PPE) such as gloves, masks, gowns, and eye protection. Employers are responsible for training all employees on standard precautions. Other safety measures include having policies and procedures in place that explain medical asepsis and standard precautions.

Surgical asepsis is obtained through sterilization. Sterilization is defined as the process of destroying all disease-causing microorganisms. Effective sterilization in the office setting is imperative in eliminating inadvertent **contamination** with disease-causing microorganisms. Selecting the type of sterilization depends on the item to be sterilized; many manufacturers suggest the best way to decontaminate and sterilize their instrumentation. Sterilization can occur by autoclave, dry heat, gas, and chemical agents. Steam is the most widely used method of sterilization.

### Sterilization Techniques

- *Autoclave:* The autoclave renders sterility by a combination of steam and pressure.
- *Dry heat:* Dry heat sterilization is accomplished by raising the temperature of surgical instrumentation to the designated temperature that renders it sterile.
- *Gas sterilization:* Sterilization by gas occurs with ethylene oxide.
- *Chemical agents:* Chemicals can be used as sterilants for certain surgical instruments. Common chemical agents are glutaraldehyde, chlorine dioxide, and sodium hypochlorite. During sterilization, it is important for all parts of the surgical instrument to be equally exposed to the sterilant. Clamps, needle holders, and scissors should be sterilized in open position. All other instrumentation should be fully emerged and sterilized according to manufacturer instructions.

### Scrubbing

Before you put sterile gloves on, you must perform a complete and careful hand washing to remove as many microorganisms as possible. A routine hand washing for medical asepsis should be performed vigorously for at least 15 seconds before and after seeing each patient, before and after eating, before and after using the restroom, before and after handling specimens or any soiled or contaminated materials, and after removing gloves. Skin carries many microbes, and a thorough hand washing for surgical asepsis, or surgical **scrub**, should be performed for two to six minutes (or the length of time recommended by the antimicrobial soap manufacturer) before taking part in any sterile surgical procedure. The purpose of the surgical scrub is to reduce the number of microorganisms and make the skin surgically clean. Just before the surgical scrub, you should put on the appropriate personal protective equipment (PPE). This can include face shield or face mask and eye protectors (goggles). The gown, gloves, and sterile drying towel should be laid out before the surgical scrub is completed. All hand and wrist jewelry must be removed prior to conducting the surgical scrub. Refer to Procedure 49–2 for instructions for performing a surgical scrub. Dry hands and forearms by grasping the sterile towel by the corner and away from the sterile field. When drying, the medical assistant must be careful not to recontaminate the skin and should not retrace any of the skin with the towel.

### Gowning

Donning a sterile gown is a must for anyone assisting is surgery. The medical assistant will be required to don a sterile gown when participating in surgery and might also be required to assist the provider in donning sterile attire (Figure 49–4). The procedures for donning a sterile gown are described in Chapter 36.

## PROCEDURE 49–2 Hand Washing for Surgical Asepsis

**PURPOSE:** To reduce the number of microorganisms on the skin and make the skin surgically clean

**EQUIPMENT:** Personal protective equipment (eye protection, mask), sterile gloves, surgical scrub agent, surgical sink, sterile dry towel

**S SKILL:** Perform a surgical scrub.

| Procedure Steps | Detailed Instructions and/or *Rationales* |
|---|---|
| 1. Don all personal protective equipment needed (eye protection, mask). | |
| 2. Lay out sterile dry towel and gloves. | |
| 3. Remove all hand and wrist jewelry. | *Jewelry harbors microbes.* |
| 4. Open surgical scrub agent and place in sink area. | (If using impregnated scrub sponge) |
| 5. Turn on water by using the automatic sensor or foot and knee controls. Wet hands and forearms, keeping hands pointed upward (during the entire procedure). | Hands should be held away from the body and higher than the elbows at all times during the procedure. |
| 6. Using the nail stick, clean under each nail. Drop the nail stick in the sink and rinse hands. | |
| 7. Wet hands and forearms up to the elbow, starting with the fingers and working down. | |
| 8. Scrub one side (hands and forearms up to the elbow), using the surgical scrub agent, starting from the fingers and working down. Rinse. | Do not go over a section that has already been scrubbed. |
| 9. Scrub the opposite side, using the same steps as in step 8. Drop the scrub brush in the sink. Rinse. The entire rinse should take between two and six minutes. | |
| 10. Turn off the water with the automatic sensor or foot and knee control. | |
| 11. Pick up the sterile dry towel, and, keeping it several inches from your body, start at the fingertips of one side and pat dry all the way up to the elbow. Repeat this procedure with the opposite side of the arm, using the opposite side of the towel. Apply sterile gloves. | Do not rub the towel back and forth. Remember to continue to hold the hands and arms pointed upward. |

## Gloving

If the provider wishes you to assist directly with the surgical procedure, sterile gloves must be worn. Dressing changes should also be performed wearing sterile gloves to protect both you and the patient. In addition, you might assist with needle biopsies, intrauterine device (IUD) insertions, and lacerations resulting from injuries. All these procedures require sterile techniques. Additional pairs of sterile gloves should be kept nearby during the surgical procedure in case of an accidental tear or puncture. Refer to Procedure 49–4 for instructions on properly putting donning sterile gloves.

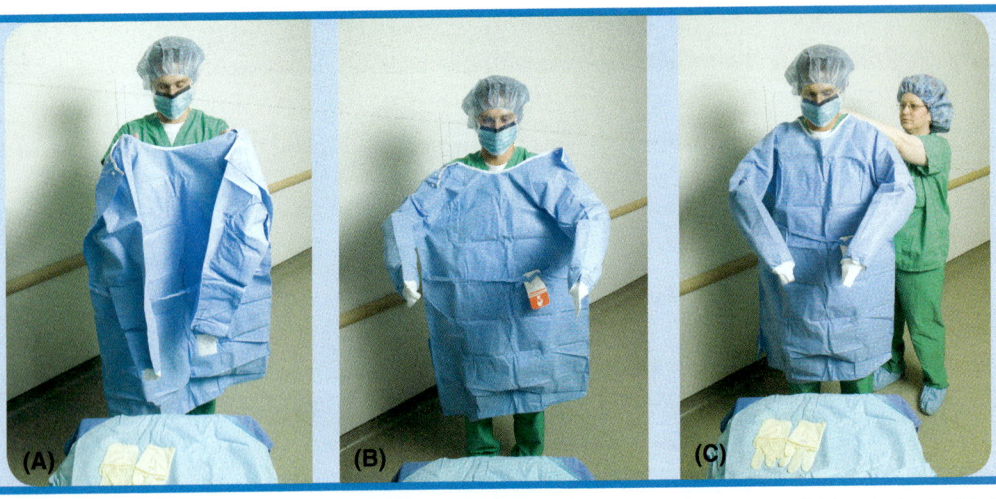


**Figure 49–4A–C:** Gowning. (A) Grasp gown by the neckline with both hands and allow it to unfold with the inside facing you. (B) Put hands and forearms into the gown without exposing the hands through the cuff. (C) An unsterile team member will assist with gown closure. *Delmar/Cengage Learning.*

## PREPARING THE PATIENT FOR MINOR SURGERY

When the patient arrives for surgery, a consent form must be completed. An example is shown in Figure 49–6. Allow the patient time to ask any questions about the procedure and answer them adequately. The patient's signature must be on the consent form, which is filed in the chart or scanned into the patient's electronic medical record (EMR). If the patient is a minor or incompetent, the person authorized to give consent must sign for the patient following an explanation of the procedure and answering any questions. The patient's vital signs should be taken, and any complaints or problems should be recorded on the patient's chart. The patient should then empty the bladder before being positioned and draped for the procedure.

## PROCEDURE 49–3 Sterile Gloving

**MEDIA LINK:** View the video, "Sterile Gloving," for this chapter on the Premium Website.

**PURPOSE:** Standing in front of a clean, clear counter surface, demonstrate the correct method of putting on sterile gloves

**EQUIPMENT:** Package of sterile gloves of proper size and biohazard waste bag. To comply with standard precautions, gloves and other protective barriers must be worn if there is any possibility of coming in contact with blood or any body fluids.

**SKILL:** Apply sterile gloves.

| Procedure Steps | Detailed Instructions and/or *Rationales* |
|---|---|
| 1. Remove your wristwatch, rings, and other jewelry from your hands and wrists and perform hand washing for surgical asepsis, following the instructions in Procedure 49–2. | |
| 2. Tear the seal and open the package of sterile gloves as you would open a book (Figure 49–5A). Place it on a clean counter surface with the cuff end toward your body. | Do not touch the inside of the package. *Hands would contaminate the inside of the sterile package.* |

| Procedure Steps | Detailed Instructions and/or *Rationales* |
|---|---|
| 3. Grasp the glove for your **dominant** hand by the fold of the cuff with the finger and thumb of your nondominant hand (Figure 49–5B). Insert your dominant hand, carefully pulling the glove on with the other hand, keeping the cuff turned back. | Dominant hand is now gloved and sterile. |
| 4. Place gloved fingers under the cuff of the other glove and insert your nondominant hand (Figure 49–5C). Put the glove on by pulling on the inside fold of the cuff (Figure 49–5D–E). Avoid touching the thumb of your dominant hand to the outside cuff of the other glove where it has been contaminated. | |
| 5. Now both hands are gloved and sterile. Place your fingers under the cuffs to smooth the gloves over the wrists and smooth out the fingers for better fit. Check for tears and holes (Figure 49–5F). | *Any break in the integrity of the glove would not maintain sterility.* |
| 6. Keep your hands above waist level. Do not touch anything other than items in the sterile field. | *Contact with any non-sterile object or surface will contaminate gloved hands, requiring removal and re-gloving.* |
| 7. Remove the gloves by pulling the glove off your dominant hand with your thumb and fingers at the palm (Figure 49–5G). Pull the glove off inside-out (Figure 49–5H). | Be careful not to touch the contaminated side of the gloves when removing. |
| 8. Slip your ungloved hand into the inside top cuff of the gloved hand (Figure 49–5I) and slip the glove off inside-out (Figure 49–5J). | |
| 9. Deposit the gloves in a biohazard waste bag if they came in contact with body fluids or other potentially infectious material. | |
| 10. Wash hands. | |

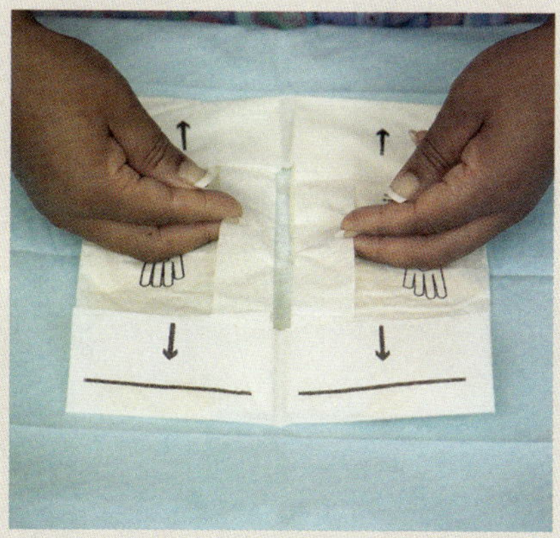

**Figure 49–5A:** Open the package by pulling on the center paper folds. *Delmar/Cengage Learning.*

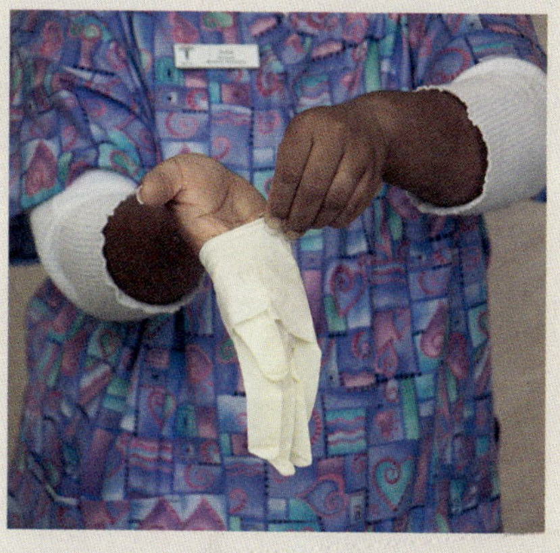

**Figure 49–5B:** Grasp the fold of the inside cuff of the gloves with the thumb and fingers of your nondominant hand. Insert your dominant hand, carefully pulling the glove on with the other hand, keeping the cuff turned back. *Delmar/Cengage Learning.*

*(continues)*

*(continued)*

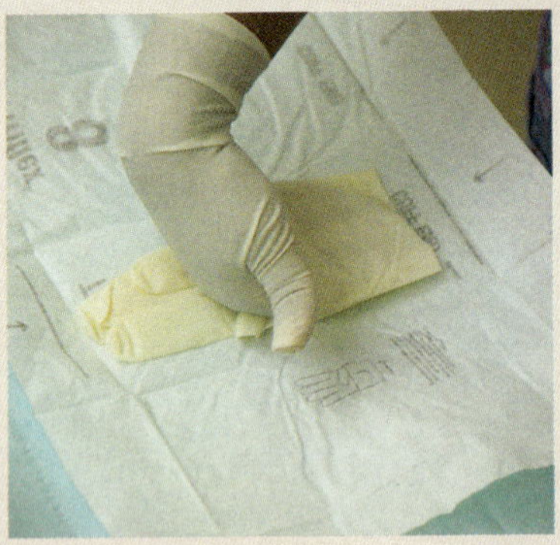

**Figure 49–5C:** Place gloved fingers under the cuff of the other glove. *Delmar/Cengage Learning.*

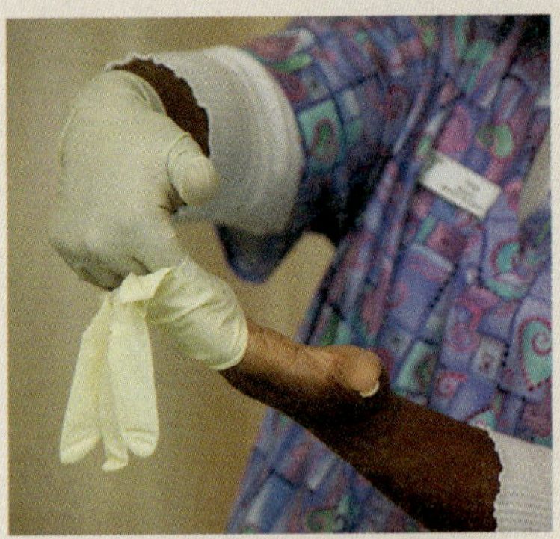

**Figure 49–5D:** With palm up, insert your nondominant hand. *Delmar/Cengage Learning.*

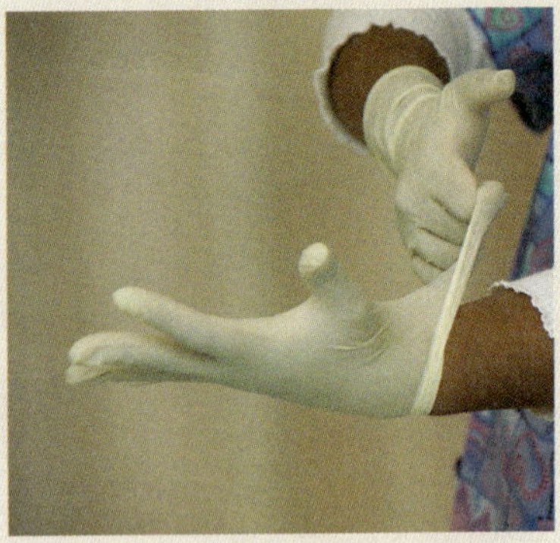

**Figure 49–5E:** Put on the glove by pulling on the inside fold of the cuff. *Delmar/Cengage Learning.*

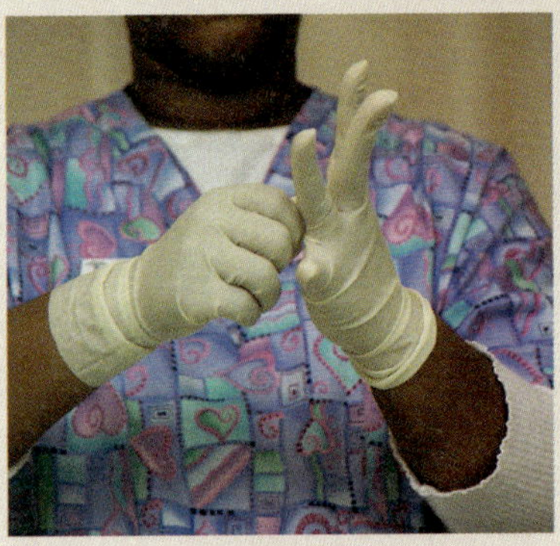

**Figure 49–5F:** Place your fingers under the cuffs to smooth the gloves over the wrists and smooth out the fingers for better fit. *Delmar/Cengage Learning.*

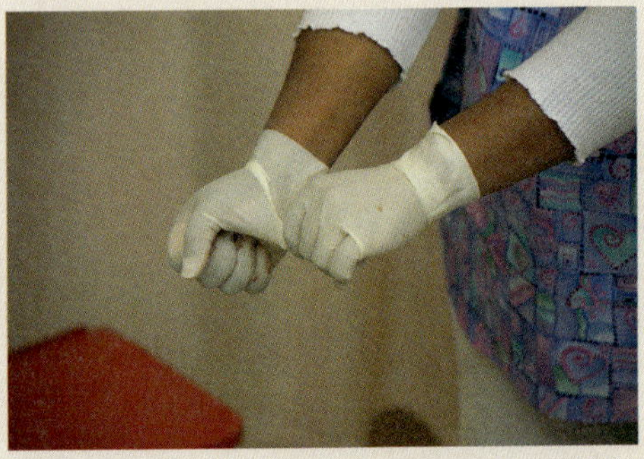

**Figure 49–5G:** Remove gloves by grasping the gloved palm of the dominant hand. *Delmar/Cengage Learning.*

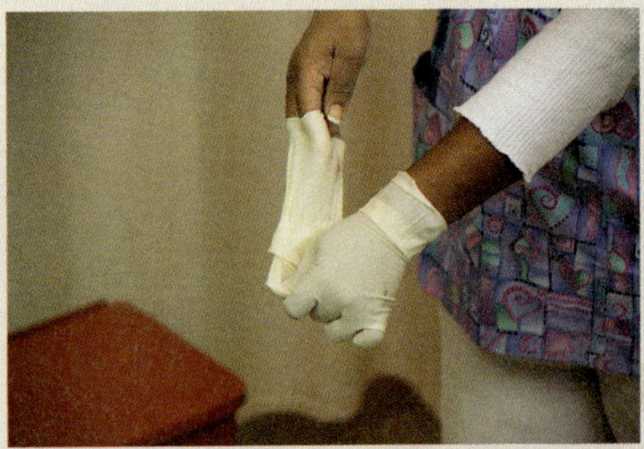

**Figure 49–5H:** Pull the glove off, turning the glove inside-out as it is being removed. *Delmar/Cengage Learning.*

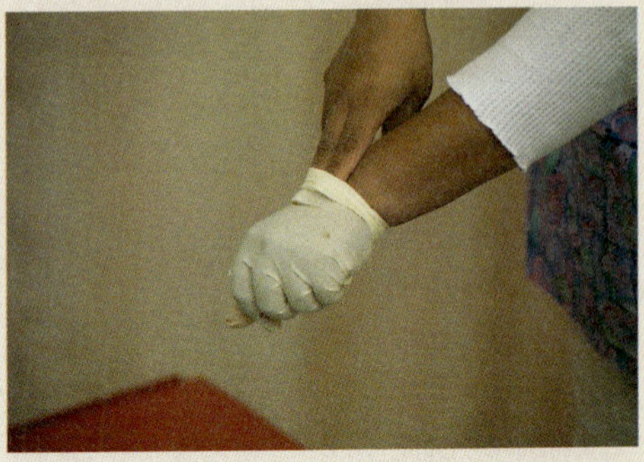

**Figure 49–5I:** Insert the ungloved hand inside the top cuff of gloved hand. *Delmar/Cengage Learning.*

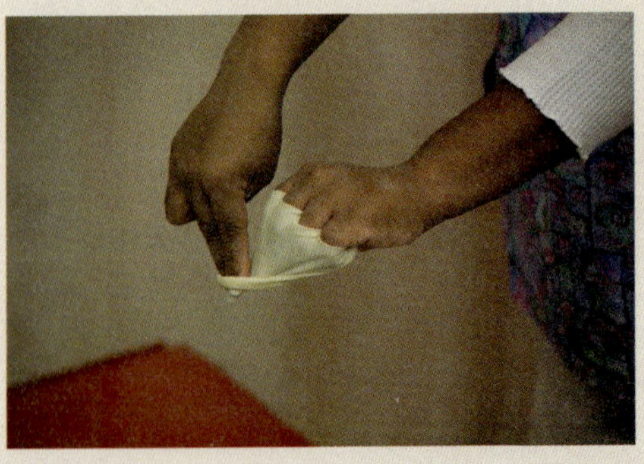

**Figure 49–5J:** Remove the glove, turning the glove inside-out as it is being removed. *Delmar/Cengage Learning.*

CONSENT TO OPERATE

Date ________ Time ________ AM PM

1. I authorize the performance upon ________
   of the following operation ________
   to be performed under the direction of Dr. ________
2. The following have been explained to me by Dr. ________
   A. The nature of the operation ________
   B. The purpose of the operation ________
   C. The possible alternative methods of treatment ________
   D. The possible consequences of the operation ________
   E. The risks involved ________
   F. The possibility of complications ________
3. I have been advised of the serious nature of the operation and have been advised that if I desire a further and more detailed explanation of any of the foregoing or further information about the possible risks or complications of the above listed operation it will be given to me.
4. I do not request a further and more detailed listing and explanation of any of the items listed in paragraph 2.

Signed ________
*(Patient or person authorized to consent for patient)*

Witness ________

**Figure 49–6:** A sample consent form for surgical procedures. *Delmar/Cengage Learning.*

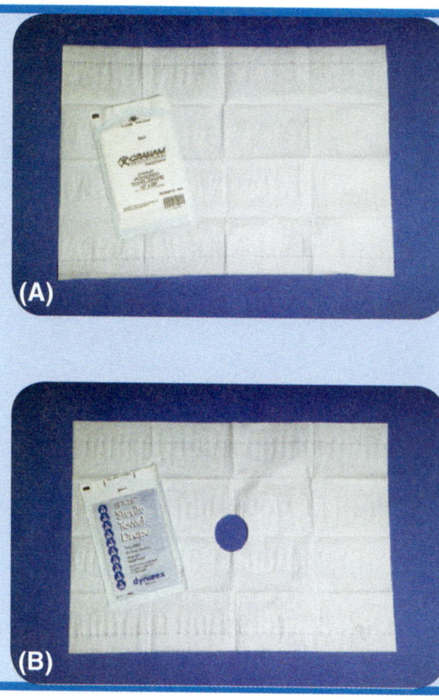

**Figure 49–7:** (A) Nonfenestrated surgical drapes and (B) Fenestrated surgical drapes. *Delmar/Cengage Learning.*

## Positioning the Patient

The patient might need to be positioned in any of a number of numerous positions for in-office surgery procedures. The position of the patient depends on the surgical site and provider preference. All the positions mentioned in Chapter 39 are suitable for minor office surgery. The following positions are the most common:

1. Horizontal recumbant or supine
2. Prone
3. Sims'
4. Fowler's
5. Knee-chest
6. Lithotomy
7. Dorsal recumbent
8. Proctologic

## Draping

Drapes are an extension of the sterile field and are designed to prevent the spread of bacteria and **strikethrough**. During surgery, drapes provide a surface on which sterile surgical supplies can be placed during surgery. Drapes can be reusable and disposable. Disposable drapes are usually the drapes of choice in a medical office. The type of drape chosen—**fenestrated** or nonfenestrated—will depend on surgical procedure, surgical site, and provider preference (Figure 49–7).

When draping the patient, the medical assistant must be careful to adhere to aseptic technique; follow these guidelines:

1. Always drape from the sterile to the unsterile.
2. Do not reach across a sterile area to drape.
3. Do not move drapes after they are placed.
4. Do not shake, flip, or fan drapes. Drapes should be unfolded and carefully placed in position.
5. Discard any drapes that become contaminated.

## Skin Preparation

Preparation of the area of skin that will be affected by the surgical procedure is called skin prep. Many providers prefer disposable skin-prep kits that contain all the necessary items for this procedure. To protect yourself and the patient from possible disease transmission, you should wear gloves during the skin prep procedure.

Because body hair encourages **microbial** accumulation, it is sometimes shaved. You must be extremely careful to avoid nicking the patient's skin (see Figure 49–8). Microorganisms can enter the body through a break in the skin, and an infection could develop from carelessness. If the skin is nicked, the provider must be notified immediately. Practice in the procedure for this skill is necessary to become proficient.

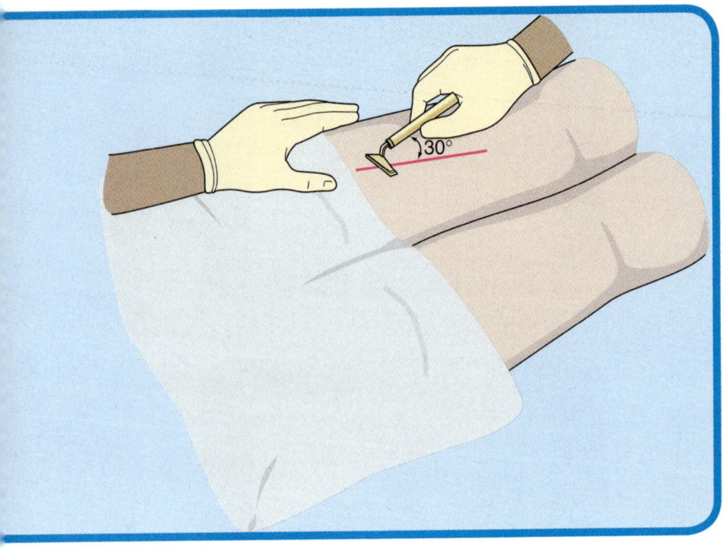


**Figure 49–8:** Angle for shaving a surgery site (or for suture insertion). *Delmar/Cengage Learning.*

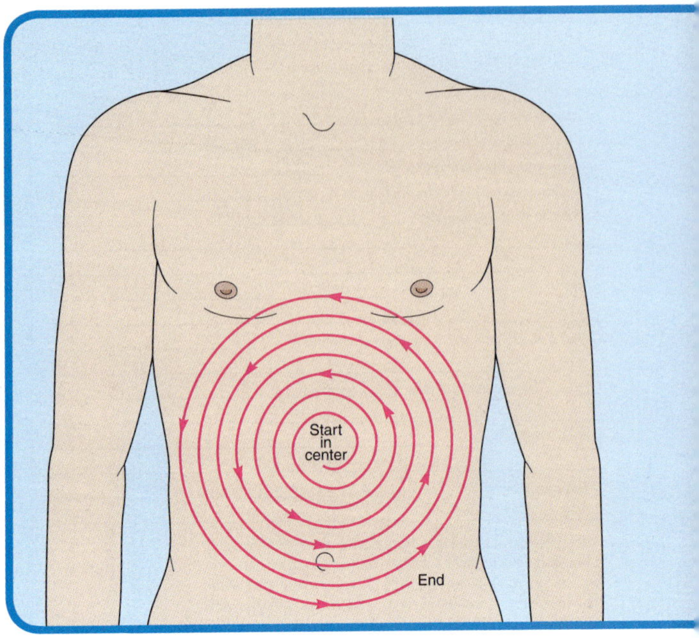


**Figure 49–9:** Apply all solutions to the skin in this circular pattern. Prepping the skin with an antiseptic solution should begin at the center of the incision site and proceed outward in one continuous circular motion as shown. *Delmar/Cengage Learning.*

The skin cannot be completely sterilized, or the cells would be destroyed, but an **antiseptic** can be used to reduce microbial growth prior to surgery. The antiseptic is applied after the skin has been shaved and properly cleansed. The solution is applied in a circular motion (see Figure 49–9), using care not to contaminate the area during the application.

When assisting with acupuncture procedures, preparation of the skin is simply to use an antiseptic such as alcohol. (If the skin is obviously dirty, wash the area with soap and water and dry it before proceeding.)

Refer to Procedure 49–4 for preparing a patient's skin for minor surgery.

## PROCEDURE 49–4 Prepare Skin for Minor Surgery

**PURPOSE:** Demonstrate each of the steps required in the skin prep procedure. *In the institutional setting, preparing the forearm might be sufficient; moreover, the shaving process can be demonstrated by using a razor with no blade.*

**EQUIPMENT:** Small basin for soap solution, 4 × 4-inch gauze squares (sponges), disposable razor, scissors, antiseptic soap solution, emesis basin for disposables, gooseneck lamp, sterile drape sheet or towels (or fenestrated drape sheet), latex or vinyl gloves, and skin antiseptic. To comply with standard precautions, gloves and other protective barriers must be worn if there is any possibility of coming in contact with blood or any body fluids.

**S SKILLS:** Prepare skin for a minor surgical procedure.

| Procedure Steps | Detailed Instructions and/or Rationales |
|---|---|
| 1. Assemble all items and wash and glove hands. | |
| 2. Introduce yourself and identify the patient. | *Speaking to the patient by name and checking the chart ensures that you are performing the procedure on the correct patient.* |

| | |
|---|---|
| B 3. Explain the procedure to the patient, ***including the rationale for why the procedure is being performed, using language the patient can understand.*** Ask the patient to remove necessary clothing and explain where the patient should put any belongings. Assist the patient if necessary. | |
| 4. Assist the patient into the proper position on the treatment table and drape with a sheet or light bath blanket as directed by the provider. | |
| 5. If appropriate, apply an absorbent towel underneath area to be shaved to catch water. Adjust the gooseneck lamp to light the area. | |
| 6. Place gauze squares in the soapy solution and use one at a time to soap the area to be shaved. After use, discard each in an emesis basin. | |
| 7. When the skin prep site is covered by scalp hair, beard, or pubic hair, use scissors to clip hair in preparation for shaving. Shave hair by placing the razor against the skin at about a 30-degree angle. | Hold the skin taut for easier shaving. Shave in the direction hair grows. Wipe soap and hair from the razor with a tissue. Swish the razor through soapy water, shake excess water from it, and shave the next area. *Use caution when clipping hair with scissors and in shaving with a razor to avoid both self-injury and harm to the patient.* |
| 8. Remove all soap and hair from the area by wetting a sterile gauze square with sterile water and wiping the area. Dry the area with sterile gauze squares. Remove the absorbent towel if used. | |
| 9. Apply antiseptic solution to the surgery site with a gauze square held by transfer forceps or disposable skin prep kit. Begin application in the center of the site and move outward in a circular motion. | *This pattern of continuous movement ensures total coverage without contamination from untreated areas.* |
| 10. Cover the prepared area with a sterile drape sheet or towel until the provider is ready to begin. | Instruct the patient not to touch the sterile field (either the sterile field of the surgical site or the instrument tray setup). |
| 11. Discard disposable items and return other items to the proper storage area. Remove gloves and wash hands. | |
| B 12. ***Attend to the patient's comfort. Patients are usually apprehensive about even minor surgical procedures. Reassurance at this time is most important.*** | |

## CHAPTER SUMMARY

- When scheduling minor surgery, advise the patient of the approximate length of time for the procedure, appropriate clothing to wear, fasting instructions, whether someone should accompany the patient and whether the patient should anticipate time off from work or arrange for home care. The patient should be given printed education materials at this time as well.
- Be sure the patient understands the procedure and the instructions regarding preoperative and postoperative care. Provide the patient with printed materials.
- Surgical instruments might have thumb or ring handles, ratchets, serrations, and teeth (see Figure 49–1).
- Most instruments are classified according to their function, including: (1) *cutting and dissecting* (scissors and scalpels), (2) *clamping and grasping* (hemostats, clamps, forceps, and needle holders), and (3) *dilating, probing, and visualizing* (retractors, scopes, specula, probes, and dilators). Review Table 49–1 for a list of common instruments used in minor surgery.
- Proper setup of the surgical tray is a vital part of the surgical process. The room where the surgery will take place and the sterile tray should be set up before the patient is escorted to the area to be prepared for the procedure.
- Surgical asepsis is obtained through sterilization, which is the process of destroying all disease-causing microorganisms. Sterilization can occur by autoclave, dry heat, gas, and chemical agents. Steam is the most widely used method of sterilization.
- Skin carries many microbes, and a thorough surgical scrub should be performed for six minutes before taking part in any sterile surgical procedure.
- It is also important to know how to apply a surgical gown and gloves properly. The medical assistant might also be required to assist the provider in donning sterile attire.
- When the patient arrives for surgery, a consent form must be completed and filed in the patient's chart. Allow the patient time to ask any questions about the procedure and answer them adequately.
- During skin prep, the affected area is cleansed and an antiseptic is applied in a circular motion. The area might also be shaved prior to cleansing if appropriate. To protect yourself and the patient from possible disease transmission, wear gloves during the skin prep procedure.

## STUDY TOOLS

| | |
|---|---|
| **Workbook** | Activities for Chapter 49 |
| **Premium Website** | |
| MEDIA LINK | View this **Media Link** for Chapter 49:<br>• Sterile Gloving |
| StudyWARE | Activities and Quizzes on the **StudyWARE™ Software** for Chapter 49 |
| | **Audio Library** of medical terms |
| | Online access to the **Critical Thinking Challenge 2.0** |
| **CourseMate** | Activities and Quizzes for Chapter 49 |
| **WebTutor** | Activities and Quizzes for Chapter 49 |

## CHECK YOUR KNOWLEDGE

1. A fenestrated sheet is one that has a(n):
   a. fold.
   b. pleat.
   c. stain.
   d. opening.
2. Autoclaved items remain sterile for ________ if they have been properly processed and protected from moisture.
   a. 3 days
   b. 30 days
   c. 3 weeks
   d. 3 months

3. To reduce the possibility of infection from a surgical procedure, skin preparation includes:
   a. cleaning the site with a soapy solution.
   b. shaving the skin.
   c. applying antiseptic solution.
   d. all of the above.
4. Before a surgical procedure can be performed, you must obtain a:
   a. signed consent form.
   b. verbal authorization.
   c. medical history.
   d. medication list.
5. The sterile tray should be set up:
   a. just before the provider enters the room.
   b. prior to the patients entering the room.
   c. 30 minutes before the procedure.
   d. while the patient is gowning.
6. The Mayo stand should be adjusted to:
   a. waist level.
   b. hip level.
   c. be level with the countertop.
   d. be level with the exam table.
7. During skin prep, avoid nicking the skin because this could cause a(n):
   a. rough surface.
   b. infection.
   c. irritation.
   d. redness.

## WEB LINKS

Integra Surgical Instruments: www.integra-ls.com/home/medical/isurgical/Miltex, Inc.: www.miltex.com

CHAPTER 8

# Preparing for Surgery

## Words to Know Challenge

**Spelling: Each line contains three spellings of a word. Underline the correctly spelled word.**

| | | |
|---|---|---|
| 1. anticeptic | antiseptic | anticeptik |
| 2. micorganism | mickroorganism | microorganism |
| 3. ratchet | rachet | rachette |
| 4. contamination | contaminition | cuntamination |
| 5. serattions | serrations | cearations |
| 6. asceptic | aseptic | aseptick |
| 7. forseps | forsepts | forceps |
| 8. microbial | microrbial | microrbital |
| 9. skrub | sgrub | scrub |

Chapter

# 9 Assisting with Minor Surgery

## OBJECTIVES

In this chapter, you will learn the following:

### KB KNOWLEDGE BASE

1. Spell and define, using the glossary at the back of the text, all the Words to Know in this chapter.
2. Describe the in-office minor surgical procedures discussed in this chapter.
3. Describe the types of anesthetics used in minor surgical procedures performed in the office.
4. List the medical assistant's duties in minor surgery performed in the office.
5. Explain the tray setup for suture removal.
6. Explain the cleanup process following an in-office minor surgery.
7. Describe important information that should be recorded on the patient's chart.

### S SKILLS

1. Demonstrate wound collection procedures.
2. Demonstrate the medical assistant's role in assisting with a minor surgical procedure.
3. Demonstrate the medical assistant's role in assisting a provider to apply sutures.
4. Demonstrate suture and staple removal.

### B BEHAVIORS

1. Apply principles of aseptic techniques and infection control.
2. Use language and verbal skills that enable patients' understanding.
3. Display sensitivity to patients' rights and feelings in collecting specimens.
4. Explain the rationale for performance of a procedure to the patient.
5. Show awareness of patients' concerns about the procedure being performed.

## WORDS TO KNOW

anesthesia
biopsy
coagulate
cryosurgery
electrocautery
excision
exudate
hemophilia
hypoallergenic
incision and drainage (I&D)
suture

## SURGICAL PROCEDURES IN THE MEDICAL OFFICE

The medical assistant might have various roles while assisting the provider with minor surgical procedures. He or she must ensure the comfort and safety of the patient and be knowledgeable enough about the procedures to assist during surgery with little or no direction, if required. Maintaining sterile technique, being knowledgeable about the provider's preferences and of the surgery being performed are critical.

Table 50–1 lists some of the common surgical procedures performed in the medical office along with some general information about each.

Outpatient, or ambulatory, surgery in recent years has become more acceptable than ever before for a number of reasons. Anesthesia has been significantly improved and causes fewer side effects in patients following surgical procedures, so patients awaken faster and easier. Also, the required time for many surgeries has decreased due to improved techniques and instruments such as the scopes used in laparoscopic surgeries. For example, an abdominal laparoscopy requires two to three very small incisions for insertion of the scope, suction, and possibly a third instrument. The gallbladder, growths, and tumors can be removed with this advanced technology. Because patients naturally feel more comfortable at home following the same-day surgery, most patients of all ages are sent home to recover and do so more rapidly than when in the hospital. Postsurgical infection rate has also declined in those patients who go home immediately following surgery. All this is highlighted by the reduced cost from the elimination of a hospital stay.

## ASSISTING WITH MINOR SURGERY

Some providers prefer to perform minor surgical procedures themselves and have the medical assistant prepare the patient, the room, and the equipment only. However, other providers like to have the medical assistant directly involved in assisting with the procedure, and those providers usually have their own preference of how the instruments are set up and what duties the medical

**TABLE 50–1 In-office Minor Surgical Procedures**

| Procedure | General Description |
|---|---|
| Laceration repair | Closing a wound or laceration by placing **sutures** or stitches or staples in the skin to hold the edges of the wound together for proper healing. |
| Sebaceous cyst removal | **Excision** of a small, painless sac containing a build-up of sebum, the secretion from a sebaceous gland. |
| **Incision and drainage (I & D)** | Incision into a localized infection, such as an abscess, to drain the **exudate** from the area. |
| **Biopsy** | Excision of a small amount of tissue for microscopic examination. Specimen must be preserved in a solution of 10% formalin until transported to the laboratory and prepared for examination. |
| Needle biopsy | Fluid or tissue cells aspirated through a needle into a syringe for microscopic examination. This specimen must also be properly preserved. |
| **Cryosurgery** | Destruction of tissue and skin lesions by using extremely cold temperatures. |
| **Electrocautery** | Removal of benign skin lesions, such as warts and skin tags, by use of electric current. This procedure is performed when a biopsy is not required and to control bleeding during a procedure. |
| Chemical destruction | Tissue destroyed by applying silver nitrate to the area. |
| Laser surgery | A concentrated laser beam (intense light beam) destroys a target area without harming the surrounding tissue. |
| Loop electrosurgical excision procedure (LEEP) | A thin, low-voltage, electrified wire loop removes abnormal cervical tissue. A vinegar (acetic acid) or iodine solution can be applied to the cervix prior to the procedure to help make abnormal cells more visible. |
| Vasectomy | The vas deferens is cut, separated, and then sealed by electrocautery or clamping. This prevents sperm from entering the semen, thus making a man sterile. |
| Circumcision | The removal of some or all the foreskin (the skin that covers the tip of the penis) from the penis. |
| Debridement | Excision of lacerated, dead, or contaminated tissue and removal of foreign matter from a wound. |

assistant is expected to perform. When assisting with a surgical procedure, it is critical to maintain strict sterile technique. A break in sterile technique or a breach of the sterile field can result in an infection for the patient.

## Anesthetics

Most in-office minor surgical procedures are performed under local **anesthesia**, which the provider administers. Local anesthesia causes a loss of sensation in a specific area of the body (the area in which the procedure will be performed) as opposed to general anesthesia, which causes a loss of sensation over the entire body (unconsciousness).

The most common local anesthetic agents are Xylocaine (lidocaine hydrochloride) and Novocain (procaine hydrochloride). The provider is the one to actually inject the anesthetic into the area, but you might be asked to hold the vial while the provider draws up the medication (Figure 50–1). The anesthetic usually begins to numb the area within approximately 5 to 15 minutes and will keep the area anesthetized for up to three hours. Some providers prefer to use an anesthetic with epinephrine additive to help constrict the blood vessels in the area, which prolongs the effect of the anesthetic.

## Specimen Collection

In procedures requiring a biopsy for analysis, carefully labeling and handling the specimen is vital. The laboratory provides a formalin solution container for preservation of the tissue specimen. This container is sterile, and the specimen must be placed directly in the solution with sterile transfer forceps. A completed lab request form must accompany the specimen for analysis.

In certain surgical procedures, such as the removal of warts or polyps, an electrocautery device may be used

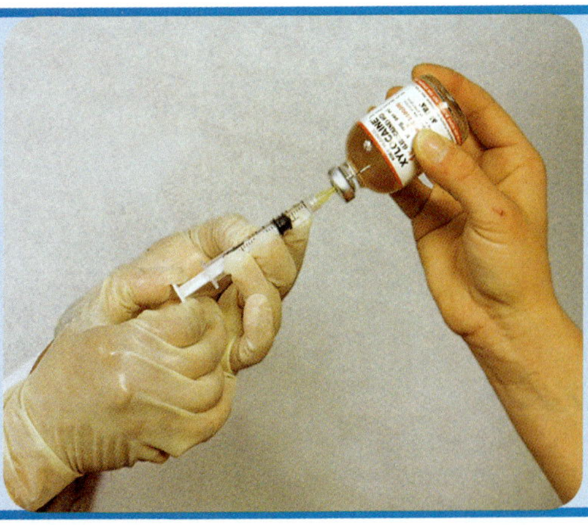

**Figure 50–1:** Hold the anesthetic solution in a convenient position so the provider can fill the syringe without contamination. *Delmar/Cengage Learning.*

### CLINICAL PEARL

A careful medical history must be taken from the patient to determine possible allergic or adverse reactions. Ask about current medications and any over-the-counter, herbal, or diet supplements taken. This helps avoid complications during and after the procedure. If the patient discloses any significant medical history or abnormality, such as **hemophilia** (a serious blood-clotting disease in which the absence of one of the necessary blood-clotting factors prevents blood from coagulating), you should bring it to the provider's attention immediately. This information should be marked in red ink on the patient's chart. Hemophilia is a sex-linked hereditary trait that occurs mostly in males. Patients who have this diagnosis must have surgery of any type *only* at a completely equipped, well-staffed medical-surgical hospital to protect their safety and well-being.

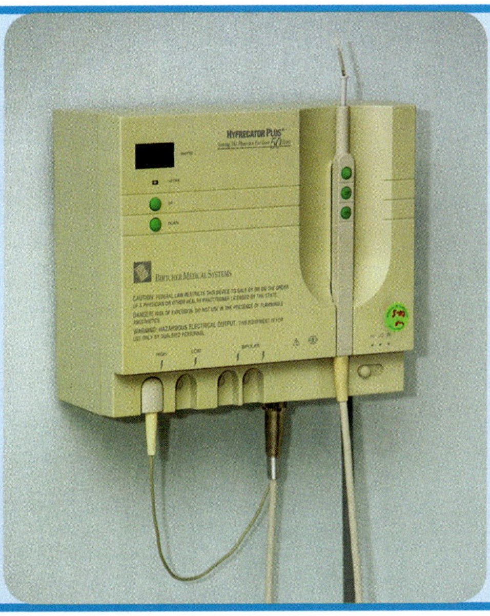


**Figure 50–2:** An electrocautery unit. *Delmar/Cengage Learning.*

(Figure 50–2). Often, this controls bleeding of the surgical site by electrocoagulation. Controlled high-frequency current is applied by the provider to the surgical area to **coagulate** the blood to close the incision. If the reusable tips are preferred by the provider for surgical procedures, they must be autoclaved to prevent possible cross-contamination. Disposable tips are available.

Another method for removing skin tags, warts, and other skin disorders and growths is by cryosurgery. Often, certain gynecologic treatments and surgical procedures are performed with this instrument. This process uses subfreezing temperature to destroy or remove tissue. Generally, the substances used are solid carbon dioxide or liquid nitrogen. It is sometimes referred to as cold cautery.

## Bandaging

Patients will present with skin sensitivities to various materials; the type of bandage the provider orders will vary and should be appropriate for the wound and for the patient's skin. For patients who are very active or who are employed in activities that could further injure or cause the wound to become dirty or wet, the wound should be wrapped in a very thick dressing to cushion and protect it and allow it to heal. Make sure you advise the patient to keep the dressing clean and dry. Remind the patient to place a plastic bag over the extremity to keep it dry during showers or baths. If the wound is on the trunk of the body, taking a shower or bath should be discouraged unless the provider has approved it. Usually, a sponge bath is preferred until the bandage comes off. This is important in minimizing the possibility of infection.

If an infection should occur, you might be asked to obtain a specimen for laboratory analysis and culture. Procedure 50–1 explains wound collection procedures. Simply use a sterile swab and insert the tip into the center of the infected area of the wound. Then transfer the swab with the specimen into the culture medium. Provide patient education regarding care of the site and when to return for a follow-up appointment. In addition, providers advise using an elastic bandage to offer more protection and support of surgical areas of the extremities, especially for pediatric and physically active patients. Application of an ACE wrap increases circulation of the area, which hastens the healing process.

# POSTOPERATIVE INSTRUCTIONS

Printed instructions should be given to the patient and explained to both the patient and family members. The patient should, of course, be given the provider's phone number and urged to phone if there are any complications or concerns. You should have a standard set of printed instructions readily available for telephone screening of those outpatient surgery patients who call in with questions or concerns. Any calls that suggest a serious problem or condition should be referred to the provider immediately. Refer to the patient education box regarding what you should caution patients about following any surgery.

## PROCEDURE 50–1 Perform Wound Collection

**PURPOSE:** To collect a wound culture while maintaining sterile technique

**EQUIPMENT:** Appropriate personal protective equipment as required by procedure, sterile gloves, sterile instrumentation, ampule, and swab

S **SKILL:** Collect a sterile wound culture.

| Procedure Steps | Detailed Instructions and/or *Rationales* |
|---|---|
| 1. Assemble all necessary supplies. | |
| 2. Introduce yourself and identify the patient. | The patient can be identified by asking his or her name and date of birth and checking the information in the chart. |
| 3. Verify the provider's orders. | |
| B 4. ***Explain the procedure and rationale for the procedure to the patient, using language the patient can understand.*** | |
| 5. Remove the sterile swab from the container. | |
| 6. Collect a sterile specimen. Roll the sterile swab in the exudate. | The swab should not touch any part of the wound except the exudate. |
| 7. Insert the sterile swab back into the container and crush the ampule. | |
| 8. Record the patient information on the container. | |
| 9. Document the procedure in the patient's chart. | |

## PATIENT EDUCATION

Usual care of patient:

1. Keep site clean and dry.
2. Place no stress on the area.
3. Drink plenty of fluids.
4. Get proper rest.
5. Eat a sensible, well-balanced diet.
6. Return for follow-up appointment.

Patients should report to the provider any of the following:

1. Unusual pain, burning, or other uncomfortable sensation
2. Swelling, redness, or other discoloration
3. Bleeding or other discharge
4. Fever above 37.7°C (100°F)
5. Nausea and vomiting
6. Any other problem or symptom

Make sure that return appointment visits are confirmed and reminder cards are given to patients before they leave the office. Phoning patients the next day is an excellent way to follow up and reassures them that you and the provider are genuinely concerned about their progress. It will also bring to the provider's attention any problems that could be eliminated early. If patients do have complaints, it is best to have the provider check the problem as soon as possible.

Follow-up visits are essential so that assessment of progress can be made by the provider and sutures or staples can be removed. Specific instructions, such as soaking or applying topical medications, will be given by the provider for certain individual cases. Providers generally instruct patients (or teach you how to instruct patients) about packing or special bandaging procedures such as with ingrown toenail removals. Providers can prescribe an analgesic for minor pain and discomfort the patient might experience following the procedure.

## DOCUMENTING SURGICAL PROCEDURES

Like all procedures, surgical procedures are to be documented in the medical record thoroughly and completed immediately. The medical record entry should include:

- *A patient identifier:* The patient's name or patient ID number can be used.
- *Informed consent:* Informed consent should be obtained from the patient before the procedure.
- *The date and time:* The date and time of the procedure should be recorded. The provider might also request the start (time of incision) and stop time of the procedure to be recorded.
- *The reason:* The provider should record in the patient chart the reason for the surgical procedure.
- *The procedure:* The provider or the medical assistant should record the procedure to be done. If the medical assistant records the procedure, it should be rechecked with the provider.
- *Specimen:* Specimen removal should be documented. The medical assistant documents what the specimen is and its source. The medical assistant also labels the specimen container with the patient's name and other patient-identifying information (name, date of birth).
- *Postoperative instructions:* The medical assistant is responsible for ensuring that the patient or his or her caregiver understands the postoperative instructions.

Procedure 50–2 lists the general steps involved when assisting with a minor surgical procedure.

## PROCEDURE 50–2 Assist with Minor Surgery

**PURPOSE:** To demonstrate (insofar as possible) each of the steps required in assisting with minor surgery

**EQUIPMENT:** Basic sterile setup: needle and syringe; needle holder; appropriate suture, scalpel handle, and blade; thumb forceps; surgical scissors; hemostats; retractor; three or four pairs of latex or vinyl gloves; gauze squares; cotton-tipped applicators; alcohol pad; fenestrated sheet or towels; towel clamps; bandages; bandage scissors; tape; ordered anesthetic; antiseptic (small glass container for antiseptic solution); plastic biohazard sharps container and waste bag (and waste receptacle); patient's chart; pen; histology request form for laboratory analysis if a biopsy is indicated; Mayo tray table; and proper lighting (extra backup sterile setup) *NOTE:* **Some of the equipment might differ according to the procedure performed.**

S **SKILL:** Demonstrate the medical assistant's role in assisting with a minor surgical procedure.

| Procedure Steps | Detailed Instructions and/or *Rationales* |
|---|---|
| 1. Wash hands. | |
| 2. Assemble the appropriate equipment and supplies. | Assemble supplies on a counter or table near a Mayo tray. Position the Mayo tray table next to the treatment table and check the condition and expiration dates of sterile items. *If an item is expired or the package shows signs of improper conditions, items might no longer be sterile.* |
| 3. Correctly set up a sterile tray, maintaining sterile technique, and cover it with a sterile drape per office policy. | Refer to Procedure 49–1 for setting up a sterile tray. |
| 4. Introduce yourself and identify the patient. | |
| B 5. ***Explain the procedure and rationale for the procedure to the patient, using language the patient can understand.*** Ensure that the patient has signed the informed consent form. Advise the patient to empty the bladder. If a biopsy is to be taken, complete a lab request form for histology analysis. | *A signature on the consent form is absolutely essential before any invasive procedure is performed.*<br>*Emptying the bladder ensures the patient's comfort during the procedure. Anxiety often results from the urge to void.* |
| 6. When the patient returns, take vital signs and record. | *Vital signs must be within acceptable limits to proceed with the procedure.* |
| B 7. Instruct the patient to disrobe as necessary for the procedure and advise where to place any belongings. Assist the patient if needed. ***Allow privacy and ask the patient to let you know when he or she is ready for positioning.*** | |
| B 8. Assist the patient to the treatment table and into the desired position for surgery. Perform a skin prep procedure. ***Give the patient support and understanding and answer any questions at this time.*** Drape the patient appropriately. | Refer to Procedure 49–4 for preparing a patient's skin for minor office surgery. |
| 9. When the provider is ready to begin the procedure, remove the sterile towel from the prepared sterile setup. Assist the provider by handing sterile gloves (if indicated) and assist with drawing up anesthesia as needed. | Use an alcohol prep to wipe the top of the anesthetic vial and hold it for the provider to draw out the amount needed. |
| 10. If you are to assist with the surgical procedure, wash hands and put on sterile gloves. Hand instruments and other sterile items to the provider as needed; mop excessive blood with gauze sponges as needed. | If additional sterile items are needed during the procedure, open the package and hand it to the provider for removal or drop it onto the center of the sterile field. |
| 11. Assist with collecting any specimen as needed by the provider. | If a biopsy is to be performed, take special care to preserve the specimen. Deposit the specimen directly into an open specimen container. Label and attach a completed laboratory requisition when the procedure is completed. |
| 12. Assist with suturing or stapling the incision as needed by the provider. | You might assist the provider in suturing the incision by clipping each individual suture after the provider ties the knot. You should perform any other assistance as directed by the provider during the procedure. |
| 13. When the surgery is completed, assist in (or perform) cleaning and bandaging the surgery site, remove gloves, and wash hands. | If the patient is allergic to adhesive, use **hypoallergenic** tape to secure the bandage. |

*(continues)*

*(continued)*

| Procedure Steps | Detailed Instructions and/or *Rationales* |
|---|---|
| B 14. ***Attend to the patient's comfort by helping the patient into a sitting position to regain balance and, when stable, from the table. Assist in dressing if necessary.*** | |
| 15. Give the patient postoperative instructions. | Instructions should include education regarding any return visit, care of surgery site, and any other orders from the provider. |
| 16. Document the procedure in the patient's chart. | |
| 17. Put on gloves and clean up the treatment area. Wash hands and restock treatment room. | Clean up treatment table, discard contaminated items in a biohazard waste bag, rinse the instruments with cold water and place in a detergent solution, remove gloves and wash hands, and restock the room. |

## APPLYING SUTURES

The term *suture* means a type of thread that joins the skin of a wound, either an accidental laceration or a surgical incision, together. A type of suture called catgut is eventually absorbed by the body and does not need to be removed (generally used in major surgeries). It is made from the intestines of sheep. Suture is also made of a material such as silk, nylon, or other manufactured substances that must be removed in a matter of days, depending on the area of the body in which they are inserted. For convenience, most providers prefer to use suture that has a needle already attached. Figures 50–3A and B shows examples of different types of suture materials and needles used in closing wounds.

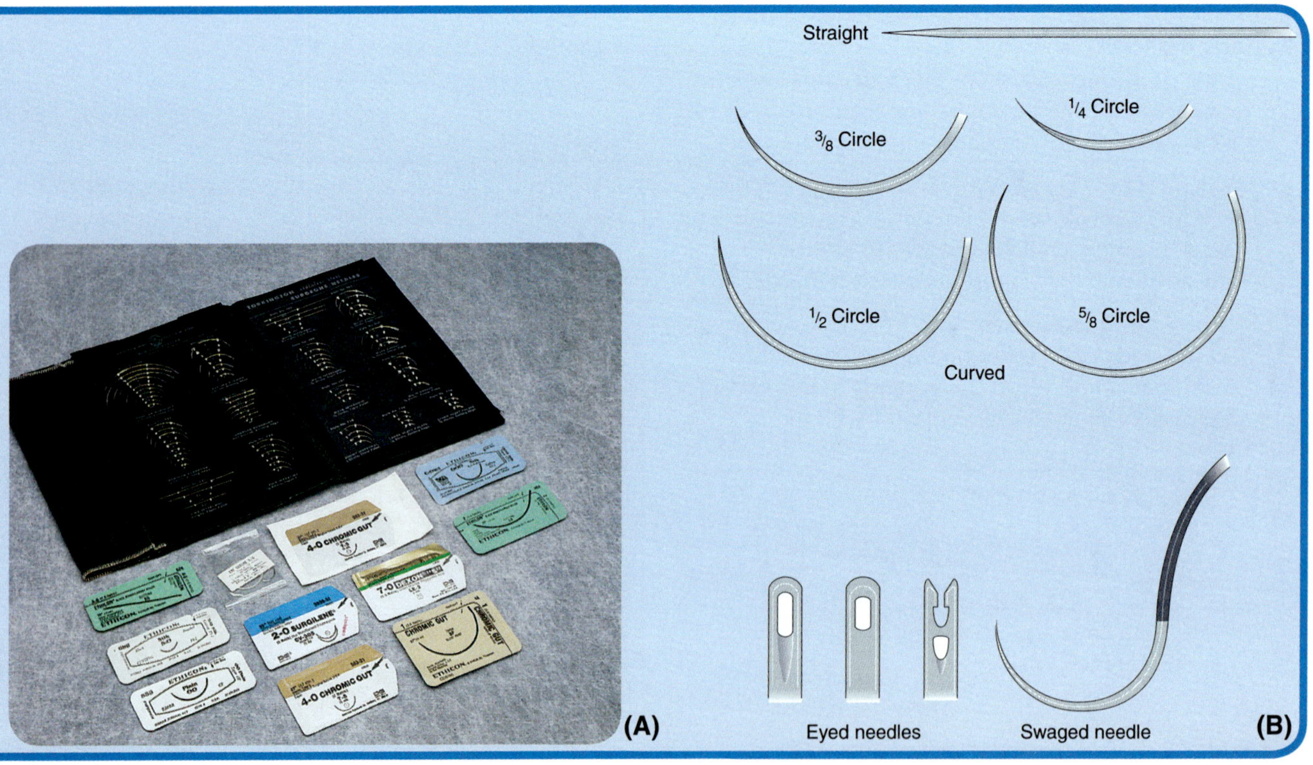


**Figure 50–3A–B:** (A) A variety of suture packs and curved and straight surgical needles. (B) Various needle shapes used in the insertion of sutures to close wounds. *Delmar/Cengage Learning.*

Most offices have a policy regarding the treatment of lacerations. If the injury is severe and might result in serious blood loss, it is usually treated in the emergency room or trauma center. However, many patients will come to their primary care physician to have a laceration sutured. Working these patients into an already full schedule can present delays for other patients waiting for scheduled appointments. Prepare the patient for the provider and assist as needed. After the suturing is complete, the provider can see other patients while you take care of the laceration patient and clean up the work area.

Your efficiency and expedient preparation of setting up the treatment room will be appreciated by both the provider and the patient in this situation. Follow the steps in Procedure 50–3 for assisting with suturing a laceration. Always make sure that you record the number of sutures (stitches) the provider inserts and the anatomical location. Go over patient education and any additional instructions from the provider before the patient leaves the office. If the patient is given instructions by the provider to redress and bandage the wound at home, show the patient how to do this. Alert patients to call with any questions or concerns.

## PROCEDURE 50–3 Assist with Suturing a Laceration

**PURPOSE:** Demonstrate each of the steps required in the procedure to assist with suturing a laceration while maintaining sterile technique

**EQUIPMENT:** Items needed for skin prep: alcohol, cotton balls, PPE, biohazard bag, gauze squares, bandages and tape, bandage scissors, antiseptic, ordered anesthetic, tetanus toxoid, patient's chart, pen; sterile items: swabs, needle and syringe, latex or vinyl gloves, fenestrated drape, ordered suture material, gauze squares, hemostats, needle holder, scissors, sharps container

S **SKILL:** Demonstrate the medical assistant's role in assisting a provider to apply sutures.

| Procedure Steps | Detailed Instructions and/or *Rationales* |
|---|---|
| 1. Wash hands and assemble all needed items, using sterile technique. | |
| 2. Introduce yourself and identify the patient. | *Speaking to the patient by name and checking the chart ensures that you are performing the procedure on the correct patient.* |
| B 3. ***Explain the procedure to the patient, using language the patient can understand and explaining the rationale for the procedure.*** Advise the patient to empty the bladder. | *Emptying the bladder ensures the patient's comfort during the procedure. Anxiety often results from the urge to void.* |
| 4. When the patient returns, take and record vital signs. | *Vital signs must be within acceptable limits to proceed with the procedure. The patient might have lost a considerable amount of blood, which could alter vital signs.* |
| B 5. Ask the patient to remove necessary clothing. Explain where the patient should place any belongings. Assist the patient if needed. ***Allow privacy if needed.*** | *The patient might experience weakness and might not feel well enough to be left alone.* |
| 6. Assist the patient into the appropriate position for skin prep of the wound. Proceed with the steps for preparing skin for minor surgery and then drape the patient appropriately. | Refer to Procedure 49–4 for preparing a patient's skin for in-office minor surgery. |
| 7. Put on PPE and sterile gloves. Arrange the instruments and other sterile items in the order the provider will use them. Remove gloves and wash hands. | *Do not reach, cough, sneeze, wave, talk, or cross over the sterile field, or it can become contaminated.* Carefully cover the sterile field with a sterile towel until the provider is ready to begin. |

*(continues)*

*(continued)*

| Procedure Steps | Detailed Instructions and/or *Rationales* |
|---|---|
| 8. When the provider is ready to begin the suturing procedure, remove the sterile towel from the prepared sterile setup. Assist the provider by handing sterile gloves (if indicated) and assist with drawing up anesthesia as needed. | Use an alcohol prep to wipe the top of the anesthetic vial and hold it for the provider to draw out the amount needed. |
| 9. If you assist with the suturing procedure, wash hands and put on sterile gloves. Hand instruments and other sterile items to the provider as needed; mop excessive blood from the wound with sterile gauze as needed. | Assist the provider by clipping each individual suture as directed by the provider. |
| 10. When the wound has been closed with sutures, assist with (or perform) cleaning and bandaging the site per the provider's orders. When bandaging is done, remove and properly dispose of gloves and wash hands. | If cleaning and bandaging the site, you might need to re-glove to keep from soiling the dressing and bandage.<br>*Some individuals are allergic to adhesive; hypoallergenic tape is then preferred.* |
| 11. Administer tetanus toxoid if ordered. | If administered, ensure that this is documented in the patient's chart as part of the entry. |
| B 12. ***Tend to the patient's needs and comfort. Assist with sitting up, getting dressed, and helping from the treatment table as needed.*** | *Allow the patient sufficient time to regain balance before standing alone because dizziness can occur.* |
| 13. Give the patient postoperative instructions. | Instruct the patient in the care of sutures and provide a return appointment for their removal. |
| 14. Document the procedure in the patient's chart. | |
| 15. Put on gloves and clean up the treatment area. Wash hands and restock treatment room. | Clean up the treatment table, discard contaminated items in a biohazard bag and sharps container, rinse the instruments with cold water and place in detergent solution, remove gloves and PPE, and dispose of them in the biohazard bag. |

## SUTURE AND STAPLE REMOVAL

Patients usually see the family or general practitioner for suture removal following laceration repair from an injury. In many offices, it is the medical assistant's responsibility to remove the sutures. It is vital to check the emergency center's report regarding the number of sutures put in so you can be sure to remove all of them.

Be sure to remove the same number of sutures as were inserted by the primary care physician. Suture that is not removed can become infected, so care in removing all the material is vital. Patients sometimes report that one or two stitches have already come out during a bandage change at home. This should also be noted on the patient's chart. Follow the steps in Procedure 50–4 for suture removal. Removal of staples is performed with a staple extractor as described in the procedure for suture removal. Check the report also for a tetanus booster and record on the patient's chart to bring the immunization record up to date. Before you remove the sutures, check the number of days the provider who put them in recommended as the time to wait before removal. Ask the provider to inspect the healing wound. After the sutures or staples have been removed, providers might order additional closure materials to cover healing incisions or lacerations (Figures 50–4A through D). A support skin closure might be necessary to keep the skin together until the wound is completely healed. The type of supportive closure should be noted on the patient's chart.

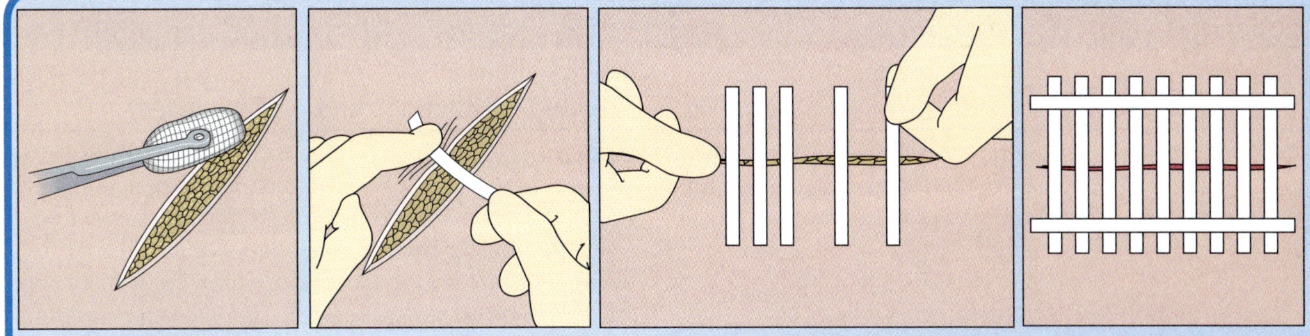


**Figures 50–4A–D:** (A) Care of an incision or wound with a closure application: Use transfer forceps with sterile gauze to apply antiseptic. (B) Apply Steri-Strip closure to the center of the incision. (C) Apply closures to each side for evenness and then fill in and cover the full wound area. If ordered, apply a topical medication and a sterile bandage. (D) For additional support, closures can also be applied parallel to the incision or wound. *Delmar/Cengage Learning.*

## PROCEDURE 50–4 Remove Sutures or Staples

**PURPOSE:** Demonstrate the steps required to remove sutures (using a mannequin or model as the patient)

**EQUIPMENT:** Sterile: thumb forceps, suture-removal scissors (or staple extractor), gauze squares, latex or vinyl gloves, cotton-tipped applicators, butterfly or Steri-Strip™ closures; skin care and documentation: antiseptic solution, hydrogen peroxide, tincture of benzoin, basin with warm soapy water, bandages, tape, towels, biohazard waste bag, sharps container, bandage scissors, patient's chart, and pen

S **SKILL:** Remove sutures from a healing laceration or incision.

| Procedure Steps | Detailed Instructions and/or *Rationales* |
|---|---|
| 1. Wash hands and assemble all needed items, using sterile technique.. | |
| 2. Introduce yourself and identify the patient. | |
| B 3. ***Explain the procedure and rationale for the procedure, using language the patient can understand,*** and answer any questions. Ask the patient about the healing condition of the incision or laceration, take vital signs, and record them on the patient's chart. | If sutures resulted from a laceration injury, ask appropriate questions regarding where and when injury occurred and when a tetanus booster was administered [file ER report in chart]. Record. |
| B 4. Ask the patient to remove necessary clothing for inspection of the healing incision. Explain where the patient should place any belongings. Assist the patient if needed. ***Allow privacy if needed.*** | |
| 5. Assist the patient to the treatment table and into the required position and drape appropriately. | |

*(continues)*

*(continued)*

| Procedure Steps | Detailed Instructions and/or *Rationales* |
|---|---|
| 6. Put on gloves and remove the bandage. Clean the incision with antiseptic solution, using cotton-tipped applicators. Advise the provider that the incision site is ready. | If the bandage has stuck to the incision (record condition of site on chart [e.g., excessive blood or drainage]), apply gauze squares that have been soaked with soapy warm water solution, or hydrogen peroxide, to the area for a few minutes to loosen the bandage from the sutures and scab. *This makes removal of the bandage easier. Pulling off a stuck bandage can reopen the wound or pull out sutures; either result would be painful.* |
| 7. After the provider orders suture or staple removal, open a sterile package containing the necessary instruments on the Mayo tray and proceed. | *Do not reach, cough, sneeze, wave, talk, or cross over the sterile field, or it can become contaminated.* Carefully cover the sterile field with a sterile towel until the provider is ready to begin. |
| For Suture Removal: | |
| 8. Grasp the knot of the suture material with thumb forceps and gently but firmly pull up, making just enough space to place the suture removal scissors to clip the suture as close to the skin as possible (Figures 50–5A and B). Pull the suture with the forceps (back) toward the healing incision so that no stress is put on it. Continue until all are removed. Count the number of sutures removed and compare with the number in the patient's chart. | *Pulling the suture away from the site could pull the incision open.*<br><br>Caution: Do not pull a suture that has been on the surface of the skin (exposed to the outside) through the path of the suture being removed, or infection can develop. |

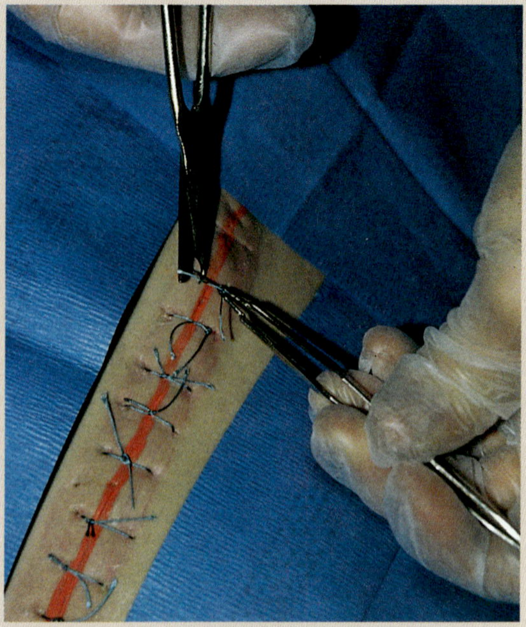

(A)

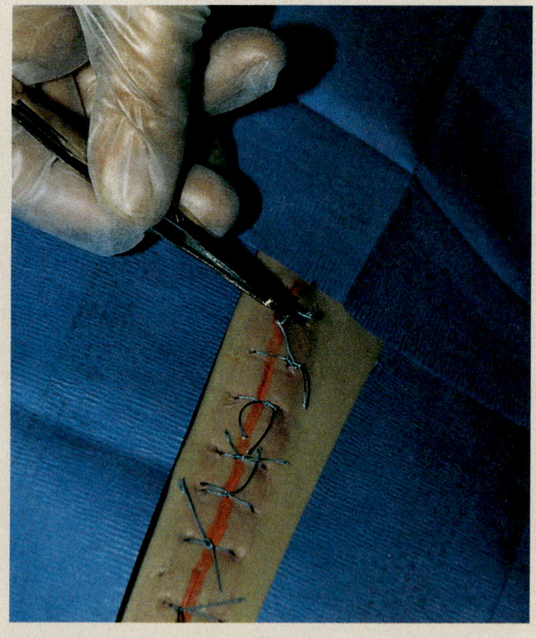

(B)

**Figures 50–5A–B:** (A) Grasp the suture knot with thumb forceps and place the curved tip of the suture-removal scissors just next to the skin under the suture and clip. (B) Gently pull the suture up and toward the incision with the thumb forceps to remove. (Pulling the suture away from the incision can pull the incision open.) *Delmar/Cengage Learning.*

| Procedure Steps | Detailed Instructions and/or *Rationales* |
|---|---|
| For Skin Staples: | |
| 9. If skin staples are to be removed, place the sterile staple extractor under a staple (one at a time) and squeeze the handles of the extractor completely closed (Figure 50–6). Lift the staple away from the skin and dispose in a sharps container. Continue until all are removed. | Explain to the patient that he or she might feel a tugging sensation. |
| 10. Apply antiseptic solution to the site and allow it to air dry. Apply Steri-Strips or a butterfly closure if necessary for support during the healing process and bandage. | |
| 11. Remove gloves and wash hands. | |
| 12. Give the patient postoperative instructions. | Instruct the patient to keep the bandage clean and dry for 24 to 48 hours or as directed by the provider. Advise the patient to avoid undue stress for the appropriate amount of time for the anatomical area. Schedule a follow-up appointment if ordered by the provider. |
| 13. Document the procedure in the patient's chart. | Document: (1) anatomical area of incision or laceration, (2) condition of site, (3) number of sutures removed, (4) type of antiseptic applied, (5) support closures applied, (6) type of bandage applied, and (7) your signature or credentials. Be sure to include the ER report if sent from the facility where the injury was treated and record the date of the tetanus booster if applicable. |
| 14. Put on gloves and clean up the treatment area. Wash hands and restock treatment room. | Clean up the treatment table, discard contaminated items in a biohazard bag and sharps container, place instruments in detergent solution after rinsing with cool water, remove gloves and PPE, and dispose of them in the biohazard bag. |

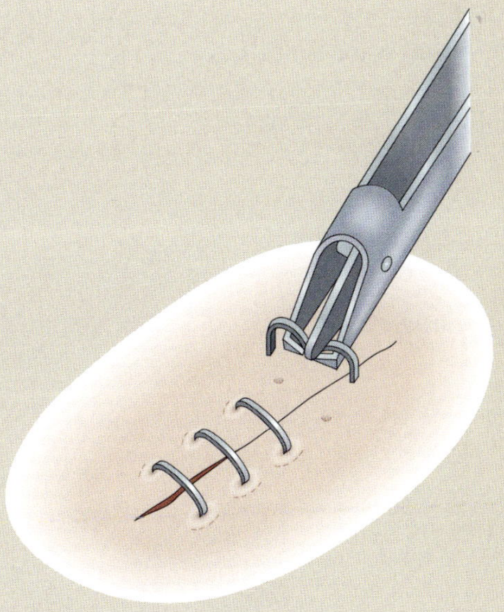

**Figure 50–6:** Removal of a staple: The staple extractor reforms the staple (clip). Then, the staple is then lifted from the incision. *Delmar/Cengage Learning.*

Advances in skin closures offer a sutureless substance applied to small lacerations. This type of closure is an adhesive material and is used frequently with children who can be frightened and thus uncooperative. A sutureless procedure is much quicker and less traumatic for the child and staff as well. Skin closures give support to the wound and offer the patient more flexibility.

### PATIENT EDUCATION

Following suture removal, patients should be advised to:

1. Keep the site dry for at least 24 hours.
2. Cover the area to keep it clean.
3. Apply supportive bandaging as needed.
4. Report any sign of infection immediately to the provider.

## CHAPTER SUMMARY

- Medical assistants should have a general knowledge of the procedures performed in their place of employment and be able to assist the provider with little or no direction. Some common procedures include laceration repair, sebaceous cyst removal, incision and drainage, biopsy, needle biopsy, cryosurgery, electrocautery, chemical destruction, laser surgery, loop electrosurgical excision procedure (LEEP), vasectomy, circumcision, and debridement.
- Most procedures are performed under local anesthesia, which the provider administers. The medical assistant might be asked to hold the vial while the provider draws up the anesthesia.
- If a biopsy is taken, careful labeling and handling of the specimen is vital. A completed lab request form must accompany the specimen for analysis.
- After a procedure, printed instructions should be given to the patient and verbally explained to both the patient and family members.
- Complete documentation includes a patient identifier, informed consent, the date and time, the reason, the procedure, any specimen collected, any postoperative instructions given, and the medical assistant's signature and credentials.

## STUDY TOOLS

| | |
|---|---|
| **Workbook** | Activities for Chapter 50 |
| **Premium Website** StudyWARE | Activities and Quizzes on the **StudyWARE™ Software** for Chapter 50 |
| | Complete the following **Competency Challenge 2.0** activity:<br>• Tuesday, 11 AM: Prepare and Assist with Procedures, Treatments, and Minor Office Surgeries |
| | **Audio Library** of medical terms |
| | Online access to the **Critical Thinking Challenge 2.0** |
| learninglab | Module 21: Minor Surgical Procedures |
| **CourseMate** | Activities and Quizzes for Chapter 50 |
| **WebTutor** | Activities and Quizzes for Chapter 50 |

## CHECK YOUR KNOWLEDGE

1. Which of the following types of anesthesia is not used in minor surgical procedures performed in the office?
   a. Local
   b. Nerve block
   c. Topical
   d. General
2. The method used to remove skin tags and warts is:
   a. electrocautery.
   b. cryosurgery.
   c. laser surgery.
   d. biopsy.
3. Local anesthesia begins to numb an area in:
   a. 30 minutes.
   b. 5–15 minutes.
   c. 1 hour.
   d. 3 hours.
4. A serious blood-clotting disease in which the absence of one of the necessary blood-clotting factors prevents blood from coagulating is:
   a. coagulitis.
   b. hemophilia.
   c. hemophilitis.
   d. angiocoagulitis.
5. A type of suture that does not need to be removed is made from:
   a. silk.
   b. nylon.
   c. catgut.
   d. all of the above.

## WEB LINKS

American Association of Medical Assistants (AAMA)
www.aama-ntl.org/

Association of Surgical Technologists (AST)
www.ast.org/

CHAPTER 9

# Assisting with Minor Surgery

## Words to Know Challenge

**Spelling: Each line contains three spellings of a word. Underline the correctly spelled word.**

| | | |
|---|---|---|
| 1. biopsy | biopsie | biopcie |
| 2. cyrosrurgery | kryosrusery | cryosurgery |
| 3. electocautery | electrocautery | elecktrocautery |
| 4. coagalate | coagulate | cogulate |
| 5. hemophilia | hemophillia | hemopilia |
| 6. anathesia | anesthesia | anathesia |
| 7. exudate | exadate | exadite |
| 8. sewture | suwture | suture |
| 9. hypoalerrgenic | hypoallergenik | hypoallergenic |
| 10. exision | excision | excison |

Chapter

# 10 Emergencies in the Medical Office

## OBJECTIVES

In this chapter, you will learn the following:

### KB KNOWLEDGE BASE

1. Spell and define, using the glossary at the back of the text, all the Words to Know in this chapter.
2. Define a medical emergency.
3. List items that might be found in a crash cart or emergency kit.
4. Explain the purpose of the universal emergency medical identification symbol.
5. State principles and steps of professional and provider CPR.
6. Discuss the importance of safety when administering CPR.
7. Explain the purpose of an AED and its capabilities.
8. Identify seven descriptive terms that describe the severity or onset of a disease or disorder.
9. List examples of emergency situations.
10. Compare and contrast symptoms of hyperglycemia and hypoglycemia.
11. Identify symptoms of a heart attack.
12. Differentiate the symptoms of heat stroke and heat exhaustion.
13. Name symptoms that might indicate damaged tissue due to cold exposure.
14. Identify the distinguishing characteristics of capillary, vein, and arterial bleeding.
15. List symptoms of internal bleeding.
16. List, in order of occurrence, the chain of events that might happen with a seizure.
17. Discuss instances when obstructed airway can occur.
18. List symptoms of shock.
19. Identify signs of possible stroke.

### S SKILLS

1. Perform an abdominal thrust on an adult victim with an obstructed airway.

## WORDS TO KNOW

acute
airway
ammonia
aspiration
cardiopulmonary resuscitation (CPR)
coma
cessation
chronic
compressions
consciousness
coroner
diabetic ketoacidosis
diaphoresis
emergency
emergency medical services (EMS)
exhaustion
flushed
frostbite
heat cramps
heat exhaustion
heatstroke
hyperglycemia
hypoglycemia
hypothermia
ingested
insulin shock

intubation
life-threatening
medical emergency
myocardial infarction
obstructed
poison
post mortem
prophylactic
seizure
severe
subtle
sudden
syncope
trauma
universal emergency medical identification
urgent

## HANDLING EMERGENCIES IN THE MEDICAL OFFICE

A provider's office must always be ready to react to an **emergency** situation. A **medical emergency** is any situation in which an individual suddenly becomes ill or injured or in circumstances calling for decided action. This can involve a patient already in the office or one brought in already experiencing problems, for example:

- A patient receives a medication or injection and has a severe reaction.
- Someone is injured just outside the office and comes in for immediate treatment.
- A patient brings in a very ill or injured family member.

Knowing how to respond and how to assist the provider in treating the individual is very important. Swift and appropriate action can affect the outcome of the situation. As a medical assistant, it is important to remember that you are not to perform at the level of **trauma** or trained medical emergency personnel, only to provide a standard of care equal to that of any person with like training and experience and within your scope of practice.

### Office Policy Manual and Documentation

Every office must identify who is responsible for recording the detailed information of an emergency situation and its handling. The office policy manual should have guidelines to follow when dealing with emergencies. An emergency plan with assigned responsibilities should be developed and made known to each employee (such as who should call 911). All staff members should be capable of administering first aid and **cardiopulmonary resuscitation (CPR)** and hold current certification in CPR. The goal for emergency care in an office is to stabilize patients to release them to their family or send them to a hospital for further treatment.

Emergencies, sudden illness, and accidents can also occur among personnel while they are working in the medical office. It is equally important to document the circumstances surrounding this type of incident. Persons experiencing at-work injuries might be eligible for benefits under workers' compensation if the injury occurred while performing job responsibilities. Employee forms can be placed in the employee's personal file and in the office personnel file. (Refer to Chapter 36 for complete instructions on filling out an OSHA 301 incident report form.)

### Emergency Supplies and Equipment

As part of the preparation for emergency care, medical offices should have the necessary supplies and equipment to handle medical emergencies that might arise. These items should be collected and set aside in a special place where they are always ready for use. This could be in the form of a small suitcase or a cart referred to as an emergency kit (Figure 55–1 A) or crash cart. Figure 55–1 B shows a crash cart in the form of a mobile cart with drawers for equipment as well as a shelf on top

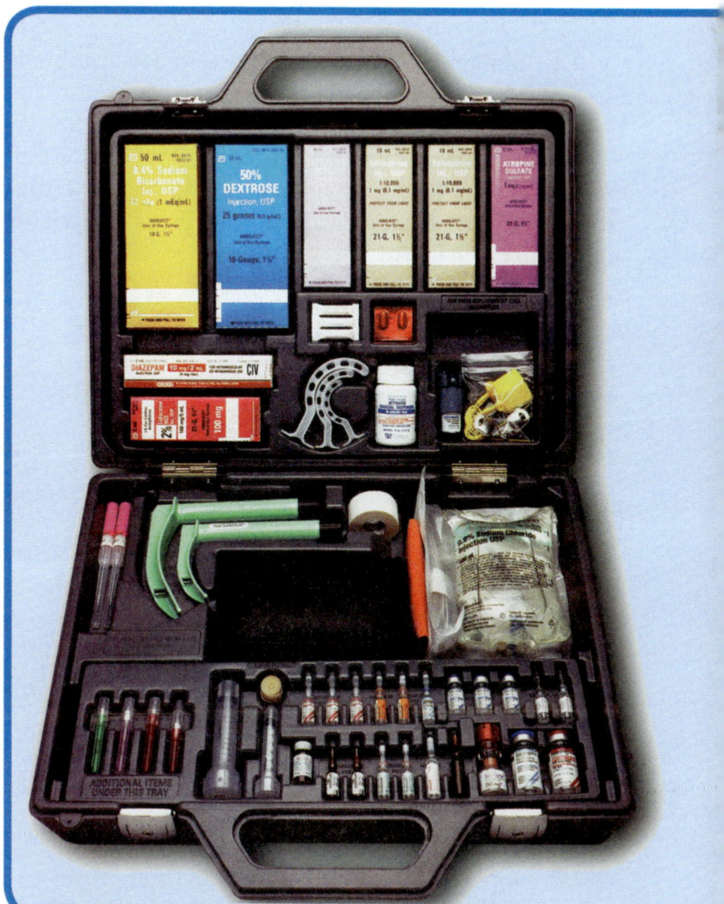


**Figure 55–1 A:** Medical emergency equipment (prepared kit). *Courtesy of Banyan International Corporation.*

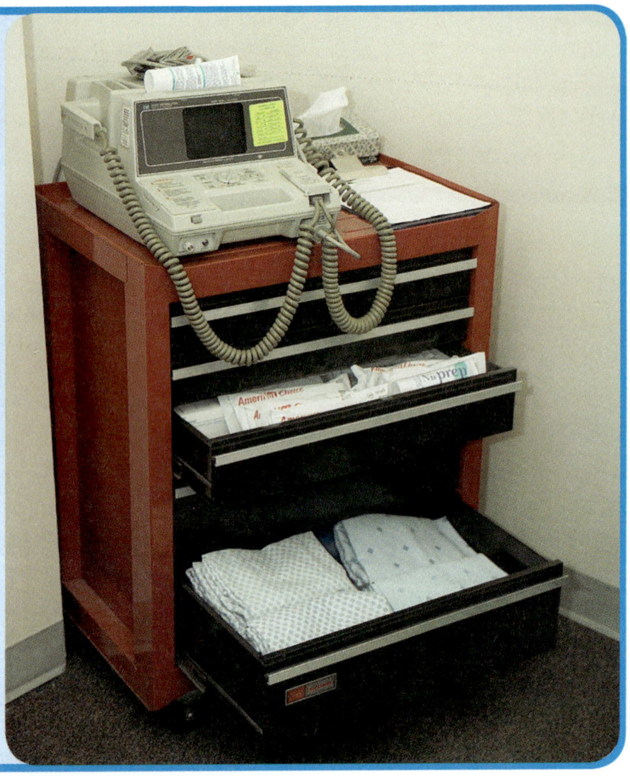

**Figure 55–1 B:** Crash cart. *Delmar/Cengage Learning.*

for a defibrillation device. All office employees should know the location of the emergency kit or crash cart and how to use the materials.

Although each practice customizes its kit or cart depending on the type of practice and the extent of emergency care it can provide, a basic list of equipment and supplies includes:

- Gloves
- Alcohol wipes
- Stethoscope
- Blood pressure cuff
- Penlight
- Aromatic spirits of **ammonia**
- Oxygen tank with flow meter and wrench for opening the tank
- Tubing, nasal cannula, and pediatric and adult masks
- Ambu bag
- Resuscitation masks in a variety of sizes
- Airways of differing sizes (nasal and oral)
- Bandage material (sterile dressings)
- Adhesive tape
- Bandage scissors
- Disposable syringes
- Tourniquets
- IV supplies: tubing and needles (butterflies and angiocaths) and fluids, including D5W, NS, D10W, and lactated Ringer's
- Medications for emergency use

**TABLE 55–1 Medications Commonly Stocked on Crash Cart**

| Emergency Medications | |
|---|---|
| • Activated charcoal | • Lidocaine |
| • Atropine | • Local anesthetics |
| • Diphenhydramine | • Nitroglycerine |
| • Epinephrine | • Phenobarbital and diazepam |
| • Furosemide | • Sodium bicarbonate |
| • Instant glucose | • Solu-Cortef™ |
| • Insulin | • Verapamil |

Table 55–1 includes some of the common medications that can be stocked on the cart.

The kit or cart should be checked regularly to be certain that all items are present and no dated material is past its expiration date. A chart attached to the cart should provide an inventory of the materials and check-off date for inspection to ensure that nothing is overlooked.

In addition, offices should be equipped with a defibrillation unit for responding to cardiac emergencies. A common type of defibrillator is the automated external defibrillator (AED), which is used in addition to CPR if the heart is in fibrillation or arrest. (These arrhythmias were explained in more detail in Chapter 47.) An AED, as well as the oxygen tank and Ambu bag (a mask with an attached inflation bag to assist breathing), should be readily accessible if needed. AED and CPR procedures are discussed later in this chapter.

## RECOGNIZING AN EMERGENCY

When severe injury or sudden critical illness occurs, a patient should have the advantages of trauma and critical care facilities as soon as possible. Often, the first hour is so important that it directly correlates with prognosis and the possibility of recovery. Being able to recognize that a situation is an emergency is the first step to providing assistance and medical attention.

Several emergency situations demand immediate medical intervention because of their severity and life-threatening consequences. Lack of breathing or heart action is fatal within a matter of minutes. The following are examples of life-threatening conditions:

- Cardiac arrest
- Respiratory arrest or great difficulty breathing
- Uncontrolled severe bleeding
- Head injury
- Poisoning
- Open chest or abdominal wound

- Shock
- Significant burns

Often the victim's actions will alert you that something is happening. The victim might yell or call out for help, moan from discomfort, be unresponsive, or present abnormal behavior. When you are an eyewitness, you can visually assess the situation and arrive at a decision.

## Responding to an Emergency

In any emergency, as a medical assistant, you will be expected to assess the situation and deliver appropriate care as directed. When emergencies occur in the office, as discussed earlier, you might follow an emergency plan developed by the office. The training you receive in procedures such as CPR, AED, obstructed airway, bandaging and splinting, stopping a bleed, and immobilizations can be the treatment you render. The first step in an emergency is to survey the scene to determine whether it is safe for you to encounter without causing harm to yourself. You will also determine the severity of the emergency and determine who needs to be treated first if more than one person is involved. This is determined by assessing the airway, breathing, and circulation of those involved, also known as conducting a primary survey. Those with the more severe injuries or ailments should be treated first.

If you should encounter an emergency situation or if you happen to come upon an unknown person who has become ill or lost **consciousness**, check for a **universal emergency medical identification** symbol (Figure 55–2). This symbol was designed by the American Medical Association (AMA) as a means for individuals with certain medical conditions to alert health care workers of their conditions when they are unable to. The tag is worn around the neck, wrist, or ankle. Some might identify the particular problem the person has; others might not. If a tag is found, the person should have an information card on his or her person, usually inside a wallet, that identifies the condition and provides some directions to follow. All patients who have conditions that could cause emergency episodes, such as heart conditions, diabetes, epilepsy, allergies, or a laryngectomy, should be encouraged to wear a universal emergency medical identification tag.

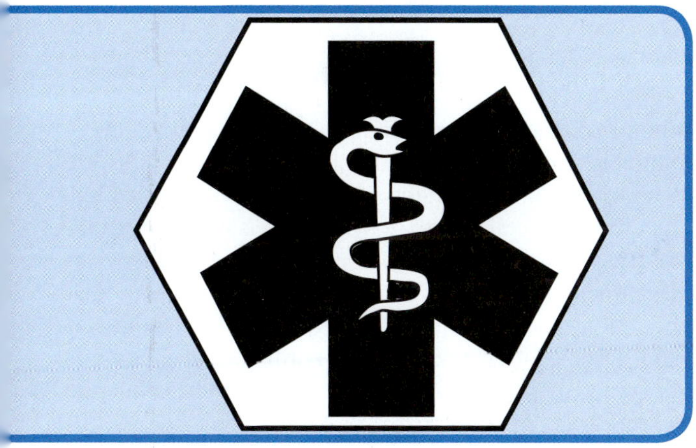

**Figure 55–2:** Universal emergency identification symbol. *Delmar/Cengage Learning.*

## Activating EMS

Activating the emergency medical services (EMS) system by telephoning 911 might also be necessary in a true emergency. Trained personnel usually provided by the police or fire departments (referred to as first responders) are generally the first to arrive on the scene. Depending on the area, emergency coverage can be provided by private ambulance services that employ trained personnel, volunteer firefighters, local law enforcement officers, or the state police.

You should know how to summon assistance in your area. If not, you may check with the office policy manual or manager to identify the appropriate service and determine what help is available and the quickest way to obtain emergency assistance. A list of all emergency numbers should be posted by every phone in the provider's office. All office staff should be aware of this information.

**CLINICAL PEARL**

Keeping a listing of emergency numbers by the phone is helpful at home as well. When an actual emergency occurs, individuals might experience difficulty finding numbers in a phone directory. Posted information saves critical time.

Some offices might place a card containing this information within the emergency kit or crash cart as well. In a situation when the provider and the medical assistant are both involved in administering first aid and there are no other office personnel present, the card could be handed to a family member to summon help.

## Documenting Emergencies

As with any medical procedure, documentation of the emergency is essential. Documenting the who, what, when, and where of the emergency is the protocol generally followed. In addition, the treatment rendered, patient education, and any follow-up for additional care will be addressed in the documentation.

Unfortunately, not all life-saving procedures are effective and occasionally the patient might expire in the office. If that happens, the local law enforcement agency that is generally on the scene will notify the **coroner** to pick up the body for **post mortem** examination. Regulations differ and are determined by local statutes. Normally, if the patient has not been examined by a provider within a fairly recent time frame, an autopsy is required to establish the cause of death to be recorded on the death certificate. If the individual was a patient, you must be certain the specifics regarding the death are recorded on the chart and notations made on additional relevant records so that no inappropriate correspondence is sent to the residence.

### Telephone Screening in an Emergency

When a patient calls the office with an emergency situation, you must listen to the caller, ask questions, and follow office policy. You might need to give the call to licensed personnel or a provider who is able to triage the situation. When a caller states there is an emergency, do not put the caller on hold. If it is a true life-threatening emergency, even a minute lost is critical. Obtain the following information:

- The victim's name
- The caller's name and phone number in case the connection is lost
- When did the problem start?
- Is the victim conscious and breathing; does the victim have a pulse?

Some situations require immediate activation of emergency medical services (EMS), for example, if the victim is not breathing or has no pulse. Check with office policy on the correct procedure to follow. Some offices instruct the caller to hang up and call 911 or the local emergency number or keep the caller on the line and have another person in the office call EMS. Either way, you must get immediate information to relay to EMS, including:

- The nature of the situation
- The location of the victim

Then continue to speak with the caller and provide any immediate assistance as appropriate:

- Reassure the caller that EMS is on the way.
- Give appropriate specific instructions in relation to the situation, such as:
  (a) If the victim has a body part pierced by an object, do not remove it.
  (b) If the victim is bleeding severely, apply pressure directly to the area.
  (c) Don't move a patient with a possible spinal injury.
- Try to stay calm and support the caller until EMS arrives and you are assured the victim is being cared for.
- Document in the patient's medical record or EHR all the information obtained and discussed.

## CPR AND AED PROCEDURES

Sudden cardiac arrest (SCA) is the total, abrupt, and unexpected loss of heart function and is a leading cause of death in the United States. According to the American Heart Association (AHA), 92% of SCA victims die before reaching the hospital; if more people knew how to perform cardiopulmonary resuscitation (CPR), more lives could be saved. Immediate CPR can double, or even triple, a victim's chance of survival (CPR Statistics, CPR & Sudden Cardiac Arrest Fact Sheet).

All medical assistants should take an approved CPR and a standard first aid course and participate in refresher courses periodically. Several organizations provide CPR training, including the AHA, American Red Cross, American Safety and Health Institute, and the National Safety Council.

Procedures are constantly being refined by these organizations, and the procedure you learn might be altered in the future, which is why it is critical to take periodic refresher courses to maintain CPR certification. In this chapter, the 2010 updates and changes to CPR and ECC (Emergency Cardiovascular Care) are discussed, but step-by-step procedures are not covered because CPR certification must be provided by one of these organizations. During your CPR training, the most up-to-date requirements will be provided along with a training manual. Adult CPR certification consists of both a written examination and a performance test-out on a mannequin similar to the one pictured in Figure 55–3. More information can be found at the organizations' Websites:

- AHA: www.heart.org
- American Red Cross: www.redcross.org
- American Safety & Health Institute: www.ahsi.org
- National Safety Council: www.nsc.org

### Responding to Cardiac Arrest

When SCA occurs, immediate action is imperative; every minute is critical. The majority of adults (80% to 90%) are in ventricular fibrillation when the initial ECG is obtained. The time from collapse to defibrillation is critical because the window of opportunity for survival of sudden cardiac arrest is very narrow. Each minute of ventricular fibrillation results in approximately 10% decrease in survival. Resuscitation is most successful if defibrillation is performed within about the first five minutes after the victim has collapsed.

Current guidelines from the AHA and Red Cross advocate immediate defibrillation of the victim using an

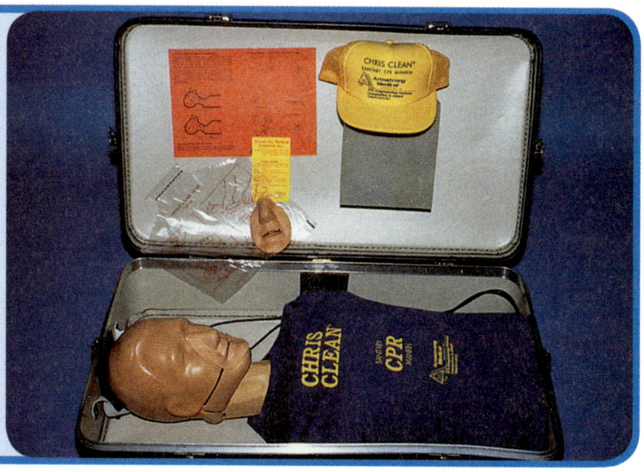


**Figure 55–3:** Chris Clean CPR training mannequin with disposable parts. *Delmar/Cengage Learning.*

AED, which provides electric stimulation to the chest. CPR should be given until an AED is available. CPR is also necessary immediately after an AED shock because most victims experience a period of no pulse after the shock. CPR and AEDs are beneficial in restoring effective heart rhythm. The chain of survival involves the following sequence of events occurring as quickly as possible:

1. Recognition of early warning signs
2. Activation of the EMS system
3. Basic CPR
4. Early defibrillation with AED
5. Intubation
6. Intravenous administration of medications

## Principles of CPR

CPR is a life-saving procedure performed when a person's breathing or heartbeat has stopped. CPR involves two elements: chest compressions and artificial respiration (mouth-to-mouth rescue breathing). The purpose is to keep oxygen flowing to the lungs and blood flowing to the brain and other vital organs until normal heart rhythm can be restored. The CPR procedure was easily remembered by applying the A-B-Cs (airway, breathing, and circulation):

- Clear the **airway**.
- Initiate rescue breathing to provide oxygen to the victim's lungs. A variety of devices are available, from the simple CPR mouth barriers and pocket masks to CPR ventilating masks and Ambu bag and masks.
- Begin chest **compressions** to restore blood circulation. Brain damage or death can occur if blood circulation stops.

However, the 2010 American Heart Association (AHA) guidelines have recommended a change in the basic life support (BLS) sequence to C-A-B (chest compressions, airway, breathing) for adults, children, and infants (excluding newborns). For information on newborns, refer to the neonatal section of the AHA guidelines. The reasoning behind this change is that the majority of cardiac arrests occur in adults, and the highest survival rates are reported when chest compressions are initiated very early on. The old sequence of A-B-C delayed the initiation of compressions while rescuers attempted to open the airway and search for a proper barrier device or ventilation equipment. This change in process should now be minimal (only the time required to deliver the first cycle of 30 chest compressions) for one-person CPR and even less when two rescuers are present. Guidelines for cardiac arrest, respiratory arrest, and obstructed airway are similar but vary according to the age of the patient. Table 55–2 includes the adult, child, and infant CPR skills.

**CLINICAL PEARL**

For the latest and up-to-date recommendations and procedures, visit the AHA Website, www.heart.org, or American Red Cross Website, www.redcross.org.

## AED Procedure

The AED is used in connection with CPR to restore cardiac function. AEDs are easily operated and can be used in the office even in the absence of the provider. They are also being installed for use by the public in many places such as shopping malls, bus stations, and airports. In a provider's office, designated personnel should be trained to operate the equipment to be prepared to respond to life-threatening emergencies. Accurate recording of time, actions, and the use of the defibrillator is very important to document emergency response and provide for risk management. Equally important is the scheduled equipment check to ensure that the battery is charged, the cables are intact, and the dated electrode package remains sealed and has not expired.

The AED can:

- Analyze the heart rhythm of a person in fibrillation or arrest.
- Recognize a shockable rhythm.
- Advise the operator through lights, text, and voice prompts if shock is indicated.
- With built-in diagnostic capability, permit life-saving intervention without the operator needing to evaluate the situation or interpret an ECG.

The AED consists of two large electrodes (pads that are placed on the patient's chest) and cables that connect to the machine. A battery package is the source of power so that the equipment can operate in any location;

## TABLE 55–2 Summary of Key BLS Components for Adults, Children, and Infants

| Component | Recommendations: Adults | Children | Infants |
|---|---|---|---|
| Recognition | Unresponsive (for all ages) | | |
| | No breathing or no normal breathing (only gasping) | No breathing or only gasping | |
| | No pulse palpated within 10 seconds for all ages (HCP only) | | |
| CPR sequence | C-A-B | | |
| Compression rate | At least 100/min | | |
| Compression depth | At least 2 inches (5 cm) | At least ⅓ AP diameter about 2 inches (5 cm) | At least ⅓ AP diameter about 1 ½ inches (4 cm) |
| Chest wall recoil | Allow complete recoil between compressions<br>HCPs rotate compressions every 2 minutes | | |
| Compression interruptions | Minimize interruptions in chest compressions<br>Attempt to limit interruptions to <10 seconds | | |
| Airway | Head tilt—chin lift (HCP suspected trauma: jaw thrust) | | |
| Compression-to-ventilation ratio (until advanced airway placed) | 30:2<br>1 or 2 rescuers | 30:2<br>Single rescuer<br>15:2<br>2 HCP rescuers | |
| Ventilations: when rescuer untrained or trained and not proficient | Compressions only | | |
| Ventilations with advanced airway (HCP) | | 1 breath every 6–8 seconds (8–10 breaths/min)<br>Asynchronous with chest compressions<br>About 1 second per breath<br>Visible chest rise | |
| Defibrillation | Attach and use AED as soon as available. Minimize interruptions in chest compressions before and after shock; resume CPR beginning with compressions immediately after each shock. | | |

**Source:** 2010 American Heart Association Guidelines for CPR and ECC.

some units have a self-contained battery. The AED is indicated when the victim is unresponsive, is not breathing, and has no pulse. Although AEDs are manufactured by various companies, and some differences exist between the different machines, there are universal steps to follow.

- Turn on the power.
- Attach the electrode pads of the AED to the victim's chest (must be against dry bare skin and might require cutting or shaving of hair. Usually, a disposable razor is with the equipment). Adult pads may be used on victims over 8 years old.
- Analyze the heart rhythm. Some machines respond automatically; others require a button to be pushed. Stop CPR. It is critical for no one to touch the victim while the rhythm is being analyzed.
- Charge the AED if so advised by the AED message; some charge automatically.
- Advise everyone to stay clear and then push the shock button if the AED so indicates. Some AED systems have been designed to deliver both adult and child shock doses. You must follow the AED instructions to select the lower (child) shock doses for children ages 1–8.
- If the victim responds, leave the electrodes in place in case of re-arrest. If no response, repeat the analysis and shock sequence.

- Continue efforts until emergency medical services arrive.

Caution is needed with the use of AED equipment in certain situations:

- For children 1 to 8 years of age, be sure to change the child key or switch and use the child pads. If this is not available, you may use the adult pads and dose.
- For infants under the age of 1, there is not enough evidence to recommend for or against the use of an AED.
- The victim must not be in water; drag the victim from the area before using.
- If the victim has an implanted pacemaker or defibrillator, place the electrode at least one inch to the side.
- Remove and wipe dry any area covered with a transdermal patch that interferes with electrode placement.

## Documenting CPR and AED Procedures

If defibrillation or CPR is performed by the provider or an employee within the office, it must be recorded on a chart. If the victim is not a patient, a new chart must be established and the incident recorded. As soon as care is provided, a doctor–patient relationship is established, and there are legal responsibilities.

## CPR for Children and Infants

CPR procedures for children and infants vary somewhat from those for adults. Children are considered to be from age 1 to puberty or about 12 to 14 years old. Infants are considered to be from newborn discharge from hospital to 1 year old.

If a rescuer is treating a child *found* in cardiac arrest, the rescuer should initially provide five cycles of CPR before attaching an AED. If the collapse is *witnessed*, the AED should be used as soon as it is available. Recall that the AED device should be dose-attenuated for children under the age of 8, and there is no recommendation for infants at this time.

With infants and children, the prime concern is usually respiratory because arrest from asphyxia is more common than cardiac arrest. Opening the airway might need to be attempted a couple of times before ventilation is successful. A single rescuer in this situation is advised first to give appropriate CPR for five cycles and then to break to summon the EMS system. The provision of CPR first is indicated because arrest from asphyxia is more common than cardiac arrest in children, and the child is much more likely to benefit from initial CPR.

CPR for children and infants also must be taught and the student evaluated for competence by an approved instructor. Providing CPR for infants uses a slightly different technique than for children. A few of the differences are mentioned here:

- When assessing the infant's consciousness, flick the bottom of the foot.
- Using a resuscitation mouthpiece, cover the infant's mouth and nose.
- Observe the infant's chest for evidence of effective breaths.
- Use the brachial artery in the arm to check for a return of the pulse (Figure 55–4).

## CPR Safety

It is realistic to believe that any emergency situation involves exposure to certain body fluids and has the potential for disease transmission. These can be minimized by using a face shield or face mask barrier device. They might provide a degree of protection. Masks without one-way valves, including the S-shaped devices, offer little if any protection and should not be considered for routine use. Obviously, **intubation** and bag compression by trained medical emergency personnel is more effective and highly desirable because it does not require personal contact.

The perceived risk of disease transmission during CPR has reduced the willingness of laypersons to provide mouth-to-mouth in unknown cardiac arrest victims. If a lone rescuer refuses to initiate mouth-to-mouth ventilation, he should at least access the EMS system, open the airway, and perform chest compressions until a rescuer

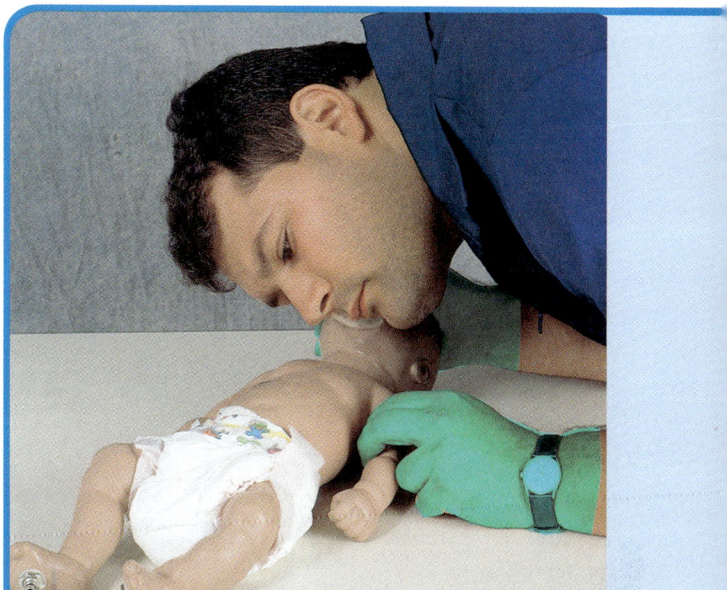

**Figure 55–4:** Check for a pulse in the brachial artery while observing for breaths. *Delmar/Cengage Learning.*

arrives who is willing to provide ventilation or until EMT or paramedics can use the necessary barrier devices.

The probability that a rescuer will become infected with HBV or HIV as a result of performing CPR is minimal. Although some incidents have been documented from blood exchange or penetration of the skin, infection during mouth-to-mouth has not been documented. HBV-positive saliva has not been shown to be infectious even to oral mucous membranes. Saliva has not been implicated in the transmission of HIV even after bites, percutaneous inoculation, or contamination of cuts and open wounds with HIV-infected saliva. The theoretical risk of infection is greater for salivary transmission of herpes simplex and airborne diseases such as tuberculosis and other respiratory infections. Rare instances of herpes simplex transmission during CPR have been reported. Rescuers with impaired immune systems might be particularly at risk of acquiring tuberculosis and should be tested initially and about 12 weeks after a known exposure. Performance of mouth-to-mouth when blood is apt to be exchanged, such as in trauma cases, does pose a theoretical risk of HBV or HIV transmission.

Public safety and health care personnel should follow the guidelines established by the CDC and OSHA. These involve the use of latex or vinyl gloves and mechanical ventilation equipment. Rescuers who themselves are ill should not perform the procedures if other methods of ventilation are available.

## COMMON EMERGENCIES IN THE MEDICAL OFFICE

Several terms describe the severity and length of time for onset of disease or illness. Some of the more common terms are:

- **Chronic**—long, drawn out, not acute. Some diseases have a slow chronic phase but can quickly change into an acute episode.
- **Subtle**—hidden, not apparent, treacherous. Often, disease conditions have a slow, hidden beginning and then quickly develop symptoms.
- **Urgent**—a situation requiring intervention as soon as can be arranged. This term may be applied to the need for care when experiencing a blocked ureter by a kidney stone.
- **Sudden**—occurring quickly and without warning. Onset of headaches or allergies can be sudden.
- **Acute**—having a rapid onset, severe symptoms, and short course. Heart attacks are an example of acute illnesses.
- **Severe**—extensive, advanced. When injuries are severe, it usually implies multiple sites and requires considerable medical attention. The term is also applied to an illness that requires aggressive action and is potentially irreversible.
- **Life threatening**—can cause death. Extensive trauma and massive circulatory or respiratory involvement that might be beyond medical intervention are deemed life threatening.

Almost any injury or illness could be manifest in most of the preceding classifications. Consider a cut that is bleeding: It could be oozing, a slow flow, a pulsating flow, or a hemorrhage that is life threatening. The following conditions are examples of disorders, diseases, or situations that can present emergency events if in an acute phase.

### Hyperglycemia and Hypoglycemia

Diabetic patients can present emergency situations by going into **diabetic ketoacidosis,** which can lead to diabetic **coma,** death, or **insulin shock** (Table 55–3). Diabetic ketoacidosis is caused by an increased amount of sugar in the blood that can occur if **hyperglycemia** is not treated. This can be caused by consuming excess carbohydrates, an infection, fever, emotional stress, or failing to take adequate insulin. The patient might complain of confusion, dizziness, weakness, or nausea. Vomiting is possible. Respiration might be rapid and deep. The skin might be dry and **flushed**. The patient's breath has a sweet or fruity odor, which might be evident some distance away. The patient can lapse into unconsciousness and die if not treated quickly. The patient should be transported to the nearest hospital for positive diagnosis and reduction of blood sugar.

Insulin shock or **hypoglycemia** can occur from an excess amount of insulin in the body. This can happen if food is not eaten regularly in measured amounts, if the patient vomits after taking insulin, after engaging in excessive exercise, or if too much insulin is taken. The patient might have muscle weakness, anxiety, mental confusion, a pounding heartbeat, hunger, and **diaphoresis**. The skin will be cold, pale, and moist. The patient might lapse into unconsciousness and have seizures. He or she should be given some form of sugar. Sweetened orange juice, sublingual sugar, or tubes of glucose are often used. The sugar should end the shock; if not, the patient must be transported at once to a hospital.

You must be alert to the possibility of diabetic ketoacidosis or insulin shock in a diabetic patient with these symptoms. If the patient can talk, ask if insulin or food has been taken. This will give you a better idea of the need for treatment of diabetic ketoacidosis or insulin shock. If the condition cannot be determined, the provider might suggest giving the patient a little sugar because insulin shock can cause irreversible brain damage. Recent studies indicate that a very small amount of sugar placed under the tongue of an unconscious person will be absorbed rapidly into the bloodstream and return the patient to consciousness.

**TABLE 55–3 Causes, Symptoms and First Aid of Diabetic Ketoacidosis and Insulin Shock**

| | Diabetic Ketoacidosis (DKA) | Insulin Shock |
|---|---|---|
| *Causes* | Too little insulin | Too much insulin |
| | Illness | Too little food or delayed meal |
| | Stress | Too much exercise |
| | | Alcohol consumption on empty stomach |
| *Symptoms* | Thirst or very dry mouth | Moist and pale, diaphoresis |
| | Frequent urination | Nervous, anxious, irritable |
| | Dry or flushed skin | Shaky |
| | Nausea, vomiting, or abdominal pain | Lightheaded |
| | Fruity odor on breath | Hungry |
| | Feeling constantly tired | Fast heartbeat, palpitations |
| | Difficult time breathing | Blurred vision |
| | Confusion or difficulty paying attention | Headache |
| | High blood glucose levels | Confusion |
| | High levels of ketones in the urine | Seizures |
| *First aid* | Keep patient warm | If conscious, give patient food or drink containing 15–20 grams of carbohydrate (sugar, honey, corn syrup, candy, orange juice, soft drink, or glucose tablets) |
| | Obtain medical help immediately | If unconscious, obtain medical help immediately |

## Fainting

The medical term for fainting is **syncope**, explained as a brief episode of unconsciousness. Fainting itself is not a disease but rather a symptom of an underlying condition or disease. A patient who feels faint should lower his or her head between the legs or lie down with his or her feet elevated to improve the blood circulation to the brain (Figure 55–5). The patient who is about to faint might be pale; perspiring; have cold, clammy skin; and complain of dizziness or nausea. An emesis basin should be handy in case the patient vomits. Each examination room should be supplied with aromatic spirits of ammonia capsules, which can be easily broken and used to arouse the patient. These should not be held directly under the nose but passed back and forth about six inches under the nose. The patient should be kept in a reclining position until fully recovered and then be gradually allowed to sit up. The patient should regain consciousness within a minute or two from a simple fainting episode; any time longer than that might require EMS activation. The provider should be alerted to examine the patient, and vital signs must be monitored to determine whether they are stabilized before allowing the patient to leave your facility. Realize that in this situation, the patient might need emotional support and reassurance.

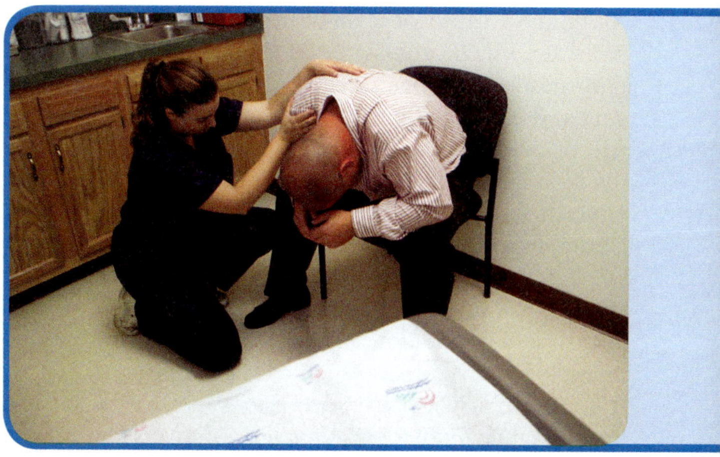

**Figure 55–5:** Assist the patient to lower the head between the legs when feeling faint. *Delmar/Cengage Learning.*

## Heart Attack

Patients might arrive at the office complaining of severe chest pain or pressure. It is extremely important for the provider to be alerted immediately to rule out whether the patient is suffering from a heart attack, otherwise known as a **myocardial infarction**, the leading cause of death for both men and women. The patient might also complain of pain radiating down one or both arms and a tightness of the chest or pain radiating into the left shoulder and jaw (mandible). The pulse is usually rapid and weak. The patient might be perspiring profusely; have cyanotic lips and fingernails; and be nauseated, anxious, and agitated and might be in denial that anything serious is occurring.

These classic symptoms were identified primarily from observation of adult males who were the subjects of research studies. However, findings now indicate that heart disease is also very prominent among women. In fact, statistics indicate that heart disease kills more women than all forms of cancer combined. In recent studies, it has been noted that women can experience symptoms somewhat differently than men. Because of this, women might not recognize they are having a coronary event and do not seek medical attention. In fact, more than 60 percent of women who suffered sudden cardiac death had no known symptoms of heart disease.

Women do experience chest pain and pressure, but they are more likely to have other symptoms as well, such as:

- Shortness of breath
- Burning sensation in the chest (often dismissed as heartburn)
- Nausea and vomiting and other flulike symptoms
- Unexplained fatigue or weakness
- Pain in the jaw, neck, shoulder, back, or ear
- Overwhelming sense of doom

A common cause of a myocardial infarction is atherosclerosis, which causes a buildup of plaque in the coronary arteries. This plaque can break away from the artery wall and cause a clot to form, which can create a blockage of one or more of the coronary arteries, restricting the blood flow to the heart and causing the heart to stop. Other heart conditions such as various arrhythmias and cardiomyopathy can also be the cause.

The first intervention is to help the patient into a sitting position and elevate his or her feet if possible. You should never allow a patient with cardiac symptoms to walk or carry objects such as a heavy purse or coat. If you have a wheelchair, use it to transport the patient to an examination room. Chapter 40 covers the procedures for safely assisting a patient from a wheelchair to an exam table and vice versa. Most cardiac patients prefer to have their head elevated, so once seated, adjust the table as needed.

The provider might want you to administer oxygen or prepare an injection for the patient. Always have the crash cart with IV equipment and emergency medications ready for the provider. If the patient has previously been diagnosed with angina and has a medication such as nitroglycerine, it should be given immediately. Many providers also recommend taking one regular-size aspirin to help dissolve any blood clot that might be present.

If oxygen administration is ordered to assist the patient to breathe more easily, a nasal cannula connected by tubing to a portable oxygen tank will be used. The tank valve is opened and the flow meter set at the amount prescribed by the provider, usually 3 to 4 liters. Feel the area adjacent to the nasal tips to ensure that oxygen is flowing. The woman in Figure 55–6 A is receiving oxygen through a nasal cannula fitted over her face with a nasal tip in each nostril. The cannula is then draped behind each ear and brought forward under the chin. An adjustable slide on the cannula can be moved toward the chin to maintain its position. Figure 55–6 B shows the tips of the cannula, which must be inserted into the nostrils. Monitor the patient's level of anxiety and effects of the oxygen. Be sure to document the use of oxygen on the patient's chart, indicating the method, amount of

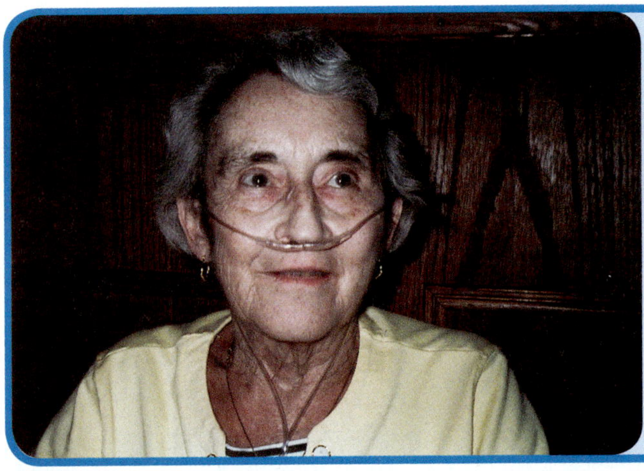

**Figure 55–6 A:** Administer oxygen by nasal cannula.
*Delmar/Cengage Learning.*

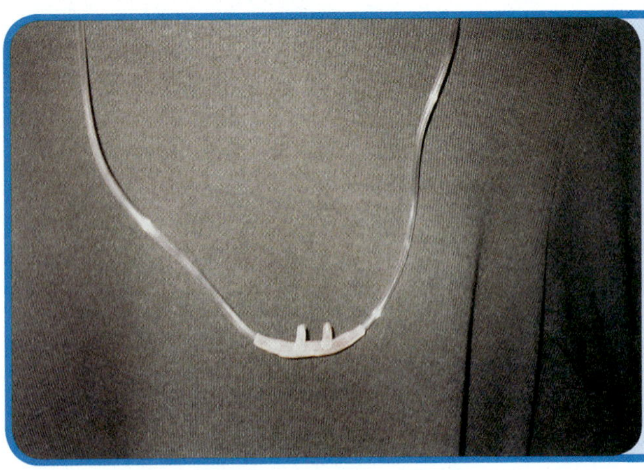

**Figure 55–6 B:** Tips of the nasal cannula.
*Delmar/Cengage Learning.*

flow, time begun, and patient's response. The provider might also order an electrocardiogram to be done immediately. Refer to Chapter 47 for the procedure of obtaining an ECG if you need to be refreshed. The emergency medical service should be summoned per the provider's request. If the provider is out of the office, summon EMS immediately on your own so the victim can be stabilized and transported to the hospital as quickly as possible. If the patient stops breathing, start rescue breathing and, if there is no pulse, start chest compressions (CPR). Time is critical in the event of a myocardial infarction. Prompt, appropriate treatment within the first hour of an attack can save lives and reduce damage.

## Heat Exposure

The patient who is exposed to high temperatures for a long period in industry or at home can suffer from **heat cramps**. These patients might have diaphoresis (excessive sweating) and should drink large amounts of water because they lose a large amount of body salt. The patient will complain of severe muscle cramps of the abdomen, arms, and legs and might also complain of faintness, dizziness, and exhaustion. First aid to replace salt is provided by giving the patient a balanced electrolyte drink such as Gatorade. The patient should lie down in a cool place. If muscle spasms are severe, IV normal saline may be given. It is important to differentiate between **heatstroke** and **heat exhaustion**.

In heat exhaustion, the skin is pale, cool, and moist and the body temperature is normal. The patient becomes overheated with profuse perspiration, usually after some form of vigorous exercise. He or she might have headaches, muscle cramps, nausea, dizziness, and fatigue. The pulse is weak and rapid, and the respirations are quiet and shallow. The patient should stop all activity, move to a cooler place, and consume cool water or sports drink. If the patient's signs and symptoms worsen or don't resolve within an hour, medical care should be sought. If the body temperature reaches 40°C/104°F, immediate medical treatment is necessary because heatstroke is probably occurring.

Heatstroke is the most severe of the heat-related problems. The patient suffering from heatstroke will have a red, dry face. The skin will be hot and dry, and the body temperature can be above 40°C/104°F. The pulse will be rapid and then gradually slow and weaken. Respirations will be rapid and hollow. The pupils of the eyes will be dilated but equal. Headache, shortness of breath, nausea or vomiting, dizziness, weakness, and dry mouth are common symptoms. Treatment is to get the individual out of the heat immediately and cool the body with cool water or wet cloths. Have the patient drink cool water or other nonalcoholic, caffeine-free beverages. EMS should be activated because this is a potentially life-threatening condition.

## Cold Exposure

**Hypothermia** occurs when your body loses heat faster than it can produce it, resulting in a dangerously low body temperature. This occurs when the body temperature drops lower than 35°C/95°F. If left untreated, respiratory and heart failure can occur and eventually lead to death. Exposure to cold weather and submersion in cold water are the usual causes of hypothermia. Common signs and symptoms include shivering, slurred speech or mumbling, confusion, weak pulse, and shallow breathing. Treatment includes bringing the patient's temperature back up to normal by bringing him or her inside, removing any wet clothing, and covering him or her with layers of blankets. EMS should be activated because this can be a life-threatening condition.

Exposure to freezing temperatures will often result in **frostbite**. The body parts most often damaged by cold are the hands, feet, ears, and nose. Symptoms that might indicate damaged tissue are a tingling sensation with numbness followed by pain and redness of the skin. If exposure is continued, the patient might complain of burning and itching. Sensation might be completely lost. The skin can be white or grayish-yellow and waxy in appearance. Severe frostbite can cause blistering and hardening of the skin. The first aid required is to warm the affected part slowly by placing it in water with a temperature of 40°C/104° to 41.7°C/107°F. This helps reduce tissue damage. Never rub frostbite; you will cause tissue damage. Hot tea or coffee will act as a stimulus and dilate blood vessels to increase circulation. The patient should *not* be allowed to smoke because of the constriction effect on the blood vessels. After warming, wrap the area loosely with sterile dressing. If feet are frostbitten, the patient must avoid the pressure of standing or walking because this causes additional damage to the tissue. If the skin turns red and has a tingling sensation as it warms, circulation is returning. If the skin remains numb or blisters, seek medical care.

## Hemorrhage

It is important to understand the different sources of bleeding and determine the seriousness of the hemorrhage. Bleeding can be of three types: arterial, venous, and capillary. The term *hemorrhage* refers to excessive, uncontrolled bleeding. Arterial bleeding produces bright red blood in spurts. If the ruptured artery is a large branch, death can occur in three minutes or less. Bleeding from a vein produces a steady flow of dark red blood. It is important to control bleeding quickly. This is best accomplished by covering the wound with a clean cloth or pad of gauze squares, if available, and exerting pressure directly on the bleeding area (Figure 55–7). The area might also require elevation to stop the bleeding. Sometimes, especially with arterial bleeding, this is not

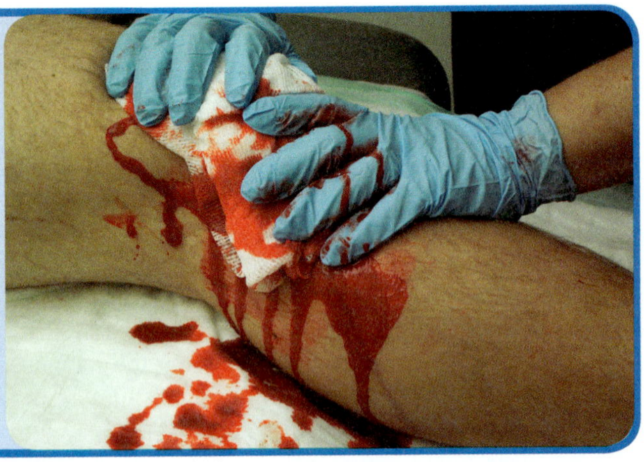

**Figure 55–7:** Applying direct pressure. *Delmar/Cengage Learning.*

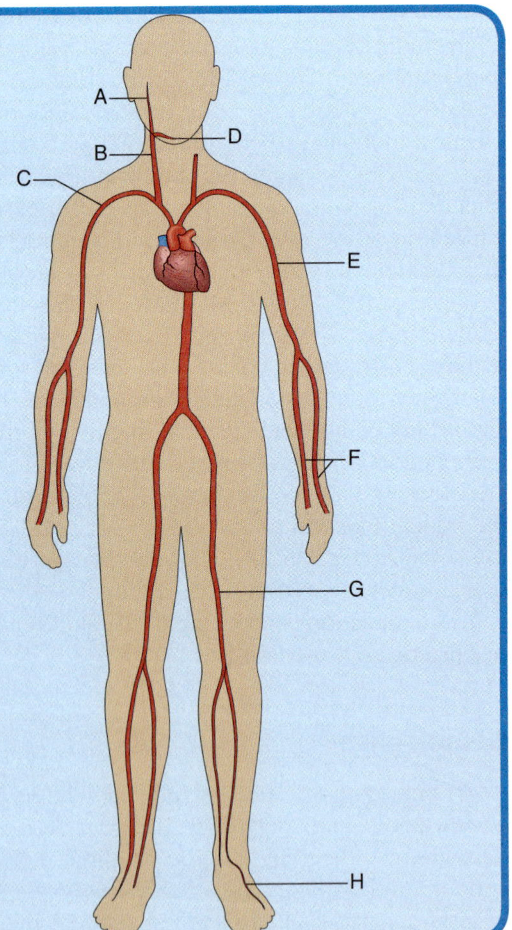


**Figure 55–8:** Pressure points. *Delmar/Cengage Learning.*

sufficient, and pressure must be exerted at the pressure point proximal to the wound to stop the flow of blood to the area (Figure 55–8). Any bleeding from capillary damage produces a steady ooze from the wound area. This type of bleeding often clots without first aid measures.

Internal bleeding causes symptoms similar to those of shock. The patient can have a rapid, weak pulse; shallow breathing; cold, clammy skin; dilated pupils; dizziness; faintness; thirst; restlessness; and a feeling of anxiety. Internal hemorrhage might need to be controlled by surgery. The patient must be kept in a recumbent position with strictly limited movement until the surgery can be performed.

Internal bleeding can be difficult to detect unless it produces symptoms or external signs. For example, the patient who coughs up bright red blood might have a lung hemorrhage, or vomiting bright red blood might indicate an ulcer has started bleeding. If the patient is vomiting what looks like coffee grounds, it could indicate chronic slow bleeding of the stomach. If the patient notices coal-black stools, a loss of blood in the intestines is probable and, if the patient has bright red rectal bleeding, it is likely to be from a lesion in the rectum or lower colon. A patient with severe abdominal pain from trauma might have internal bleeding from a ruptured organ such as a kidney, liver, or spleen. Internal bleeding that causes symptoms of shock and produces pain probably requires surgical intervention to correct. Slow bleeding, when the cause has been determined, can be treated with medication and, if intestinal, by altering the diet to allow the area to heal. In addition, a hemorrhage that occurs with the rupture of various types of aneurysms is discussed in Chapter 30.

Epistaxis (nosebleed) can be the result of excessively dry air over a prolonged period, hypertension, injury, or simply blowing the nose too hard (see Chapter 25). First aid for epistaxis is to elevate the head and pinch the nostrils closed for at least six minutes. Keep the patient in a sitting position with the head tilted forward so that the blood will not trickle down the throat unseen. The use of a cold compress over the nasal area or on the back of the neck can be helpful. A piece of gauze can be placed between the lips and gums with pressure against this area for several minutes. Specially treated gauze is best for nasal packing because it is less difficult to remove. A provider should be consulted if bleeding is not easily controlled. Sometimes, the addition of humidity to the air will relieve the patient who has recurrent epistaxis.

Another common bleeding condition that can present to the office is that of a pregnant patient experiencing vaginal bleeding. It is necessary to determine the kind of flow. If bleeding is heavy, the patient should lie down immediately with feet elevated, and emergency medical services should be called. If there has been a discharge of clots or tissue substance, this should be collected and sent along with the patient to the hospital for possible analysis. Your employer will let you know the protocol on how to handle these types of emergencies.

## Poisoning

Poison can be **ingested**, absorbed, inhaled, injected, or acquired from bites and stings. Poisoning can occur from a medication overdose. It can be accidental or intentional. If someone calls regarding a possible ingestion of **poison**, always obtain the patient's name, age, sex, and weight and ask what was taken, how much was taken, and the time it was taken. Learn the location and the telephone number of the local poison control center, which is staffed with registered nurses, pharmacists, and providers 24 hours a day, seven days a week, so that you can direct callers to the best source of help. The poison control center will determine what the treatment should be.

Children are often the victims of ingested poisonings. They will swallow pills, detergent, household cleaners, painting supplies, and drain cleaners and eat plants. Usually, the evidence is nearby, such as opened pill bottles, pills on the floor or loose in a purse, spilled liquids on clothing and the floor, opened containers, and pieces of plant material. If the poisoning is not discovered quickly, symptoms such as nausea, stomach cramps, shallow breathing, drowsiness, skin color change, and even unconsciousness can occur. Remember, the poison control center is your prime source of information. Follow its instructions to provide the appropriate care. If the provider or treatment center advises examining the patient, instruct the caller to bring in the material ingested and a sample of anything vomited, if possible, so an analysis can be made to verify what was swallowed.

Poisoning by inhalation can be caused by cleaning fluids and sprays used in a poorly ventilated area. Carbon monoxide poisoning can be caused by a faulty exhaust system in an automobile or home heating system. Poisoning by injection is usually the result of drug abuse. The patient might exhibit symptoms ranging from confusion to excitement to hallucinations to convulsions. These poisonings usually require the EMS system to be activated.

## Seizures (Convulsions)

A **seizure** is a severe, involuntary contraction of muscles that first causes the patient to become rigid and then to have uncontrollable movements. Seizures can occur when the patient has high body temperature, head injuries, brain disease, or a brain disorder such as epilepsy. The patient becomes unconscious and can be injured during the seizure. The face and lips can become cyanotic, and the patient might stop breathing. He or she might also lose bladder and bowel control and bite the tongue. When the seizure has stopped, the patient might be confused and complain of headache and **exhaustion**.

During the convulsive phase, your main goal is to prevent injury to the patient. If the patient is in the upright position when the seizure occurs, ease him or her to the floor. Do not restrain movement and move any objects out of the way that might cause injury. Do not force any object between the patient's teeth, or it could cause vomiting, **aspiration**, or spasm of the larynx. If mucus or saliva is present, turn the head to the side to prevent choking. If the victim is not breathing, open the airway with the head-tilt or jaw-thrust maneuver. Allow the patient to rest or sleep after the seizure is over. Document the length of the seizure and any other pertinent information. Provide emotional support as the patient regains composure because this situation can cause the person to feel embarrassed. If the seizure is due to the condition of status epilepticus (continuous seizure), EMS must be activated because this is a life-threatening condition. Administration of oxygen and antiseizure medication might be necessary; therefore, alert the provider immediately.

## Obstructed Airway

One of the most common medical emergencies is an **obstructed** airway. The most usual cause in adults is food aspirated while eating. This occurs when partially chewed food is sucked into the trachea when talking, laughing, or coughing while eating. Children, on the other hand, can get toys, toy parts, buttons, candy, or a variety of other objects caught in their throat and obstruct their airway. Pieces of food are also a problem for children; the most dangerous food is the hot dog, because if fed in a small sliced portion, it's just the right shape to cause choking.

**CLINICAL PEARL**

Most people are familiar with the dangers of plastic wrapping and bags because of all the warning labels, but one of the most common airway obstructers is the latex balloon. Safety authorities believe no young child should have a balloon unless it is made of Mylar. Children ages 4 to 8 require supervision if playing with or trying to inflate latex balloons.

The obstruction, if complete, must be cleared away immediately because brain damage can result in about four minutes from lack of oxygen. A person who is choking usually places his or her hand at the throat, which is the universal distress signal (Figure 55–9). This is called conscious choking. The individual might not be able to cough or speak and will simply fall from the chair if

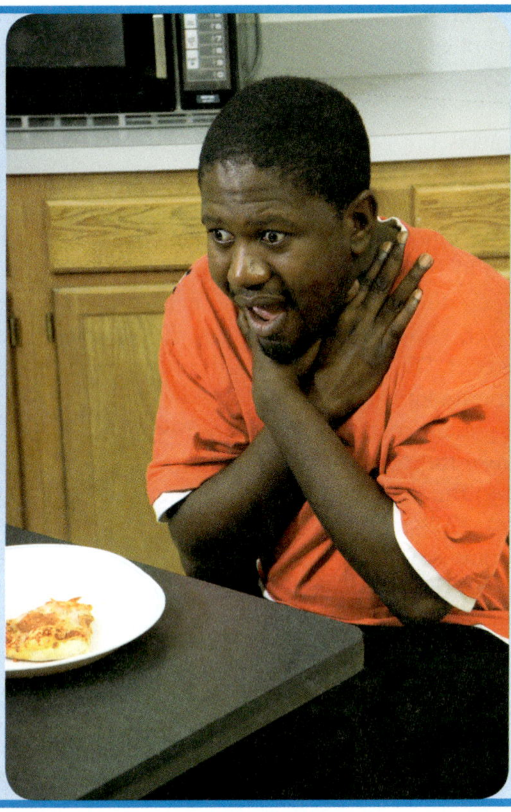

**Figure 55–9:** Universal distress signal. *Delmar/Cengage Learning.*

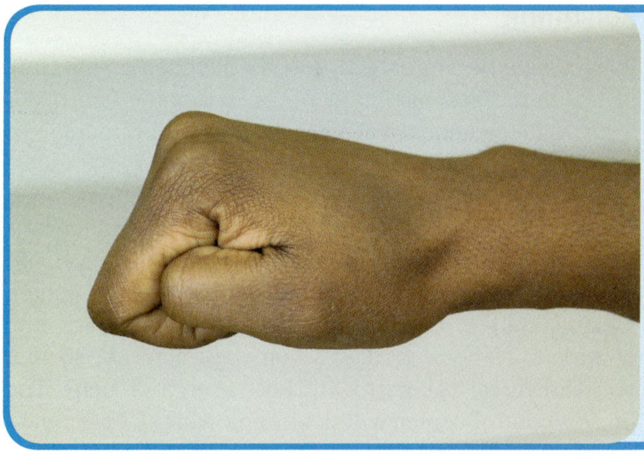

**Figure 55–10 A:** Fist with thumb flexed. *Delmar/Cengage Learning.*

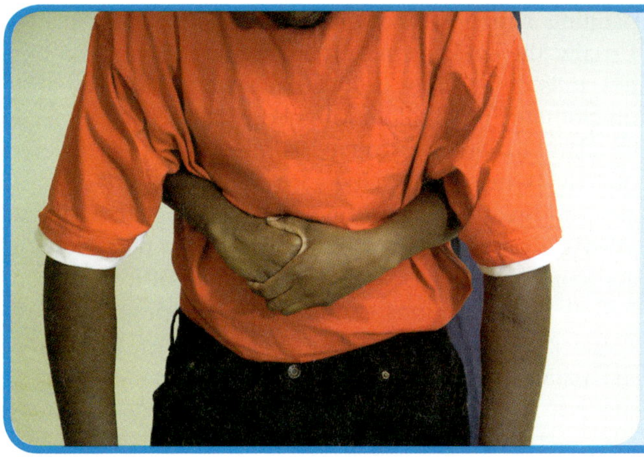

**Figure 55–10 B:** Hand placement for abdominal thrust. *Delmar/Cengage Learning.*

nothing is done. You should always ask the patient, "Are you choking?" and watch for a response such as the universal distress signal before attempting any intervention.

Chest thrusts, back blows or slaps, or abdominal thrusts are effective for relieving an obstructed airway in conscious adults and children older than 1 year of age, although injuries have been reported with the abdominal thrust. There is insufficient evidence to determine which should be used first. These techniques should be applied in rapid sequence until the obstruction is relieved; more than one technique might be needed. Unconscious victims should receive CPR. The finger sweep should be used in the unconscious patient with an obstructed airway only if solid material is visible in the airway. There is insufficient evidence for a treatment recommendation for an obese or pregnant patient with an obstructed airway. For the abdominal thrust method, while standing behind the victim, reach around the waist. Clench one hand to make a fist, and grasp your fist with the other hand. Place the thumb side of the fist against the midline of the victim's abdomen between the waist and the rib cage (Figure 55–10 A and B). Thrust your fist inward and upward in quick, firm movements to move air out of the lungs with enough force to dislodge the obstruction.

A choking victim who is alone can use the abdominal thrust with his or her own fist or thrust against a chair back or any hard object of appropriate height (Figure 55–11).

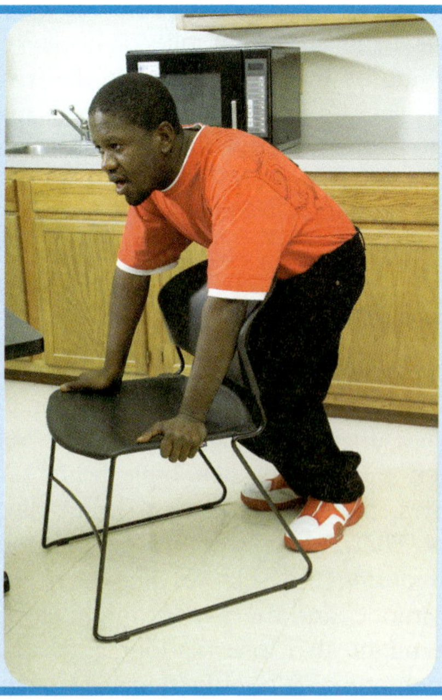

**Figure 55–11:** Self-administered abdominal thrust. *Delmar/Cengage Learning.*

If a patient is in an advanced stage of pregnancy or is very obese, abdominal thrusting is not possible. A chest thrust can be used to dislodge the material. If the patient is standing, from the back, place your arms around the victim directly under the axillae. Using the abdominal clenched-fist technique, place your thumb over the sternum; place your other hand over the fist, and give firm thrusts, pulling straight back toward yourself.

If the thrusts have dislodged the obstruction but have not expelled it from the victim's mouth, then a finger sweep is performed. Open the victim's mouth by tilting the head back with one hand and moving the jaw forward to lift the tongue away from the back of the throat. Insert an index finger along the inside of the cheek and sweep deeply into the mouth in a hooking action. Be careful not to push an obstruction deeper into the throat. If it is possible to dislodge an obstruction, be sure to remove it from the mouth. If dentures are worn, it is helpful to remove them. If the patient has vomited, it is extremely important to turn the patient on his or her side to keep an open airway and prevent aspiration of material into the lungs.

**CLINICAL PEARL**

**Important**

- *Do not* try to remove an object that is stuck in the victim's throat; you might push it farther into the airway. Only if it is lying within the mouth should it be removed.
- If the heart stops, *do not* begin CPR chest compressions until the airway is open.

Follow the steps in Procedure 55–1 to perform an abdominal thrust on an adult victim with an obstructed airway. The procedure is written for an office setting, but obstructed airway incidents usually occur in restaurants, at parties, and other places where food is being eaten.

## PROCEDURE 55–1 Perform an Abdominal Thrust on an Adult Victim with an Obstructed Airway

**MEDIA LINK**: View the video, "Abdominal Thrusts," for this chapter on the Premium Website.

**PURPOSE:** To dislodge an object obstructing the airway and restore breathing

**EQUIPMENT:** Disposable gloves and resuscitation mouthpiece

**SKILL:** Perform an abdominal thrust on a adult victim with an obstructed airway.

| Procedure Steps | Detailed Instructions and/or *Rationales* |
|---|---|
| 1. Observe the victim using the universal distress signal. | |
| 2. Ask, "Are you choking?" If yes, ask, "Can you speak?" | A weak cough, a wheezing breath sound, and inability to speak are signs of obstruction. |
| 3. Get into position behind the victim. | *The victim can become worse and go into unconsciousness at any time; this position allows you to perform the maneuver as well as lower the patient to the floor.* |
| 4. Extend your arms around the victim's abdomen and locate his or her umbilicus with the index finger of one hand. With the other hand, make a fist with your thumb bent outward. Place the thumb against the abdomen just above the umbilicus. | |
| 5. Place your other hand over the fist. | |
| 6. Keep your thrusts in the soft high abdominal area to avoid injury to the rib cage and sternum. Give an abdominal thrust by forcefully pulling up and back quickly. | *Force pushes the abdominal organs up against the diaphragm to force out air and the obstruction. Note*: If the patient is pregnant or obese, perform chest thrusts instead of abdominal thrusts. |

*(continues)*

*(continued)*

| Procedure Steps | Detailed Instructions and/or *Rationales* |
|---|---|
| 7. If this is unsuccessful, repeat thrusts until the obstruction is expelled or the victim loses consciousness. | |
| 8. If the victim becomes unresponsive and falls to the floor, position him or her on his or her back and activate the emergency response system by calling 911, open the airway, remove the object if you see it, and begin CPR. | *The victim can go into respiratory and cardiac arrest if the obstruction remains.* |
| 9. Every time you open the airway to give breaths, open the victim's mouth wide and look for the object. If you see it, remove it; if not, continue CPR. | |
| 10. After the victim has resumed breathing and the heart is beating or EMS services have taken over the rescue, remove your gloves and the mouthpiece and dispose of them in the biohazard waste container. | |
| 11. Document the procedure. | |

### Charting Example

| | |
|---|---|
| 6/24/XX<br>1:25 PM | Pt. sitting in reception room began choking on piece of candy. Complete airway obstruction. Notified Dr. Green, EMS called. Given multiple abdominal thrusts; candy was expelled. Breathing and heart rate restored. Patient evaluated by Dr. Green to ensure that no complications resulted from abdominal thrusts.<br>G. Jenks, CMA(AAMA) |

## Special Considerations for Infants

An infant or toddler experiencing a blocked airway will have difficulty breathing, coughing, and crying and might display cyanosis. The recommended AHA and Red Cross course of action is:

1. Place the baby face-down on your forearm, which is extended on your thigh (Figure 55–12). You might also kneel or sit with the infant on your lap to do this.
2. The head should be lower than the body and supported by your hand.
3. With the heel of your other hand, deliver five backslaps, forcefully, in the middle of the back between the infant's shoulder blades.
4. If this is unsuccessful, turn the infant face up; support the head and neck. Keep the head lower than the trunk.
5. Place two fingers on the midsternal area just below the nipple line.
6. Give five quick downward chest thrusts; deliver chest thrusts at a rate of about one per second (Figure 55–13).
7. Continue with five back blows and five chest thrusts until the object is dislodged or the infant becomes unconscious.
8. If unsuccessful, call out for help to notify EMS.
9. If no help arrives, give the infant CPR for one minute and then call 911 yourself.
10. Continue CPR until assistance arrives.

Some additional information:

- Even if the procedure is successful and infant seems fine, check with the provider for further instructions.
- If you can *see* the object, try to remove it with your finger.
- *Do not* try to grasp the object and pull it out if the infant is conscious.
- *Do not* perform the procedure on an infant who stops breathing for other reasons, such as asthma, swelling in the throat, head injury, or an infectious process.

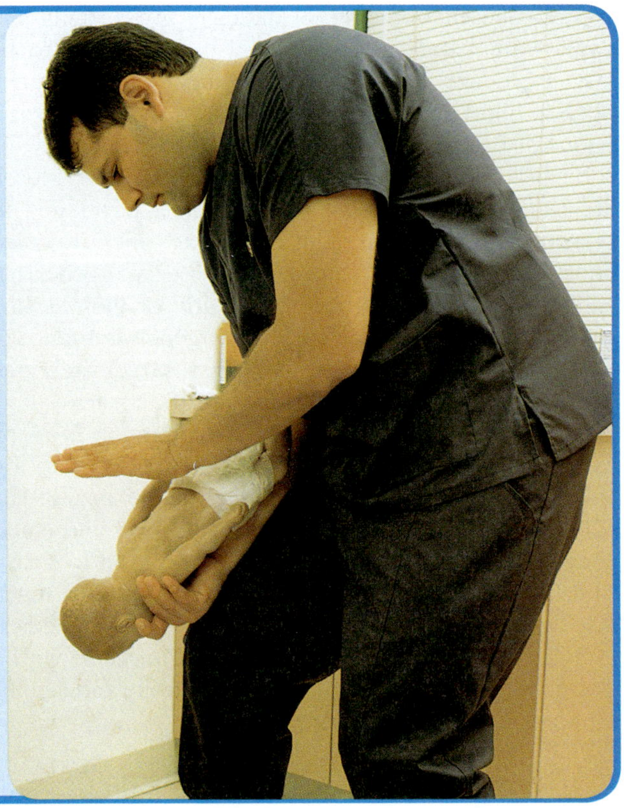

**Figure 55–12:** Back blows on an infant. *Delmar/Cengage Learning.*

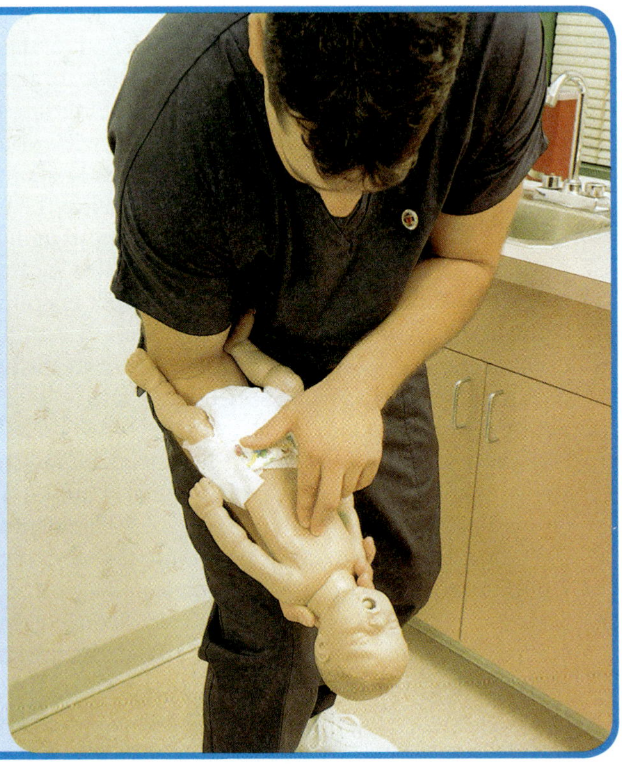

**Figure 55–13:** Infant chest thrusts. *Delmar/Cengage Learning.*

## Accidental, Allergic, and Drug-Induced Distress

Respiratory problems can also arise from other conditions such as:

- A patient suffering from severe edema of the vocal cords as a result of an allergic reaction to food or stings of bees or wasps must be hospitalized as quickly as possible.
- The victim of a drowning must receive rescue breathing immediately. This can be given before the patient is taken from the water if there is help to support the patient while resuscitation is given. A person surviving drowning needs to be hospitalized for follow-up observation.
- Poisoning by toxic gases, such as carbon monoxide, or suffocation can also require immediate rescue breathing.
- A person having an asthma attack might have great difficulty breathing. The provider must determine the treatment needed, but you can be helpful by attempting to calm the patient. Emotional upset often starts an asthma attack.
- Some medications can cause a slowing or **cessation** of breathing.
- Electric shock can cause respiratory paralysis. The victim must be moved away from the source of the electricity by indirect means (never touch the victim) and then be given rescue breathing and CPR if necessary.

## Shock

Shock can be associated with many kinds of injuries and is a serious depressor of vital body functions. Symptoms include a rapid, thready, weak pulse; shallow, rapid respirations; dilated pupils; ashen color; and cool, clammy skin. All of these result from decreased blood volume because of diminished cardiac output causing a drop in blood pressure. It is possible for shock to cause death even when the injury causing the shock is not life threatening. First aid measures include placing the patient in a recumbent position with feet elevated unless there is a head injury, in which case the patient is kept flat. If the patient has difficulty breathing or has a chest injury, the head and shoulders should be elevated. It is best to place a blanket under and over the patient to maintain body warmth but not to overheat.

Shock can be caused by various circumstances. It can be associated with a heart attack or respiratory collapse. It frequently follows trauma or physical injury. Extensive burns, electrical shock, hemorrhage, near drowning, and severe infection can all result in shock. Another type, an anaphylactic shock, is an acute allergic reaction to a foreign substance, which can include certain foods, beestings, or injections of therapeutic or **prophylactic** substances. The patient might have dyspnea, cyanosis, and seizures. Epinephrine and oxygen should be immediately available for use by the provider or by the medical assistant under the direction of the provider. No patient should be given an allergy injection and then be allowed to leave the office immediately because anaphylactic shock can result from these injections. Patients can also have severe reactions to penicillin, aspirin, serums, vaccines, local anesthetics, salicylates, and X-ray contrast media.

### Stroke

The common term for a cerebrovascular accident (CVA) is stroke. A CVA is the result of a ruptured blood vessel in the brain or an occlusion of a blood vessel. The patient might have a light stroke with very little damage or a more extensive one with immediate paralysis in the form of sagging muscles on one side of the face or the inability to use an arm or leg. One entire side of the body might be paralyzed. The patient might complain of numbness. The pupils of the eyes might be unequal in size. The patient might have mental confusion, slurred speech, nausea, vomiting, or difficulty in breathing and swallowing. Control of urine and bowels can also be lost. Avoid any unnecessary movement of the patient. Keep in mind that the patient who appears to be unconscious or is unable to speak might be able to hear what is being said. If a patient is experiencing a CVA, loosen the clothing and be sure the patient is positioned to prevent choking on excess saliva. Strokes are now called brain attacks and are considered to be emergency situations. The patient who exhibits any of the warning signs of stroke needs immediate emergency assistance to ensure optimal recovery. Remember, approximately one third of patients with a major stroke die as a result of the condition. Quick, appropriate intervention in many cases limits damage caused by blood vessel occlusion and helps restore patients to the prior state of health. The AHA has adapted a series of actions for EMS and emergency personnel to take to evaluate and react to stroke similar to those for cardiac response. It involves initial field evaluation criteria, rapid transportation, medical evaluation, CT scan interpretation, and injection with a clot-dissolving drug if it is an ischemic stroke and actions for acute hemorrhage if not.

## CHAPTER SUMMARY

- It is critical for medical office personnel to be ready to react to an emergency situation. A medical emergency is any situation in which an individual suddenly becomes ill or has an injury or circumstances calling for decided action.
- As part of your preparation for emergency care, the office should have the necessary supplies and equipment to handle any emergency that might come under your care. These items should be collected and set aside in an emergency kit or crash cart, where they will always be ready for use.
- A universal emergency medical identification symbol was designed by the AMA as a means for individuals with certain medical conditions to alert health care workers of their conditions when they are unable to.
- CPR is a life-saving procedure performed when a person's breathing or heartbeat has stopped. CPR involves two elements: chest compressions and artificial respiration (mouth-to-mouth rescue breathing).
- AED units are used in addition to CPR if the heart is in fibrillation or arrest and permits life-saving intervention without the operator needing to evaluate the situation or interpret an ECG. The AED unit is computerized and can analyze the heart rhythm of a person in fibrillation or arrest; recognize a shockable rhythm; and advise the operator through lights and voice prompts if shock is indicated.
- It is realistic to believe that any emergency situation involves exposure to certain body fluids and has the potential for disease transmission. These can be minimized by using a face shield or face mask barrier device. They can provide a degree of protection.
- Several terms describe the severity and length of time for onset of disease or illness: *chronic*, *subtle*, *urgent*, *sudden*, *acute*, *severe*, *life threatening*. Being familiar with the terms will help you establish what your steps will be for preparing and directing the patient.
- Diabetic ketoacidosis, insulin shock, fainting, heart attack, heat and cold exposures, hemorrhaging, poisoning, seizures, obstructed airway, shock, and stroke are common emergencies you might encounter. Understanding the proper protocol to handle each of these conditions, and being able to distinguish symptoms and characteristics of each, is essential in your role as a medical assistant.
- Hyperglycemia is caused by an increased amount of sugar in the body, whereas hypoglycemia is caused by an excess amount of insulin. Being able to recognize the differences in symptoms will assist you in notifying the provider so proper treatment can be given.
- Severe chest pain or pressure, pain radiating down one or both arms, and a tightness of the chest or pain radiating into the left shoulder and jaw (mandible) might indicate symptoms of a heart attack. The pulse is usually rapid and weak. The patient might be perspiring profusely; have cyanotic lips and fingernails; be nauseated, anxious, and agitated; and in denial that anything serious is occurring.

- In heat exhaustion, symptoms such as cool, pale, moist skin with a normal body temperature occur usually after some form of vigorous exercise. The patient becomes overheated with profuse perspiration and might have headaches, muscle cramps, nausea, dizziness, fatigue with a pulse that is weak and rapid, and respirations that are quiet and shallow.
- Heatstroke symptoms include a red, dry face with hot and dry skin. The body temperature can be above 40°C/104°F, and the pulse will be rapid but then gradually slow and weaken. Respirations will be rapid and hollow. The pupils of the eyes will be dilated but equal. Headache, shortness of breath, nausea or vomiting, dizziness, weakness, and dry mouth are common symptoms.
- Symptoms that might indicate damaged tissue (frostbite) are a tingling sensation with numbness followed by pain and redness of the skin. If exposure is continued, the patient might complain of burning and itching. Sensation can be completely lost. The skin might be white or grayish-yellow and waxy in appearance.
- Arterial bleeding produces bright red blood in spurts. Bleeding from a vein produces a steady flow of dark red blood. Any bleeding from capillary damage produces a steady ooze from the wound area.
- Internal bleeding causes symptoms similar to those of shock. The patient can have a rapid, weak pulse; shallow breathing; cold, clammy skin; dilated pupils; dizziness; faintness; thirst, restlessness; and a feeling of anxiety. External signs can include coughing or vomiting up bright red blood or vomiting what looks like coffee grounds. In addition, coal-black stools, bright red rectal bleeding, and severe abdominal pain are other symptoms.
- A seizure is a severe involuntary contraction of muscles that first causes the patient to become rigid and then to have uncontrollable movements. The patient becomes unconscious and can be injured during the seizure. The face and lips can become cyanotic, and the patient might stop breathing. He or she might also lose bladder and bowel control and bite the tongue. When the seizure has stopped, the patient might be confused and complain of headache and exhaustion.
- Obstructed airway most often occurs in adults when food is aspirated while eating. This occurs when partially chewed food is sucked into the trachea when talking, laughing, or coughing while eating. Children, on the other hand, can get toys, toy parts, buttons, candy, or a variety of other objects, in addition to food, caught in their throat and obstruct their airway.
- Shock symptoms include a rapid, thready, weak pulse; shallow, rapid respirations; dilated pupils; ashen color; and cool, clammy skin.
- Signs of a possible stroke can include immediate paralysis in the form of sagging muscles on one side of the face or the inability to use an arm or leg. One entire side of the body might be paralyzed. The patient might complain of numbness. The pupils of the eyes might be unequal in size, and the patient might present mental confusion, slurred speech, nausea, vomiting, or difficulty in breathing and swallowing. Control of urine and bowels can also be lost.

## STUDY TOOLS

| | |
|---|---|
| **Workbook** | Activities for Chapter 55 |
| **Premium Website** MEDIA LINK StudyWARE | View this **Media Link** for Chapter 55:<br>• Abdominal Thrusts |
| | Activities and Quizzes on the **StudyWARE™ Software** for Chapter 55 |
| | Complete the following **Competency Challenge 2.0** activity:<br>• Thursday, 11 AM: Prepare for Emergencies |
| | **Audio Library** of medical terms |
| | Online access to the **Critical Thinking Challenge 2.0** |
| **CourseMate** | Activities and Quizzes for Chapter 55 |
| **WebTutor** | Activities and Quizzes for Chapter 55 |

## CHECK YOUR KNOWLEDGE

1. This unit is computerized and can analyze the heart rhythm of a person in fibrillation or arrest, recognize a shockable rhythm, and advise the operator through lights and voice prompts if a shock is indicated.
   a. ECG
   b. AED
   c. EMS
   d. Ambu bag
2. The most immediate information you need to relay to EMS includes:
   a. the nature of the situation and the address of the victim's location.
   b. the victim's name.
   c. the caller's name and phone number in case the connection is lost.
   d. when the problem started.
3. When distinguishing the severity and length of time for onset of disease or illness, which of the following common terms describes having rapid onset, severe symptoms, and a short course?
   a. Chronic
   b. Subtle
   c. Acute
   d. Life threatening
4. In which of the following emergency situations should the patient be given some form of sugar to help alleviate the situation?
   a. Diabetic ketoacidosis
   b. Hyperglycemia
   c. Diaphoresis
   d. Hypoglycemia
5. The signs of a patient having heat exhaustion would be:
   a. pale, cool, and moist skin and normal body temperature.
   b. hot and dry skin and body temperature possibly above 40°C/104°F.
   c. a weak pulse and shallow breathing, body temperature dropping lower than 35°C/95°F.
   d. white or grayish-yellow skin waxy in appearance.
6. Symptoms that might include shortness of breath; a burning sensation in the chest; nausea and vomiting; unexplained fatigue or weakness; and/or pain in the jaw, neck, shoulder, back, or ear could indicate:
   a. heart attack.
   b. stroke.
   c. shock.
   d. seizure.
7. If an obstructed airway is complete, the object must be removed immediately, within ________, to prevent brain damage from lack of oxygen.
   a. 30 seconds
   b. 2 minutes
   c. 4 minutes
   d. 6 minutes
8. Coughing up what appears to be coffee grounds can indicate:
   a. lung hemorrhage.
   b. a chronic slow bleed of the stomach.
   c. epistaxis.
   d. an ulcer has started bleeding.

## WEB LINKS

American Academy of Emergency Medicine: www.aaem.org

American Heart Association: www.heart.org

Mayo Clinic: www.mayoclinic.com

National Institutes of Health: www.nih.gov

U.S. National Library of Medicine: www.nlm.nih.gov

American Red Cross: www.redcross.org

National Center for Emergency Medicine Informatics: www.ncemi.org

## RESOURCES

Beebe, R., and Funk, D. (2010). *Fundamentals of Emergency Care* (3rd ed.). Clifton Park, NY: Delmar Cengage Learning.

*BLS for Healthcare Providers: Guidelines for CPR and ECC (2005)*. (2006). Dallas, TX: American Heart Association.

CPR & Sudden Cardiac Arrest (SCA) Fact Sheet. "CPR Statistics." www.heart.org/HEARTORG/CPRAndECC/WhatisCPR/CPRFactsandStats/CPR-Statistics_UCM_307542_Article.jsp. (Retrieved 10/12/2010)

Estes, M. E. Z. (2010). *Health Assessment & Physical Examination* (3rd ed.). Clifton Park, NY: Delmar Cengage Learning.

Heller, M., and Veach, L. (2009). *Clinical Medical Assisting: A Professional, Field Smart Approach to the Workplace.* Clifton Park, NY: Delmar Cengage Learning.

Lindh, W., Pooler, M., Tamparo, C., and Dahl, B. (2010). *Delmar's Comprehensive Medical Assisting Administrative and Clinical Competencies* (4th ed.). Clifton Park, NY: Delmar Cengage Learning.

Simmers, L. (2009). *Diversified Health Occupations* (7th ed.). Clifton Park, NY: Delmar Cengage Learning.

Wellness Letter. (2000). *Is It a Heart Attack? If You're a Woman, Will You Know?* Berkeley: University of California.

CHAPTER **10**

# Emergencies in the Medical Office

## Words to Know Challenge

**Spelling: Each line contains three spellings of a word. Underline the correctly spelled word.**

| | | |
|---|---|---|
| 1. asperation | aspirashun | aspiration |
| 2. diaphoresis | diephoresis | diaforesis |
| 3. profalatic | frofalytic | prophylactic |
| 4. exhaustion | eghaustion | egaustion |
| 5. ammonea | ammonia | amoania |
| 6. seezure | seazure | seizure |
| 7. cessation | sessation | cesation |
| 8. coraner | coriner | coroner |
| 9. intubation | entubation | intobacion |
| 10. poision | poison | poisen |
| 11. sincope | syncape | syncope |
| 12. resuscitation | resesutation | recessatation |

**Matching: Match the term in column I to its definition in column II.**

| | COLUMN I | COLUMN II |
|---|---|---|
| ____ | 1. Chronic | A. Extensive, advanced |
| ____ | 2. Subtle | B. Requires intervention as soon as possible |
| ____ | 3. Urgent | C. Can cause death |
| ____ | 4. Sudden | D. Long, drawn out, not acute |
| ____ | 5. Acute | E. Provides vital health information |
| ____ | 6. Severe | F. Injury |
| ____ | 7. Life-threatening | G. The act of reviving |

(continues)

| Answer | Term | | Definition |
|---|---|---|---|
| E | 8. Universal emergency medical ID | | H. Rapid onset, severe symptoms, short course |
| F | 9. Trauma | | I. Unexpected occurrence needing immediate action |
| G | 10. Resuscitation | | J. Another term for heart attack |
| N | 11. Bandage | | K. Hidden, not apparent |
| J | 13. Myocardial infarction | | L. Period after death |
| I | 14. Medical emergency | | M. Occurring quickly, without warning |
| L | 15. Post mortem | | N. A dressing |

Chapter 11

# First Aid for Accidents and Injuries

## OBJECTIVES

In this chapter, you will learn the following:

### KB KNOWLEDGE BASE

1. Spell and define, using the glossary at the back of the text, all the Words to Know in this chapter.
2. Identify four pieces of information that can help you evaluate the severity of an illness or injury when screening a patient over the phone.
3. Describe how to remove foreign bodies from the eyes and ears.
4. Compare and contrast the various types of fractures.
5. Discuss the treatment for animal and human bites.
6. Describe the symptoms of an allergy to stings.
7. Name the three types of burns and give examples of each.
8. Explain the classifications of burns and the treatment for each.
9. Explain the effects of cold and heat applications.
10. Identify and describe the various types of wounds.
11. Explain to the patient the proper care of bandages.

### S SKILLS

1. Demonstrate the proper method of cleaning a wound.
2. Demonstrate application of a tube gauze bandage.
3. Demonstrate application of a spiral bandage.
4. Demonstrate application of a figure-eight bandage.
5. Demonstrate application of a cravat bandage to the head.

### B BEHAVIORS

1. Apply critical thinking skills in performing patient assessment and care.
2. Use language and verbal skills that enable patients' understanding of the procedure being performed.
3. Concepts of effective communication.

## WORDS TO KNOW

abrasion
anaphylactic
avulsion
chemical
cravat
electrical
foreign body
friction
immobilize
incision
laceration
molten
puncture
rabies
shock
splinter
superficial
thermal
wound

## ACCIDENTS AND INJURIES

Knowing what to do when an accident or injury occurs is very helpful not only in your professional life but also in your personal life. When you have a basic understanding of first aid, you can respond quickly and efficiently to sudden incidents without becoming overly anxious or upset. As you come in contact with injury incidents, you will learn when they can be handled with simple first aid and when they require the assistance of a provider or advanced emergency medical services. Recall that many illnesses and injuries can occur in varying degrees of severity. As an example, consider a burn. A burn confined just to the skin surface may be managed without medical assistance unless it covers extensive body surface, whereas, a relatively small area of burn can require medical attention if it extends into underlying tissue. If you are ever unsure of the severity of an injury, it is always better to seek medical assistance or advanced emergency services than to underestimate the severity and care needed.

Keep in mind what you learned in Chapter 55 about recognizing and responding to an emergency. When screening patients over the phone, you need specific information before you can determine whether the situation warrants emergency medical care, an office visit, or management at home. Ask the caller to give you a brief history of the victim's situation, the nature of the initial injury or accident, the time the accident occurred or the illness began, and a description of the victim's current condition. Unlike cardiac or respiratory arrest, which always requires emergency response, the sudden accidents and injuries discussed in this chapter might or might not require the same level of response. The decision to seek emergency response depends on the extent and severity of the condition and the reaction or response of the individual. After obtaining the facts, you can respond appropriately as directed.

## COMMON INJURIES

There are common injuries you might encounter for which your facility must provide treatment. In some cases, the initial care might be delivered and the patient might then need to be sent to the hospital or specialist for further treatment. Common injuries you might see include foreign bodies within various body areas, dislocations and fractures, strains and sprains, and a variety of wounds that need treatment. Many of these injuries tend not to be life-threatening; however, always be prepared for the occasional injury that needs to be treated as an emergency.

### Foreign Bodies

**Foreign bodies** are substances or objects that become lodged in any part of the human body. Common foreign bodies are dirt, metal shavings, and eyelashes to the eyes; small objects such as beads placed by children in the ears and nose; items accidentally swallowed; and splinters and fishhooks in the skin. Foreign bodies require immediate attention by the provider to prevent further damage.

It is fairly common for a speck of dirt, soot from a fire, or an eyelash to lodge in the eye, for example. Always wash your hands before touching the eyes. A foreign body under the lower lid can usually be seen easily and can be removed with a bit of cotton or a fold of tissue moistened with water. If a foreign body is under the upper lid, it might be possible to remove it by pulling the upper lid down over the lower lid. If this procedure is not successful, it might be necessary to grasp the eyelashes and carefully turn back the upper lid over a cotton swab (Figure 56–1).

An object located under the upper lid may also be removed with a folded piece of moistened sterile gauze. If the material cannot be removed easily or is on the cornea, try flushing with large amounts of water to dislodge it (see Chapter 40). Any object imbedded on the cornea must be removed by the provider. Until the object can be removed, the object must be stabilized by covering both eyes with a sterile compress to help keep the injured eye from moving, which will cause discomfort and additional irritation. The eyes move together, so covering only the injured eye could do more harm than good. If the object is protruding, try covering the eyes with Styrofoam or plastic cups and hold in place with a gauze wrap. This will prevent the object from being pushed deeper into the eye. In addition, warn the patient not to rub the affected eye, which would only embed the object deeper into the cornea. When chemicals, either liquid or powder, get in the eyes, use a sterile eye irrigation solution to dilute and neutralize the chemical.

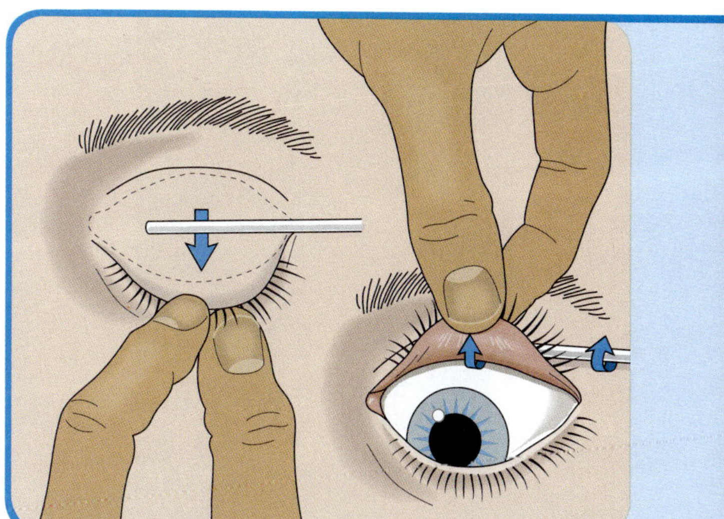

**Figure 56–1:** Remove a foreign body from upper eyelid by turning the eyelid back over a cotton-tipped swab or the stem of a wooden kitchen match. *Delmar/Cengage Learning.*

This solution should be continuously dripped into the eye for 20 minutes. Pre-packed solutions should be kept in the provider's office for emergency use. If a sterile solution is not available, use any clean tap or bottled water to flush the eye. Eye injuries should be evaluated by a provider as soon as possible.

First aid for an object lodged in the ear consists of placing several drops of warm olive oil, mineral oil, or baby oil into the ear and pulling back on the earlobe to straighten the external canal while the head is tilted toward the unaffected side (Figure 56–2). Then let the oil run out and see whether the object comes out with it. Never try to dig an object out of the ear; damage can be done to the external canal or tympanic membrane. If first aid measures are not successful, a provider should examine the patient.

Children are notorious for putting things, such as beans, pebbles, buttons, or marbles, in their ears or up their noses. Instilling oil in the ear when there are large, smooth objects to be removed might make them more difficult to grasp and retrieve. Often, these can be removed from the nose with forceps or irrigated out of an ear by directing water against the wall of the external canal. (Refer to Chapter 40 on ear irrigation.) However, water should never be used with any object, such as beans or peas that would swell, thereby causing pain and making removal much more difficult.

You might get a call from a parent who is frightened because a child has swallowed a small object. It is best for the provider to perform an X-ray examination such as a fluoroscopic exam to see whether the object is actually in the stomach. If the object is not sharp, it might pass through the intestinal tract and be eliminated in the stool.

**Splinters** can generally be removed with a sterile needle and splinter forceps in the office. The skin should be washed with soap and water. Lift the end of the exposed splinter with the sterile needle and it remove it by grasping with a pair of sterile splinter forceps. If a splinter or thorn is under a fingernail, it is best to have a provider remove it. After the splinter or thorn is removed, the area should again be washed with soap and water; apply antibiotic ointment and cover with an adhesive bandage.

Another common injury involving a foreign body is that of an embedded fish hook. One of the hazards of fishing, or of being around individuals who are casting for fish, is that hooks can become embedded in fingers, backs, scalps, or any part of the anatomy that is exposed. It is best for a provider to use a local anesthetic for such removal. When the area is numb, the provider can push the barb on through the flesh and then cut if off with a pair of nipper pliers (Figure 56–3). After this is done, you can back out the remainder of the hook. Another possibility is to cut off the shank of the hook and pull out the barbed end. After the hook is removed, the area should be carefully cleaned with an antimicrobial soap or solution; apply antibiotic ointment and a dry dressing. As with any injury, a tetanus toxoid booster might be needed if it has been longer than five years since the last booster. The provider might also prescribe an antibiotic.

## Strains and Sprains

Strains are the result of overuse of a muscle or group of muscles or when a muscle or tendon is overextended by stretching. They can be caused by improper lifting or

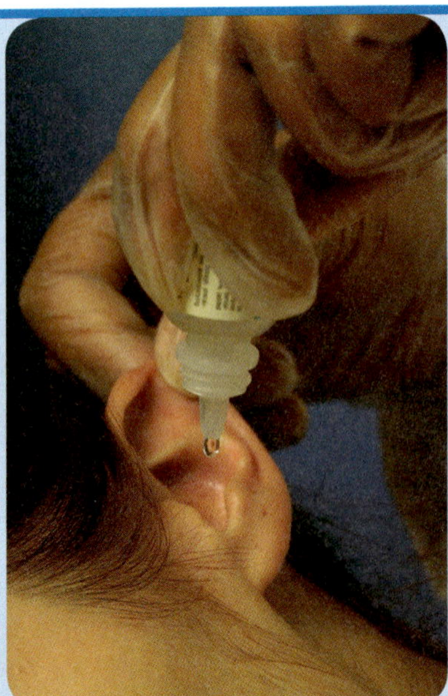

**Figure 56–2:** After the patient's head is tilted to the side, pull back on the ear to straighten the external canal and instill ear drops. *Delmar/Cengage Learning.*

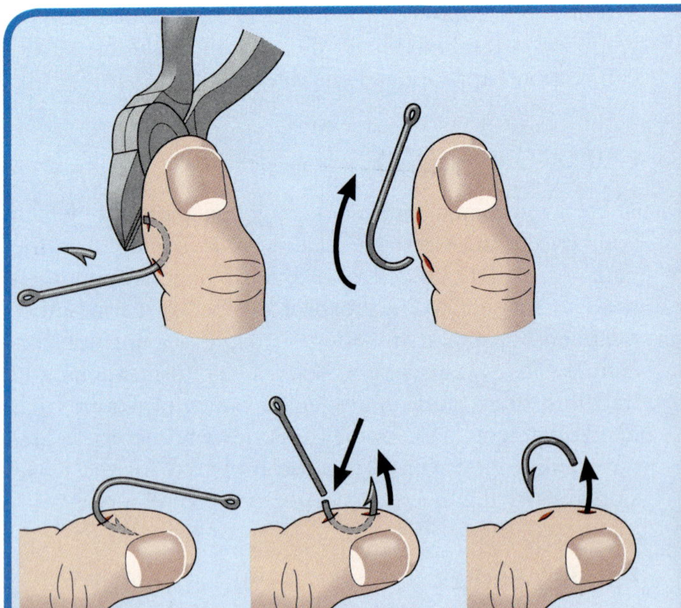

**Figure 56–3:** Fish hook removal by (A) cutting the barb or (B) cutting the shank. *Delmar/Cengage Learning.*

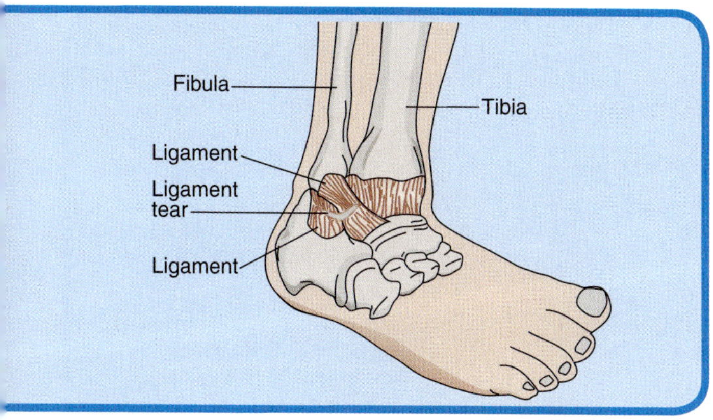


**Figure 56–4:** In an ankle sprain, one or more of the ligaments can be torn or stretched. *Delmar/Cengage Learning.*

by slipping while moving a heavy object. Muscle strain is common after engaging in any strenuous activity that you are not accustomed to doing (Figure 56–4).

Sprains occur when muscles, tendons, or ligaments surrounding a joint are torn. They are usually the result of overuse or trauma from twisting the joint and are sometimes so severe that a fracture can also occur. A common site is the ankle.

First aid for both sprains and strains is to rest the injured muscles in a comfortable position and use what is known as RICE (rest, ice, compression, elevation) or a newer term, PRINCE (protection, rest, ice, NSAIDS or acetaminophen, compression, and elevation) method. Protect the injury by using some form of support mechanism such as an ACE bandage or ankle stirrup if an ankle is involved. Rest the involved area. If a lower extremity is involved, the patient might want to use crutches until the area is pain free. Ice the area for the first 48 to 72 hours or until the swelling is reduced. Non-steroidal medications (NSAIDS) such as ibuprofen or acetaminophen can be used for pain and swelling. Compression can be accomplished with the ACE wrap or ankle brace if an ankle injury (refer to Procedure 56–4 on applying an elastic bandage); be sure the supportive device is not too loose or tight. Elevate the injured area for approximately two to three days, making sure to elevate the involved area higher than the heart.

### Dislocations

At least half of all dislocations involve the shoulder, but dislocations are possible at any freely moving joint. When a bone end slips out of the socket or when the capsule surrounding a joint is stretched or torn, a dislocation is likely to occur. There is usually severe pain and obvious deformity of the joint area and possible loss of function of the affected limb. There is also noticeable swelling. Dislocations are best treated by a provider. The only first aid measure is to **immobilize** the dislocation during the trip to the medical office or hospital. Treat all sprains, strains, and dislocations as if they are a fracture. The injured extremity should be carefully supported in the position in which it was found to avoid additional injury. This involves splinting from the joint above to the joint below the injury. With a shoulder involvement, this probably involves immobilizing the affected arm by wrapping it to the body for support. (Refer to Chapter 57 for applying an arm sling.)

### Fractures

Fractures are breaks in a bone caused by trauma or bone disease. There are several types of fractures; however, they are all classified as either open or closed (Figure 56–5). In a *closed* or *simple fracture*, there is no open wound. In an *open* or *compound fracture*, there is an open wound. First aid for an open fracture is to control bleeding and to splint without moving the bone ends. The patient might also need to be treated for **shock**. Check the pulse and motor and sensory reflexes (PMS). Capillary refill of the distal area to all fracture sites on an injured limb will be impaired. To ensure good perfusion and unimpaired neurological function, treatment must be administered as soon as possible. A fracture can be accurately diagnosed only by an X-ray unless bone ends can be seen in an open wound or a severe deformity is present. A provider is the only person who should attempt to straighten, or reduce, a fracture. Refer to Table 56–1 for a description of the various types of fractures.

## BITES AND STINGS

Bites and stings are common occurrences that seem more likely in the summertime.

Bites can occur from animals (both pets and strays) and humans. They can be **superficial** or can break the skin, causing a **puncture** or **laceration**. Stings come from, bees, wasps, hornets, and other insects and can present very minimal symptoms such as swelling, redness, and itching or be life threatening.

### Animal Bites

An animal bite can tear skin and cause a bruise. The bite is dangerous because of the possibility of infection or **rabies**. The **wound** should be thoroughly cleansed with an antiseptic soap and rinsed well with water. The area should be bandaged and immobilized, and the patient should be examined by a provider as soon as possible. The bite must be reported to the police or local health authorities, who will examine the animal for rabies. Generally, the animal should be held for observation for at least 15 days to see whether it is rabid. The decision must be made regarding the use of anti-rabies serum, depending on what is known about the animal and what type of animal it is. If the skin is broken and

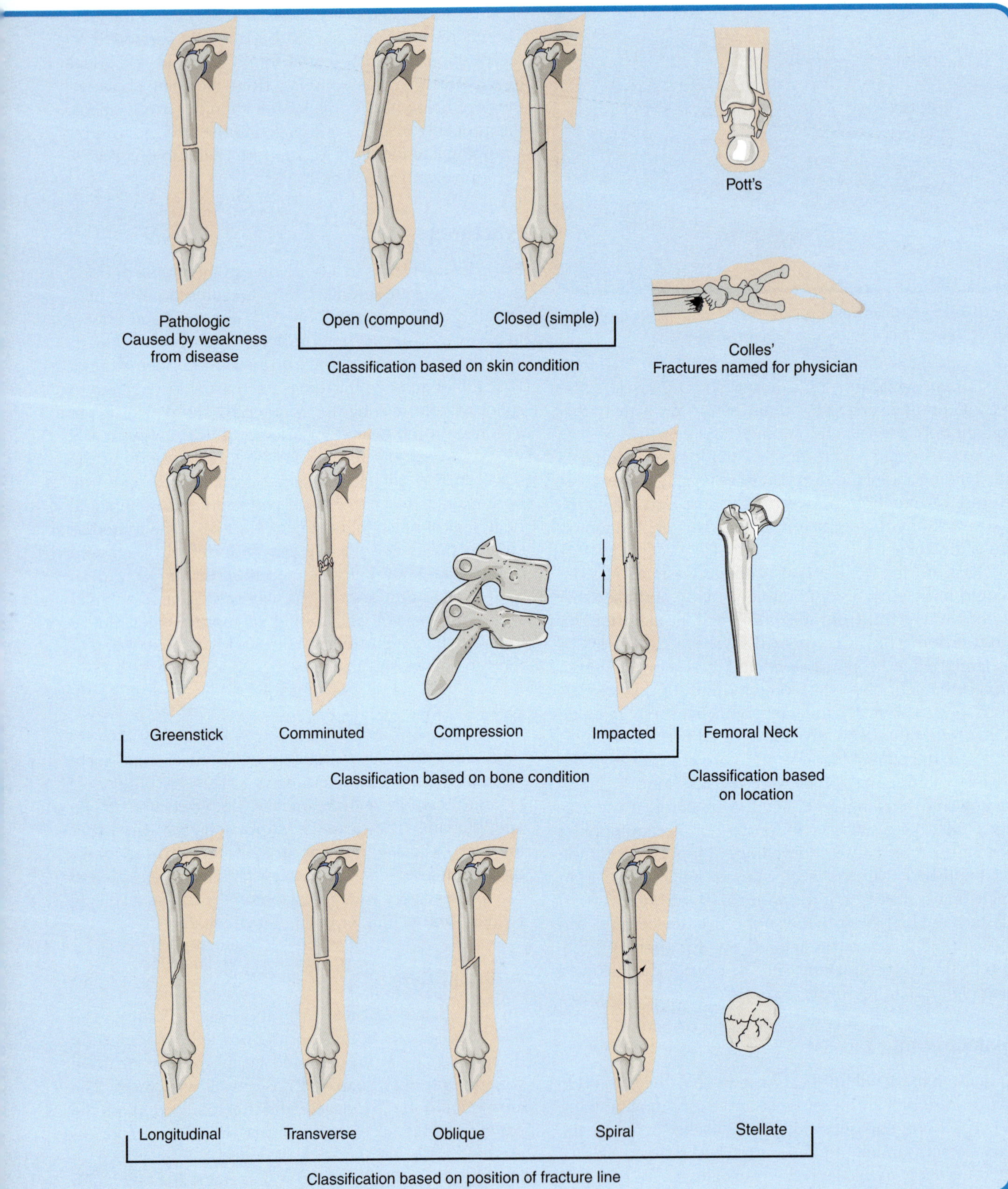


**Figure 56–5:** Types of fractures. *Delmar/Cengage Learning.*

**TABLE 56–1 Types of Fractures**

| Name | Description |
|---|---|
| Greenstick (incomplete) | Bone partially bent and partially broken; often occurs in children |
| Closed (simple, complete) | Skin intact over the fracture; bone is completely broken into two or more pieces. |
| Transverse | Fracture crosses the bone at a 90° angle to the bone's axis |
| Oblique | A diagonal fracture of a bone |
| Open (compound) | Open wound over the ends of the fractured bones; often an end of the bone is visible |
| Impacted | One bone fragment is wedged into the other bone fragment |
| Comminuted | Crushing or splintering of the bone |
| Spiral | Fracture spirals around a long bone; occurs as the result of the bone twisting |
| Depressed | Fragments or portions of the bone pressed down into the skull; can be into the brain and surrounding tissue |
| Colles | Fracture of the distal end of the radius bone in the wrist |
| Potts | Fracture of the lower part of the fibula with serious injury of the lower tibial articulation, usually a chipping off of a portion of the medial malleolus or rupture of the medial ligament |

the animal cannot be tested, anti-rabies serum should be used. When the animal can be observed and is found to be free of rabies, no serum is necessary.

Bites can also result in a laceration and need suture repair. Generally, when children are bitten on the face, arms, or hands, the provider will refer them to a plastic surgeon for repair with minimal scarring.

In some areas of the world, snakebites occur. A snakebite will show a two-fang wound. Recommended first aid is to cleanse the area to remove any surface venom with antibacterial soap and water and immobilize the victim. If the bite is located on an extremity, try to maintain the extremity *below* the level of the heart. Do not cut into the wound or attempt to suck out venom. Do not apply cold packs or ice or apply a tourniquet.

## Human Bites

A human bite that breaks the skin also needs to be cleaned with antibacterial soap and water, and the patient should be seen by a provider. Concern regarding human bites because of HIV and hepatitis B is also an issue. Although the transmission of HIV is not likely (the only way HIV could be transmitted in this manner is if the bite breaks the skin and the person doing the biting has bleeding gums), it is a possibility. Patients who have sustained such a bite from another person should be advised to have injections to be immunized against hepatitis B. With all bites, a tetanus injection must be administered to the patient if he or she has not received one within five years.

## Stings

Bees, wasps, and hornets cause deaths every year. If the victim is not sensitive to the sting, the result can be only a painful swelling with redness and itching. When several stings are received at one time, the victim can become quite ill and might develop severe hives or generalized edema. When a patient is severely allergic to stings, the sting can cause acute illness. The patient can become restless, complain of headache, have shortness of breath, or have mottled blueness of the skin. When shortness of breath is not apparent, the victim can appear to be in shock and have severe nausea, vomiting, and bloody diarrhea. The severely allergic patient should always have a special emergency kit known as an EpiPen, which is a self-administered epinephrine injection, close at hand when a sting is possible (Figure 56–6). If anaphylactic shock is evident, epinephrine should be given as a lifesaving measure. (Refer to Chapter 55 for a discussion about **anaphylactic** shock and stings.)

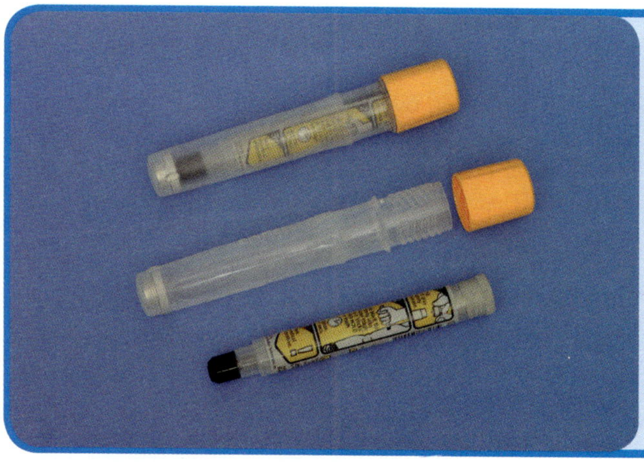

**Figure 56–6:** EpiPens. *Delmar/Cengage Learning.*

A honeybee leaves the stinger in the skin, and it should be immediately removed by scraping it out carefully with a credit card or other rigid object. This is usually the only treatment needed. You can make a paste of baking soda and water to be applied to the area or apply an anti-itch cream, lotion, or gel such as Benadryl. Never grasp the stinger with your fingers or a tweezers because that would inject more of the venom. Wasps, hornets, and yellow jackets retain their stingers and can unfortunately sting repeatedly; therefore, no stinger can be removed.

## BURNS

According to the American Burn Association, there are one million burn injuries in the United States and an estimated 45,000 hospitalizations per year. Extensive burns require painful treatment and a long period of rehabilitation. They often result in permanent disfigurement and physical and emotional problems.

### Types of Burns

Burns are basically of three types: **thermal**, **chemical**, and **electrical**, with thermal being the most common.

- *Thermal*—Caused by residential fires; automobile accidents; playing with matches; accidents with gasoline, space heaters, or firecrackers; scalding water from the stove or tub; and coming in contact with curling irons, stoves, or clothing irons. Some childhood burns, such as from cigarettes, can be traced to deliberate abuse. Sunburn occurs from overexposure to the sun.
- *Chemical*—From contact with, ingestion, inhalation, or injection of acids or alkalines.
- *Electrical*—Occur after contact with faulty electrical wiring, a child chewing on an electrical cord, or from downed high-voltage power lines. Although rare, an electrical burn can also come from a lightning strike.

### Classification of Burns

Burns are classified by three methods. One is by the percentage of body surface area (BSA) involved in the burn. The Rule of Nines illustrated in Figure 56–7A and the Lund and Browder chart in Figure 56–7B are methods to estimate the size of the burn. These methods establish a standard by which all injuries can be estimated. The Lund and Browder chart is more specific and has a way to estimate areas for different age groups because body proportions are quite different for infants and small children as compared with adults.

A familiar classification reflects the extent of burn as a relationship to the layer of skin involved and is estimated from one to four degrees (Figure 56–8). A first-degree burn (also called a superficial burn) involves an injury primarily to the epidermis, resulting in reddening of the skin and moderately severe pain. A sunburn or contact with boiling water or steam can cause this type of burn (Figure 56–9A). A second-degree burn (also called a partial-thickness burn) involves the epidermis and part of the dermis. The leakage of plasma and electrolytes from the capillaries damaged by the burn into the surrounding tissues raises the epidermis to form blisters and results in mild to moderate edema and pain (Figure 56–9B). Third- or fourth-degree burns (also called full thickness burns) involve the epidermis, dermis, and subcutaneous skin layers, including fat and muscle tissue (Figure 56–9 C). No blisters appear, but white, leathery tissue and thrombosed vessels are visible. Although most providers have combined the third- and fourth-degree burns into the same category and consider them third-degree burns, some use the term *fourth-degree burn* for burns involving all layers of the skin, muscle, and bone. This can result from an industrial injury such as contact with **molten** metal.

Another classification of burns measures the severity of a burn by a combination of two methods. It correlates the burn's depth with its size (BSA) to determine its severity, which is then classified as a minor, moderate, or major burn.

- A *minor* burn has less than 2% of BSA at the third-degree level and burns on less than 15% for adults and 10% for children at the second-degree level.
- A *moderate* burn is when third-degree burns cover 2% to 10% of BSA; second-degree burns cover from 15% to 25% on adults or over 10% on children.
- A *major* burn is when a third-degree burn covers more than 10% of BSA or second-degree burns cover more than 25% in adults or 20% in children; burns of the hands, feet, or genitalia are also major burns; burns that are complicated by fractures, affect poor-risk patients, or are electrical are also major burns.

The classification of burns is at the discretion of the provider or the treatment facility involved.

### Treatment of Burns

The treatment of burns depends on the classification of the burn, although the first priority is to stop the burning process. Treat first-degree burns with cold water and a dressing to protect the area. Applying cold water

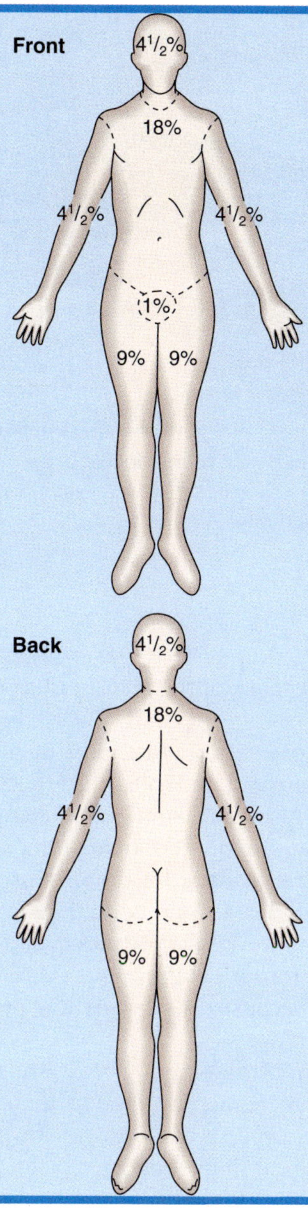


**Figure 56–7A:** Diagram for use in calculating the extent of burns or other injuries for an adult. *Delmar/Cengage Learning.*

to the area should stop the pain and might even keep the burn from progressing into deeper tissue layers. Encourage a victim of severe sunburn to soak in a tub of cool water and drink large amounts of fluids. Patients who are on photosensitive drugs need to be warned about their increased danger from exposure to the sun and the need to wear protective sunscreen and clothing. Pharmacists generally place a warning label on the prescription bottles containing these drugs. The application of butter or ointments is contraindicated for two reasons: it will hold in the burn and cause more pain, and it will be painful to remove when the burn is evaluated and treated. In addition, butter contains salt, which would be

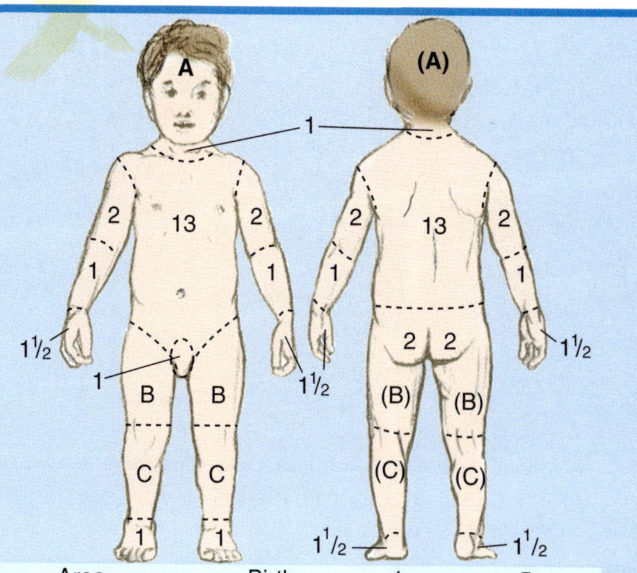


| Area | Birth | 1 yr | 5 yr |
|---|---|---|---|
| A (head) | 19 | 17 | 14 |
| B (one thigh) | 6 1/2 | 7 1/2 | 9 |
| C (one leg) | 6 | 6 | 6 |

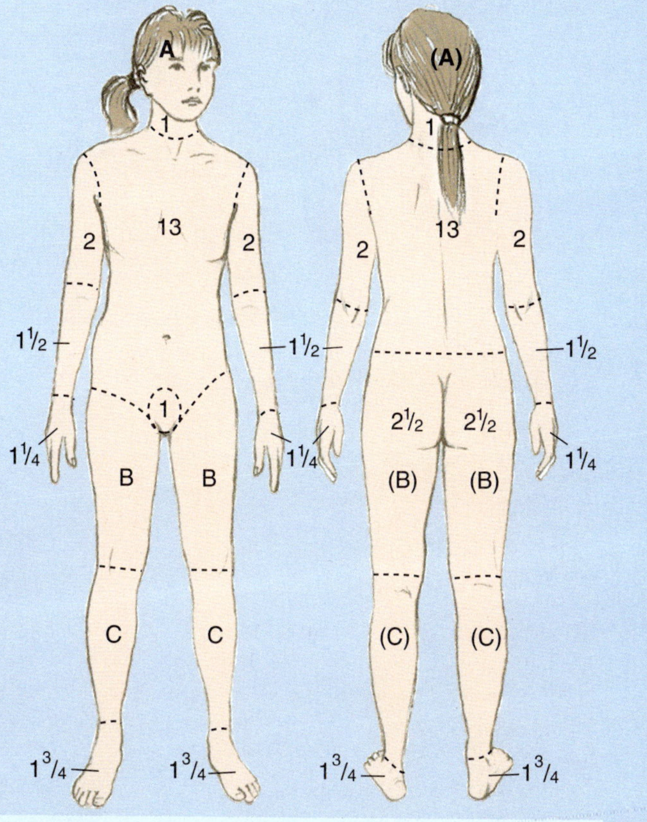


| Area | 10 yr | 15 yr | Adult |
|---|---|---|---|
| A (head) | 11 | 9 | 8 |
| B (one thigh) | 8 1/2 | 9 | 9 |
| C (one leg) | 6 | 6 1/2 | 7 |

**Figure 56–7B:** Lund and Browder chart. *Delmar/Cengage Learning.*

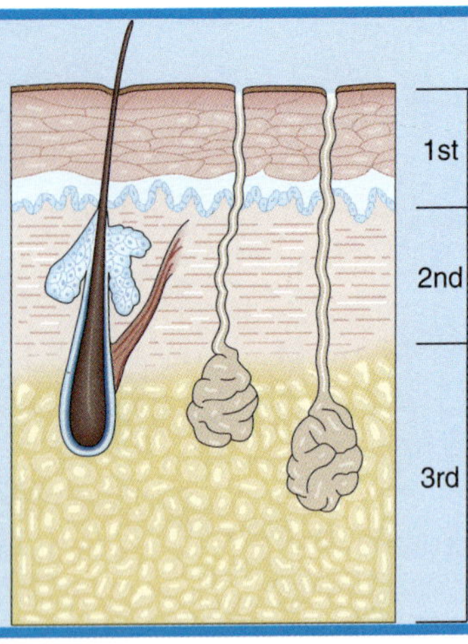


**Figure 56–8:** Layers of skin. *Delmar/Cengage Learning.*

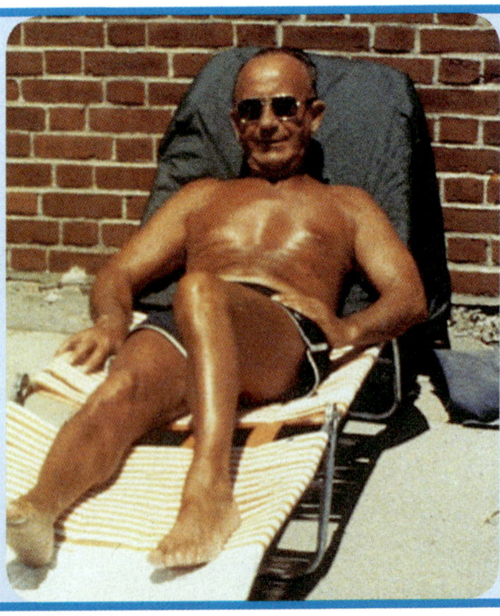

**Figure 56–9A:** First-degree burns involve the top layer of skin. *Courtesy of the Phoenix Society of Burn Survivors, Inc.*

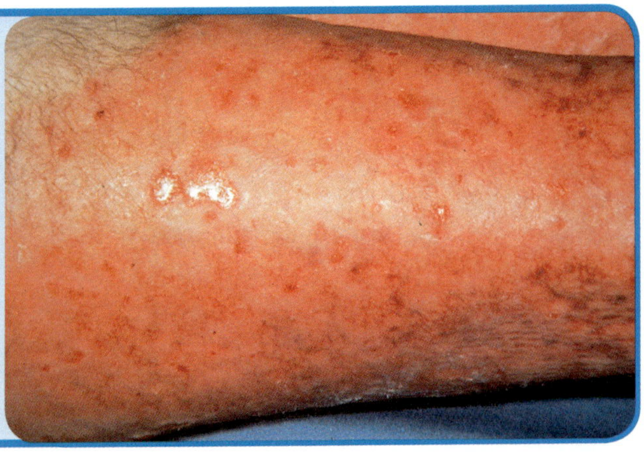

**Figure 56–9B:** Second-degree, or partial-thickness burns affect the top layers of skin. The healing process is slower, and scarring can occur. *Courtesy of the Phoenix Society of Burn Survivors, Inc.*

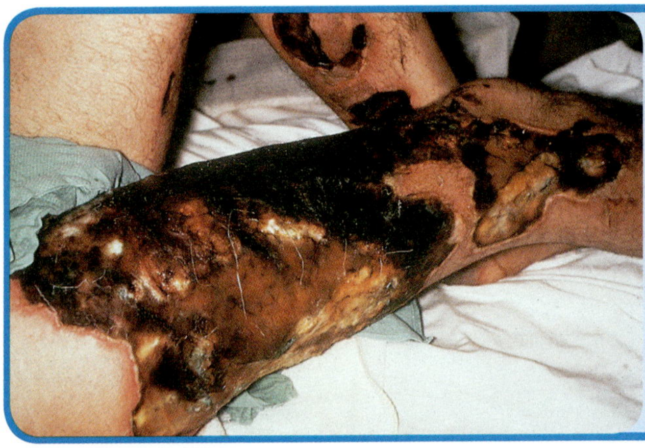

**Figure 56–9C:** Third- and fourth-degree burns are the most serious, affecting or destroying all layers of skin in addition to the fat, muscle, bones, and nerves. *Courtesy of the Phoenix Society of Burn Survivors, Inc.*

very painful if the skin surface was broken. Ice is also contraindicated because of the chance of frostbite to the damaged tissue.

In second-degree burns, first aid can include treatment for shock, removal of any jewelry because edema might be severe, providing ample amounts of liquid to drink, and covering the burned area with a sterile dressing. Healing can be facilitated if the blisters are opened by the provider under aseptic conditions and the area covered with a sterile dressing. Patients should be cautioned to refrain from breaking blisters and peeling the skin themselves because this leaves the area open to infection.

Third- and fourth-degree burns should receive immediate medical treatment. If more than 10 percent of the BSA is involved, it is considered a major burn and requires surgical intervention, IV fluids for fluid replacement, medication for pain, and probably tetanus antitoxin or a toxoid booster shot if it has been longer than five years since the patient has received one. The only first aid that is appropriate is to cover the burned area with sterile dressings and treat the patient for shock. Remember to avoid applying a dressing to second- and third-degree burns with any material that could adhere to the area because it will cause pain and tissue damage when it has to be removed. No attempt should be made to remove clothing that is in contact with the burn. The patient will need surgical care to remove the burned fabric, clean the area, and dress the wound.

## Treating Electrical and Chemical Burns

When burns are caused by electricity or chemicals, other factors must be considered before first aid can be given. An electrical burn results from contact with electrical wiring, power lines, or lightning. The first concern is to remove the victim from the source of electricity—but only *after* the electrical source has been turned off. This situation requires evaluation. If the electrical source is from the wiring within a home, the main electrical supply coming into the house can be shut off at the electrical box, thereby making rescue safe. If the electrical source is power lines, the electric company must be summoned. If the person and the electrical source are in a wet area, keep in mind that electricity conducts well through water. If you come in contact with the water, you could receive a severe shock or be electrocuted. EMS personnel have been electrocuted trying to rescue people from situations involving downed wires and water. Because of this potential for a lethal accident, policy states that they must summon the electric company or the fire department to deal with the electrical source prior to any rescue attempt.

If the voltage is of a sufficient amount, it is possible for the victim to suffer circulatory and respiratory arrest, which necessitates administering CPR and obtaining advanced medical care. The everyday electrical burn is treated like any other burn; however, the extent of the damage might not be readily observable. Electrical burns can cause extensive internal damage along the conduction pathway, which can take a few days to manifest itself. Persons struck by lightning need CPR and immediate emergency treatment. They might have the hallmark ferning markings on their body, which are characteristic of lightning burns. They might, too, have extensive internal damage and, if they were standing when struck, have extensive burns to the soles of the feet where the lightning exits the body.

Chemical burns are treated by removing any clothing from the burn area and then immediately flooding the area with water for at least 15 minutes. A dry chemical should first be brushed off carefully before flushing the patient's skin because some chemicals, such as lime, are activated by water. Following the flooding of water, chemical burns, like all other burns, should be covered with a sterile dressing. A chemical burn of the eye should be flooded with water continuously for at least 20 minutes. A provider should always examine eye burns immediately.

## APPLYING HEAT AND COLD TREATMENTS

In the treatment of injuries, providers often order the application of a heat or cold pack. The provider will give specific instructions concerning the length of time and where to apply the treatment.

Many offices and clinics today use disposable heat and cold packs because of their convenience (Figure 56–10).

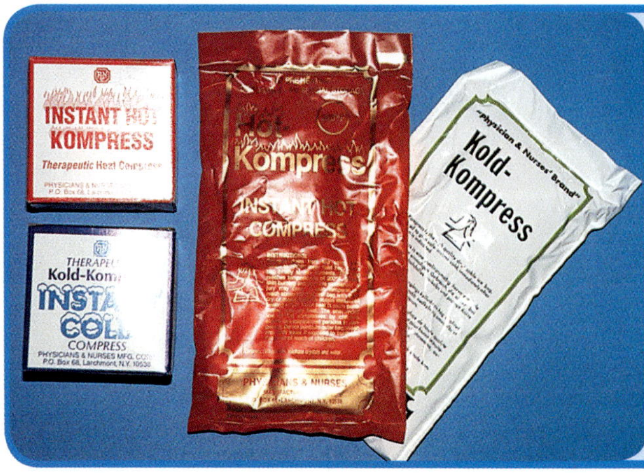


**Figure 56–10:** Hot and cold packs. *Delmar/Cengage Learning.*

These plastic packs contain chemicals that are activated by either squeezing the bag or mixing the contents to produce cold or by bending a metal disc to initiate heat. Many of these disposable packs are reusable by boiling or freezing them, which is of further convenience to the patient. When using these packs, it is recommended for them to be placed in a cloth covering or a disposable towel to protect the skin. If the provider requests moist heat or cold treatment, you should use a clean, moist cloth towel between the plastic pack and the skin. Moisture facilitates conduction to tissues. Moist heat is less likely to cause burns of the skin, and it provides deeper penetration to tissues. Unless otherwise ordered by the provider, the pack should be left in place for 20 minutes at a time. Generally, the standard instruction is on for 20 minutes and off for 10. This may be repeated to increase circulation, but constant hot or cold is never advised.

The application of cold decreases bacterial growth, body temperature, and local circulation temporarily. It also is a temporary anesthetic, relieves inflammation, helps control bleeding, and reduces swelling. The average temperature is between 10°C and 26.7°C (50°F and 80°F). Cold applications are used in burns, sprains, strains, and bruises and in the initial treatment of injuries to the eye.

Heat applications are used to increase tissue temperature, circulation, and rate of healing. When heat is applied to an injured area, pain decreases. The average temperature is between 40.6°C and 49°C (105°F and 120°F). Heat treatments relieve congestion in deep muscle layers and visceral organs and muscle spasms. The heat dilates blood vessels, which helps increase circulation and reduce localized swelling *after* the initial 48 to 72 hours of cold treatment following the injury.

## WOUNDS

It is important to know the characteristics of and be able to identify and treat many types of wounds. **Abrasions** involve a scrape of the epidermis with dots of blood and possibly the presence of foreign material such as dirt or gravel (56–11). First aid is to clean the area carefully with soap and water, apply an antiseptic solution or ointment, and cover with a dressing. If the abrasion resulted from contact with rusty metal or an unusually dirty object, an injection of tetanus toxoid or antitoxin might be required.

An **avulsion** is when the skin is torn off and the wound is bleeding profusely. Avulsions generally occur on limbs and appendages such as fingers, toes, hands, arms, and legs. Often, they occur during a motor vehicle accident or when a body part gets caught in machinery. Clean the wound with soap and water and replace the skin flap in its original position. Apply pressure to control the bleeding. When the bleeding has stopped, apply a pressure bandage.

A wound caused by a sharp object that leaves a clean cut is called an **incision** and can need sutures to close (Figure 56–12). Some people prefer to use tape Steri-Strips for closure rather than sutures if the wound is not too long and not in an area that bends. The area must be carefully cleaned with soap and water, and an antiseptic can be applied before covering with a sterile dressing.

A laceration is a tearing of body tissue and is more difficult to clean and suture properly (Figure 56–13). Special care must be taken to avoid infection. In the first aid care of an incision or laceration, the first concern must be control of bleeding. Apply direct pressure to the wound area and elevate the extremity. If direct pressure is not effective, apply indirect pressure on the appropriate pressure point.

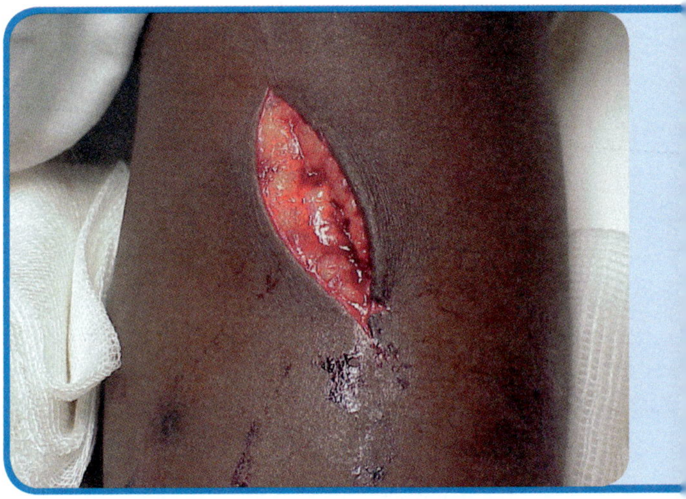

**Figure 56–12:** Incision. *Delmar/Cengage Learning.*

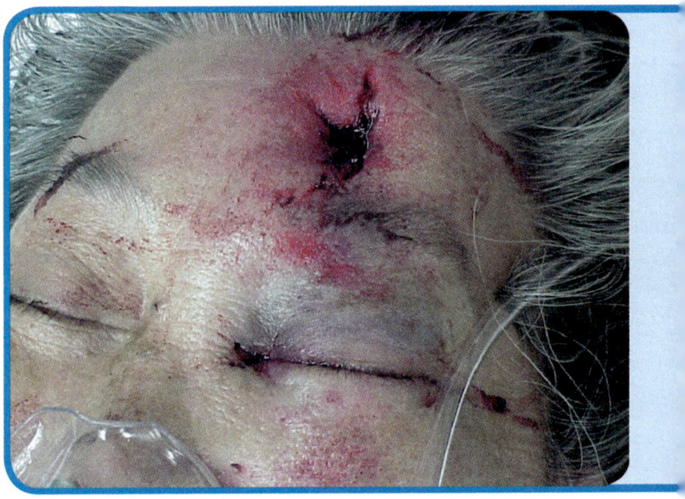

**Figure 56–13:** Laceration. *Delmar/Cengage Learning.*

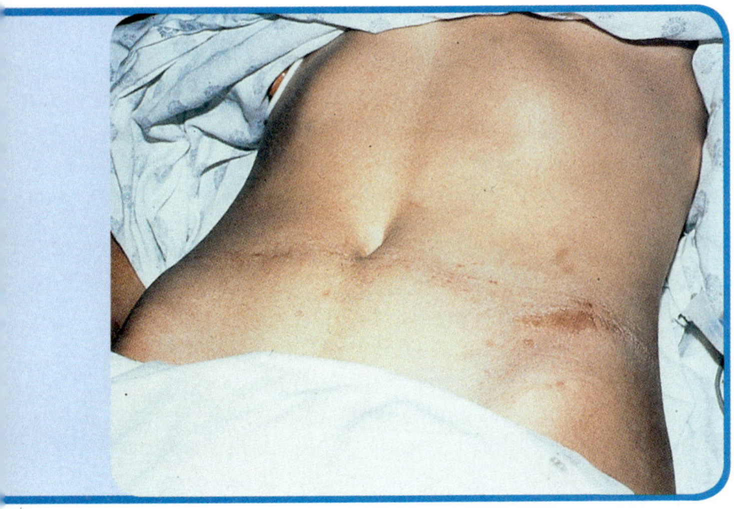

**Figure 56–11:** Abrasion. *Delmar/Cengage Learning.*

A puncture wound is one made with a pointed object, such as an ice pick, knife, or nail (Figure 56–14). First aid is to clean the wound area and, if necessary, enlarge the hole with a probe to allow for irrigation with antiseptic solutions. A puncture wound can also be the result of an animal or human bite, as mentioned earlier. It is usually possible to identify the type of bite by looking at the shape of the wound. A human bite is identified by the shape of the denture and needs to be cleaned carefully.

### Cleaning Wounds

Human skin cannot be sterilized, but the microorganisms that might be harmful can be washed off the skin's surface

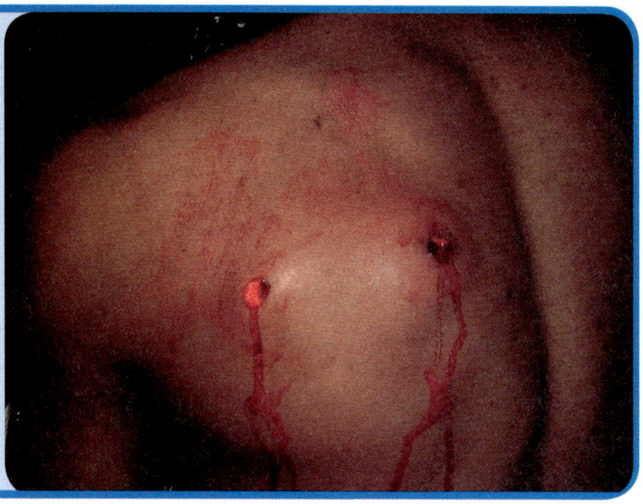

**Figure 56–14:** Puncture. *Delmar/Cengage Learning.*

with Betadine or other antimicrobial solution, water, and **friction**. Applying an antiseptic following the washing makse the skin essentially germ free. The procedure of cleaning a wound is usually the responsibility of the medical assistant and is presented in Procedure 56–1.

When the wound does not bleed excessively and does not involve tissues below the skin, the area can be thoroughly cleaned. If a wound is superficial and will heal well with simple cleaning and protection from contamination, sutures are unnecessary. Soaking the wound area in an antiseptic solution might be necessary if debris is ground in. This helps loosen the debris and make the cleaning process easier. Some clean cuts can be closed with adhesive Steri-Strips or butterfly closures, depending on the length, depth, and severity of the wound.

## PROCEDURE 56–1 Clean Wound Areas

**MEDIA LINK:** View the video, “Clean Wound Areas,” for this chapter on the Premium Website.

**PURPOSE:** To remove blood, debris, and surface microorganisms from the area of injury

**EQUIPMENT:** Basin, antibacterial solution (Betadine), warm water, sterile gauze sponges, sterile sponge forceps, gloves, sterile water, irrigation syringe, biohazard and regular waste receptacle, bandage and tape, patient chart or EHR, pen

**SKILL:** Demonstrate the proper method of cleaning a wound.

| Procedure Steps | Detailed Instructions and/or *Rationales* |
|---|---|
| 1. Assemble the equipment and materials, wash hands, and put on gloves. | |
| 2. Introduce yourself, identify the patient, and ***explain the procedure, using language the patient can understand.*** | *Ensures that you are performing the procedure on the correct patient. Giving patients an explanation helps allay any fears about the procedure.* |
| 3. Grasp several gauze sponges with sponge forceps. | |
| 4. Dip the sponges into warm detergent water. | Make certain the water is at a comfortable temperature. |
| 5. Wash the wound and wound area to remove microorganisms and any foreign matter. | Be careful not to injure the patient further with the instrument. Clean the wound area with sponges only, working from the inside to 2 or 3 inches around the wound as you would for a surgical prep. If there is a lot of debris on the wound, you might soak the wound in an antibacterial solution first. *This prevents bringing microorganisms from the surrounding skin into an open wound.* |
| 6. Discard the sponges in proper waste receptacle. | Unless the sponges are soaked or dripping with blood or body fluids, a regular receptacle is used. |

*(continues)*

*(continued)*

| Procedure Steps | Detailed Instructions and/or *Rationales* |
|---|---|
| 7. Irrigate the wound thoroughly with sterile water. | |
| 8. Blot the wound dry with sterile gauze and dispose of the gauze in the proper waste receptacle. | |
| B 9. ***Call the provider to inspect the wound and assist as needed with treatment.*** | |
| 10. Apply a sterile dressing and bandage it in place (Figure 56–15). | The provider might order an antibiotic ointment to be applied; this not only helps prevent infection but keeps the wound from sticking to the bandage. |
| B 11. ***Instruct patient in how to care for the bandage and to watch for signs of circulation impairment and infection.*** | The patient should be told to watch for redness, swelling, and sensation of pain or fever. Typed instructions should be given to the patient for follow-up care. |
| 12. Clean up the work area. | Place all used materials and gloves in the proper waste receptacle for safe disposal. |
| 13. Wash hands. | |
| 14. Document. | |

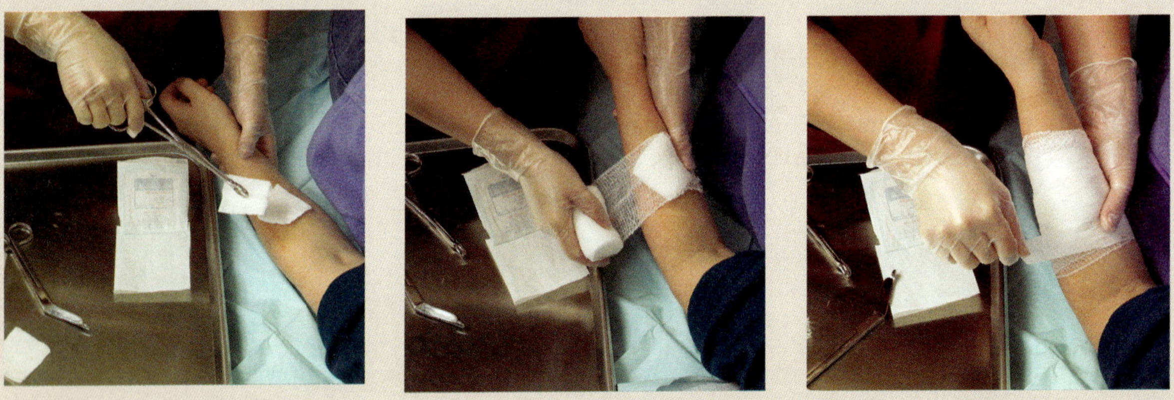

**Figure 56–15:** Apply sterile gauze and bandage in to place. *Delmar/Cengage Learning.*

## Charting Example

| | |
|---|---|
| 65-3-XX<br>1:25 pm | Extensive wound over knee and lateral surface of right leg from fall off bicycle onto gravel area by road. Also jagged 10 cm laceration from broken glass fragment. Wound cleansed thoroughly with antibacterial solution and water. Two glass fragments removed and wound closed with four sutures by provider. Sterile dressing, antibiotic ointment, and bandage applied. Patient given follow-up instructions and patient education provided. Patient tolerated procedure well.<br>S. Davis, RMA(AMT) |

When bleeding has been severe, no attempt should be made to clean the area because it can restart the bleeding. Because the patient will need additional medical care, it can be cleaned then. A pressure bandage should be applied securely and the patient taken for emergency medical care immediately. (A pressure bandage usually consists of multiple layers of gauze squares or pads tightly fastened to the skin with tape or bound with a roller bandage or ACE bandage. If such a patient comes to your office, wait for instructions from the provider before removing the pressure dressing. You will be responsible for having a suture set up for use when the provider is ready. You might question the patient or a relative to find out what caused the wound and how large and deep it is. You should also inquire about the most recent tetanus immunization booster and record the information on the patient's chart. The general rule is for the patient to have a tetanus injection every 10 years; however, for an injury, the requirement changes to every five years. The provider will write the orders for the necessary immunizations. You should not proceed with any medication or injection until the order has been written by the provider.

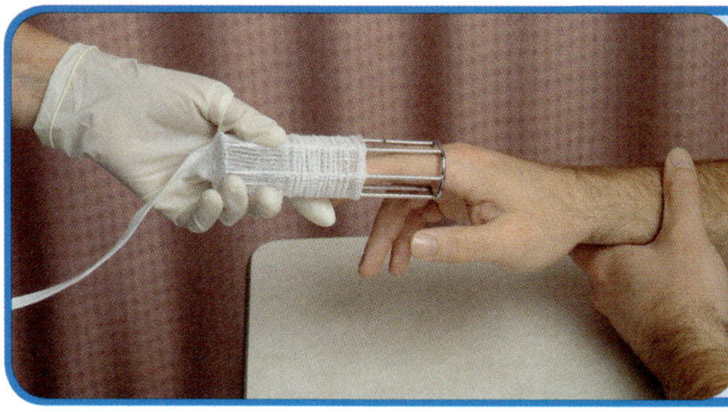

**Figure 56–16A:** The cylindrical applicator is placed over the finger. *Delmar/Cengage Learning.*

## Bandaging Wounds

After the provider has treated the wound, it might become your responsibility to apply the dressing. You must also educate the patient to keep the bandage clean and dry and to watch for signs of infection such as redness, pain, and drainage. He or she should be advised to contact the provider if any of these signs occur. The following illustrations and procedures are guidelines to care for the patient satisfactorily.

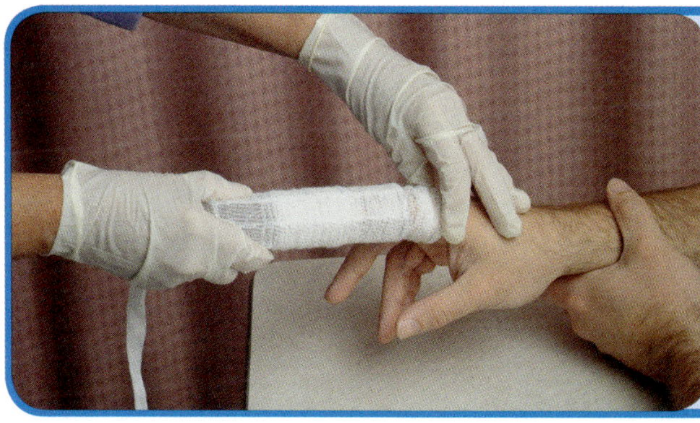

**Figure 56–16B:** Gauze is stretched over the finger. *Delmar/Cengage Learning.*

### Tube Gauze Bandage

The easiest and probably quickest way to bandage arms, legs, fingers, and toes is with a tubular gauze bandage. Use an appropriately sized cylindrical cage applicator. The amount of tube gauze you expect to use is stretched over the applicator and placed over the extremity. By manipulating the cylinder around the extremity, grasping the tube gauze, withdrawing the cylinder, twisting the gauze, and repeating the sequence, a snug gauze bandage can be placed over the dressing (Figures 56–16A–C). Refer to Procedure 56–2 for applying a tube gauze bandage.

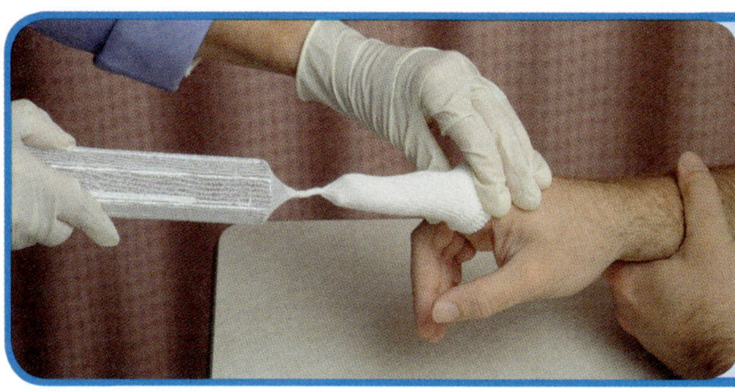

**Figure 56–16C:** The applicator is pulled off, leaving the bandage. *Delmar/Cengage Learning.*

### Spiral Bandage

An injury on the arms or legs requires the dressing to be held in place with a spiral bandage. Refer to Procedure 56–3 for applying a spiral bandage.

## PROCEDURE 56–2 Apply a Tube Gauze Bandage

**PURPOSE:** To cover a wound or hold a bandage in place on an appendage such as a finger, toe, arm, or leg

**EQUIPMENT:** Scissors, dressing, adhesive tape, tube gauze bandage, applicator, gloves, a waste container, patient chart or EHR, pen

**S SKILL:** Demonstrate application of a tube gauze bandage.

| Procedure Steps | Detailed Instructions and/or *Rationales* |
|---|---|
| 1. Assemble the equipment and materials, wash hands, and put on gloves. | |
| B 2. Introduce yourself, identify the patient, and ***explain the procedure, using language the patient can understand.*** | *Ensures that you are performing the procedure on the correct patient. Giving patients an explanation helps allay any fears about the procedure.* |
| 3. Choose an applicator that is larger than the appendage to be bandaged. | |
| 4. Cut an appropriate amount of tubular bandage to be applied and slide onto the applicator. | A general rule is to cut three times the applicator size. |
| 5. Slide the applicator over the appendage. (*Apply first layer.*) | Start at the proximal end of the appendage, hold the bandage in place, and then directly pull the applicator approximately 1 inch past the distal end. |
| 6. Turn the bandage gauze one complete turn. | |
| 7. Next, slide the applicator toward the proximal end of the appendage. | |
| 8. Repeat application process until area is completely covered. | |
| 9. Anchor bandage at the proximal end and secure with tape. | Some providers might want you to secure the bandage by tying off the gauze at the wrist. Do this by:<br>a. Cut the excess bandage from the finger and take the end of the bandage diagonally across the back of the hand to the wrist.<br>b. Circle the wrist once or twice.<br>c. Tie off or tape it at the wrist or tape it in place. |
| B 10. ***Instruct patient in how to care for the bandage and to watch for signs of circulation impairment and infection.*** | The patient should be told to watch for redness, swelling, and sensation of pain or fever. Typed instructions should be given to the patient for follow-up care. |
| 11. Clean up area and dispose of used supplies. | |
| 12. Wash hands. | |
| 13. Document. | |

### Charting Example

| | |
|---|---|
| 1-12-XX<br>1:25 PM | A tubular gauze bandage and antibiotic ointment applied to the right index finger. Patient education provided on how to keep the bandage clean and dry and to watch for signs of infection. Follow-up appointment scheduled for dressing change and wound recheck in 48 hours. J. Finelli, RMA(AMT) |

## PROCEDURE 56–3 Apply a Spiral Bandage

**MEDIA LINK:** View the video, "Spiral Bandage," for this chapter on the Premium Website.

**PURPOSE:** To apply a spiral bandage *NOTE*: This procedure describes how to apply a dressing to a wound and then cover it with a bandage.*

**EQUIPMENT:** Bandage, adhesive tape, scissors, sterile dressing, a waste container, patient chart or EHR, pen

**S SKILL:** Demonstrate application of a spiral bandage.

| Procedure Steps | Detailed Instructions and/or *Rationales* |
|---|---|
| 1. Assemble the equipment and materials, wash hands, and put on gloves. | |
| B 2. Introduce yourself, identify the patient, and ***explain the procedure, using language the patient can understand.*** | *Ensures that you are performing the procedure on the correct patient. Giving patients an explanation helps allay any fears about the procedure.* |
| 3. Carefully open a dressing, without contaminating it, and place it over the wound area. | (*Omit step 3 to eliminate dressing application.) |
| 4. Anchor the bandage by placing the end of the bandage on a bias at the starting point (see Figure 56–17A). | |
| 5. Encircle the part, allowing the corner of the bandage end to protrude (see Figure 56–17B). | CAUTION: Take care not to wrap extremities straight around because it impedes circulation to the distal part of the extremity. |
| 6. Turn down the protruding tip of the bandage (see Figure 56–17C). | |
| 7. Encircle the part again (see Figure 56–17D). | |
| 8. Continue to encircle the area to be covered with spiral turns spaced so that they do not overlap (see Figure 56–17E). | |
| 9. If a closed spiral bandage is desired, overlap spiral turns until the dressing is completely covered (see Figure 56–17F). | |
| 10. Complete the bandage by taping it in place (see Figure 56–17G). | |
| B 11. ***Instruct patient in how to care for the bandage and to watch for signs of circulation impairment and infection.*** | The patient should be told to watch for redness, swelling, and sensation of pain or fever. Typed instructions should be given to the patient for follow-up care. |
| 12. Clean the area and discard contaminated materials and gloves in a proper waste receptacle. | |
| 13. Wash hands. | |
| 14. Document. | |

*(continues)*

*(continued)*

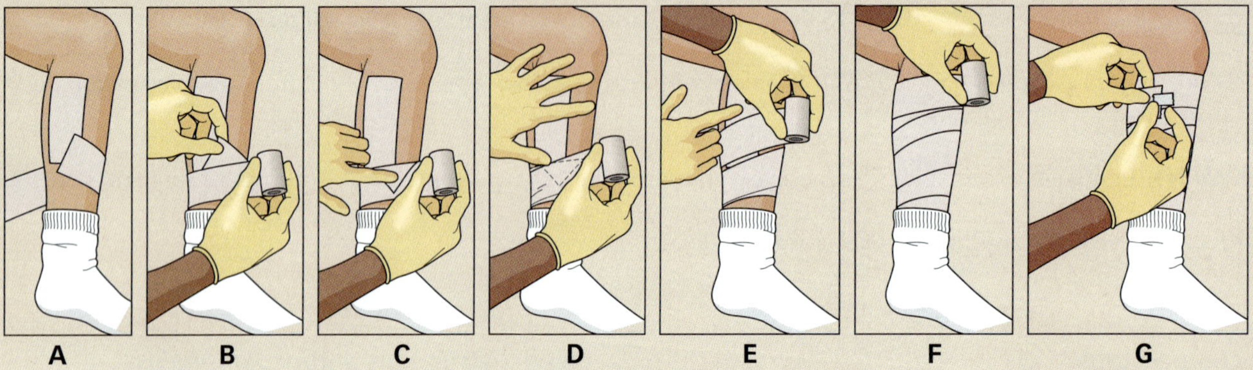


**Figure 56–17A–G:** Application of a spiral bandage. *Delmar/Cengage Learning.*

## Charting Example

| | |
|---|---|
| 4-18-XX<br>1:25 PM | Open spiral bandage applied over dressing on left lower leg. Patient education provided on how to keep the bandage clean and dry and to watch for signs of infection. Follow-up appointment scheduled for dressing change and wound recheck in 48 hours. C. Spatz, CMA(AAMA) |

## Figure-Eight Bandage

A wound on the palm or back of the hand may be protected with a dressing and a figure-eight bandage (Figure 56–18). Refer to Procedure 56–4 for applying a figure-eight bandage.

## Cravat Bandage

When applying a dressing to the forehead, ears, or eyes, a **cravat** can hold the dressing in place (Figure 56–19). Refer to Procedure 56–5 for applying a cravat bandage.

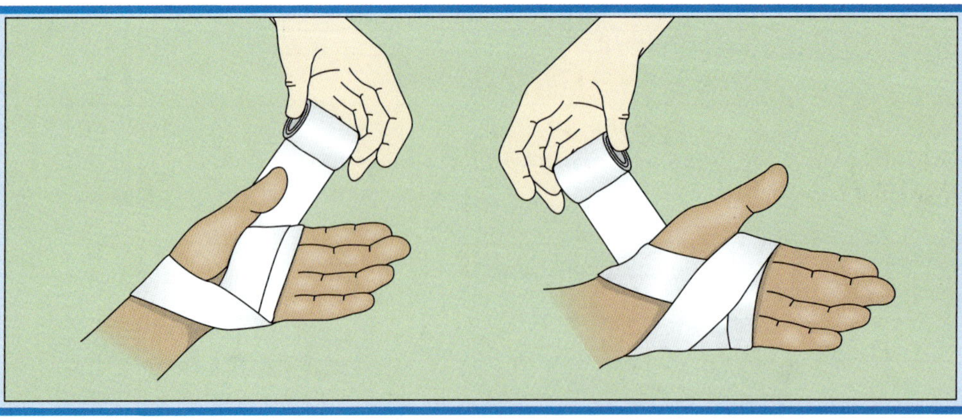

**Figure 56–18:** Figure-eight bandage to hand and wrist. *Delmar/Cengage Learning.*

## PROCEDURE 56–4 Apply a Figure-Eight Bandage

**MEDIA LINK:** View the video, "Figure-Eight Bandage," for this chapter on the Premium Website.

**PURPOSE:** To apply a figure-eight bandage *NOTE*: This procedure describes how to apply a dressing to a wound and then cover it with a bandage.*

**EQUIPMENT:** Sterile dressing, bandage, gloves, scissors, tape, a proper waste receptacle, patient chart or EHR, pen

S **SKILL:** Demonstrate application of a figure-eight bandage.

| Procedure Steps | Detailed Instructions and/or *Rationales* |
|---|---|
| 1. Assemble the equipment and materials, wash hands, and put on gloves. | |
| B 2. Introduce yourself, identify the patient, and ***explain the procedure, using language the patient can understand.*** | *Ensures that you are performing the procedure on the correct patient. Giving patients an explanation helps allay any fears about the procedure.* |
| 3. Apply a dressing over the wound. | (*Omit step 3 to eliminate dressing application.) |
| 4. Anchor the bandage with one or two turns around the palm of the hand. | |
| 5. Roll the gauze diagonally across the front of the wrist and in a figure-eight pattern around the hand. | |
| 6. Cut the gauze and tape at the wrist. | Caution: Do not impair circulation. |
| B 7. ***Instruct patient in how to care for the bandage and to watch for signs of circulation impairment and infection.*** | The patient should be told to watch for redness, swelling, and sensation of pain or fever. Typed instructions should be given to the patient for follow-up care. |
| 8. Discard contaminated materials and gloves in a proper waste receptacle. | |
| 9. Wash hands. | |
| 10. Document. | |

### Charting Example

| | |
|---|---|
| 6-14-XX<br>1:25 PM | Figure-eight bandage applied to right hand. Patient education provided on how to keep the bandage clean and dry and to watch for signs of infection. C. Spatz, CCMA |

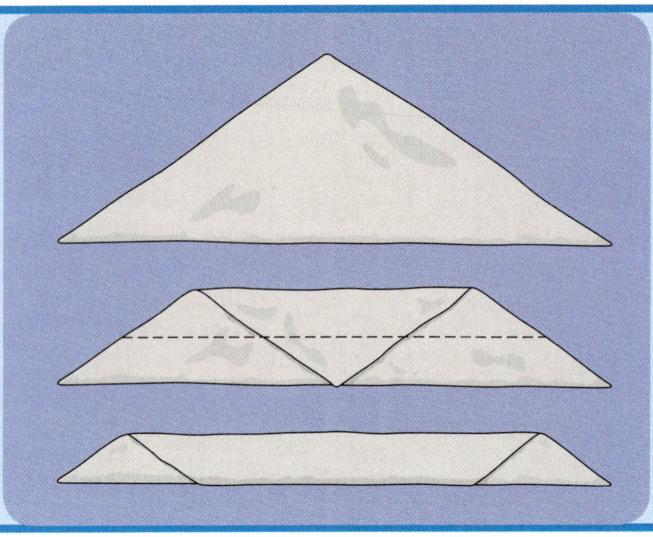

**Figure 56–19:** Folding a triangular bandage to make a cravat bandage. *Delmar/Cengage Learning.*

## PROCEDURE 56–5 Apply a Cravat Bandage to Forehead, Ear, or Eyes

**PURPOSE:** To apply a cravat bandage to the head *NOTE*: This procedure explains how to apply a dressing to a wound and then cover it with a cravat bandage.*

**EQUIPMENT:** Sterile dressing, cravat bandage, gloves, a proper waste receptacle, patient chart or EHR, pen

S **SKILL:** Demonstrate application of a cravat bandage to the head.

| Procedure Steps | Detailed Instructions and/or *Rationales* |
|---|---|
| 1. Assemble the equipment and materials, wash hands, and put on gloves. | |
| B 2. Introduce yourself, identify the patient, and ***explain the procedure, using language the patient can understand.*** | *Ensures that you are performing the procedure on the correct patient. Giving patients an explanation helps allay any fears about the procedure.* |
| 3. Apply a dressing over the wound. | (*Omit step 3 to eliminate dressing application.) |
| 4. Place the center of the cravat over the dressing. | |
| 5. Take the ends around to the opposite side of the head and cross them. Do not tie. | |
| 6. Bring the ends back to the starting point and tie them (Figure 56–20). | |
| B 7. ***Instruct patient in how to care for the bandage and to watch for signs of circulation impairment and infection.*** | The patient should be told to watch for redness, swelling, and sensation of pain or fever. Typed instructions should be given to the patient for follow-up care. |
| 8. Discard the contaminated materials and gloves in a proper waste receptacle. | |
| 9. Wash hands. | |
| 10. Document. | |

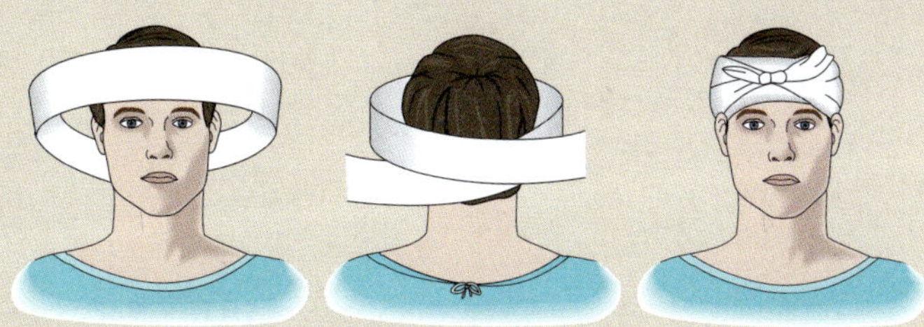

**Figure 56–20:** Applying a cravat bandage to the head. *Delmar/Cengage Learning.*

### Charting Example

| | |
|---|---|
| 8-28-XX<br>1:25 PM | Cravat bandage applied over dressing on head. Patient education provided on how to keep the bandage clean and dry and to watch for signs of infection. C. Spatz, CCMA |

## CHAPTER SUMMARY

- When deciding whether the situation warrants emergency medical care, an office visit, or management at home, ask the caller to give you a brief history of the victim's situation, the nature of the initial injury or accident, the time the accident occurred or the illness began, and a description of the victim's current condition.
- Remove a foreign body under the lower eyelid with a bit of cotton or a fold of tissue moistened with water. If a foreign body is under the upper lid, remove it by pulling the upper lid down over the lower lid. If this procedure is not successful, it might be necessary to grasp the eyelashes and carefully turn back the upper lid over a cotton swab.
- Placing several drops of warm olive oil, mineral oil, or baby oil into the ear and pulling back on the earlobe to straighten the external canal, letting the oil run out to see whether the object will come out with it is first aid for an object lodged in the ear.
- Being able to compare and contrast fractures and having knowledge of the various types will help you assist the provider and the patient.
- With animal and human bites, the wounds must be thoroughly cleansed with an antiseptic soap and rinsed well with water. The area should be bandaged and immobilized, and the patient should be examined by a provider as soon as possible to determine further treatment.
- Acute illness can occur in patients that are severely allergic to stings. The patient might become restless, complain of headache, have shortness of breath, or have mottled blueness of the skin. When shortness of breath is not apparent, the victim might appear to be in shock and have severe nausea, vomiting, and bloody diarrhea.
- Burns are classified by three methods: the percentage of body surface area (BSA) involved in the burn, the Rule of Nines, and the Lund and Browder chart. These methods establish a standard by which all injuries can be estimated.
- Hot and cold pack applications are often used in the treatment of injuries. The provider will give specific instructions concerning the length of time and where to apply the treatment.
- Wounds can be caused by trauma or surgical procedures. Open wounds are abrasions, avulsions, incisions, lacerations, and punctures, and closed wounds are contusions. You should be able to identify the wound type and provide patient teaching to identify infection of a wound.

## STUDY TOOLS

| | |
|---|---|
| **Workbook** | Activities for Chapter 56 |
| **Premium Website** | |
| MEDIA LINK | View these **Media Links** for Chapter 56:<br>• Clean Wound Areas<br>• Spiral Bandaging<br>• Figure-Eight Bandaging |
| StudyWARE | Activities and Quizzes on the **StudyWARE™ Software** for Chapter 56 |
| | Complete the following **Competency Challenge 2.0** activity:<br>• Thursday, 11 AM: Emergency Procedures |
| | **Audio Library** of medical terms |
| | Online access to the **Critical Thinking Challenge 2.0** |
| learninglab | Module 23: First Aid and Responding to Emergencies |
| **CourseMate** | Activities and Quizzes for Chapter 56 |
| **WebTutor** | Activities and Quizzes for Chapter 56 |

## CHECK YOUR KNOWLEDGE

1. With all human bites, a tetanus injection must be administered to the patient if he or she has not received one within:
   a. one year.
   b. five years.
   c. seven years.
   d. 10 years.
2. At least half of all dislocations involve which of the following body parts?
   a. Shoulder
   b. Wrist
   c. Ankle
   d. Knee
3. A ________ leaves the stinger in the skin, and it should be removed immediately by scraping it out carefully with a credit card or other rigid object.
   a. wasp
   b. hornet
   c. yellow jacket
   d. honeybee
4. Partial-thickness burns are also referred to as:
   a. first-degree burns.
   b. second-degree burns.
   c. third-degree burns.
   d. fourth-degree burns.
5. When using the PRINCE method on a strain or sprain, the injury should be treated with a cold pack for the first __________hours.
   a. 12–24
   b. 24–36
   c. 24–48
   d. 48–72
6. Which of the following types of wounds involves the skin being torn off and the wound bleeding profusely?
   a. Laceration
   b. Avulsion
   c. Abrasion
   d. Puncture
7. This type of fracture involves an open wound.
   a. Simple
   b. Closed
   c. Compound
   d. Both a and b are correct

## WEB LINKS

American Academy of Emergency Medicine: www.aaem.org

American Red Cross: www.redcross.org

National Center for Emergency Medicine Informatics: www.ncemi.org

National Institutes of Health: www.nih.gov

U.S. National Library of Medicine: www.nlm.nih.gov

WebMD: www.webMD.com

## RESOURCES

Beebe, R., and Funk, D. (2010). *Fundamentals of Emergency Care* (3rd ed.). Clifton Park, NY: Delmar Cengage Learning.

Estes, M. E. Z. (2010). *Health Assessment & Physical Examination* (3rd ed.). Clifton Park, NY: Delmar Cengage Learning.

Heller, M., and Veach, L. (2009). *Clinical Medical Assisting: A Professional, Field Smart Approach to the Workplace*. Clifton Park, NY: Delmar Cengage Learning.

Lindh, W., Pooler, M., Tamparo, C., and Dahl, B. (2010). *Delmar's Comprehensive Medical Assisting Administrative and Clinical Competencies* (4th ed.). Clifton Park, NY: Delmar Cengage Learning.

CHAPTER 11

# First Aid for Accidents and Injuries

## Words to Know Challenge

**Spelling: Each line contains three spellings of a word. Underline the correctly spelled word.**

| | | |
|---|---|---|
| 1. anafalactic | anaphylactic | aniphylactic |
| 2. avulsion | evulsion | avulzion |
| 3. cravat | cravet | cravette |
| 4. moltan | molten | moltin |
| 5. superficiel | superficial | superfisual |
| 6. thermel | theremal | thermal |

**Matching: Match the term in column I to its definition in column II.**

| | COLUMN I | COLUMN II |
|---|---|---|
| I | 1. Abrasion | A. Smooth cut |
| H | 2. Chemical | B. A brisk rubbing |
| G | 3. Electrical | C. A hole |
| B | 4. Friction | D. A tear |
| F | 5. Immobilize | E. An injury |
| D | 6. Incision | F. To prevent from moving |
| A | 7. Laceration | G. Having a current |
| C | 8. Puncture | H. Acid or alkaline substance |
| K | 9. Foreign body | I. A scrape or scratch |
| L | 10. Rabies | J. State of very low blood pressure, rapid pulse, pallor |
| J | 11. Shock | K. Not normally found in the location; splinter, dirt |
| M | 12. Splinter | L. Transmitted by an animal bite |
| E | 13. Wound | M. Thin, sharp piece of wood |

# Appendix A
## Measurements and Abbreviations

### CONVERTING MEASUREMENTS

| LENGTH | Centimeters | Inches | Feet |
|---|---|---|---|
| 1 centimeter | 1.000 | 0.394 | 0.0328 |
| 1 inch | 2.54 | 1.000 | 0.0833 |
| 1 foot | 30.48 | 12.000 | 1.000 |
| 1 yard | 91.4 | 36.00 | 3.00 |
| 1 meter | 100.00 | 39.40 | 3.28 |

| VOLUMES | Cubic Centimeters | Fluid Drams | Fluid Ounces | Quarts | Liters |
|---|---|---|---|---|---|
| 1 cubic centimeter | 1.00 | 0.270 | 0.033 | 0.0010 | 0.0010 |
| 1 fluid dram | 3.70 | 1.00 | 0.125 | 0.0039 | 0.0037 |
| 1 cubic inch | 16.39 | 4.43 | 0.554 | 0.0173 | 0.0163 |
| 1 fluid ounce | 29.6 | 8.00 | 1.000 | 0.0312 | 0.0296 |
| 1 quart | 946.0 | 255.0 | 32.00 | 1.000 | 0.946 |
| 1 liter | 1000.0 | 270.0 | 33.80 | 1.056 | 1.000 |

| WEIGHTS | Grains | Grams | Apothecary Ounces | Pounds |
|---|---|---|---|---|
| 1 grain (gr) | 1.000 | 0.064 | 0.002 | 0.0001 |
| 1 gram (gm) | 15.43 | 1.000 | 0.032 | 0.0022 |
| 1 apothecary ounce | 480.00 | 31.1 | 1.000 | 0.0685 |
| 1 pound | 7000.00 | 454.0 | 14.58 | 1.000 |
| 1 kilogram | 15432.0 | 1000.00 | 32.15 | 2.205 |

### RULES FOR CONVERTING ONE SYSTEM TO ANOTHER

#### Volumes

Grains to grams—divide by 15
Drams to cubic centimeters—multiply by 4
Ounces to cubic centimeters—multiply by 30
Minims to cubic millimeters—multiply by 63
Minims to cubic centimeters—multiply by 0.06
Cubic millimeters to minims—divide by 63
Cubic centimeters to minims—multiply by 16
Cubic centimeters to fluid ounces—divide by 30
Liters to pints—divide by 2.1

### Weights

Milligrams to grains—multiply by 0.0154
Grams to grains—multiply by 15
Grams to drams—multiply by 0.257
Grams to ounces—multiply by 0.0311

### Temperature

Multiply centigrade (Celsius) degrees by $\frac{9}{5}$ and add 32 to convert Fahrenheit to Celsius.
Subtract 32 from the Fahrenheit degrees and multiply by $\frac{5}{9}$ to convert Celsius to Fahrenheit.

## COMMON HOUSEHOLD MEASURES AND WEIGHTS

| | |
|---|---|
| 1 teaspoon | = 4–5 mL or 1 dram |
| 3 teaspoons | = 1 tablespoon |
| 1 dessert spoon | = 8 mL or 2 drams |
| 1 tablespoon | = 15 mL or 3 drams |
| 4 tablespoons | = 1 wine glass or ½ gill |
| 16 tablespoons (liq) | = 1 cup |
| 12 tablespoons (dry) | = 1 cup |
| 1 cup | = 8 fluid ounces or ½ pint |
| 1 tumbler or glass | = 8 fluid ounces or 240 mL |
| 1 wine glass | = 2 fluid ounces, 60 mL |
| 16 fluid ounces | = 1 pound |
| 4 gills | = 1 pound |
| 1 pint | = 1 pound |

## MEDICAL SYMBOLS

| | | | |
|---|---|---|---|
| O | pint | ′ | foot, minute |
| # | pound, number | ″ | inch, second |
| ℞ | recipe, prescription | ° | degree |
| ♂ | male | % | percent |
| ♀ | female | × | multiply |
| $\bar{s}$ | without | ÷ | divide |
| $\bar{c}$ | with | = | equals |
| – | minus, negative, alkaline reaction | ∞ | infinity |
| $\overline{aa}$ | equal parts | ↑ | increase |
| | | ↓ | decrease |

## ABBREVIATIONS

| | |
|---|---|
| a, aa | of each |
| abd | abdomen |
| a.c. | before meals |
| ad lib | as desired |
| A & P | anterior and posterior |
| aq | aqueous, water |
| | |
| b.i.d., BID | twice a day |
| bm, BM | bowel movement |
| BP, B/P | blood pressure |
| BUN | blood urea nitrogen |
| | |
| $\bar{c}$ | with |
| C | Celsius, centigrade |
| Ca | calcium |
| cap | capsule |
| CBC | complete blood count |
| CC | chief complaint |
| CCU | coronary care unit |
| CHF | congestive heart failure |
| CNS | central nervous system |
| c/o | complains of |
| $CO_2$ | carbon dioxide |
| comp | compound |
| COPD | chronic obstructive pulmonary disease |
| CPR | cardiopulmonary resuscitation |
| CSF | cerebrospinal fluid |
| CVA | cerebrovascular accident |
| cysto | cystoscopy |
| | |
| D & C | dilatation and curettage |
| Dil, dil | dilute |
| DOA | dead on arrival |
| DOB | date of birth |
| DPT | diphtheria, pertussis, tetanus |
| dx, Dx | diagnosis |
| | |
| ECG | electrocardiogram |
| EEG | electroencephalogram |
| EENT | eye, ear, nose, throat |
| EKG | electrocardiogram |
| elix | elixir |
| ER | emergency room |
| ext. | extract |
| | |
| F | fahrenheit |
| F | female |
| FBS | fasting blood sugar |
| FH | family history |
| fl | fluid |
| fl. oz. | fluid ounce |
| Fx | fracture |
| | |
| GB | gallbladder |
| GI | gastrointestinal |
| gm | gram |
| GP | general practitioner |
| gtt, Gtt, gtts | drop, drops |
| GU | genitourinary |
| GYN | gynecology |
| | |
| H, h | hour |
| HCL | hydrochloric acid |
| Hgb | hemoglobin |

| | |
|---|---|
| HPI | history present illness |
| Hx | history |
| ICU | intensive care unit |
| I & D | incision and drainage |
| IM | intramuscular |
| inj | injection |
| I & O | intake and output |
| IPPB | intermittent positive pressure breathing |
| IT | inhalation therapy |
| IUD | intrauterine device |
| IV | intravenous |
| IVP | intravenous pyelogram |
| k | potassium |
| KUB | kidney, ureter, and bladder |
| lat | lateral |
| lb | pound |
| liq | liquid |
| LLQ | left lower quadrant |
| LMP | last menstrual period |
| LUQ | left upper quadrant |
| M | male |
| mm | millimeter |
| MS | multiple sclerosis |
| NB | newborn |
| neg | negative |
| NKA | no known allergies |
| no. | number |
| noct | at night |
| NPO | nothing by mouth |
| N & V | nausea and vomiting |
| OB | obstetrics |
| OD | overdose |
| OP | outpatient |
| OR | operating room |
| os | mouth |
| oz | ounce |
| Path | pathology |
| PBI | protein bound iodine |
| p.c. | after meals |
| Peds | pediatrics |
| per | through, by |
| PID | pelvic inflammatory disease |
| PKU | phenylketonuria |
| PO, p.o. | by mouth |
| prn | as desired, needed |
| pro time | prothrombin time |
| Psych | psychiatry |
| pt | patient |
| pulv | powder |
| Px | physical examination |
| q | every |
| q (2, 3, 4) h | every (2, 3, 4) hours |
| qh | every hour |
| q.i.d., QID | four times a day |
| qns | quantity not sufficient |
| qs | quantity sufficient |
| qt | quart |
| R | right |
| Ra | radium |
| RBC | red blood cells |
| REM | rapid eye movement |
| rep | let it be repeated |
| R/O | rule out |
| ROM | range of motion |
| ROS | review of systems |
| Rx | prescription, take |
| $\bar{s}$ | without |
| sig | instructions, directions |
| SOB | shortness of breath |
| sol | solution |
| solv | solvent |
| s.o.s. | distress signal |
| sp. gr. | specific gravity |
| stat | immediately |
| syr. | syrup |
| T | temperature |
| T & A | tonsillectomy and adenoidectomy |
| tab | tablet |
| TIA | transient ischemic attack |
| t.i.d. | three times a day |
| tinct. | tincture |
| TPR | temperature, pulse, respiration |
| TUR | transurethral resection |
| UA | urinalysis |
| ung. | ointment |
| URI | upper respiratory infection |
| UTI | urinary tract infection |
| VD | venereal disease |
| VS | vital signs |
| WBC | white blood cells |
| WNL | within normal limits |
| wt., Wt. | weight |

# Glossary

**ABHES** Accrediting Bureau of Health Education Schools.
**abandonment** to desert, to give up entirely.
**abbess** a mother superior; a woman who is the head of an abbey of nuns.
**abbreviations** shortened form.
**abdomen** the cavity in the body between the diaphragm and the pelvis.
**abdominal** pertaining to the abdomen.
**abdominopelvic** pertaining to the anterior body cavity below the diaphragm.
**abduction** to move away from the midline.
**ablation** a surgical procedure using a resectoscope inserted into the uterus through the cervix.
**abortion** the termination of pregnancy; spontaneous or induced.
**abrasion** an injury caused by rubbing or scraping off the skin.
**abrupt** sudden; blunt, curt.
**absolute** free as to condition, unlimited in power.
**absorb** to suck or swallow up, to drink in.
**abstinent** refraining from use; being away from.
**absurd** contrary to sense or reason.
**abuse** to maltreat; to use wrongly.
**accelerator** increasing action or function.
**acceptance** agreeing verbally or in writing to the terms of a contract, which is one of the requirements of an enforceable contract.
**accept assignment** Provider agrees to accept the insurer's payment as payment in full for the service provided.
**accommodation** the process of the lens changing shape to permit close vision.
**account** record of all transactions made on an individual's financial record that lists debits, credits, and balance
**account history** the past financial record.
**accountant** one who keeps, audits, and inspects the financial records of individuals or businesses.
**accounting formula** The formula which is considered the basis for all financial accounting, which is assets minus liabilities equals net worth.
**accounts payable (A/P)** The total amounts owed by the practice to suppliers and other service providers for regular business operating expenses, such as medical office supplies and equipment, office rental space, utilities (gas and electric, water, telephone and/or internet services), and office staff salaries.
**accounts receivable (A/R)** money owed to the practice by patients.
**accounts receivable (A/R) ratio** The total dollar amount of the outstanding payments or claims due to the office from patients and customers.
**accreditation** a process in which an educational institution or program establishes credibility or legitimacy by complying with predetermined standards.
**accreditation** the assignment of credentials; approval given for meeting established standards.
**accredited** certified as being of a speciﬁced quality; accepted as valid.
**Accrediting Bureau of Health Education Schools (ABHES)** An accrediting body that provides programmatic accreditation for medical assisting and other healthcare programs.
**accumulated** to pile up; collect; gather.
**accuracy** correctness, exactness.
**accurate** correct, exact, without error.
**accurate and precise testing (APT)** refers to a standard for performing laboratory procedures to ensure reliability of results.
**acetylcholine** a hormone released at the parasympathetic and skeletal nerve endings.
**Achilles' tendon** a tendon attaching the gastrocnemius muscle of the leg to the heel.
**achromatic** a condition of total color blindness.
**acidosis** a disturbance of the acid–base balance of the body.
**acne valgaris** a skin condition characterized by inflammation of sebaceous glands and producing pimples.
**acquaintance** the state of knowing a person or subject.
**acquire** to gain by one's own efforts or actions; to get.
**acquired immunodeficiency syndrome (AIDS)** a viral disease that renders the immune system ineffective.
**acquisition** acquired by one's own efforts.
**acromegaly** a chronic condition characterized by enlargement of bones of the extremities and some bones of the head; thickening of facial soft tissues.
**acronym** a word formed from the initial letters of each major word in a term.
**action potential** the temporary electrical charge within a cell.
**activate** to make active or more active.
**active listening** participation in the conversation with another by paraphrasing words and phrases or giving approving or disapproving nods.
**acuity** refers to the sharpness or clearness of vision or hearing.
**Acupuncture** A procedure used to treat pain by inserting extremely thin, sterilized needles, sometimes electrified with low-voltage, along the network of 12 body meridians (channels) to connect the different levels from the organs to the skin.
**acupuncture** involves the insertion of needles at various points in the body to treat disease or relieve pain.
**acute** sharp, severe; having a rapid onset, severe symptoms, and a short course; not chronic.
**acute glomerulonephritis** the rapid onset of inflammation of the glomerulus of the kidney.
**acute phase** a period of increased symptoms and severity of the disease.
**acute renal failure** the sudden cessation of kidney function.
**adapt** the act of or the result of adjusting to a new circumstance or change.
**addiction** the state of being governed or controlled by a habit, as with alcohol or drugs.
**additive** a substance deliberately added to a material to fulfill some specific purpose such as enhancing taste or color or prolonging shelf life.
**additive effect** The combined actions of two or more drugs are the same as the sum of each action individually.
**adduction** to draw together toward the midline.
**adenitis** inflammation of lymph nodes or a gland.
**adequate** equal to the requirement or occasion, sufficient.
**adhere** to stick fast, become firmly attached; to be devoted to.
**adjective** a word added to (modifying) a noun to quantify or limit it.
**adjustment** credit entry made on an account to decrease a balance owed to the medical office; may be due to insurance, professional discounts, write-offs, or to correct bookkeeping errors
**adjustments** changes to fit or bring into harmony.

**administer** to manage; to conduct, as in business.
**administrative** duties that manage or direct activities; in medical assisting, refers to tasks other than clinical in nature; front office duties.
**Administrative Simplification Compliance Act (ASCA)** identifies limited situations where paper claim forms may be submitted for payment (rather than electronic submission); signed into law on December 27, 2001 as Public Law 107-105.
**administrative skills** skills that help to manage the business affairs of a medical practice and includes two categories—administrative procedures and practice finances.
**admissions clerk** a person who processes information and forms for a patient who will be entering the health facility.
**adrenal** pertaining to the adrenal glands, which sit atop each kidney.
**adrenaline** an internal secretion derived from the adrenal glands; can be commercially prepared from animal glands; acts as a stimulant.
**adrenocorticotropic hormone (ACTH)** a hormone secreted by the anterior lobe of the pituitary gland.
**advance beneficiary notice (ABN)** Document used to notify a Medicare beneficiary that it is either unlikely that Medicare will pay or certain that Medicare will not pay for the service they are going to be provided. Beneficiaries are required to sign this document if they wish to have the service with the understanding that they will be responsible for payment.
**advance directives** a living will; a document, written in advance, that states the patient's wishes regarding end-of-life care.
**advantageous** beneficial, profitable.
**adverb** a word added to (modifying) a verb, an adjective, or another adverb.
**adverse** opposed to; unfavorable.
**advocacy** Defending or supporting the rights or interests of another. In healthcare, specifically referring to those rights or interests of a patient or other vulnerable party.
**advocate** one who pleads for or defends a cause or a person.
**advocate** Someone who speaks for another person.
**aerobe** a microorganism that can live and grow only in the presence of oxygen.
**afebrile** without fever.
**affiliate** to unite, to join, or become connected.
**agar** a dried mucilaginous substance, or gelatin, extracted from algae, used as a culture medium.
**agent** one that acts or has the power or authority to act for another.
**aggression** pushiness, assuming the offensive without cause; forcefulness.
**aging of accounts** dividing accounts into categories according to the amount of time since the first billing date.
**agonist** A drug that binds to a receptor in order to produce or trigger a response.
**airborne** transported or carried through the air.
**Al-Anon** a support group for family members of alcoholics.
**alateen** a support for teenagers with an alcoholic parent.
**albino** a person who lacks pigment in the skin, hair, and eyes, either partial or total; a person with albinoism.
**alcohol** a liquid generated by the fermentation of sugar and other carbohydrates.
**alcoholic** an individual who uses alcohol to excess.
**Alcoholics Anonymous** an organization formed to assist alcoholics to refrain from the use of alcohol.
**alcoholism** a chronic, progressive, and potentially fatal disease characterized by tolerance and physical dependency on the ingestion of alcohol.
**aldosterone** a mineralocorticoid hormone secreted by the adrenal cortex.
**alignment** being in proper position.
**alimentary canal** the intestinal tract, from the esophagus to the rectum, and accessory organs.
**allege** to state positively but not under oath and without proof; to affirm.
**allergens** any substance which causes an allergic reaction.
**allergic rhinitis** inflammation of the nose caused by an allergy.
**allergist** a physician specializing in the care of patients with allergies.
**allergy** an altered or acquired state of sensitivity; abnormal reaction of the body to substances normally harmless.
**allosteric protein** a protein found in erythrocytes that transports oxygen in the blood; hemoglobin.
**alopecia** the loss of hair; baldness.
**Alpha-Fetoprotein Screening (AFP)** a blood test during pregnancy to detect birth defects.
**alpha search** look by alphabetical order.
**alternative** different from the usual or conventional.
**alternative therapy** a therapy that is used in place of conventional therapy—often this therapy is experimental or has not been approved as a credible therapy.
**altrusim** unselfish concern for the welfare of others.
**alveoli** microscopic air sacs in the lung.
**amber** orange/yellowish color.
**amblyopia** lazy eye; a condition characterized by the inward turning of the affected eye.
**ambulate** to walk, not be confined to bed.
**ambulatory** refers to walking, being mobile.
**amenity** pleasantness, pleasant ways, civilities.
**amenorrhea** absence of menses; without menstruation.
**American Academy of Professional Coders (AAPC)** An organization that promotes professionalism and encourage and support education, networking, and certification in the medical billing and coding areas.
**American Association of Medical Assistants (AAMA)** A professional organization for medical assistants that certifies medical assistants and provides continuing education opportunities.
**American Medical Technologists (AMT)** A professional organization that provides credentialing opportunities for medical assistants and continuing education opportunities.
**ammonia** strong-smelling inhalants used to revive a person who has fainted; also known as ammonia inhalants or spirits of ammonia.
**amnesia** loss of memory.
**amniocentesis** the use of a needle to withdraw amniotic fluid from the amniotic sac.
**amniotic** pertaining to the amniotic fluid within the amniotic membrane surrounding the fetus.
**amphetamine** a central nervous system stimulant, often referred to as an upper.
**amplifier** a device on an electrocardiograph that enlarges the ECG impulses.
**ampule** a small glass container that can be sealed and its contents sterilized.
**amputate** to cut off, remove a part.
**anaerobe** a microorganism having the ability to live without oxygen.
**anal** pertaining to the anus or outer rectal opening.
**analysis** the examination of anything to determine its makeup; a description of the process or the examination, point by point.
**analytical** characterized by a method of analysis, a statement of point-by-point examination.
**anaphylactic** a severe and rapid multisystem allergic reaction.
**anaphylaxis** a hypersensitive reaction of the body to a foreign protein or a drug; the term implies symptoms severe enough to produce serious shock, even death.
**anatomic** pertaining to the anatomy or structure of an organism.
**anatomical** the position with the human body upright, facing forward, with the palms facing toward the front of the body.
**anatomical position** the position with the human body upright, facing forward, with the palms facing toward the front of the body.
**anatomy** the study of the physical structure of the body and its organs.
**anchor** the attachment of a skeletal muscle; the wrapping at the start of a gauze or elastic bandage.

**anemia** a deficiency of red blood cells, hemoglobin, or both.
**aneroid** operating without a fluid; when used in reference to a sphygmomanometer, measuring by a dial instead of a mercury column.
**anesthesia** without sensation, with or without loss of consciousness.
**anesthesiologist** one who studies anesthiology.
**anesthesiology** the study of anesthesia.
**anesthetic** an agent that produces insensibility to pain or touch, either generally or locally.
**anesthetize** to cause a loss of sensation, loss of consciousness.
**aneurysm** a widening, external dilation caused by the pressure of blood on weakened arterial walls.
**angina** pain and oppression radiating from the heart to the shoulder and left arm; a feeling of suffocation.
**angiography** a radiologic study of an artery using a radiopaque medium.
**angioplasty** an invasive procedure to alter the interior of a blood vessel.
**angle** the inclination of two straight lines that meet in a point.
**annotate** to provide with explanatory notes.
**annotating** to provide critical or explanatory notes.
**annuity** a sum of money to be received yearly, either in a lump sum or by installments.
**anorexia (nervosa)** loss of appetite; with anorexia nervosa, loss of appetite for food not explainable by disease, which may be a part of psychosis.
**anorexic** one suffering from anorexia.
**antagonist** A drug that blocks the actions of a receptor or its intended ligand.
**antagonize** to annoy; to arouse opposition.
**antecubital** the inner surface of the arm at the elbow.
**anteflexed** abnormal bending forward.
**anterior** before or in front of.
**anteverted** a forward placement.
**antibody** a protein substance carried by cells to counteract the effect of an antigen.
**antibody-mediated** humoral immunity; when antibodies and complement work together to destroy antigens.
**anticipate** to predict, based on experience and training, situations or events that may be likely to occur, that may or may not require intervention.
**anticipation** expect, forsee.
**anticoagulant** a substance that prohibits the coagulation of blood.
**antigen** any immunizing agent that, when introduced into the body, may produce antibodies.
**antihistamine** a class of drugs used to counteract allergic reactions or cold symptoms.
**antiseptic** an agent that will prevent the growth or arrest the development of microorganisms.
**antitoxin** a protein that defends the body against toxins.
**anuria** the absence of urine.
**anus** the external opening of the anal canal.
**anxiety** a condition of mental uneasiness arising from fear or apprehension.
**aorta** the main trunk of the arterial system of the body.
**apex** the point, tip, or summit of anything; in reference to the heart, the point of maximum impulse of the heart against the chest wall.
**Apgar** refers to a method for assessing the condition of newborns.
**apical** referring to the apex.
**apnea** the absence of breathing.
**aponeurosis** extension of connective tissue beyond a muscle in round or flattened tendons; a means of insertion or origin of a flat muscle.
**apostrophe** a punctuation mark showing the absence of a letter or letters or possession.
**apothecaries** An early term for pharacist.
**apothocary** one who dispenses drugs and medicines.
**appearance** outward or visible persona that a person gives to other individuals.
**appearance** outward show.
**appendectomy** the excision of the appendix.
**appendicitis** inflammation of the appendix.
**appendicular** pertaining to the limbs or things that append (attach) to other parts.
**appointment** an engagement; a meeting at a particular time.
**apprehension** anticipation of something feared, dread; a mental conception.
**apprenticeship** a training or learning period; study under the guidance of a skilled, experienced worker.
**apprenticeship** a period of time when one is bound by agreement to learn some trade or craft.
**apprise** to inform.
**appropriate** correct, suitable.
**aqueous humor** a watery, transparent liquid that circulates between the anterior and posterior chambers of the eye.
**arachnoid** a delicate, lacelike membrane covering the central nervous system.
**arbitrary** depending on will or whim, self-willed; depending on choice or discretion.
**ardently** eagerly, passionately, intensely.
**areola** a ringlike coloration about the nipple of the breast.
**aromatherapy** the use of essential oils from plants for a therapeutic effect.
**arrhythmia** without rhythm; irregularity.
**arteriography** a radiologic study of an artery using a radiopaque medium.
**arterioles** small blood vessels connecting arteries with capillaries.
**arteriosclerosis** a degeneration and hardening of the walls of arteries.
**artery** a blood vessel carrying blood away from the heart, usually filled with oxygenated blood.
**arthritis** inflammation of a joint.
**articulate** to join together, as in a joint.
**artifact** something extraneous to what is being looked for. activity that causes interference on EKGs.
**artificial insemination** the mechanical placement of semen containing viable sperm into the vagina.
**ascending** referring to that portion of the colon that ascends from the lower right quadrant to the upper right quadrant of the abdomen.
**ascertain** to make certain.
**ascites** an abnormal accumulation of fluid in the abdomen.
**ASCLS** American Society for Clinical Laboratory Science.
**asepsis** a condition free of organisms.
**aseptic technique** means of performing tasks without contamination by organisms.
**aseptic technique** The process of maintaining sterility throughout a surgical procedure.
**asphyxiation** suffocation, loss of consciousness as the result of too little oxygen and too much carbon dioxide.
**aspiration** removal by suction.
**assault** physical harm; a violent attack.
**assertive** Confident, persistent manner of communicating one's thoughts and ideas, in a positive manner.
**assess** to determine, to appraise the condition or state.
**assets** anything owned that has exchange value, all the entries on a balance sheet that show the property or resources of a person or business.
**associate's degree** a degree granted by a junior college at the end of a two-year course.
**asthma** an allergic reaction to a substance resulting in wheezing, shortness of breath, and difficulty in breathing.
**astigmatism** blurring of the vision caused by an abnormal curvature of the cornea.
**asymmetry** lack of same size, shape, and position of parts or organs on opposite sides.
**atelectasis** lack of air in the lungs caused by the collapse of the alveoli of the lungs.
**atherosclerosis** fatty degeneration of the walls of the arteries.
**atmosphere** any surrounding influence.
**atria** the upper chambers of the heart.
**atrial depolarization** the excitement and contraction caused by the SA node at the beginning of the cardiac cycle.
**atrioventricular** see **AV node.**

**atrium** cardiac auricle; the upper chamber of the heart.
**atrophy** wasting away of a muscle.
**attachment** the point at which something attaches or originates.
**attenuated** diluted; to reduce virulence of a pathogenic organism.
**at the time of service (ATOS)** when service is rendered; real time.
**attitude** state of thought or feeling.
**attribute** quality or characteristic; to give credit for.
**atypical** deviated from normal.
**audible** loud enough to be heard.
**audiometer** a device to measure the degree of hearing ability.
**audiometry** testing of the hearing sense.
**audit** inspection.
**audit trail** a record of transaction that identifies which what person or persons and at what time and day an electronic record was accessed in order to maintain accountability for the security of the information as it is accessed.
**auditory** pertaining to the sense of hearing; the external canal of the ear.
**augmented** refers to leads 4, 5, and 6 of the standard 12-lead ECG tracing; these leads are of different voltage.
**aural** the ear; temperature measurement using tympanic infrared scanner.
**auscultate** to listen for sounds produced by the body.
**auscultation** the process of listening for sounds within the body.
**authorization** the giving of authority.
**authorize** to give permission.
**autoclave** a pressurized device designed to heat aqueous solutions above their boiling point to achieve sterilization. It was invented by Charles Chamberland in 1879.
**autoimmune** a condition wherein the person's antibodies react against their own normal tissues.
**autologous** given by oneself.
**automated teller machine (ATM)** a banking machine operated by inserting a credit or bank card and entering a personal identification number (PIN) code. Deposits, transfers, withdrawals, and other banking functions can be performed at the ATM location 24 hours a day, seven days a week.
**automation** behavior in an automatic or mechanical fashion.
**autonomic** spontaneous; the part of the nervous system concerned with reflex control of bodily functions.
**autonomous** self-governing.
**autonomy** independence or freedom of an individual's will; the right to choose
**autotrophs** microorganisms that feed on inorganic matter.
**auxiliary** to provide aid.
**AV node** atrioventricular node; the beginning of the bundle of his in the right atrium; nerve fibers responsible for the contraction of the ventricles.
**avulsion** an injury in which a body structure is forcibly detached
**axial** pertaining to the spinal column, skull, and rib cage of the skeleton.
**axilla** the underarm area, armpit.
**axillary** referring to the underarm area.
**axon** an extension from a nerve cell.
**ayurvedic** the traditional healing system of India that may be the oldest formal medical system in the world.
**ayuredic medicine** traditional healing system of India that addresses mental and spiritual well-being and physical health. ayurveda identifies three types of energies that are present in all things: vata, pitta, and kapha and believe that imbalances in any of these areas can cause disease.

**bacteria** unicellular microorganism concerned with the fermentation and putrefaction of matter; disease-causing agent.
**balance** to bring into or keep in equilibrium; to have equal weight and power.
**balance sheet** Also known as a "statement of financial position" that reveals a company's assets, liabilities and owner's equity (net worth).
**bandage** a piece of cloth used to hold a dressing in place, to support a body part; provide compression, or to protect from external contamination.
**bankruptcy** the state of being bankrupt, being legally declared unable to pay debts.
**barbiturate** a sedative or hypnotic drug, also known as a downer.
**barrier** to prevent access; bar passage.
**barter** to give one thing in exchange for another.
**bartholin's glands** two small mucous glands, situated one on each side of the vaginal opening at the base of the labia minora.
**baseline** the initial information on which additional data is based.
**basophil** a granulated white blood cell.
**battery** any illegal beating of another person.
**behaviors** a term used to describe professional characteristics or attitudes that are expected in particular professions.
**beneficence** the doing of good for another; the act of caring
**benefits** anything that promotes or enhances well-being.
**benign** nonmalignant; not cancerous.
**benign hypertrophy** nonmalignant enlargement.
**bereavement** sadness as a result of death of a loved one.
**bereavement time** time that an employee can take off when a family member or very close friend dies.
**beriberi** a disease resulting from lack of vitamin B, thiamine.
**Beyond a reasonable doubt** being sure of a criminal defendant's guilt to a moral certainty.
**Biases** A person's slant toward a particular belief.
**biceps** the muscle of the upper arm that flexes the forearm.
**biconvex** the curving out on both sides.
**bicuspid** heart valve between the left atrium and left ventricle, also known as the mitral valve.
**biennially** happening once in 2 years.
**bile** a secretion of the liver; a greenish-yellow fluid with a bitter taste.
**bilirubin** a yellow breakdown product of normal heme catabolism. its levels are elevated in certain diseases, and it is responsible for the yellow color of bruises and the brown color of feces.
**bimanual** two-handed; with both hands.
**bimonthly** occurring once in 2 months.
**binge** a spree; to overindulge, such as with alcohol or food.
**binocular** pertaining to the use of both eyes; possessing two eyepieces as with a microscope.
**biochemistry** a science concerned with the chemistry of plants and animals.
**biofeedback** a method, usually with the help of electronic equipment, that enables a person to learn to control otherwise involuntary bodily functions.
**biofeedback** a method that enables a person, usually with the help of electronic equipment, to learn to control otherwise involuntary bodily functions.
**biohazard** organism, or substance derived from an organism, that poses a threat to (primarily) human health.
**biohazardous** any material that has been in contact with body fluid and is potentially capable of transmitting disease.
**biopsy** excision of a small piece of tissue for microscopic examination.
**birthday rule** a means to identify primary responsibility in insurance coverage.
**bizarre** odd, unusual, strikingly out of the ordinary.
**bladder** a membranous sac or receptacle for a secretion; the gallbladder, urinary bladder.
**bleb** an elevation of the epidermis; a blister; in the lungs refers to a bubble-like structure from destroyed alveoli.
**bloodborne** capable of being transported in blood.
**blood pressure** the amount of force exerted by the heart on the blood as it pumps the blood through the arteries.
**body mass index (BMI)** a measure of body fat that is the ratio of the weight of the body in kilograms to the square of its height in meters.
**body mechanics** the use of appropriate body positioning when moving and lifting objects to avoid injury.
**body surface area (BSA)** refers to the total surface of the human body.
**bolus** a mass of masticated food ready to be swallowed.

**bonding** the attachment of two persons; the relationship between a parent and a baby.
**bookkeeper** one who records the accounts and transactions of a business.
**booster** a subsequent injection of immunizing substance to increase or renew immunity.
**bowel** refers to intestines.
**bowman's capsule** part of the renal corpuscle; surrounds the glomerulus of the nephron.
**brachial** refers to the brachial artery in the arm; the artery used in measuring blood pressure.
**brachytherapy** a type of radiation therapy that places radioactive isotopes in or near the tumor.
**bradycardia** slow heart rate.
**braille** printing for the blind, using a system of raised dots.
**brain scan** a diagnostic test using a scanner to measure radioisotopes within the brain.
**breach** violation of a law, contract, or other agreement.
**brochure** a small pamphlet or booklet of information.
**bronchi** the primary divisions of the trachea.
**bronchiole** small terminal branches of the bronchi that lack cartilage.
**bronchitis** inflammation of the mucous membranes of the bronchial tree.
**bruit** an adventitious sound of venous or arterial origin heard on auscultation; usually refers to the sound produced by the mixing of arterial and venous blood at dialysis shunts.
**BSA** see **body surface area.**
**buccal** the mouth; oral cavity.
**bulbourethral glands** two small glands, one on each side of the prostate gland, terminating in the urethra by way of a duct.
**bulimia nervosa** a condition characterized by alternating periods of overeating followed by forced vomiting and the use of laxatives to remove food from the body.
**bundle** a number of things bound together.
**bunion** a bursa with a callus formation.
**bursa** a sac or pouch in connective tissue chiefly around joints.
**business associate agreement (BAA)** an agreement with a company that ensures the company understands the person's expectations as to what the company will do with the privileged information they will have access to and the consequences of an inappropriate disclosure.

**CAAHEP** Commission on Accreditation of Allied Health Education Programs.
**caduceus** the wand of hermes or mercury; used as a symbol of the medical profession.
**caduceus** a medical symbol depicted by a staff with a serpent coiled around its shaft
**calculate** to compute.
**calculator** an electronic or mechanical device for the performance of mathematical computations.
**calculi** commonly called stones; usually composed of mineral salts.
**calibration** a set of graduated markings to indicate values.
**callus** in fractures, refers to the formation of new osseous material around the fracture site.
**calorie** a unit for measuring the heat value of food.
**calyces** two or more calyx.
**calyx** the cuplike division of the kidney pelvis.
**cancellation** to strike out by crossing with lines; marking a postage stamp or check or to delete an appointment or event.
**cancellous** a latticework structure, as the spongy tissue of bone.
**cancer** a malignant tumor or growth; specifically the hyperplasia of cells with infiltration and destruction of tissue.
**cancerous** refers to a malignant growth.
**cannula** a tube or sheath enclosing a trocar (triangular bore needle); after insertion, the trocar is removed.
**capacity** having the mental competency to make health care decisions, or execute a will at the time the will was signed and witnessed. The decision-maker must understand the nature of the decision and be aware of the potential risks.
**capillary** a microscopic blood vessel connecting arterioles and venules.
**capitation** a structure of payment based on the number served.
**caption** heading, title, or subtitle.
**carbohydrate** an organic combination of carbon, hydrogen, and oxygen as a sugar, a starch, or cellulose.
**carbon dioxide** a gas found in the air, exhaled by all animals; the chemical formula is $CO_2$.
**carbon monoxide** a colorless, odorless, poisonous gas caused by the incomplete combustion of carbon.
**carboxyhemoglobin** combined carbon monoxide and hemoglobin in red blood cells.
**carbuncle** a staphylococcal infection following furunculosis, characterized by a deep abscess of several follicles with multiple draining points.
**carcinoembryonic antigen** a tumor marker that can be detected in the blood when tested.
**carcinogen** cancer-causing agent.
**carcinoma** a malignant tumor from epithelial tissue.
**cardiac** pertaining to the heart.
**cardiac sphincter** the muscle that encircles the esophagus where it enters the stomach.
**cardinal signs** principal signs: temperature, pulse, respiration, and blood pressure.
**cardiologist** a physician specializing in the care of patients with diseases of the heart.
**cardiology** the study of the heart and its diseases.
**cardiopulmonary resuscitation (CPR)** a combination of rescue breathing and chest compressions delivered to victims thought to be in cardiac arrest
**cardiovascular** pertaining to the heart and blood vessels.
**caregiver** the person responsible for another's care and well-being.
**carotid** pertaining to the carotid artery.
**carpal** bone of the wrist.
**carpal tunnel syndrome (CTS)** the symptoms associated with the entrapment of the median nerve within the carpal bones and the transverse ligament at the wrist.
**carrel** a small, partitioned space.
**carrier** one who carries, transports; with insurance, it's the company who provides the policy.
**cartilage** a strong, tough, elastic tissue forming part of the skeletal system; precalcified bone in infants and young children.
**CAT scan** see **computerized transaxial tomography.**
**cataract** an opacity of the lens of the eye resulting in blindness.
**catarrhal** pertaining to inflammation of mucous membranes; causing severe spells of coughing with little or no expectoration.
**catarrhal stage** inflammation of the mucous membranes.
**catastrophic** of great consequence; disastrous.
**categorize** to arrange by class or kind; to place like things together.
**catheterization** to insert a catheter into a cavity (for example, urinary bladder to remove urine) to remove body fluid.
**caudal** pertaining to any taillike structure.
**caustic** capable of burning; an agent that will destroy living tissue.
**cauterize** to burn with an electrical cautery or chemical substance.
**cautery** an iron or caustic used to burn tissue.
**cavities** a hollow space, such as within the body or organs.
**cecum** the beginning of the ascending portion of the large intestine that forms a blind pouch at the junction with the small intestine.
**celiac disease** dilation of the small and large intestines.
**cell** structural and functional unit of all living organisms; sometimes called the building block of life.
**cell-mediated** direct cellular response to antigens.

**cell membrane** the structure that surrounds and encloses a cell.
**central** situated at or related to a center.
**centrifuge** a machine for the separation of heavier materials from lighter ones through the use of centrifugal force.
**centriole** an organelle within the cell.
**cerebellum** lower or back brain below the posterior portion of the cerebrum.
**cerebral** pertaining to the cerebrum of the brain.
**cerebrospinal** referring to the brain and spinal cord.
**cerebrospinal fluid** the liquid that circulates within the meninges of the spinal cord and ventricles and meninges of the brain.
**cerebrovascular accident** a stroke; hemorrhage in the brain.
**cerebrum** the largest part of the brain. It is divided into two hemispheres with four lobes in each hemisphere.
**certificate** a written declaration of some fact.
**certificate of completion** a document awarded upon fulfillment of a program's criteria.
**certificate of waiver** refers to a list of basic laboratory tests that may be performed in the physician's office by nonlaboratory personnel.
**certification** written declaration.
**certified** holding a certificate; being certificated; guaranteed in writing.
**Certified Clinical Medical Assistant (CCMA)** credential given by the National Healthcare Association(NHA) after eligible candidates pass the certification exam.
**Certified Medical Administrative Assistant (CMAA)** credential given by the National Healthcare Association(NHA) after eligible candidates pass the certification exam.
**Certified Medical Assistant, CMA (AAMA)** the credential given by the American Association of Medical Assistants (AAMA) to eligible candidates that pass the CMA(AAMA) examination.
**certified ophthalmic technician (COT)** a person trained and certified in diagnostic testing procedures and limited examination of the eye.
**cerumen** waxlike brown secretion found in the external auditory canal.
**cervical** pertaining to the neck portion of the spinal column; also to the entrance into the uterus.
**cervicitis** an inflammation of the cervix of the uterus.
**cervix** the entrance into the uterus.
**cesarean** surgical removal of an infant from the uterus.
**cessation** ceasing or discontinuing.
**chaos** a state of complete confusion; disorder.
**charge slip** see encounter form.
**charting** the recording of observations, subjective and objective findings, diagnostic procedures, treatments, and other pertinent data in the patient file.
**chemical** a simple or compound substance used in chemical processes.
**chemotherapy** the use of chemical agents in the treatment of disease, usually associated with cancer therapy.
**cheyne-stokes** a breathing pattern characterized by alternating periods of apnea and hyperventilation.
**chief complaint** the main reason for seeking medical care.
**Chief complaint, History, Examination, Details, Drugs/Dosages, Assessment, and Return visit (CHEDDAR)** Acronym that provides a structured charting method for data acquired during a routine healthcare visit; it encourages more detailed of the information obtained during the patient interview and examination.
**chiropractic** a system of healing based upon the theory that disease results from a lack of normal nerve function; treatment by scientific manipulation and specific adjustment of body structures, such as the spinal column.
**chiropractor** a health care provider who uses chiropractic methods to treat patients.
**chlamydia** a sexually transmitted disease caused by a bacteria that lives as an intracellular parasite.
**chloroform** a liquid compound that yields a gas that dulls pain and causes unconsciousness.
**cholecystectomy** surgical removal of the gallbladder.
**cholecystolithiasis** an abnormal presence of stones in the gallbladder.
**cholelithiasis** stones in the gallbladder.
**cholenergic** nerve fibers capable of secreting acetylcholine.
**cholera** an acute, specific, infectious disease characterized by diarrhea, painful cramps of muscles, and a tendency to collapse.
**cholesterol** a sterol present in the tissues which contributes to heart disease when elevated; transported in the blood plasma of all animals.
**chorionic gonadotropin** a hormone detectable in the urine of a pregnant female soon after conception.
**choroid** the vascular coat of the eye between the sclera and the retina.
**chromosome** structures within the cell's nucleus that store hereditary information.
**chronic** continuing a long time, returning; not acute.
**chronic glomerulonephritis** the slow, progressive destruction of the glomerulus of the kidney.
**chronic leukemia** a form of leukemia characterized by insidious onset and slower progress.
**chronic obstructive pulmonary disease (COPD)** a syndrome characterized by chronic bronchitis, asthma, and emphysema, or any combination of these conditions, resulting in dyspnea, frequent respiratory infections, and thoracic deformities from attempting to breathe.
**chronic renal failure** the end result of the progressive loss of kidney function.
**chronologic** the arrangement of events, dates, etc., in order of occurrence.
**chyme** the mixture of partially digested food and digestive secretions found in the stomach and small intestines during digestion of a meal.
**cilia** hairlike projections from epithelial cells, as in the bronchi.
**circulatory** refers to the circulatory system; the process of blood flowing through the vessels to all the cells of the body.
**circumcision** surgical removal of the foreskin of the penis.
**circumference** the distance around a circle; with mensurations, the measurement of the head.
**circumversion** rotation of an extremity in a circular motion.
**cirrhosis** an interstitial inflammation with hardening of the tissues of an organ, especially the liver.
**civil law** pertaining to the rights of private individuals; legal proceedings concerning rights that are not criminal.
**clarity** clearness, absence of cloudiness.
**classified** arranged in a group or classification according to some system.
**clause** part of a sentence with a subject and a predicate.
**claustrophobia** an abnormal fear of being in enclosed or confined places.
**clavicle** the collar bone, articulating with the sternum and scapula.
**clearinghouse** a private or public company that often serves as the middleman between physicians and billing groups, payers and other health care partners for the transmission and translation of electronic claims information into the specific format required by payers
**CLIA** see **Clinical Laboratory Improvement Amendments.**
**clinical** based on observation; in medical assisting, pertains to duties considered "back office"; not administrative in nature.
**clinical diagnosis** identification of a disease by history, laboratory findings, and symptoms.
**Clinical Laboratory Improvement Amendments (CLIA)** legislation dealing with the operation of a clinical laboratory.
**clinical skills** these are skills that are an extension of the provider's responsibilities and can be divided into fundamental practices, diagnostic procedures and patient care.
**clitoris** an erectile organ located at the anterior junction of the labia minora.

**clonal** the duplicated copy; with immunity it is the cells produced to attack antigens.
**clone** an exact copy.
**CMS-1500 form** the standard claim form designed by the centers for medicare and medicaid services to submit physician services for third-party (insurance companies) payment
**coagulation** lessening of the fluidity of a liquid substance; clotting or curdling.
**coccyx** the tailbone; the last four bones of the spine.
**cochlea** the snail-shaped portion of the inner ear.
**coercion** to force or compel; to restrain or constrain by force.
**coinsurance** a percentage that a patient is responsible for paying for each service after the deductible has been met.
**coitus** sexual intercourse between a man and a woman.
**colitis** inflammation of the colon.
**collaborate** to work together.
**collateral** subordinate, secondary; property deposited as security for a loan.
**colleague** an associate at work, usually one of similar status.
**collections ratio** a formula that determines how efficiently and timely an office is collecting payments for services rendered by the physicians.
**colon** the large intestine.
**colorimeter** an instrument used for measuring the amount of pigments and determining the amount of hemoglobin in the blood.
**colostomy** incision of the colon for the purpose of making a more or less permanent opening.
**colposcopy** a diagnostic examination to visualize the cervix through a colposcope.
**coma** an abnormal deep stupor from which a person cannot be aroused by external stimuli.
**coma scale** refers to the Glascow Coma Scale used to determine level of consciousness.
**combining forms** in medical terminology, the word root with a combining form vowel (usually an "o") that aids in making the word pronounceable, particularly when adding a suffix that begins with a consonant.
**comminuted** a crushed bone fracture with many fragments.
**commiserate** to feel or express sympathy or pity for.
**Commission on Accreditation of Allied Health Education Programs (CAAHEP)** an accrediting body that provides programmatic accreditation for medical assisting and other healthcare programs.
**common bile duct** a duct carrying bile from the hepatic and cystic ducts to the duodenum.
**Common law** the traditional unwritten law of england, based on custom and usage, which began to develop over a thousand years before the founding of the united states. today, almost all common law has been enacted into statutes with modern variations by all the states except louisiana, which is still influenced by the napoleonic code. in some states, the principles of common law are so basic they are applied without reference to statute.
**commonality** people in general; a body corporate or its membership.
**communicable** capable of being transmitted from one person or species to another, also known as contagious.
**communication** the act of communicating; information given; a means of giving information.
**comorbidity** a condition that exists along with the primary diagnosis of a patient.
**compatible** able to be mixed or taken together without destructive changes (as in blood typing and cross-matching); matching; not opposed to.
**compensate** to make amends; be equivalent to.
**compensation** anything given as an equivalent or to make amends; pay.
**compensatory damages** damages recovered in payment for actual injury or economic loss, which does not include punitive damages (as added damages due to malicious or grossly negligent action).
**competency** demonstrated capability, being able; a task to achieve.
**competent** fit, able, capable.
**complement** a group of about 20 inactive enzyme proteins present in the blood.
**complementary** something that will add to or make another thing complete or whole.
**complete blood count** a test requested by a doctor or other medical professional that gives information about the cells in a patient's blood; also known as a CBC; amongst the most commonly performed blood tests in medicine.
**complexity** the state of being complicated.
**compliance** consent; conformity to formal or official requirements.
**complicated** not simple, involved; having many parts; not easy to solve.
**complimentary** express appreciation; given without charge.
**complimentary therapy** therapy used in addition to traditional therapies.
**compose** to form by putting together, creating.
**compound** not simple, composed of two or more parts; with fractures, refers to bone fragments piercing the skin externally.
**comprehensive** covering all areas; inclusive.
**compression** to exert force against, press.
**Computed Transaxial Tomography (CAT)** computed axial tomography, a medical imaging method employing tomography in which digital geometry processing is used to generate a three-dimensional image of the internals of an object from a large series of two-dimensional x-ray images taken around a single axis of rotation.
**computer** a mechanical, electric, or electronic device that stores numerical or other information and provides logical answers at high speed to questions bearing on that information.
**computerized** to store in a computer; to put in a form a computer can use; to bring computers into use to control an operation.
**Computerized Axial Tomography (CAT)** a series of x-ray views of the body used to construct a three-dimensional picture.
**conceal** to hide, to keep secret, to withhold, as information.
**conceive** to become pregnant; the uniting of the sperm and ovum.
**conception** the union of the sperm of a male and the egg of a female; fertilization.
**conceptualize** to form a concept, thought, notion, or understanding.
**concise** condensed, short.
**condenser** part of a microscope substage that regulates the amount of light directed on a specimen.
**confidential** revealed in confidence; secret information.
**confidential** being prudent and conscious—especially in regards to speech.
**Confidential Communication Preference (CCP) form** a form a patient signs which authorizes other individuals to receive information regarding the patient's care. Individuals not listed will not be permitted to receive or ask for such information.
**confidentiality** to be held in confidence; a secret.
**confinement** restriction within certain limits.
**confirmation** making firm or sure; convincing proof.
**confirmed** verified or ratified.
**confirmed** Verification of authenticity
**conflict** a clash of opinions or interests; a fight or struggle; an inner moral struggle; to come into opposition.
**confrontation** to stand face to face with.
**congenital** existing at birth.
**congestive heart failure** a complex condition of inadequate heart action with retention of tissue fluids; may be either right- or left-side failure, or both.
**congratulations** to express pleasure; a recognition of accomplishment.
**conjunction** meeting; a word that connects.

**conjunctiva** a mucous membrane that lines the eyelids and covers the anterior sclera of the eyeball.
**connective** that which connects or binds together; one of the five main tissues of the body.
**connotations** something implied or suggested.
**consciousness** awareness, full knowledge of what is in one's own mind.
**consecutive** following in order, successive.
**consecutively** a series of things that follow each other.
**conserve** to keep from damage or loss; to maintain.
**consideration** a vital element in the law of contracts, consideration is a benefit which must be bargained for between the parties, and is the essential reason for a party entering into a contract. consideration must be of value and is exchanged for the performance or promise of performance by the other party.
**constipation** a sluggish action of the bowel; usually refers to an excessively firm, hard stool that is difficult to expel or lack of a bowel movement over a time.
**constrict** to narrow; to become smaller because of contraction of a sphincter muscle.
**contact dermatitis** inflammation and irritation of the skin caused by contact with an irritating substance.
**contagious** catching; able to be transmitted by contact.
**contaminate** to place in contact with microorganisms.
**contemporary** happening or existing at the same time; a person living at the same time as another.
**content** the matter dealt with in a field of study; matter contained.
**context** the part of a written or spoken statement that surrounds a particular word or passage and can clarify its meaning.
**continuity of care** the delivery of services provided to a person that proceeds without a lapse or interruption, with the intended purpose of maintaining a level of health and treatment
**contraception** against conception.
**contract** to draw together, reduce in size, or shorten.
**contraction** the muscle action of the uterus during labor; in spelling and punctuation, the shortening of a word by the omission of one or more letters, which are replaced with an apostrophe.
**contracture** permanent shortening or contraction of a muscle.
**contradiction** to deny; to assert to the contrary of.
**contrast** to show difference; in radiology, refers to a radiopaque medium used to outline body organs.
**contrast media** a substance used to enhance the visibility of structures or fluids within the body for medical imaging
**contributory** giving a share; helping toward a result.
**contributory factors** Additional components that can be considered when selecting an evaluation and management code: time, nature of presenting problem, counseling and coordination of care.
**Control** testing of machines and testing kits in the laboratory to detect any deficiencies prior to testing patient specimens.
**controversial** open to dispute; relating to discussion of opposing views.
**conventional** growing out of custom; not spontaneous.
**convey** to impart, as an idea; to transfer.
**convulsion** attack of involuntary muscular contractions often accompanied by unconsciousness.
**cooperate** to work together.
**coordination** a state of harmonious adjustment or function.
**coordination of benefits** when both spouses have health care insurance, the policy provision that limits benefits to 100% of the cost; also known as dual coverage.
**coordinator** a person who works for harmonious functioning of parts or agents toward the production of a desired result.
**COPD** see **chronic obstructive pulmonary disease.**
**cornea** the transparent extension of the sclera that lies in front of the pupil of the eye.
**coronal** the plane dividing the body into front and back portions.
**coronal (plane)** a line drawn through the side of the body from head to toe, making a front and back section.
**coronary** referring to the arteries surrounding the heart muscle; also refers to a "heart attack," which involves the coronary arteries.
**coroner** an official who investigates a sudden, suspicious, or violent death to determine the cause. In some communities this position has been replaced by the medical examiner.
**corpus luteum** the yellow body that develops in the ruptured graafian follicle after the ovum has been discharged.
**correspondence** communication by the exchange of letters.
**cortex** the outer portion of the kidney.
**corticosteroids** hormones used to treat inflammation.
**cost ratio** a formula that demonstrates a cost of a specific procedure or service.
**cost-benefit analysis** an analysis which allows for program evaluation by demonstrating whether the benefits received will outweigh its costs.
**COT** see **certified ophthalmic technician.**
**countershock** (in cardiology) a high-intensity, short-duration, electric shock applied to the area of the heart, resulting in total cardiac depolarization.
**courteous** polite, considerate, and respectful in manner and action.
**CPT** see **Current Procedural Terminology.**
**cramp** a spasmodic, painful contraction of a muscle or muscles.
**cranial** pertaining to the cranium or skull.
**cranium** the skull; the eight bones of the head enclosing the brain; generally applied to the 28 bones of the head and face.
**cravat** a triangular bandage, folded lengthwise; it may be used as a circular, figure-eight, or spiral bandage to control bleeding or to tie splints in place
**credit balance** occurs when the amount paid is greater than was due or the account is being paid in advance of service provided.
**crenated** notched or scalloped, as the crenated condition of blood corpuscles.
**cretinism** a congenital condition caused by the lack of the hormone thyroxin.
**criminal law** of, involving, or having the nature of a crime.
**crisis** the turning point of a disease; a very critical period; an emergency situation.
**criterion** a standard of criticism or judgment (plural: criteria).
**critical thinking** using deductive reasoning to examine a problem or issue from a variety of different angles in order to arrive at the most appropriate conclusion and using that information in order to guide behaviors.
**critique** a critical examination of a thing or situation, to determine its nature, worth, or conformity to standards.
**crohn's disease** an inflammation of the GI tract with debilitating symptoms.
**cross-match** a blood test used to ensure compatibility of the donor to the recipient when transfusing blood.
**crutches** staffs with a cross-piece at the top to place under the arms of a lame person.
**cryosurgery** the use of a substance at subfreezing temperature to destroy or remove tissue.
**cryptorchidism** failure of the testicles to descend into the scrotum.
**CTD** see **cumulative trauma disorder.**
**CTS** see **carpal tunnel syndrome.**
**cultivate** to form and refine; to improve.
**culture** a method of growing a microbial organism to determine what it is, its abundance in the sample being tested, or both. It is one of the primary diagnostic methods of microbiology.
**cumulative trauma disorder (CTD)** an injury resulting from repetitive movement of a body part.
**curette** an instrument to scrape material from a cavity.

**currency** any form of money.
**current** happening now; of the present time; the latest information.
**Current Procedural Terminology (CPT)** a numerical listing of procedures performed in medical practice; a standardized identification of procedures. Published by the american medical association.
**curriculum** a course of study at a school or university.
**cushing's syndrome** a disorder resulting from the hypersecretion of glucocorticoids from the adrenal cortex.
**cusp** a sharp point or apex.
**customarily** by custom, the usual course of action under similar circumstances.
**cyanosis** a bluish discoloration of the skin caused by lack of oxygen.
**cyst** a bladder; any sac containing fluid.
**cystic** pertaining to a cyst; of disease, refers to a condition with multiple cysts.
**cystic fibrosis** a disease condition of fibrous tumors that have undergone cystic degeneration, accumulating fluid in the interspaces; also known as fibrocystic disease.
**cystitis** inflammation of the urinary bladder.
**cystoscope** an instrument for examining the interior of the urinary bladder.
**cystoscopy** a diagnostic procedure performed with a cystoscope that allows a provider to look at the inside of the bladder and urethra, collect urine samples, and examine the prostate gland; it also enables biopsies to be taken or small stones to be removed by way of a hollow channel in the cystoscope.
**cytokine** a nonantibody protein of the immune system that regulates immune response.
**cytologist** one who studies cells and interprets slides.
**cytology** the study of cell life and cell formation.
**cytoplasm** cellular matter, not including the nucleus of a cell.
**cytotechnologist** a laboratory specialist who prepares and examines tissue cells to study cell formation.
**cytotoxic** capable of destroying cells.

**DACUM** an acronym for "design a curriculum."
**daltonism** the inability to distinguish between red and green.
**data** facts from which conclusions can be inferred.
**date of birth (DOB)** the date a person is born, including the month, day, and year.
**date of service (DOS)** the calendar date a service begins or is provided.
**Daysheet** Form used for recording all daily financial transactions of charges made and payments received; also called a daily journal
**D & C** see **dilatation and curettage.**
**DEA** see **Drug Enforcement Administration.**
**debilitated** weakened; impaired the strength of.
**debit** to deduct, to charge.
**debit balance** Occurs when the amount paid is less than the total due
**débridement** to clean up or remove, as is done with damaged tissue around a wound.
**decibel** a unit of measure to express the degree of loudness of sound.
**decimal** numbers that are expressed as a fraction of a part using 10 as its base number; it also refers to the period used to separate a whole number from a fraction, as in 10.2, otherwise read as "ten and two-tenths."
**decline stage** becoming less intense, subsiding; a period of time when the symptoms of disease start to disappear.
**dedicated** committed to; set apart for a special use.
**deductible** an amount to be paid before insurance will pay.
**deductions** to deduct or subtract; remove, take away.
**defamation** to slander, or to attack the reputation of an individual or group.
**defecate** to pass stool or move bowels.
**defendant** the party sued in a civil lawsuit or the party charged with a crime in a criminal prosecution.
**defibrillation** to cause fibrillation to end; restore to normal action.
**defibrillator** a device designed to deliver an electric shock to a patient, in an effort to stop pulseless ventricular fibrillation or ventricular tachycardia.
**dehydration** withdrawal of water from the tissues naturally or artificially.
**delegation** a person or group of persons officially elected or appointed to represent another or others; to entrust power
**delete** to remove, erase.
**delirium tremens** a psychic disorder involving hallucinations, both visual and auditory, found in habitual users of alcohol.
**deltoid** the muscle of the shoulder.
**demeanor** behavior; bearing.
**demography** the study of population statistics concerning births, marriage, death, disease, and many other indicators.
**dendrite** an extension from a nerve cell.
**denial** a refusal to believe or accept; disowning.
**denomination** a category or classification of currency.
**denominator** The bottom number of a fraction.
**denote** to indicate, to mean.
**dental assistant** a health care worker employed by a dentist to perform management and clinical functions and provide chairside assistance.
**dental hygienist** a licensed health care provider who is trained to x-ray and perform prophylactic treatments on teeth.
**dentist (DDS)** a licensed health provider who cares for the teeth, repairing and replacing as needed.
**deoxyribonucleic acid (DNA)** material within the chromosome that carries the genetic information.
**dependable** that which may be relied upon.
**dependence** that on which one depends; reliance.
**dependent** person covered under a subscriber's insurance policy.
**dependent children** (please remove from key terms list)
**depict** to represent by a picture; portray.
**depleted** consumed, emptied, exhausted.
**deposit** to entrust money to a bank or other institution.
**deposit record** a record of a financial deposit that is given by the bank to the customer at the time of the deposit.
**deposit slip** a slip accompanying a bank deposit and containing an itemized list of checks or cash deposited, the date, and the depositer's signature.
**deposition** testimony given under oath.
**depressant** a drug that causes a slowing down of bodily function or nerve activity.
**depressed** a state of depression, a period of low spirits; referring to a fracture, usually a fracture of the skull where bone fragments are driven (depressed) inward.
**deprivation** to be deprived; without; having to do without or unable to use.
**dermatitis** an inflammation of the skin, often the result of an irritant.
**dermatologist** a physician who specializes in the diseases and disorders of the skin.
**dermatology** the study of the skin and its diseases.
**dermis** true skin.
**descending** refers to the portion of the large intestine from the splenic flexure to the sigmoid.
**description** a word picture.
**desensitization** the process of making an individual less susceptible to allergens.
**desensitizing** a process of exposing a patient to small levels of an allergen to gradually build up a nonallergic reaction.
**design** working plan; layout; sketch.
**designate** to point out; indicate; appoint.
**detection** find out or discover.
**detrimental** harmful, injurious.
**deuteranopia** the difficulty in differentiating between the shades of green and bluish reds and some neutral shades.
**devastate** to lay waste, plunder, destroy.
**development** the advancement of abilities and knowledge.

**dextrose** a simple sugar, also known as glucose.
**diabetes mellitus** a metabolic disease caused by the body's inability to use carbohydrates.
**diabetic** one afflicted with the condition diabetes.
**diabetic coma** a diabetic emergency that can be fatal if not treated promptly and properly.
**diabetic ketoacidosis** a complication of diabetes that occurs when the body cannot use sugar (glucose) as a fuel source because the body has no insulin or not enough insulin, and fat is used instead. Byproducts of fat breakdown, called ketones, build up in the body
**diagnostic** referring to measures that assist in the recognition of diseases and disorders of the body.
**diagnostic-related group (DRG)** method of determining reimbursement from medical insurance according to diagnosis on a prospective basis.
**dialysis** removal of the products of urine from the blood by passage of the solutes through a membrane.
**diaphanography** a type of transillumination used to examine the breast, using selected wavelengths of light and special imaging equipment.
**diaphoresis** profuse sweating.
**diaphragm** the muscle of breathing that separates the thorax from the abdomen.
**diarrhea** frequent bowel movements, usually liquid or semisolid.
**diarthrosis** a movable joint; another word for synovial.
**diastole** the relaxation phase of the heartbeat; the period of least pressure.
**dictation** spoken words; recorded voice communication.
**dietician** one who is trained in dietetics, which includes nutrition, and in charge of the diet of an institution.
**differential** refers to determining the number of each type of leukocyte in a cubic millimeter of blood.
**diffuse** to scatter or spread.
**diffusion** a process whereby gas, liquid, or solid molecules distribute themselves evenly through a medium.
**digestion** the process by which food is broken down, mechanically and chemically, in the gastrointestinal tract and converted into absorbable forms.
**digestive** pertaining to digestion.
**digitally** pertaining to or resembling a finger or toe, as an examination using a finger or fingers.
**digital rectal exam (DRE)** examination performed by the provider to check for abnormalities of organs or other structures in the pelvis and lower abdomen.
**dilate** to enlarge, expand in size; to increase the size of an opening.
**dilation and curettage (D & C)** dilation of the cervix and scraping of the interior lining of the uterus.
**dimpling** a condition characterized by indentations in the skin.
**diphtheria** an acute infectious disease characterized by the formation of a false membrane on any mucous surface, usually in the air passages, interfering with breathing.
**diplomate** an advanced status of medical practice.
**direct payment** payment made directly to the physician by the insurance company.
**disability** a legal incapacity.
**disaster** an occurrence inflicting widespread destruction and distress.
**disciplinary** designed to correct or punish breaches of conduct.
**discipline** self-control, conduct, system of rules.
**disclose** to uncover, reveal.
**discoid** a type of lupus that is confined to the skin; also called cutaneous.
**discreet** wisely cautious, prudent.
**discrepancy** inconsistencies; variances.
**discretion** the use of judgment, prudence.
**disease** sickness, illness, ailment.
**disinfection** the process of applying antimicrobial agents to non-living objects to destroy microorganisms.
**dislocation** the displacement of a part; usually refers to a bone temporarily out of its normal position in a joint.
**dispense** to distribute; to deal out in portions.
**dispense as written (DAW)** Phrase indicating that substitutions for generics or similar medications are not allowed by the prescriber
**displacement** the transfer of emotions about one person or situation to another person or situation.
**disposition** the act or manner of putting in a particular order; arrange.
**dissect** to cut into parts for examination; to separate.
**distal** farthest from the center, from the medial line, or from the trunk.
**distend** to become inflated, to stretch out.
**distinctive** unmistakable, different from anything else.
**distort** to misrepresent; to twist out of usual shape.
**distributive justice** the act of assigning or allotting
**diversion** the act of diverting or turning aside.
**diverticulitis** inflammation of the diverticula.
**diverticulum** a sac or pouch in the walls of a canal or organ, particularly the colon.
**dividend** The result of dividing one number by another.
**divisor** The number used to divide into another number.
**divulge** to make public; to make known; reveal.
**DNA** see **deoxyribonucleic acid.**
**doctorate** a postgraduate degree conferred following extensive course work, an individual research project, and the writing of a dissertation; a PhD.
**Doctor of Medicine (MD)** an individual who has met all the requirements in the state to become licensed as a medical doctor.
**Doctor of Osteopathic Medicine (DO)** a doctor licensed by the state to practice medicine. These practitioners place special emphasis on the body's musculoskeletal and nervous systems, preventive medicine, and holistic patient care, and patient education.
**Doctorate** Persons that hold doctoral degrees have attained advanced knowledge through higher education in disciplines such as nursing, mathematics, education, chemistry, philosophy, and so on and have the right to be addressed as doctor.
**doctrine** the principles of any branch of knowledge; a belief held or taught.
**documentary** presenting facts without inserting fictional matter.
**documentation** refers to both the act of preparing, or the evidence created when a healthcare professional records, information regarding a patient during the course of assessment and treatment; can be handwritten or electronically.
**domestic** not foreign; private.
**dominant** strongest; prevailing, the prime or main.
**dominant gene** the prevailing gene.
**dorsal** pertaining to the back.
**dorsal recumbent** body position in which the patient is on his or her back, face up, legs separated, knees flexed with feet flat.
**dorsalis pedis** a pulse point palpable on the instep of the foot.
**dosimeter** a device which measures exposure to ionizing radiation, such as x-rays, alpha rays, beta rays, and gamma rays.
**double-entry bookkeeping system** an accounting method in which each financial transaction is recorded in two accounts; equal debits and credits are recorded for each transaction
**douche** an irrigation of the vagina.
**dowel** a round piece of wood.
**downcoding** A practice of third-party payers in which the benefits code has been changed to a less complex or lower cost procedure than was reported.
**downtime** refers to being offline; computer failure; time when nothing is scheduled.
**dribbling** uncontrolled leakage of urine from the bladder.

**drill** disciplined repetitious exercises as a means of perfecting a skill or procedure.
**droplet** a very small drop.
**droplet infection** a disease that results from contamination with water-based microorganisms.
**Drug Enforcement Administration (DEA)** a division of the federal government responsible for the enforcement of laws regulating the distribution and sale of drugs.
**dual** referring to two; having two parts.
**duodenum** the first segment of the small intestine.
**dura mater** the outer membrane covering the brain and spinal cord.
**duration** the amount of time a thing continues.
**dwarfism** a condition caused by inadequate growth hormone during childhood.
**dysmenorrhea** painful menstruation.
**dysplasia** precancerous cells; with cervix are precursors to cervical cancer.
**dyspnea** difficult or labored breathing.
**dyspneic** difficulty in breathing.
**dystrophy** progressive atrophy or weakening of a part, such as the muscles.
**dysuria** painful urination; difficulty in urination.

**ECG or EKG** see **electrocardiogram.**
**echocardiography** ultrahigh-frequency sound waves directed toward the heart to evaluate function and structure of the organ.
**echoes** reflections of sound.
**ectopic** in an abnormal position; in pregnancy refers to the embryo or fetus being outside the uterus.
**eczema** a noncontagious skin disease characterized by dry, red, itchy, and scaly skin.
**edema** a condition of body tissues containing abnormal amounts of fluid, usually intercellular; may be local or general.
**effacement** the thinning out of the cervix during labor.
**efficiency** the ratio of energy expended to results produced.
**ejaculation** the expulsion of seminal fluid from the male urethra.
**ejaculatory duct** the duct from the seminal vesicle to the urethra.
**elaborate** to improve by successive operations; to work out in detail.
**elasticity** ability to return to shape after being stretched.
**electrical** charged with electricity; run by electricity.
**electrocardiogram (EKG, ECG)** a graphic record of the electric currents generated by the heart; a tracing of the heart action.
**electrocardiogram technician (ECG tech)** a person trained in obtaining electrocardiograms, a record of cardiac impulses.
**electrocardiograph** a machine for obtaining a graphic recording of the electrical activity of the heart.
**electrocautery** an apparatus used to cauterize tissue with heat from a current of electricity.
**electrocoagulation** coagulation of tissue by means of a high-frequency electric current.
**electrode** an instrument with a point or a surface that transmits current to the patient's body.
**electroencephalography (EEG)** recording of the electric currents generated by the brain; a tracing of brain waves.
**electrolyte** a substance that, in solution, conducts an electric current.
**electromagnet** a soft iron core that temporarily becomes a magnet when an electric current flows through a coil surrounding it.
**electromagnetic** a specialized field of radiology that involves the use of both electrical and magnetic fields for diagnosis of disease processes.
**electromagnetic radiation** rays produced by the collision of a beam of electrons with a metal target in an x-ray tube.
**electromyography** the insertion of needles into selected skeletal muscles for the purpose of recording nerve conduction time in relation to muscle contraction.
**electron** a minute particle of matter charged with the smallest known amount of negative electricity; opposite of proton.
**electronic** operated by the use of electrons.
**Electronic Claims Tracking (ECT)** computer software designed for monitoring insurance claims
**Electronic Data Interchange (EDI)** Refers to the exchange of routine business transactions from one computer to another in a standard format, using standard communications protocols
**Electronic health record (EHR)** aggregate electronic record of health-related information on an individual that is created and gathered cumulatively across more than one health care organization and is managed and consulted by licensed clinicians and staff involved in the individual's health and care.
**Electronic Media Claims (EMC)** A flat file format used to transmit or transport claims
**Electronic medical record (EMR)** the electronic record of health-related information for an individual that is created, gathered, managed, and consulted by licensed clinicians and staff that is maintained through a single organization involved in the individual's health and care.
**elements** substances in their simplest form; the basic building blocks of all matter.
**elicit** to draw out, to derive by logical process.
**elimination** to remove, get rid of, exclude; also to pass urine from the bladder or stool from the bowel.
**elite** choice, superior, select.
**ellipses** a mark or series of marks used in writing or printing to indicate an omission, especially of letters or words.
**emaciation** to become abnormally thin; the loss of too much weight.
**emancipated minor** no longer under the care, custody, or supervision of a parent or guardian.
**embolism** the presence of an obstruction in a blood vessel.
**embolus** a circulating mass in a blood vessel; foreign material that obstructs a blood vessel.
**embryo** the first 8 weeks of development after fertilization.
**emergency** an unexpected occurrence or situation demanding immediate action.
**Emergency Medical Services (EMS)** A group that provides out-of-hospital acute medical care and/or transport to definitive care to patients experiencing a medical emergency
**emergency medical technician (EMT)** an individual trained to respond in emergency situations and provide appropriate initial medical treatment.
**emergency preparedness** Preparing for the first and immediate response to any type of hazard or emergency event.
**Emergent** Arising suddenly and unexpectedly.
**emesis** to vomit.
**emetic** medication that induces vomiting.
**Empathetic** Putting yourself in another person's shoes
**empathy** sympathetically trying to identify one's feelings with those of another.
**emphysema** a chronic lung disease characterized by overdistention of the alveolar sacs and inability to exchange oxygen and carbon dioxide.
**empirically** based on observations or experiment.
**empyema** exudate (pus) within the pleural space of the chest cavity.
**enact** to make into law.
**Encoder** software application that allows searching or browsing within CPT, HCPCS, ICD-9-CM code sets, and Medicare coding guidelines.
**encompass** to surround, enclose.
**encounter** to meet, unexpectedly or by chance.
**Encounter form** a record of information obtained during a health care visit, usually a preprinted document, that designates what services and/or procedures are performed and at what level of acuity those services should be billed. Also called a charge slip.

**encounter form** Document used to record the services provided to a patient; also known as a superbill.
**encounter form** Form listing the procedures that are performed in that medical office, with their respective codes; also called superbill or charge slip
**endocardium** the serous membrane lining of the heart.
**endocervical** the lining of the canal of the cervix.
**endocrine** a gland that secretes directly into the blood stream.
**endocrinologist** a physician specializing in the diseases and disorders of the endocrine system.
**endocrinology** the study of the endocrine or ductless glands of internal secretion.
**endocytosis** a cellular process to bring large molecules of material into the cytoplasm of the cell.
**endometrium** the mucous membrane lining of the uterus.
**endoplasmic reticulum** an organelle within the cytoplasm of a cell.
**endorse** to approve, recommend, or sponsor.
**endorsement** the act of endorsing; approving.
**Endorsement** when a physician gains licensure in a particular state as a result of passing the national board examination.
**endoscope** an instrument consisting of a tube and optical system for observing the inside of an organ or cavity.
**enema** the instillation of fluid into the rectum and colon.
**engorge** to fill with blood to the point of congestion; to devour or engulf.
**enhance** to intensify, improve.
**enthusiasm** intense interest; zeal; passion.
**entity** a thing having reality.
**enucleation** surgical excision of the eyeball.
**enumerate** to count separately, name one by one.
**enunciate** to speak or pronounce clearly.
**envelope** to enclose completely with a cover; a paper container for a letter.
**environment** surroundings.
**enzyme** a complex chemical substance produced by the body, found primarily in the digestive juices, that acts upon food substances to break them down for absorption.
**eosinophil** a white blood cell or cellular structure that stains readily with the acid stain eosin; specifically an eosinophilic leukocyte.
**epidemic** affecting many persons at one time.
**Epidemic** a disease affecting large numbers of individuals in a population
**epidermis** the outer layer of the skin; literally *over the true skin*.
**epididymis** a convoluted tube resting on the surface of the testicle that carries sperm from the testicle to the vas deferens.
**epigastric** pertaining to the area of the abdomen over the stomach.
**epiglottis** a cartilagenous lid that closes over the larynx when swallowing.
**epilepsy** a chronic disease of the nervous system characterized by convulsions and often unconsciousness.
**epinephrine** a hormone produced by the adrenal medulla.
**epiphysis** a portion of bone not yet ossified; the cartilagenous ends of the long bones that allow for growth.
**episiotomy** an incision in the perineum to avoid tearing during childbirth.
**epistaxis** nosebleed; hemorrhage from the nose.
**epithelial** pertaining to a type of cell or tissue that forms the skin and mucous membranes of the body.
**equity** the value of property beyond the total amount owed on it.
**equivalent** equal to in value, size, or effect.
**erectile** refers to tissue that is capable of erection, usually caused by vasocongestion.
**ergonomics** the applied science of being concerned with the nature and characteristics of people as they relate to design and activities with the intention of producing more effective results and greater safety.
**erythema** diffuse redness over the skin because of capillary congestion and dilation of the superficial capillaries.
**erythrocyte** a red blood cell (RBC).
**erythropoiesis** the formation of red blood corpuscles.
**eschar** slough, especially after a cauterization.
**esophagus** a collapsible tube from the pharynx to the stomach, through which pass the food and water the body ingests.
**essential** necessary; when referring to blood pressure, indicates an elevation without apparent cause.
**e-statement** An electronic bank statement sent via email from the bank to the customer's email address; a paperless bank statement.
**esthetic** relating to the principles of beauty and taste.
**estrogen** a female hormone produced by the ovaries.
**ether** a colorless liquid used to produce unconsciousness and insensibility to pain.
**ethical** right, according to the principles of ethics.
**ethics** standards of conduct and moral judgement.
**ethics** a system of moral principles; the rules of conduct in respect to a particular class of actions
**ethnicity** Demographic term that indicates with what societal group a patient identifies himself/herself.
**etiology** the study of the cause of disease.
**etiquette** conventional rules for correct behavior.
**euphoria** a feeling of well-being, elation.
**eustachian tube** refers to the tube of the middle ear that connects to the pharynx.
**evacuants** a medication that promotes emptying of the bowels.
**evacuate** to empty, especially the bowels.
**evacuated** Withdrawal; to remove; to make empty.
**evacuation** withdrawal, to remove, to make empty.
**evaluation** assessment; judgment concerning the worth, quality, significance, or value of a situation, person, or product.
**eversion** the movement of the sole of the foot away from the median plane.
**evoke** to call forth or up; summon; elicit.
**excretion** the process of expelling material from the body.
**exemplify** to show by example.
**exempt** excluded; not liable; freedom from duty or service; privileged.
**exemption** freed from or not liable for something to which others are subject.
**exfoliate** to scale off dead tissue.
**exhale** to breathe out.
**exhaustion** extreme fatigue.
**exocrine** a gland that secretes substances through a duct into the body.
**exocytosis** a cellular process that moves materials within the cell to the outside.
**exogenous** originating outside an organ or part.
**exophthalmia** abnormal protrusion of the eyeball.
**Exophthalmos** (NOTE: Exophthalmus is already in the glossary as exophthalmia. It can be spelled exophthalmos, exophthalmus or exophthamia).
**exorcism** the act of expelling an evil spirit.
**expectorate** to spit, to expel mucus or phlegm from the throat or lungs.
**expedient** suitable means for achieving or attaining a purpose or end; of immediate advantage, convenient.
**expedite** to hasten.
**expended** spent or used, as with money or energy.
**expenditure** Actual payment of cash or cash-equivalent for goods or services, or a charge against available funds in settlement of an obligation as evidenced by an invoice, receipt, voucher, or other such document.
**experience** observation or practice resulting in knowledge; knowledge gained by seeing and doing.
**expertise** special knowledge or skill.
**expiration** the expulsion of air from the lungs in breathing.
**explicit** clearly and definitely expressed; unambiguous; leaving no room for questions.

**express** to utter; to make known in words or by action.
**expressed** said in words or by action.
**extend** movement of a joint to increase the angle of that joint.
**extensive** having a wide range.
**extensor** the muscle of a muscle team that extends a part, allowing the joint to straighten.
**external** the outermost part of the body.
**externship** a supervised employment experience in a qualified health care facility as part of the educational curriculum.
**extinguish** to put out; put an end to.
**extinguisher** a device for putting out fire.
**extracellular** outside the cell.
**extract** a substance distilled or drawn out of another substance.
**extremes** The highest or lowest level of a math function on an interval.
**extremities** the terminal parts of the body—the arms, legs.
**extrinsic** originating from outside one's self; motivation coming from factors outside of an individual
**exudate** pus; the collection of purulent material in a cavity.
**exudative** pertaining to any fluid that filters from the circulatory system into lesions or areas of inflammation.
**eyewash** a device using water to remove foreign material from the eyes, usually in emergency situations.

**facility** a building; in medical situations, a building for the care and treatment of patients.
**facsimile** an exact copy.
**facultative** able to live under conditions of temperature or oxygen supply that vary; having the capability to adapt to more than one condition, as a facultative anerobe.
**failure to thrive (FTT)** A description applied to infants and children whose current weight or rate of weight gain is significantly below that of other children of similar age and sex.
**faith** belief in the doctrines of religion; a firm belief in something for which there is no proof.
**fallopian tube** the ovaduct; the passageway for the ova from the ovary to the uterus.
**familial** pertaining to the same family.
**family practice** one which cares for patients of all ages and all conditions not requiring specialization.
**fascia** a fibrous membrane covering, supporting, and separating muscles; may also unite the skin with underlying tissue.
**fast** to abstain from food; without food or water.
**fatal** causing death.
**fax** a message that is transmitted over phone lines and printed by the recipient's equipment.
**feasible** possible; practicable.
**febrile** pertaining to a fever.
**fecal** pertaining to feces.
**feces** stool, bowel movement.
**Federal law** legislation enacted by Congress and signed by the President.
**fee-for-service** Payment for each service that is provided.
**fee schedule** listing of allowable charge.
**Felonies** crimes sufficiently serious to be punishable by death or a term in state or federal prison.
**femoral** pertaining to the artery that lies adjacent to the femur.
**femoral point** the pressure point on the femoral artery.
**femur** the thigh bone of the leg.
**fenestrated** having a window or opening.
**fertilization** impregnation of the ovum by the sperm; conception.
**fetal** pertaining to a fetus, pregnancy beyond the third month.
**fetal alcohol syndrome** a group of birth defects in infants born to mothers who persisted to consume alcohol during gestation.
**fetal monitor** a device to access fetal heart beat.
**fetus** an embryo after 8 weeks of gestation.
**fibrillation** the quivering of muscle fibers; ineffective, rapid but weak heart action.
**fibroid** a tumor made up of fibrous and muscular tissue.
**fibrosis** abnormal formation of fibrous tissue.
**fibula** a long bone in the leg from the knee to the ankle.
**filtration** the movement of solutes and water across a semipermeable membrane as a result of a force, such as gravity or blood pressure.
**financial records** Records that reflect the financial status of the medical office or business.
**fiscal** of or pertaining to finances in general.
**fissure** an ulcer, split, crack, or tear in the tissue.
**fistula** an abnormal tubelike passage from a normal cavity or an abscess to a free surface.
**flatulence** the existence of flatus or intestinal gas.
**flatus** intestinal gas.
**flex time** refers to the practice of permitting work hours within a range of time.
**flexed** bent, as at a joint.
**flexibility** easily bent, compliant, yielding to persuasion.
**flexible** the ability to adapt to circumstances; ability to flex and bend; nonrigid.
**flexible sigmoidoscope** A scope used for a flexible sigmoidoscopy exam to evaluate the lower part of the large intestine (colon).
**flexible spending account (FSA)** Pre-tax funds set aside for use in payment of medical services and supplies not covered by insurance.
**flexor** the muscle of a muscle team that bends a part.
**flora** plant life as distinguished from animal life; plant life occurring or adapted for living in a specific environment, as flora in the intestines.
**flu** an abbreviation for the word influenza; a respiratory or intestinal infection.
**fluoroscope** a device consisting of a fluorescent screen in conjunction with an x-ray tube to make visible shadows of objects interposed between the screen and the tube.
**flushed** sudden reddish coloration of the skin.
**follicle** a small excretory duct or sac or tubular gland; a hair follicle.
**folliculitis** a staphylococcal infection of a hair follicle.
**Fomite** An object (such as clothing, towels, or utensils) that may harbor a disease agent, and is also capable of transmitting it.
**Food and Drug Administration (FDA)** The government agency responsible for regulating the approval of medications, foods, cosmetics and certain supplements.
**forceps** an instrument used to grasp tissue and to clamp blood vessels.
**foreign (body)** anything that is not normally found in the location; usually refers to dirt, splinters, etc.
**foreskin** loose skin covering the end of the penis.
**forge** to imitate, especially to counterfeit, as a signature.
**formaldehyde** a colorless, pungent gas used in its liquid form to harden tissue for pathologic study, or as a germicide, disinfectant, or preservative, according to the strength of the solution.
**formalin** wood alcohol containing 40% formaldehyde.
**fortitude** courageous endurance.
**fovea centralis** a depression in the posterior surface of the retina that is the place of sharpest vision.
**Fowler's** a full or partial sitting examination position.
**fraction** A numerical expression of the number of portions of a whole by using the number of portion over the designated whole number, as in 1/8 or "one-eighth."
**fracture** the sudden breaking of a bone.
**fraudulent** characterized by cheating and deceit; obtained by dishonest means.
**frequency** the need to void urine often, though usually only a small amount at one time.
**friction** resistance of one surface to the motion of another surface rubbing over it.
**fringe (benefits)** benefits included in or added to the salary paid, such as health insurance, retirement fund, etc.

**frontal** anterior; the forehead bone; refers to the plane drawn through the side of the body from the head to the foot.
**frostbite** A condition where localized damage is caused to skin and other tissues due to extreme cold
**functional** practical, working, useful.
**fundus** that portion of an organ most remote from its opening; with uterus, the body of the uterus above the openings of the fallopian tubes.
**Funduscopy** Examination of the fundus of the eye.
**fungus** a vegetable, cellular organism that subsists on organic matter, such as bacteria or mold; a disease condition that causes growth of fungal lesions on the surface of the skin.
**furuncle** the medical term for a boil.

**gait** manner of walking.
**gallbladder** a small sac suspended beneath the liver that concentrates and stores bile.
**galley proofs** printed matter in preliminary form, to be corrected.
**galvanometer** an instrument that measures current by electromagnetic action.
**gamete** a germ cell; any reproductive body.
**ganglion** a mass of nerve tissue that receives and sends out nerve impulses.
**gangrene** a form of necrosis; the putrefaction of soft tissue.
**gastric** pertaining to the stomach.
**gastrocnemius** the large muscle in the calf of the leg.
**gastroenterologist** a physician specializing in the care of patients with diseases and disorders of the gastrointestinal tract.
**gastroenterology** the study of the stomach and intestines and their diseases.
**gastrointestinal (GI)** pertaining to the stomach and intestines.
**gastrointestinal (GI) system** also called the digestive tract, alimentary canal, or gut, the system of organs within multicellular animals that takes in food, digests it to extract energy and nutrients, and expels the remaining waste.
**gastroscopy** examination of the stomach with a gastroscope.
**gatekeeper** one who regulates access to someone or something; in insurance, a primary care physician who coordinates the patient's referral to specialists and hospital admissions.
**gauge** the size of a needle bore; the smaller the number the larger the needle bore.
**gene** a substance within the chromosome that dictates heredity.
**general equivalence mappings (GEMs)** provide forward and backward mapping between the ICD-9 and ICD-10 coding systems.
**General Skills** The skills that are necessary regardless whether working in a clinical or administrative capacity. They include legal functions, communication skills, the ability to deliver education and operational functions.
**Generalist** Medical assistants work as a generalists when they perform both clinical and administrative duties in addition to general responsibilities.
**generate** to produce, as heat, ideas, power.
**generic** general; characteristic of a genus or group.
**genetic** pertaining to the genes.
**genital herpes** fluid-filled lesions on the external genitalia, which are contagious upon direct contact.
**genitalia** the external sexual organs.
**genogram** a graph of family health history.
**genucubital** pertaining to the elbows and knees; the knee-elbow position.
**genupectoral** pertaining to the knees and chest; the knee-chest position.
**geriatrics** the study and treatment of the diseases of old age.
**gerontologist** a physician specializing in the care of the aged.
**gestation** period of intrauterine fetal development.
**gestational diabetes** form of diabetes found in pregnant women.
**gigantism** a condition resulting from the overproduction of growth hormone during childhood.
**glance** a quick look or view.
**glaucoma** a disease of the eye characterized by increased intraocular pressure.
**glomerulonephritis** inflammation of the glomerulus of the nephron of the kidney.
**glomerulus** the microscopic cluster of capillaries within the Bowman's capsule of the nephron.
**glucohemoglobin** sugar in the blood.
**glucose** a colorless or yellow, thick, syrupy liquid obtained by the incomplete hydrolysis of starch; a simple sugar.
**gluteus maximus** the large muscle of the buttocks.
**glycohemoglobin** test that indicates the average blood sugar over the past 2 months.
**glycosuria** sugar in the urine.
**glycosylation** the process of adding sugars to proteins or lipids.
**goiter** an enlargement of the thyroid gland.
**Golgi apparatus** an organelle within the cytoplasm of a cell.
**gonadotropic** related to stimulation of the gonads.
**gonads** the sex glands, the ovaries in the female and the testicles in the male.
**gonorrhea** a venereal disease of the reproductive organs, which is highly contagious upon direct contact.
**gooseneck lamp** a light fixture with a flexible portion that allows adjustment.
**graafian follicle** the vesicle in which ova are matured and which releases them when ripened.
**graft** a constructed part.
**Gram negative** bacteria that take on a pink color with Gram staining process.
**Gram positive** bacteria that take on a purple color with Gram staining process.
**greenstick** an incomplete fracture, occurring in children.
**grillwork** a bar-like device, usually constructed of heavy metal; an open grating for a door or window.
**groin** the depression between the thigh and the trunk of the body; the inguinal region.
**gross** exclusive of deductions; total; entire.
**gross anatomy** refers to the study of those features that can be observed with the naked eye by inspection and dissection.
**Gross negligence** carelessness which is in reckless disregard for the safety or lives of others, and is so great it appears to be a conscious violation of other people's rights to safety; more than simple negligence or mistake; less than intentionally evil.
**guaiac** a solution used to test for the presence of occult blood in the stool.
**guaiac test paper** a screening agent to test for hidden blood.
**guarantee** assurance that something will be done as specified; a pledge.
**guarantor** a person who makes or gives a guarantee or pledge, often to pay another's debt or obligation in the event of default.
**Guardian** a person who has been appointed by a judge to take care of a minor child or incompetent adult personally and/or manage that person's affairs.
**guilds** associations of persons engaged in the same trade or calling for mutual protection.
**Guilds** an association of persons engaged in a common trade or calling for mutual advantage and protection. Medicine was divided into three guilds during the seventeen hundreds; Surgeons, barbers and apothecaries.
**GYN** see **gynecology.**
**gynecologist** a physician specializing in the care of diseases and disorders of women, particularly the genital organs.
**gynecology (GYN)** the study of diseases of the female, particularly of the organs of reproduction.

**haemophilus** bacterial strains that grow best in hemoglobin.
**hallucinogen** a substance that causes hallucinations.
**hamstring** a group of muscles of the posterior thigh.

**handicap** to hinder; those who are physically disabled or mentally retarded.
**hangover** the malaise that follows ingestion of a considerable amount of alcohol.
**harassment** continual annoyance; persecution.
**harbor** place of protection; in health care, surfaces that allow microorganisms to hide and grow.
**hard copy** information printed on a solid surface, such as paper, instead of displayed on a CRT screen or stored on a disk.
**hardware** the visible parts of a computer system (keyboard, disk drive, monitor, and printers).
**harmonious** having parts combined in a proportionate, orderly, or pleasing arrangement; being peaceable or friendly.
**hazard** danger; risk.
**HCFA** Health Care Financing Administration.
**health** a state of complete physical and mental or social well-being.
**health maintenance organization (HMO)** a type of managed care operation that is typically set up as a for-profit corporation with salaried employees.
**health reimbursement arrangement (HRA)** an account with employer contributions used to pay for medical expenses.
**health savings account (HSA)** a tax-sheltered savings account, with contributions from the employer and employee, which can be used to pay for medical expenses.
**healthcheck** a federally mandated Medicaid program for health care of children up to 21 years of age.
**heart block** a condition in which impulses from the SA node fail to carry over to the AV node, resulting in a slow heart rate and a different rate of contraction between the upper and lower heart chambers.
**heart murmur** a sound produced by the leakage of blood through a heart valve.
**heartburn** a burning sensation beneath the breastbone, usually associated with indigestion.
**heat cramps** Painful, brief muscle cramps that occur during exercise or work in a hot environment; muscles may spasm or jerk involuntarily
**heat exhaustion** A condition whose symptoms may include heavy sweating and a rapid pulse, as a result of the body overheating
**heat stroke** A severe condition caused by impairment of the body's temperature-regulating abilities, resulting from prolonged exposure to excessive heat and characterized by cessation of sweating, severe headache, high fever, hot dry skin, and in serious cases collapse and coma
**height** the vertical length of an object or person.
**hematocrit** an expression of the volume of red blood cells per unit of circulating blood.
**hematologist** a physician specializing in the care of patients with disorders and diseases of the blood and blood-forming organs.
**hematology** the study of the blood and its diseases.
**hematoma** a tumor or swelling that contains blood.
**hematuria** blood in the urine.
**hemodialysis** a process whereby blood is passed through a thin membrane and exposed to a dialysate solution to remove waste products.
**hemoglobin** the combination of a protein and iron pigment in the red blood cells that attracts and carries oxygen in the body.
**hemolysis** dissolution; the breaking down of red blood cells.
**hemophilia** hereditary condition, transmitted through sex-linked chromosomes of female carriers; affects males only, causing inability to clot blood.
**hemorrhage** abnormal discharge of blood either internally or externally from venous, arterial, or capillary vessels.
**hemorrhoidectomy** surgical excision of hemorrhoidal tissue.
**hemorrhoids** varicose veins of the anal canal.
**hemostat** a type of forceps.
**hemothorax** blood within the pleural space of the chest cavity.
**heparin** a substance formed in the liver that inhibits the coagulation of blood.
**hepatic** pertaining to the liver.
**hepatitis** inflammation of the liver.
**hepatitis A** An acute infectious disease of the liver caused by a virus that is transmitted by contaminated food or water or by direct person-to-person contact
**hepatitis B** acute infection of the liver transmitted through blood or body fluids.
**herbal** pertaining to plants, particularly to their medicinal qualities.
**hernia** a projection of a part from its normal location.
**herniorrhaphy** the surgical repair of a hernia.
**herpes simplex** the medical term for fever blister, an acute viral infection of the face, mouth, or nose.
**herpes zoster** the medical term for shingles, an acute viral infection of the dorsal root ganglia.
**hesitancy** difficulty in starting a urine stream.
**heterosexual** sexual attraction toward the opposite sex.
**heterotrophs** microorganisms that feed on organic matter.
**HHS** U.S. Department of Health and Human Services.
**hiatus** pertains to a herniation of the stomach through an opening or hiatus.
**HIB/hib** *Hemophilus influenzae* type B.
**hiccough** (also hiccup) a result of the spasmodic closing of the epiglottis and spasm of the diaphragm.
**hiccup** see **hiccough.**
**high-power field (hpf)** refers to microscope lens.
**hilum** the recessed area of the kidney where the ureter and blood vessels enter.
**hinge** a type of joint.
**Hippocratic oath** refers to the oath taken by a doctor bonding him to observe the code of medical ethics contained in the oath by Hippocrates in the 4th century.
**Hippocratic Oath** A code of behavior that doctors are to follow.
**histamine** a substance normally present in the body.
**histologist** (histotechnologist) a person engaged in the study of the microscopic structure of tissue.
**histology** the study of cells.
**histoplasmosis** a fungal infection caused by an organism found in bird and bat droppings.
**histotechnologist** a laboratory specialist who prepares tissues for microscopic examination and diagnosis.
**HL7 protocol** Health Level Seven protocol, the standard for exchanging information between medical applications.
**holistic** considering the whole or entire scope of a situation.
**Holter monitor** a device that attaches electrodes to a patient's chest for the purpose of obtaining a 24-hour ECG tracing in an accessory tape recorder.
**homeopathy** a system of medical practice that treats a disease by the administration of minute doses of a remedy that would in healthy persons produce symptoms similar to those of the disease.
**Homeopathy** a 200-year-old system of medicine based on the Law of Similars. This means that if a dose of a substance can cause a symptom, that same substance in minuscule amounts can cure the symptom.
**homeostasis** maintenance of a constant or static condition of internal environment.
**homosexual** sexual attraction toward the same sex as oneself.
**honesty** the state of being truthful, trustworthy; genuine.
**horizontal** not vertical; flat and even; level; parallel to the plane of the horizon.
**hormone** a chemical substance secreted by an organ or gland.
**hospice movement** an organization dedicated to providing care with dignity people who are terminally ill.
**Hospitalist** work with patients admitted to the hospital. These individuals work in many different departments and reduce the load of hospital visits for the primary care provider and specialist.

**hourly wage** amount of wages paid to an employee per hour; a varying amount of income depending on hours worked
**hostility** unfriendliness, enmity.
**human chorionic gonadotropin (hCG)** a hormone produced in pregnancy that is made by the embryo soon after conception.
**human immunodeficiency virus (HIV)** a retrovirus that causes acquired immunodeficiency syndrome (AIDS), a condition in humans in which the immune system begins to fail, leading to life-threatening opportunistic infections.
**human organism** the collective higher individual resulting from the organization of cells, tissues, organs, and organ systems.
**humble** modest, unassuming.
**humerus** the long bone of the upper arm.
**humor** something that is designed to be amusing or comical.
**humoral** antibody-mediated immunity.
**hyaline membrane disease** a condition resulting from incomplete development of the respiratory system in premature infants.
**hydrocele** the accumulation of fluid in the scrotum.
**hydrochloric acid** a digestive juice found in the stomach.
**hygiene** the study of health and observance of health rules.
**hygienist** one who provides health-related services, such as dental procedures.
**hymen** a membranous fold partially or completely covering the vaginal opening.
**hyperglycemia** increase of blood sugar, as in diabetes.
**hyperopia** a defect of vision so that objects can only be seen when they are far away; farsightedness.
**hypersensitive** oversensitive; abnormally sensitive to a stimulus of any kind.
**hypertension** elevated blood pressure.
**hyperthermia** higher than normal temperature.
**hyperthyroidism** a condition caused by excessive secretion of the thyroid glands.
**hypertonic** having a higher concentration of salt than found in a red blood cell.
**hyperventilation** excessive deep and frequent breathing.
**hyphen** a punctuation mark used to divide or create compound words.
**hypnosis** a state that resembles sleep but is induced by suggestion.
**hypoallergenic** unlikely to cause an allergic reaction.
**hypochondriac** pertaining to the upper outer regions of the abdomen below the thorax; also someone with a morbid fear of disease, resulting in abnormal concern about one's health.
**hypogastric** referring to an abdominal area in the middle lower third of the abdomen.
**hypoglycemia** deficiency of sugar in the blood.
**hypotension** abnormally low blood pressure.
**hypothalamus** a structure of the brain between the cerebrum and the midbrain; lies below the thalamus.
**hypothermia** below normal body temperature.
**hypothyroidism** a condition caused by a marked deficiency of thyroid secretion.
**hypotonic** having a lower concentration of salt than found in a red blood cell.
**hypoxia** a lack of oxygen.
**hysterectomy** surgical removal of the uterus.
**hysteroscopy** a procedure using the hysteroscope to view the endometrium of the uterus.

**ICD** see **International Classification of Diseases.**
**I & D** see **incision and drainage.**
**identification** anything by which a person or thing can be identified.
**idiopathic** disease without recognizable cause.
**idle** uninvolved; doing nothing.
**ileocecal** the valve between the end of the small intestine and the cecum.
**ileostomy** a surgical opening from the ileum onto the abdominal wall.
**ileum** the last section of the small intestine.
**iliac** the edge or crest of the pelvic bone.
**ilium** the hip bone.
**illegible** impossible to read.
**illicit** improper; unlawful; not sanctioned by custom or law; illegal.
**illuminating** enlightening; throwing light on.
**imaging** a representation or visual impression produced by a lens, mirror, etc.
**immobilize** to keep out of action or circulation; stationary.
**immune** protected or exempt from a disease.
**immunization** becoming immune or the process of rendering a patient immune.
**immunoassays** a biochemical test that measures the level of a substance in a biologic liquid, typically serum or urine, using the reaction of an antibody or antibodies to its antigen.
**immunodeficiency** lacking the components necessary to mount an immune response.
**immunoglobulin** a large protein molecule that assists in the immune response.
**immunologic** pertaining to immunology.
**immunology** a broad branch of biomedical science that covers the study of all aspects of the immune system in all organisms.
**immunosuppressed** a condition wherein the immune system has been overpowered and cannot function adequately.
**impacted** refers to a fracture where the broken ends are jammed together.
**impaction** a collection of hardened feces in the rectum that cannot be expelled.
**impending** to be at hand or about to happen.
**implant** something implanted into tissue; a graft; artificial part.
**implement** a tool or instrument for doing something; to put into effect.
**implementation** put into effect.
**implication** involvement, bringing into connection.
**implied** hinted, suggested.
**impotence** inability of a male to obtain or maintain an erection.
**impulse** a charge transmitted through certain tissues, especially nerve fibers and muscles, resulting in physiologic activity.
**inappropriate** not appropriate, out of place.
**incident report** a report giving detailed information about an emergency situation and how it was handled.
**incineration** burn, setting afire.
**incision** cut.
**incision and drainage (I & D)** cutting into for the purpose of providing an exit for material, usually a collection of pus.
**inclined** leaning or tending toward.
**income statement** A statement that demonstrates the profit and expenses for a given month and also includes year-to-date information for a given year.
**incompetent** not capable; not legally qualified; deficient.
**incomprehensible** beyond belief, not to be grasped by the mind.
**incongruous** lacking harmony or agreement.
**incontinent** unable to control the bladder or bowel.
**increments** becoming greater; amount of increase; gain.
**incubation** the interval between exposure to infection and the appearance of the first symptom.
**incus** the anvil, the middle bone of the three in the middle ear.
**indemnity** to compensate for damage done or loss caused.
**independent practice association (IPA)** An association of independent physicians, or other organization that contracts with independent physicians, and provides services to managed care organizations on a negotiated per capita rate, flat retainer fee, or negotiated fee-for-service basis.
**indexing** A system of cross-referencing information contained in office files so that the data may be searched using different characteristics as the query term.
**Indication** The intended purpose or reason for using a particular medication.

**indigent** needy, poor, destitute.
**indigestion** difficulty in digesting food.
**induction** the process of causing or producing; to bring on.
**inevitable** unavoidable, destined to occur.
**infarction** infiltration of foreign particles; material in a vessel causing coagulation and interference with circulation.
**infectious** capable of producing infection; denoting a disease in the body caused by the presence of germs; tending to spread to others.
**infectious mononucleosis** a disease seen most commonly in adolescents and young adults, characterized by fever, sore throat, leg and muscle soreness and fatigue (symptoms of a common cold or allergies). Mononucleosis is caused by the Epstein-Barr virus (EBV).
**inferior** below, under.
**inferior vena cava** the large vein that carries deoxygenated blood from the lower half of the body into the heart.
**infertility** inability to achieve conception.
**infirmity** illness, disease.
**inflict** to strike, to cause punishment.
**influenza** an acute illness characterized by fever, pain, coughing, and general upper respiratory symptoms.
**informed consent** agreement to do something or to allow something to happen only after all the relevant facts are known.
**infrared** pertaining to those invisible rays just beyond the red end of the visible spectrum that have a penetrating heating effect.
**infusion** to instill; introduction of a substance into a vein.
**ingested** to eat.
**inguinal** referring to the region where the thigh joins the trunk of the body; the groin.
**inguinal canal** a passageway in the groin for the spermatic cord in the male.
**inguinal hernia** the presence of small intestine in the inguinal canal.
**inhale** to breathe in.
**initial** the first; beginning; the first letter of each of a person's names.
**initiate** to get something started, begin.
**initiative** the action of taking the first step; ability to originate new ideas.
**innate** inborn; inherent.
**innate** characteristics that are inherent or natural, while others must be learned.
**inoculating loop** a laboratory instrument used to transfer organisms from one source to another.
**inorganic** not living; occurring in nature independently of living things.
**inseminate** to impregnate with semen.
**insertion** the place where a muscle is attached to the bone that it moves.
**insidious** hidden, not apparent.
**insignificant** unimportant; petty; of little or no value.
**insomnia** abnormal inability to sleep.
**inspect** to examine closely.
**inspection** the first part of a physical examination; close observation.
**inspiration** to breathe in, inhale.
**instill** to slowly drop liquid onto a surface or into a cavity.
**institute** to originate as a custom.
**insufficient** not as much as needed.
**insulin** a hormone secreted by the islets of langerhans in the pancreas.
**insulin shock** a condition of excess insulin or lack of blood sugar.
**insurance** a contract to guarantee compensation for a specified situation.
**intact** unbroken, undamaged.
**intangible** that which cannot be touched, easily defined, or grasped.
**integrity** soundness of character; honesty in particular.
**integumentary** the skin; a covering.
**integumentary system** the largest organ system by surface area, comprising skin, hair, nails, and sweat glands and their products (sweat and mucus). It distinguishes, separates, and protects. the name derives from the latin *integumentum*, which means "a covering."
**intellectualization** to employ reasoning to avoid confrontations or stressful situations.
**intelligence** the ability to learn or understand.
**interaction** to act upon one another.
**intercede** to mediate, plead on behalf of another.
**intercostal** between the ribs.
**interference** confusion of desired signals caused by undesired signals, as in artifacts on an ECG.
**interferon** a lymphokine that helps regulate the activities of macrophages and natural killer cells.
**interjection** a part of speech; an exclamation.
**interleukin** a substance that is a messenger between leukocytes.
**intermediate** in the middle.
**intermittent** stopping and starting again at intervals.
**intermuscular** within the muscle.
**internal** the innermost part(s) of the body.
**internal revenue service** the division of federal government charged with implementing tax laws and collecting taxes.
**International Classification of Diseases (ICD)** a comprehensive listing of diseases and disorders of the human body.
**interneurons** neurons connecting sensory to motor neurons.
**internist** a physician specializing in the care of patients with internal diseases.
**internship** a time following graduation wherein practice of the profession is performed.
**interpersonal** between persons.
**interpret** to explain, translate; to determine the meaning.
**interpretive** computerized analysis of ECG tracings.
**interval** time between events; space.
**intervention** taking action to modify, hinder, or change an effect.
**interventional hysterosalpingography** a diagnostic examination to evaluate the fallopian tubes.
**intervertebral** between the vertebrae.
**interview** a meeting between two people where one asks questions of the other.
**intestine** the alimentary canal extending from the pylorus of the stomach to the anus.
**intimidate** to make afraid, to frighten.
**intimidation** to make afraid; to deter with threats.
**intolerance** an adverse effect of a medication that is not related to an immune response.
**intoxicated** a condition caused by the overindulgence in alcoholic beverages.
**intracellular** within the cell.
**intracellular leukemia** should not be a key term (only *leukemia* should be a key term)
**intradermal** within the skin.
**intramuscular (IM)** type of injection administered into a muscle.
**intraocular** within the eyeball.
**intrauterine device (IUD)** an object inserted into the uterus to prevent pregnancy.
**intravenous** to insert into the vein.
**intravenous pyelography (IVP)** the insertion of a radio-paque material into the vein for the purpose of x-raying the kidneys and ureters.
**intricate** complicated, complex, elaborately interwoven.
**intrinsic** belonging to one's self inherently; motivation coming from within an individual
**intubation** insertion of a tube into the larynx for entrance of air.
**intuition** the immediate knowing or learning of something without the conscious use of reasoning.
**inunction** the process of administering drugs through the skin.
**invasive (procedure)** diagnostic methods involving entry into living tissue.
**inventory** an itemized list of goods in stock.
**inversion** the movement of the sole of the foot toward the median plane.
**in vivo** that which takes place inside an organism.
**invoice** a document that includes itemization of goods and purchases or services provided together with the charges and terms of the agreement.
**involuntary** independent of or even contrary to will or choice.

**iodine** a nonmetallic element belonging to the halogen group.
**ipecac** an emetic; causes vomiting.
**iris** the colored, contractible tissue surrounding the pupil of the eye.
**irrational** lacking the power to reason; senseless.
**irreconcilable** cannot be brought into agreement.
**irrelevant** not pertinent, not to the point.
**irreparable** damaged beyond possibility of repair.
**irrigate** to wash out with a liquid.
**ischemia** temporary and localized anemia caused by obstruction of the circulation to a part.
**ischium** posterior and inferior portion of the hip bone.
**ishihara** refers to an eye test to determine color vision.
**islets of langerhans** clusters of cells in the pancreas.
**isotonic** having the same concentration of salt as found in a red blood cell.
**issue** to send forth; to put into circulation.
**IVP** see **intravenous pyelography.**

**Jaeger** a system for measuring near vision acuity.
**Jaeger chart** an eye chart is used for reading up close and for determining near vision.
**jaundice** a yellowish discoloration of the sclera and skin due to the presence of bile pigments in the blood.
**jejunum** the middle segment of the small intestine, which measures approximately 8 feet in length.
**jeopardize** to put at risk.
**job description** a combination of skills and behaviors expected of an employee; effectively fulfill the responsibilities in a designated work position.
**joint commission** refers to the agency that has oversight for hospitals adhering to regulations that allow them to bill for medicare reimbursement for medical services provided
**journal** a record of happenings; a diary.
**journalizing** entries on the daily log.
**judgment** a decision; ability to make the right decisions.
**jurisdiction** the authority given by law to a court to try cases and rule on legal matters within a particular geographic area and/or over certain types of legal cases.

**keloid** an overgrowth of new skin tissue; a scar.
**ketone (acetone)** products of metabolism generated from carbohydrates, fatty acids, and amino acids in humans.
**key components** the major factors to be considered when selecting an evaluation and management code: history, exam, medical decision making.
**keying** pressing a lever or button, as on a typewriter, with the finger to operate the machine.
**kidney** a bean-shaped organ that excretes urine and is located retroperitoneally, high in the back of the abdominal cavity.
**knee-chest** body position in which the patient kneels on the exam table with buttocks elevated, back straight, and chest resting on the table
**knowledge base** a term used to describe the theoretical portion of an educational program.
**KUB** kidneys, ureters, and bladder; refers to a radiologic study.
**kyphosis** a convex curvature of the spine; humpback.

**L & A** light and accommodation.
**labia majora** the two large folds of adipose tissue lying on each side of the vulva of the female; external genitalia.
**labia minora** the two mucocutaneous folds of membrane within the labia majora.
**laboratory technician** a health care worker who performs specialized chemical, microscopic, and bacteriologic tests of blood, tissue, and body fluids.
**laboratory** a room or building in which scientific tests or experiments are conducted.
**laceration** a cut or tear.
**lacrimal** pertaining to tears; the glands and ducts that secrete and convey tears.
**Lamaze** a program or method of managing labor during birth.
**laminectomy** the removal of a portion of the vertebral posterior arch.
**lancet** a sharp, pointed instrument used to pierce the skin to obtain a capillary blood sample.
**laryngeal** pertaining to the larynx.
**laryngectomy** surgical removal of the larynx or voice box.
**laryngitis** inflammation of the vocal cords.
**larynx** the voice box.
**lateral** pertaining to the side.
**latissimus dorsi** the large muscle of the back.
**lavage** the washing out of a cavity.
**laxative** a substance that induces the bowels to empty.
**ledgers** the principal account books of a business establishment, containing the credits and debits.
**legible** easy to read, readable.
**legislating** the act of exercising the power and function of making laws that have the force of authority by virtue of their origin by a state legislature or US Congress.
**legionnaires' disease** an acute bronchopneumonia.
**leisure** spare or free time, away from the pressure and responsibilities of work.
**lens** a part of the eye that bends or refracts images onto the retina.
**lesion** an injury or wound; a circumscribed area of pathologically altered tissue.
**lethal** deadly; capable of causing death.
**lethargic** sluggishness, apathy.
**leukemia** a disease characterized by a great excess of white blood cells; it exists in a lymphatic and myelogenous form; it is often fatal, especially in adults.
**leukocyte** a white blood cell.
**leukocyte esterase** a urine test for the presence of white blood cells and other abnormalities associated with infection.
**liability** anything to which a person is liable, responsible, legally bound.
**liaison** intercommunication between two entities.
**license** a legal permit to engage in an activity.
**licensed practical nurse (LPN)** an individual trained in basic nursing techniques, to provide direct patient care under the supervision of an RN or physician.
**life-threatening** used to describe diseases or conditions where the likelihood of death is high
**ligament** fibrous tissue that connects bone to bone.
**ligation** to tie off; the process of binding or tying.
**limbs** refers to the arms and legs.
**limited** to restrict; to hold within fixed bounds.
**limited check** a check that will be marked void if written for more than a certain amount. This type of check is often used for payroll or insurance payments.
**listlessness** lack of desire, interest.
**liter** a unit of measure; 1,000 mL or approximately 1 quart.
**lithotomy** an examination position wherein the patient lies upon the back with thighs flexed upon the abdomen and legs flexed upon the thighs.
**lithotripsy** destruction of stone; stonecrusher.
**liver** the largest gland in the body, located in the upper right quadrant of the abdomen beneath the diaphragm.
**living will** advance directive; a document, written in advance, that states the patient's wishes regarding end-of-life care.
**LMP** last menstrual period.
**longevity** a long duration of life; lasting a long time.
**longitudinal fissure** the deep cleft between the two hemispheres of the cerebrum.
**lordosis** abnormal anterior curvature of the lumbar spine.
**low-power field (lpf)** refers to microscope lens.
**lubb dupp** sounds made by the heart.
**lumbar** pertaining to the back, specifically to the five vertebrae above the sacrum.

**lumbar puncture** the insertion of a needle between the vertebrae in the lumbar area for the purpose of withdrawing spinal fluid.
**lumen** the space within an artery, vein, or capillary; the space within a tube.
**lung** the organ of respiration, located within the thoracic cavity.
**lupus erythematosus** a chronic autoimmune disease that causes changes in the immune system.
**luteinizing** a hormone effect that causes ovulation and progesterone in the female and sperm production and testosterone in the male.
**lyme disease** a disease caused by a spirochete that is carried by the deer tick.
**lymph** a body fluid formed within the tissue spaces and circulated throughout the body.
**lymphatic system** a network of transparent vessels carrying lymph fluid throughout the body.
**lymphedema** excess lymph fluid in the tissues.
**lymphocyte** a type of white blood cell.
**lymphokine** a cytokine produced by a T-cell.
**lymphokine leukemia** should not be a key term (only *leukemia* should be a key term)
**lymphoma** a tumor of the lymphatic tissue. NOTE: This is a new word to be inserted into the Words to Know and added to the glossary.
**lysosomes** an organelle within the cytoplasm of the cell.

**macrophage** a phagocytic cell that destroys antigens.
**macule** a discolored spot or patch on the skin neither elevated nor depressed.
**magnet therapy** a therapy which involves placing small magnets close to the skin in order to correct an imbalance.
**magnetic** having the properties of a magnet, able to attract.
**magnetic resonance imaging (MRI)** a diagnostic test using magnetic waves to visualize internal body structures.
**magnify** to make something look larger than it really is.
**mailable** a standard for judging written correspondence as satisfactory for sending.
**maintenance** to preserve; the act or work of keeping something in proper condition.
**malaise** a feeling of discomfort or uneasiness.
**malignant** a cancerous growth; tumor.
**malinger** to pretend illness to escape dealing with a situation or obligation.
**malleus** the largest of the three bones of the middle car, also called the hammer.
**malnutrition** lack of necessary or proper food substances in the body.
**mammary glands** the breasts.
**mammogram** an x-ray of the breast.
**mammography** the process of using low-dose x-rays to examine the human breast. It is used to look for different types of tumors and cysts.
**management** the act, manner, or practice of managing, handling, or controlling something.
**managerial accounting** the study and analysis of financial data as it applies to operational issues within a company. also known as cost accounting.
**mandate** an order of authorative command; instruction.
**manifestation** act of disclosing; revelation; display.
**manipulation** the passive movement of a joint to determine the range of flexion and extension.
**manipulation therapy** any treatment or procedure involving the use of the hands; additional manual skills used by osteopathic physicians.
**marginal** close to the lower limit of acceptability.
**marrow** the soft tissue in the hollow of long bones.
**massage** manipulation of tissues for therapeutic purposes by rubbing, kneading, or tapping with the hands.
**masses** a multitude; a large number of people.
**mastectomy** surgical removal of a breast.
**master** refers to a reference document used to compare other similar documents or values to, as in a master patient list, or an original document saved to a file which can be copied or modified as needed.
**materials safety data sheet (MSDS)** printed materials that come with hazardous chemicals that provide basic information to the safety and health of the user.
**matrix** a format for establishing a time schedule for appointments.
**maturation index (MI)** a measurement of cellular maturity.
**maturation** refers to a stage of cellular development.
**maturity** a state of full development.
**meaningful use** with reference to healthcare records, this term is used by government agencies to refer to the way in which medical record information is employed in order to provide a means for improving patient care and patient outcomes through evaluating treatment patterns and verifying necessity of medical procedures performed.
**means** the average which is derived by adding up all the values of a given series and dividing by the number of values.
**measles** a highly contagious disease characterized by the presence of maculopustular eruptions.
**mechanical** pertaining to machinery.
**medial** pertaining to the middle or midline.
**medicaid** a government health care program.
**medical assistant** an integral member of the health care delivery team, qualified by education and experience to work in the administrative office, the examining room and the physician office laboratory.
**medical emergency** an injury or illness that is acute and poses an immediate risk to a person's life or long-term health
**medical malpractice** an act or continuing conduct of a physician or hospital that does not meet the standard of professional competence and results in provable damages to the patient.
**medical necessity** services or supplies that are needed for the diagnosis or treatment of your medical condition and meet accepted standards of medical practice.
**medication order** instructions written by a licensed provider for administration of a medication to a patient
**medicare** a federal health program for paying certain medical expenses of the aged.
**medigap** refers to situations not covered by medicare insurance.
**medulla** the inner section of the kidney.
**medulla oblongata** enlarged portion of the spinal cord; the lower portion of the brainstem.
**melanin** a pigment that gives color to the skin, hair, and eyes.
**melanocytes** cells that produce the pigment of the skin, melanin.
**membrane** a thin, soft, pliable layer of tissue that lines a tube or cavity or covers an organ or structure.
**menarche** the first menstrual period.
**meniere's disease** a disorder of the ear characterized by nausea, vomiting, tinnitus, and hearing loss.
**meninges** the membranes covering the brain and spinal cord.
**meningitis** inflammation of the meninges of the brain and/or spinal cord.
**meniscus** a concave level of fluid in a tube or cylinder.
**menopause** the permanent cessation of menstruation.
**menorrhagia** excessive menstrual flow, hemorrhage.
**menstruation** periodic discharge of bloody fluid from the uterus.
**mensuration** the process of measuring.
**mercury** a liquid metal used in measurement devices such as thermometers and sphygmomanometers; chemical symbol, Hg.
**merit** to deserve reward or praise; excellence.
**mesentery** a peritoneal fold connecting the intestine to the posterior abdominal wall.

**metabolism** the successive transformations to which a substance is subjected from the time it enters the body to the time it or its decomposition products are excreted, and by which nutrition is accomplished and energy and living substance are provided.
**metabolized** the successive transformation of a substance from the time it enters the body to the time it or its decomposition products are excreted, and by which nutrition is accomplished and energy and living substance are provided.
**metacarpal** pertaining to the five bones of the hand between the wrist and the phalanges.
**metastasis** movement of cancer cells from one part of the body to another.
**metastasize** the process whereby malignant cells leave the primary lesion and migrate to another location.
**metatarsal** the five bones of the feet between the instep and the phalanges.
**methodical** systematic, following a plan or method.
**metric system** a system of measurements that uses the base function of ten.
**MI** see **myocardial infarction.**
**microbes** organisms that are microscopic (too small to be visible to the human eye).
**microbial** related to microbes.
**microfiche** a sheet of microfilm capable of accommodating and preserving a considerable number of book pages in reduced form.
**microfilming** using a machine to put copies of written data such as a patient file into a smaller, storable format.
**microhematocrit** packed cell volume (PCV) that measures the proportion of blood volume that is occupied by red blood cells.
**microorganism** a microscopic living body not perceivable by the naked eye.
**microscopic** visible only with a microscope.
**microscopic anatomy** an area of study that deals with features that can be seen only with a microscope.
**micturtion** the passing of urine.
**midbrain** that portion of the brain connecting the pons and the cerebellum.
**midlevel practitioner** healthcare providers such as a nurse practitioner or physician's assistant. they are able to examine patients, order diagnostic tests and prescribe certain types of medications. activities for midlevel practitioners are usually directed and/or dictated by a supervising physician.
**midline** the middle.
**midsagittal** an imaginary vertical plane made by dividing the body down the middle, creating equal right and left sides; also known as the midline.
**migraine** a severe headache with characteristic symptoms.
**mineralocorticoid** a biologic principle of the adrenal cortex involved in regulating body fluid and electrolytes.
**minute** a measurement of time equal to 60 seconds; very small, tiny.
**misalignment** out of alignment; not straight.
**misdemeanor** a lesser crime than a felony, punishable by a fine and/or county jail time for up to one year.
**misspelled** to spell incorrectly.
**mitochondria** an organelle within the cytoplasm of the cell.
**mitosis** the division of a cell.
**mitral** the valve in the heart between the chambers of the left side, also known as the bicuspid.
**mobile banking** a banking method that allows the bank customer to perform banking actions on his or her cell phone or other mobile device.
**mobility** quality of being mobile; easy to move.
**modifier** changes; limits the meaning.
**modifies** changes the form or quality of; alters slightly.
**molten** melted.
**monilia** a family of parasitic fungi or molds.
**moniliasis** an infection of the mucous membranes by yeastlike fungi.
**monitor** to oversee or observe.
**monoclonal** a laboratory-produced hybrid cell that produces antibodies.
**monocular** possessing a single eyepiece, as with a microscope.
**monocyte** single nucleated cells that leave the blood and enter into tissues to become macrophages.
**monogamous** an exclusive relationship between two people.
**monokine** a cytokine produced by macrophages or monocytes.
**monotone** a single, unvaried tone; having the same pitch; a tiresome sameness.
**mons pubis** a pad of fatty tissue and coarse skin overlying the symphysis pubis in the female.
**moral** a principle of right and wrong in conduct.
**moral** pertaining to distinction of "right" and "wrong"
**morality** right living; virtue.
**mores** folkways that, through general observance, develop the force of a law.
**morphology** a branch of biology dealing with the form and structure of organisms.
**motor** refers to the nerves that permit the body to respond to stimuli.
**mouth** the oral cavity; can also refer to the opening to organs.
**MRI** see **magnetic resonance imaging.**
**mucosa** pertaining to mucous membrane.
**MUGA** see **multiple-gated acquisition scan.**
**multi-provider clinic** group practices, which consists of three or more physicians who share a facility for the purpose of practicing medicine.
**multi-skilled** having more than one skill area for employment.
**multichannel** refers to the capability of ECG equipment of processing impulses from multiple leads.
**multiple-gated acquisition scan (MUGA)** a diagnostic test to evaluate the condition of the myocardium of the heart.
**mumps** an acute contagious disease characterized by inflammation of the parotid gland and other salivary glands.
**murmur** a soft blowing or rasping sound heard on auscultation of the heart.
**muscle team** a pair of skeletal muscles, one that flexes and one that extends the joint.
**muscle tone** a state of muscle contraction in which a portion of the fibers are contracted while others are at rest.
**muscle** a type of tissue composed of contractile cells or fibers that effect movement of the body.
**muscular** pertaining to muscles.
**musculoskeletal** pertaining to the muscular and skeletal systems.
**mutation** a change in an inheritable characteristic; cellular change caused by an influence.
**myelin** a fatlike substance forming the principal component of the myelin sheath of nerve fibers.
**myelography** an x-ray examination of the spinal cord following an injection of a radiopaque material.
**myocardial infarction (MI)** blockage of a coronary artery that interrupts the flow of blood to the heart muscle.
**myocardium** the muscle layer of the heart.
**myometrium** the muscular structure of the uterus.
**myopia** a defect in vision so that objects can only be seen when very near; nearsightedness.
**myxedema** a condition resulting from the hypofunction of the thyroid gland.

**nagel's rule** a method of predicting the anticipated date of delivery when pregnant.
**narcolepsy** overwhelming attacks of sleep that the victim cannot inhibit; sleeping sickness.
**narcotic** a drug capable of producing sleep and relieving pain or inducing unconsciousness and even death, depending upon the dosage.
**nasal** pertaining to the nose.
**nasal speculum** an instrument permitting visualization of the inside of the nasal cavity.

**national center for competency testing** a national certifying organization which certifies medical assistants and other healthcare professionals after successful completion of a certification exam.
**National Certified Medical Assistant (NCMA)** the credential given by the National Center for Competency testing to successful candidates that pass the NCMA exam.
**National Certified Medical Office Assistant (NCMOA)** the credential given by the National Center for Competency testing to successful candidates that pass the NCMOA exam.
**National Healthcare Association** NHA provides products and services to health care professionals, including continuing education, program development, career and networking services, as well as 10 certification exams for several allied health care area, including Certified Clinical Medical Assistant (CCMA) (and Certified Medical Administrative Assistant (CMAA).
**National Provider Identifier (NPI)** the name of the standard unique health identifier for health care providers
**naturopathy** a multidisciplinary approach to health care based on the belief that the body has the power to heal itself.
**naturopathy** a multidisciplinary approach to health care based on the belief that the body has power to heal itself. Treatment is based on assessment of the correct diet, rest, relaxation, exercise, fresh air, clean water, and sunlight the patient is receiving.
**nausea** an inclination to vomit.
**needle holder** instrument used to hold a suture needle during the suturing process.
**needlesticks** unintentional injury that occurs in the course of handling injection materials used for medication administration
**negate** to deny the existence or truth of.
**neglect** to ignore or pay no attention to; to leave uncared for.
**negligent** guilty of neglect; lacking in due care or concern; act of carelessness.
**negotiable** capable of being discussed and terms arranged.
**neoadjuvant** new attachment process; giving chemotherapy prior to surgery to shrink the tumor before removal.
**neonate** a newborn infant.
**neoplasm** a new growth.
**neoplastic** new abnormal tissue formation; cancer-related.
**nephrologist** a physician specializing in the diseases and disorders of the kidney.
**nephrology** the study of the kidney and its diseases.
**nephron** the structural and functional unit of the kidney.
**nephrotic syndrome** term applied to renal disease of whatever cause characterized by massive edema, proteinuria, and usually elevation of serum cholesterol and lipids.
**nerve** a group of nervous tissues bound together for the purpose of conducting nervous impulses.
**nervosa** loss of appetite for food not connected with a disease; part of a psychosis.
**net** remaining after all deductions have been made; to clear as profit.
**net worth** assets minus liabilities, that demonstrates the value of a business.
**neurilemma** a thin membranous sheath enveloping a nerve fiber.
**neurologist** a physician specializing in the diseases and disorders of the nervous system.
**neurology** the study of the nervous system and its diseases.
**neuron** a nerve cell.
**neurosurgery** surgical procedures performed on the nervous system.
**neutrophil** a granulated white blood cell.
**nicotine** a poisonous alkaloid extracted from tobacco leaves.
**nit** the egg of a louse or other parasitic insect.
**nitrite** a urine test that is positive in urinary tract infections from the presence of bacteria reducing nitrates to nitrite.
**nocturia** having to void at night.
**node** a knot, knob, protuberance, or swelling.
**nomenclature** a system of technical or scientific names.
**nominal** too small to be considered, or a very small amount.
**nomogram** representation by graphs, diagrams, or charts of the relationship between numerical variables.
**non compos mentis** general legal term for all forms of mental illness.
**nonchalant** unconcerned, indifferent.
**noninvasive procedurer** a diagnostic method not requiring entry into body tissue.
**nonpathogen** an organism that does not produce a disease.
**nonspecific urethritis** inflammation of the urethra in males and vaginitis or cervicitis in females caused by bacteria or an allergy to substances used by a sexual partner.
**norepinephrine** a hormone secreted by adrenal medulla in response to sympathetic stimulation.
**normal saline** a solution with the same salt content as that found within a red blood cell.
**no show** term used to describe a visit in which a patient fails to present for examination without giving the provider advance notice.
**noun** the name of anything, such as a person, place, object, occurrence, or state.
**NREM (non–rapid eye movement)** a stage of sleep in which the sleeper does not experience rapid eye movement. In a healthy young adult, NREM sleep usually accounts for 75%–90% of sleep time.
**nuclear** pertaining to the nucleus of an atom.
**nuclear medicine** the branch of medicine that uses radionuclides in the diagnosis and treatment of disease.
**nuclear medicine technologist** an individual trained in the specialized field of operating cameras that detect and map the radioactive drug in a patient's body to create diagnostic images.
**nucleolus** a structure found within the nucleus of the cell.
**nucleus** the vital body in the protoplasm of a cell.
**numerator** the top number of a fraction.
**numeric** denoting a number or system of numbers.
**nurse anesthetist** is an RN that is certified to administer anesthesia.
**nurse assistant (NA)** a person trained to assist nurses and attend to patients.
**nurse midwife** a nurse trained in the delivery of babies.
**nurse midwife** a professional RN who has had extensive training and experience in labor and delivery.
**nurse practitioner** a midlevel practitioner that is able to examine patients, order diagnostic tests and prescribe certain types of medications. Usually supervised by a physician but may work independently in some states.
**nurse practitioner** an RN with advanced clinical experience and education in a special branch of practice.
**nurture** to care for, train, or educate.
**nutrition** refers to edible material, food, things that nourish.
**nutritionist** a member of the health care team who studies and applies the principles and science of nutrition.

**obese** weighing more than 30% of ideal body weight.
**objective** the end toward which action is directed; of a disease symptom, perceptible to persons other than the one affected; on a microscope, a lens or series of lenses.
**obligate** to bind legally or morally.
**obligation** responsibility; a moral, social, or legal tie.
**obliterate** to blot out; leave no trace; destroy.
**observant** quick to notice, watchful.
**obsolete** out of use, discarded, no longer useful.
**obstetrician** a physician who specializes in the care and treatment of women during pregnancy and childbirth.

**obstetrics** the branch of medicine dealing with women during pregnancy, childbirth, and postpartum.
**obstructed** blocked.
**obturator** anything that obstructs or closes a cavity or opening; refers to that internal portion of an examining instrument that facilitates the introduction of the instrument into the body and is then withdrawn, permitting visualization of the internal area.
**occipital** pertaining to the back part of the head, the posterior lobe of the cerebrum.
**occlude** to close up, obstruct.
**occluder** a device to block viewing when conducting an eye examination.
**occult** obscure; hidden.
**occulta** obscure; hidden.
**occupational medicine** diagnosing and treating disease or conditions arising from occupational circumstances.
**Occupational Safety and Health Administration (OSHA)** an agency of the United States Department of Labor. It was created by Congress under the Occupational Safety and Health Act, signed by President Richard M. Nixon, on December 29, 1970. Its mission is to prevent work-related injuries, illnesses, and deaths by issuing and enforcing rules (called standards) for workplace safety and health.
**occupational therapist (OT)** a health care worker involved in the use of purposeful activity with individuals who are limited by physical injury or illness, psychosocial dysfunction, developmental or learning diabilities, poverty and cultural differences, or the aging process to maximize independence, prevent disability, and maintain health.
**occupational therapy assistant (OTA)** a person trained to assist an occupational therapist.
**Ocular** (1) eyepiece of a microscope; (2) Pertaining to the eye
**O.D.** oculus dexter, or right eye.
**Offer** a specific proposal to enter into an agreement with another; an offer is an essential component of an enforceable contract.
**office manager** (business office manager) an individual responsible for the overall operation of the medical office.
**ointment** a salve; a fatty, soft substance having antiseptic or healing properties.
**olfactory** pertaining to the sense of smell.
**oliguria** scanty production of urine.
**oncogenes** a gene in a tumor cell.
**oncologist** a doctor who has been specially trained in the study of tumors and cancer.
**oncology** the branch of medicine dealing with tumors, usually malignant.
**online banking** The practice of making bank transactions or paying bills electronically via the Internet.
**on-site** at the location.
**operating information** the information that is needed on a day-to-day basis in order for a company to conduct business.
**ophthalmic** pertaining to the eye.
**ophthalmic technician (OT)** an individual trained for assisting ophthalmologists with patients as well as procedures associated with the eyes.
**ophthalmologist** a physician specializing in the diseases and disorders of the eye.
**ophthalmology** the study of the eye and its diseases.
**opportunistic** seizing the opportunity; taking advantage of the situation.
**opposition** action against, resistance.
**optic** pertaining to the eye or sight.
**optic disc** the blind spot where the optic nerve exits from the retina of the eye.
**optometrist** a person who measures the eye's refractive power and prescribes correction of visual defects when needed.
**oral** pertaining to the mouth.
**orbital** refers to the cavity within the skull where the eye is located.
**organ** a part of the body constructed of many types of tissue to perform a function.
**organ of Corti** terminal acoustic apparatus in the cochlea of the inner ear.
**organelles** functional structures within the cytoplasm of a cell.
**organic** pertaining to or derived from animal or vegetable forms of life.
**organizational ethics** the standards by which an organization will hold itself accountable to proper conduct
**origin** the beginning or source of anything; of muscles, the anchor.
**orthopedics** the branch of medicine dealing with the structure and function of bones and muscles.
**orthopedist** a physician who corrects deformities and treats diseases and disorders of the bones, joints, and spine.
**orthopnea** respiratory condition in which breathing is possible only in an erect sitting or standing position.
**orthostatic** standing; concerning an erect position.
**O.S.** oculus sinister, or left eye.
**os** pertains to a mouth or opening.
**oscilloscope** an instrument that displays a visual representation of electric variations on the fluorescent screen of a cathode ray tube.
**OSHA** U.S. Occupational Safety and Health Administration.
**osmosis** the process of diffusion of water or another solvent through a selected permeable membrane.
**osseous** bonelike, concerning bones.
**osteopathy** any bone disease; also refers to a school of medicine based on the belief that the bony fragment of the body largely determines the structural relations of its tissues.
**osteoporosis** a condition resulting from a decrease in the amount of calcium stored in the bone.
**OTA** see **occupational therapy assistant.**
**OTC** see **over the counter.**
**otic** pertaining to the ear.
**otitis** inflammation of the ear; can be referenced to the external, middle, or internal ear.
**otorhinolaryngologist** a physician specializing in diseases and disorders of the ear, nose, and throat.
**otorhinolaryngology** the study of the ear, nose, and larynx and their diseases.
**otosclerosis** condition characterized by progressive deafness caused by the fixation of the stapes of the middle ear.
**outsourcing** an arrangement by which a task, operation, or job that could be performed by employees within a company is instead contracted to another company.
**O.U.** oculus uterque, or each eye.
**ovary** the female gonad, which produces hormones causing the secondary sex characteristics to develop and be maintained.
**over-the-counter (OTC)** referring to accessible, nonprescription drugs.
**overdraft** an amount beyond what is currently in the account.
**ovulation** the periodic ripening and rupture of a mature graafian follicle and the discharge of the ovum.
**ovum** an egg, the female gamete or reproductive cell.
**oxalate** a salt of oxalic acid.
**oxygen** a colorless, odorless, tasteless gas found in the air; chemical symbol, $O_2$.
**oxygenate** combine or supply with oxygen.

**pacemaker** the SA node of the heart; also refers to an artificial device that initiates heartbeat.
**pallor** lack of color, paleness.
**palpate** to feel; to examine by touch.
**palpation** the technique of examination using the fingers or hands.
**pancreas** an organ that secretes insulin and pancreatic digestive juice.
**pancreatitis** inflammation of the pancreas.
**pandemic** epidemic over a large region; epidemic in many regions.
**panic value** an important indicator on a lab test that indicates immediate notification of the health care provider.
**pantomime** motions or gestures used for expressive communication.
**papanicolaou (Pap) smear** a test to detect cancer cells in the mucus of an organ.
**papillae** small protuberances or elevations, such as the taste buds of the tongue.
**papillary muscles** muscular attachments to the undersides of the heart valves from the walls of the ventricles, which open the valves during the relaxation phase of the heartbeat.

**papule** red, elevated area on the skin.
**parabasal** beside, near, an accessory to the base or lower part.
**paralytic ileus** paralysis of the intestinal wall with symptoms of acute obstruction.
**paramedic** health care providers who provide emergency and supportive medical care; have additional training beyond EMT status.
**parameter** quantity to which an arbitrary value may be given as a convenience in expressing performance or for use in calculations.
**parasite** an organism that lives in or on another organism without rendering it any service in return.
**parasympathetic** a division of the autonomic nervous system.
**parathyroid** small endocrine glands located close to the thyroid gland.
**parenteral** other than by mouth.
**parietal** a central portion of the cerebrum located on each side of the brain.
**paroxysmal** a sudden attack of a disease; fit of acute pain, passion, coughing, or laughter.
**paroxysmal stage** occurring repeatedly; recurrent symptoms.
**partnership** two or more physicians that have a legal agreement to share in the total business operation of the practice.
**patella** the kneecap.
**pathogen** any microorganism or substance capable of producing a disease.
**pathologic** a condition caused by a disease.
**pathologist** a physician specializing in the interpretation and diagnosis of changes caused by disease in tissues and body fluids.
**pathology** the study of the nature and cause of disease.
**pathophysiology** the study of mechanisms by which disease occurs, the responses of the body to the disease process, and the effects of both on normal function.
**patience** calm in waiting, endurance without complaint.
**patient care technician (PCT)** a health care worker who uses both nursing and medical assisting skills to provide patient care in a hospital setting.
**patient centered medical homes** a team-based model of care led by a personal physician who provides continuous and coordinated care throughout a patient's lifetime to maximize health outcomes.
**patient education** Information, instructions and cautions provided to a patient intended to ensure and advance his or her safety, health and/or recovery from injury or illness.
**patient portal** a component of an Electronic Health Records (EHR) system that allows patients to communicate with their medical office electronically, to request lab results, referrals, appointments, and in some instances communicate with doctors via email.
**Patient Protection and Affordability Act** a bill passed in 2010 intended to expand access to health insurance, provide additional consumer protections and reduce costs of health care.
**patronize** to treat condescendingly.
**payee** a person to whom money is paid.
**PCT** see **patient care technician**.
**PDR** *Physician's Desk Reference.*
**peak flow** the maximum rate of air flow out of the lungs during forced expiration; used especially for monitoring lung capacity of individuals with asthma.
**pectoralis major** the principal muscle of the chest wall.
**pediatric** the branch of medicine dealing with the care of children and their diseases.
**pediatrician** a physician specializing in the diseases and disorders of children.
**pediatrics** the branch of medicine dealing with the care of children and their diseases.
**pediculosis** the scientific name for lice.
**peer** equal; usually refers to someone of similar standing or status.
**peer review** assessment by other physicians or scientists in the same field.
**pelvic** pertaining to the pelvis.
**penis** the male external sex organ.
**peptic** pertaining to digestion; can also refer to an ulcer of the upper digestive tract.
**per capita** for each person.
**perceive** to become aware of through the senses; to understand.
**percentage** rate or proportion of each hundred.
**percentage** rate or proportion of each hundred.
**percentile** any value in a series dividing the distribution of its members into 100 groups of equal frequency.
**perception** awareness through the senses; the receipt of impressions; consciousness.
**percussion** tapping the body lightly but sharply to determine the position, size, and consistency of an underlying structure.
**percussion hammer** a hard, rubber-surfaced instrument used to test tendon reflex action.
**performance** to execute an undertaking; an action; success in working.
**performance objectives** statements on a resume which identify a person's specific knowledge, skills, or behaviors
**perfusion** passing of a fluid through spaces; the act of pouring over or through.
**pericarditis** inflammation of the pericardium, the covering of the heart.
**pericardium** the membranous sac that covers the heart.
**perineum** the region between the vagina and anus of the female and the scrotum and anus of the male.
**periodic** occurring, appearing, or done again and again, at regular intervals.
**periodical** appearing at regular intervals of time.
**periosteum** the fibrous membrane covering the bone except at the articulating surfaces.
**peripheral** pertaining to a portion of the nervous system; an item attached to a computer system.
**peristalsis** a progressive, wavelike muscular movement that occurs involuntarily in the urinary and digestive system.
**peritoneal** pertaining to the peritoneum.
**peritoneum** the membrane that lines the abdominal cavity and covers the abdominal organs.
**permeable** capable of being penetrated; allowing entrance.
**pernicious anemia** a severe anemia characterized by progressive decrease in the production of red blood cells.
**perplexing** troubling with doubt, puzzling.
**PERRLA** an acronym meaning pupils equal, regular, react to light and accommodation.
**persecute** treat badly; do harm to again and again; pursue to injure.
**perserverance** the act of continuing steadfastly, especially in the face of discouragement.
**personal protective equipment (PPE)** protective clothing, goggles, or gloves designed to protect the wearer's body or clothing from contamination by blood or other potentially infectious materials for job-related occupational safety and health purposes.
**personality** the personal or individual qualities that make one person different from another.
**perspective** a view of things, or facts, in which they are in the right relations.
**pertinent** having to do with what is being considered; relevant or to the point.
**pertussis** an acute infectious disease characterized by a paroxysmal cough, ending in a whooping inspiration.
**petechiae** small, purplish, hemorrhagic spots on the skin.
**petition** a written plea in which specific court action is sought.
**petty** small, having little value, mean, narrow-minded.
**petty cash** a small amount of cash available for small business expenses used for postage stamps, inexpensive office supplies, and small charitable donations, usually maintained in a locked container.
**pH** a measure of acidity or alkalinity.
**phagocyte** a white blood cell that engulfs and destroys antigens.

**phagocytosis** ingestion and digestion of bacteria and particles by phagocytes.
**phalanges** bones of the fingers and toes.
**phalanx** any one of the bones of the fingers or toes.
**phantom limb** an illusion following amputation of a limb that the limb still exists.
**pharmaceutical** concerning drugs or pharmacy.
**pharmacist (RPH)** a licensed health care provider who prepares and dispenses drugs.
**pharmacology** the study and practice of compounding and dispensing medical preparations.
**pharmacy technician (PT)** an assistant to a pharmacist who prepares and in some situations administers medication.
**pharynx** the throat; that portion of the alimentary canal between the mouth and the esophagus.
**phenylalanine** an amino acid of a protein.
**phenylketonuria (PKU)** a genetic disorder resulting from the body's failure to oxidize an amino acid, perhaps because of a defective enzyme.
**phimosis** a narrowing of the opening of the foreskin of the penis.
**phlebitis** inflammation of a vein.
**phlebotomist** a health care worker who specializes in obtaining blood samples.
**photocopy** a photographic reproduction of written matter made by a special device.
**photophobia** sensitive to light; avoiding light.
**photosensitivity** inability to tolerate light due to medication effects or illness
**physical** pertaining to the body; also used for the examination of the body.
**physical medicine** the branch of medicine dealing with the treatment of disorders and diseases with mechanical devices, as in physical therapy.
**physical therapist (PT)** one who is licensed to assist in the examination, testing, and treatment of physically disabled or handicapped people through the use of special exercise, application of heat or cold, use of sonar, and other techniques.
**physician** a medical doctor; one skilled in the practice of medicine.
**physician's assistant (PA)** a person trained in certain aspects of the practice of medicine to provide assistance to the physician.
**physician assistant** a midlevel practitioner that is able to examine patients, order diagnostic tests and prescribe certain types of medications. Usually supervised by a physician.
**Physicians' Desk Reference (PDR)** one of the reference books that lists information about medications.
**physician's office laboratory (POL)** a designated room in the physician's office where laboratory procedures and tests are performed by qualified persons.
**physiology** the study of the function of the cells, tissues, and organs of the body.
**pia mater** innermost of the three meninges of the brain and spinal cord.
**pigment** any coloring matter.
**pineal body** a small endocrine gland attached to the posterior part of the third ventricle of the brain.
**pinocytosis** the process whereby a cell engulfs large amounts of liquid.
**pitch** the frequency of vibrations of sound that enable one to classify sound on a scale from high to low.
**pitfall** trap or hidden danger.
**pituitary** a small endocrine gland attached to the base of the brain; the "master" gland.
**PKU** see **phenylketonuria.**
**placebo** an inactive substance that is given as a medicine for its suggestive effect.
**placebo effect** refers to the fact that some people respond favorably to a known ineffective treatment because they believe it is working.
**placenta** the structure through which the fetus obtains nourishment during pregnancy; the afterbirth.
**plague** a deadly epidemic or pestilence.
**Plague** potentially infectious life-threatening diseases, usually transmitted by bites of rodent fleas to humans
**Plaintiff** the party who initiates a lawsuit by filing a complaint with the clerk of the court against the defendant(s) demanding damages, performance and/or court determination of rights.
**planes** a flat or relatively smooth surface; points of reference by which positions or parts of the body are indicated.
**plasma** the liquid part of the lymph and blood.
**platelet** a type of cell found in the blood that is required for clotting.
**pleura** a serous membrane that covers the lungs and lines the thoracic cavity.
**pleurisy** inflammation of the pleura.
**plexuses** a network of nerves.
**plight** unfavorable situation or distressed condition.
**plural** the form of a term that indicates more than one.
**pneumoencephalography** an x-ray examination of ventricles and subarachnoid spaces of brain following withdrawal of cerebrospinal fluid and injection of air or gas via a lumbar puncture.
**pneumonia** inflammation of the lung caused primarily by microbes, chemical irritants, vegetable dust, or allergy.
**pneumonitis** an inflammation of the lungs, also known as pneumonia.
**pneumonoconiosis** a respiratory condition caused by inhalation of dust particles from mining or stone cutting.
**pneumothorax** a collection of air or gas in the pleural cavity that displaces lung tissue.
**podiatrist** (chiropodist) a person trained to diagnose and treat diseases and disorders of the feet.
**podiatry** the branch of medicine dealing with disorders of the feet.
**poison** a substance that, if taken internally or applied externally, is a threat to life.
**POL** see **physician's office laboratory.**
**policy** a high-level overall plan; general principles of an organization.
**polio** (poliomyelitis) an acute, infectious, systemic disease that causes inflammation of the gray matter of the spinal cord.
**polling** pertains to obtaining an unauthorized FAX transmission.
**polycystic kidney disease** a condition of multiple cysts in the kidney.
**polycythemia** an excess of red blood cells.
**polyneuralgia** pain in many nerves.
**polyp** a tumor with a pedicle, especially on mucous membranes, such as in the nose, rectum, or intestines.
**polyuria** excessive secretion and discharge of urine.
**pons** a portion of the brainstem connecting the medulla oblongata and cerebellum with upper portions of the brain.
**popliteal** pertains to the area in back of the knee.
**portal** pertaining to the portal circulation of blood from impaired internal organs to the liver for processing before entering the inferior vena cava.
**positive** strongly affirmative.
**positron emission tomography (PET scan)** a form of imaging permitting visualizing the physiologic function of the body.
**post mortem** pertaining to or occurring during the period after death; common term for autopsy.
**posted** to transfer charges from the day sheet to patient account records.
**posterior** toward the rear or back or toward the caudal end.
**postmark** a dated cancellation of a stamp by the post office that also identifies the place of posting.
**postoperative (post-op)** after or following a surgical procedure.
**postpartum** the period following delivery of a baby.
**postscript (PS)** an addition to a letter written after the writer's name has been signed.
**posture** the position and carriage of the body as a whole.
**potential** possible; ability to develop into actuality.

**power of attorney** a legal document authorizing a person to act as another's attorney, legal representative, or agent.
**PPM** see **provider-performed microscopy.**
**practice management system (PMS)** computer system used to keep and generate the records and reports of the practice.
**Practice Management Software (PMS)** a type of medical office software that provides the medical office the electronic component to deal with day-to-day financial operations of a medical practice, and frequently includes the ability for appointment scheduling, patient registration, charge and payment posting, and insurance and billing.
**practicum** a supervised employment experience in a qualified health care facility as part of the educational curriculum; also known as an externship.
**practitioner** one who practices the profession of medicine.
**preauthorization** prior approval of insurance coverage and necessity of procedure.
**precancerous** a state just prior to the development of cancer.
**precautions** care beforehand; a preventive measure.
**precise** exact; definite; very accurate.
**precision** exactness, accuracy.
**precordial** pertaining to that area of the chest wall over the heart for the placement of ECG chest leads.
**preferred provider organization (PPO)** an organization of physicians who network together to offer discounts to purchasers of health care insurance.
**prefix** a word component added to the beginning of a word root or combining form that typically modifies the remaining part of the term.
**pregnancy** the condition of being with child.
**preliminary** coming before, leading up to.
**premium** the amount paid or payable (for example, an insurance policy premium).
**prenatal** the period before birth.
**preoperative (preop)** the preparatory period preceding surgery.
**Preponderance of the evidence** the greater weight of the evidence required in a civil (non-criminal) lawsuit for the trier of fact (jury or judge without a jury) to decide in favor of one side or the other. this preponderance is based on the more convincing evidence and its probable truth or accuracy, and not on the amount of evidence.
**preposition** a word that shows the relationship of an object to some other word in the sentence.
**presbycusis** impairment of acute hearing in old age.
**presbyopia** a defect of vision in advancing age involving loss of accommodation.
**prescribe** to lay down as a rule or direction; to order or advise the use of.
**prescription** a written direction for the preparation of a medicine.
**prevention** the act of keeping something from coming to pass; to hinder.
**preventive** tending to prevent or hinder; something used to prevent disease.
**primary** occurring first in time, development, or sequence; earliest.
**primary diagnosis** the main reason a patient is seen or cared for during an encounter.
**prioritize** to arrange in order of importance.
**priority** preference; state of being first in time, place or mark.
**privacy officer** the person designated by a healthcare organization, whether hospital system or private practice, who handles and oversees the maintenance of protected health information.
**pro tem** acting as (a temporary position); for the time being.
**Problem-Oriented Medical Record (POMR)** A system of recordkeeping used to collect specific pieces of information regarding a patient during a healthcare visit, such as patient profile, chief complaint, review of systems, physical examination, laboratory reports, chronic problems, medication and preventive care lists, and patient education.
**process** to treat or prepare by some method.
**processor** performing a whole sequence of actions or operations.
**proclivity** an inclination or predisposition toward something.
**procrastination** intentionally delaying action of something that should be done; to postpone.
**procrastinator** one who intentionally delays or postpones action.
**proctological** body position that requires the use of a proctologic examination table; the patient kneels on knee board of the table, bends at the hips and rests the chest on the table. the head is supported by a headboard.
**proctology** the study of the rectum and anus and their diseases.
**proctoscope** an instrument for the inspection of the rectum.
**proctoscopy** instrumental inspection of the rectum.
**procure** to get or obtain.
**procurement** to obtain; acquire.
**product** the result of multiplying two numbers together.
**productivity** the amount of work accomplished in a period of time.
**professional** conforming to the technical or ethical standards of a profession.
**professional ethics** a framework of evaluating conduct applicable to members of a given profession
**professionalism** professional status, methods, character, or standards.
**proficiency testing (PT)** the measurement of acquired knowledge and skills; a means of assessing the competency of someone or of something.
**proficient** well advanced in an art, occupation, skill, or branch of knowledge; unusually knowledgeable.
**profit sharing** a system by which employees receive a share of the profits of a business enterprise.
**progesterone** a hormone secreted by the graafian follicle following the expulsion of the ovum.
**programmed** arranged; planned; a sequence of actions performed by a computer.
**progress notes** record of the continuing progress and treatment of a patient.
**progress report** an upgrading of current findings.
**project** to produce and send forth with clarity and distinctness.
**projection** a defense mechanism of trying to blame another for one's own inadequacies.
**prolapse** dropping of an internal part of the body; usually refers to uterus or rectum.
**prominent** conspicuous, outstanding.
**promissory** containing a pledge to pay.
**prompt** to urge to action, to inspire.
**prone** a position, lying horizontal with the face down.
**pronoun** a word used instead of a noun, to indicate without naming.
**proofread** reading of printed proofs to discover and correct errors.
**property right** the entitlement to anything that is owned by a person or entity. Property is divided into two types: "real property," which is any interest in land, real estate, growing plants or the improvements on it, and "personal property," which is everything else.
**prophylactic** preventing disease.
**proportion** another way of saying fraction.
**proprietary** privately owned and managed and run as a profit-making organization.
**proprietorship** the amount by which assets exceed liabilities.
**prosecution** in criminal law, the government attorney charging and trying the case against a person accused of a crime, or a common term for the government's side in a criminal case.
**prostaglandins** a group of chemical substances secreted by mast cells or basophils that constricts smooth muscles in some organs.

**prostate** a gland of the male reproductive system that surrounds the proximal portion of the urethra.

**prostatectomy** excision of part or all of the prostate gland.

**prosthesis** an artificial replacement of a missing body part.

**protanopia** a problem in which the perception of reds and sometimes yellow and green become confusing.

**protected health information (PHI)** confidential health information that is protected under Health Insurance Portability and Accountability Act (HIPAA).

**protein (albumin)** a normal substance found in serum but when found in urine means the presence of an excess of serum proteins excreted in the urine rather than reabsorbed by the renal tubules; a nutrient found in foods such as eggs, meat, fish, legumes, and soy products that provides energy to the body.

**prothrombin** chemical substance existing in circulating blood which aids in the clotting process.

**protocol** a plan of treatment, usually experimental, used to determine effectiveness of new treatments or medications.

**protozoan** a single-cell animal.

**Provider** is an individual licensed to examine, diagnose and prescribe treatment to patients seeking assistance.

**Provider** the person that oversees the patient's healthcare. Often a physician, physician's assistant or nurse practitioner.

**provider-performed microscopy (PPM)** refers to microscopic procedures done in the physician's office laboratory.

**provisions** the act of providing; something provided for the future; a stipulation.

**proximal** nearest the point of attachment.

**proxy** one who has authority to vote or act for another; a certificate of authorization to vote.

**prudent** careful; wise in practical affairs.

**pruritic** pertaining to an itching sensation.

**pruritus** severe itching.

**pruritus ani** itching around the anus.

**PS** see **postscript.**

**psoriasis** a chronic inflammatory disease characterized by scaly patches.

**psychedelics** hallucinogenic drugs.

**psychiatrist** a physician specializing in the diseases and disorders of the mind, including neuroses and psychoses.

**psychiatry** the branch of medicine dealing with the diagnosis, treatment, and prevention of mental illness.

**psychological** of the mind; mental.

**psychologist** a person specializing in the study of the structure and function of the brain and related mental processes.

**psychology** the study of mental processes, both normal and abnormal, and their effects upon behavior.

**psychoneuroimmunology** a science studying the connection between the brain, behavior, and immunity.

**psychopathic** concerning or characterized by a mental disorder.

**psychosis** mental disturbance of such magnitude that there is personality disintegration and loss of contact with reality.

**psychosomatic** pertaining to interrelationships between the mind or emotions and body.

**psychotherapy** the treatment of disease by hypnosis, psychoanalysis, and similar means.

**PT** see **pharmacy technician** or **proficiency testing**.

**ptosis** a drooping or dropping of an organ or part, for example the eyelid or the kidney.

**puberty** the period of life at which one becomes functionally capable of reproduction.

**pubic** pertaining to the middle section of the lower third of the abdomen, also referred to as the hypogastric.

**pulmonary** concerning or involving the lungs.

**pulmonary edema** the presence of interstitial fluid in the lung tissue.

**pulmonary embolis** a blockage in the pulmonary artery or one of its branches.

**pulse deficit** the difference between the pulse rate measured radially and apically.

**pulse oximetry** measuring the oxygen saturation of arterial blood in a subject by utilizing a sensor attached typically to a finger, toe, or ear to determine the percentage of oxyhemoglobin in blood pulsating through a network of capillaries and that typically sounds an alarm if the blood saturation becomes less than optimal.

**pulse pressure** difference between the systolic and diastolic measurements.

**pulse** throbbing caused by the regular alternating contraction and expansion of an artery.

**punctual** prompt; being on time.

**punctuality** a desirable trait of being on time for appointments, work, etc.

**punctuation** standardized marks in written matter to clarify meaning.

**puncture** a hole made by something pointed.

**Punitive damages** damages awarded in a lawsuit as a punishment and example to others for malicious, evil or fraudulent acts.

**pupil** the contractible opening in the center of the iris for the transmission of light.

**purge** to empty; to cleanse of impurities; clear.

**Purkinje** network of fibers found in the cardiac muscle that carries the electrical impulses resulting in the contraction of the ventricles.

**pustular** pertaining to a collection of pus that has accumulated in a cavity formed by the tissue on the basis of an infectious process.

**pustule** small elevation of the skin filled with lymph or pus.

**pyelonephritis** inflammation of the kidney, pelvis, and nephrons.

**pyloric** pertaining to the opening between the stomach and the duodenum.

**pyrogen** capable of producing fever.

**QNS** quantity not sufficient.

**quackery** the pretense to knowledge or skill in medicine.

**quad-base** refers to a cane with four "feet."

**quadrant** one of four regions, as of the abdomen, divided for identification purposes.

**quadriceps femoris** a large muscle on the anterior surface of the thigh that is composed of four separate muscles.

**qualifications** a quality or attainment that fits a person for a place or position.

**quality assurance (QA)** inclusive policies, procedures, and practices as standards for reliable laboratory results that includes documentation, calibration, and maintenance of all equipment, quality control, proficiency testing, and training.

**quality control (QC)** inclusive laboratory procedures as standards to provide reliable performance of equipment, including test control samples, documentation, and analyzing statistics for diagnostic tests.

**Rabies** an acute viral disease of the nervous system of warm-blooded animals; usually transmitted by the bite of a rabid animal

**radial** referring to the radial artery or pulse taken in the radial artery.

**radiation** the emission and diffusion of rays; a product of x-ray and radium.

**radioactive** capable of emitting radiant energy.

**radioactive agents** agents used to diagnose certain medical problems or treat certain diseases.

**radiograph** a record produced on a photographic plate, film, or paper by the action of x-ray or radium.

**radiologist** one who diagnoses and treats disease by the use of radiant energy.

**radiology** the study of radiation and its uses.

**radiology technician** an individual trained in the administration of x-rays.

**radionuclides** a type of atom used in nuclear medicine for the diagnosis and treatment of disease.

**radiopaque** impenetrable to the x-ray or other forms of radiation.

**radius** a long bone of the forearm.

**rales** an unusual sound heard in the bronchi on examination of respirations.

**ramification** a subdivision or consequence.
**random** by chance; without plan.
**range of motion (ROM)** refers to the degree of movement of the body's joints and extremities.
**rapport** relationship characterized by harmony and cooperation.
**ratchet** locking mechanism of an instrument
**rational** based on reasoning, sensible.
**rationalization** to explain on rational grounds, to devise plausible explanations for one's acts.
**RAST** short for radioallergosorbent test, a blood test used to determine what a person is allergic to. This is different from a skin allergy test, which determines allergy by the reaction of a person's skin to different substances.
**Raynaud's phenomenon** a symptom of lupus characterized by fingers that turn white or blue in the cold.
**reactivity** rate of nuclear disintegration in a reactor.
**reagent** a substance involved in a chemical reaction.
**realm** kingdom or empire, as used in text.
**reason rule** refers to the purpose or reason for doing a test or procedure, an insurance company criteria for reimbursement.
**receipt** a written acknowledgement that something has been received.
**reception** the fact or manner of being received; a social gathering.
**receptionist** one employed to greet telephone callers, visitors, patients, or clients.
**receptor** peripheral nerve ending of a sensory nerve that responds to stimuli.
**recessive gene** apparently suppressed in crossbred offspring in preference for a characteristic from the other parent.
**recipient** one who receives.
**reciprocity** mutual exchange, especially the exchange of special privilege.
**Reciprocity** a physician who has been licensed in one state and wishes to move to another state may be granted a license by reciprocity if it is determined that the original licensure requirements are equal to or more stringent to the requirements of the new state.
**reconcile** process to bring checkbook and bank statement into agreement.
**rectal** referring to the rectum.
**rectocele** the protrusion of the posterior vaginal wall and anterior wall of the rectum through the vagina.
**rectum** the lower part of the large intestine between the sigmoid and the anal canal.
**recumbent** lying down.
**recurrent** returning at intervals.
**reduce** to restore the ends of a fractured bone to their usual relationship.
**redundant** extra, not needed, repetitive.
**reference** a source of information or authority.
**reference points** in communication, the sum total of values, culture, education, and experiences that an individual holds that affect the way that a message is received.
**referral** sending a patient to a provider of a different specialty for treatment beyond the scope of practice for the initial practitioner
**reflective communication** an interactive communication process in which the receiver uses verbal "mirroring" to restate what the sender has said for optimal clarification by all parties.
**reflex** an involuntary response to a stimulus.
**reflexology** massaging of the hands or feet based on the belief that pressure applied to specific points on these extremities benefits other parts of the body.
**reflux** a return or backward flow.
**refractive** the degree to which a transparent body deflects a ray of light from a straight path.
**regimen** regulation of diet, sleep, exercise, and manner of living to improve or maintain health.
**register** a formal or official recording of items, names, or actions; a record of money that has been spent.
**registered** legally certified or authenticated.
**Registered Medical Assistant, RMA (AMT)** the credential the American Medical Technologists (AMT) issues to eligible candidates, which successfully pass the RMA examination.
**registered nurse (RN)** an individual trained through formal training in the field of nursing.
**registry** a list of persons qualified in a particular area of expertise.
**regression** a defense mechanism of retreating to the thoughts and actions of an earlier, "safer," age.
**regulate** control or direction.
**regulations in the POL** standards set for quality assurance and quality control in the physician's office laboratory to ensure reliable diagnostic tests.
**regulatory** to control according to a rule; to adjust so as to make work accurately.
**rehabilitate** to put back in good condition; to restore.
**rehabilitation centers** facilities that assist in developing appropriate socialization skills, family and community reintegration, and increased independence.
**rehabilitative therapy** treatment that offers the highest level of patient care and programs that will enhance the physical, psychological, and emotional health of the population served in most of these facilities.
**reimbursement** to pay back or compensate for money spent, or losses or damages incurred.
**reiterate** to say or do again.
**rejuvenate** to make young again; to give youthful qualities to.
**relapse** recurrence of a disease or symptoms; returning to a previous condition.
**reliable** dependable, can be relied upon.
**reluctant** marked by unwillingness.
**rely** to depend on, to trust.
**REM (rapid eye movement)** a stage of sleep in which the sleeper experiences rapid eye movement. In a healthy young adult, REM sleep accounts for 10%–25% of sleep time.
**remedy** anything that relieves or cures a disease.
**remission** a period that is disease- and symptom-free.
**remote** from a distance; far removed in time and place; indirect.
**renal** pertaining to the kidney.
**renal failure** loss of function of the kidneys' nephrons.
**renal threshold** the concentration at which a substance in the blood normally not excreted by the kidney begins to appear in the urine.
**render** to present or to deliver, as a service or statement.
**renovate** restore; to make new again.
**repolarization** reestablishment of a polarized state in a muscle or nerve fiber following contraction or conduction of a nerve impulse.
**repression** to force painful ideas or impulses into the subconscious.
**reproductive** concerning reproduction.
**reputable** having a good reputation; well thought of.
**res ipsa loquitur** the thing speaks for itself.
**residency** physician training period in a specialty field of medicine.
**residual barium** barium remaining in the intestinal tract following evacuation at the completion of x-ray studies.
**residual** pertaining to that which is left as a residue.
**resistance** opposition, ability to oppose.
**resonance** quality of the sound heard on percussion of the chest; the intensification and prolongation of a sound by reflection or by vibration of a nearby object.
**resource** a source of support or supply.
**respectful** showing respect; honoring; treat with consideration.
**respiration** the taking in of oxygen and its use in the tissues and the giving off of carbon dioxide.
**respiratory therapy technician** a person trained to perform procedures of treatment that maintain or improve the ventilatory function of the respiratory tract.
**respiratory** pertaining to respiration.

**respite** a temporary cessation of something that is painful or tiring; to delay, postpone.
**respondeat superior** let the master answer.
**restricted** limited; only for a certain group.
**resumé** a summary, especially of work experiences.
**resuscitation** an emergency first aid procedure for a victim of cardiac arrest. It is part of the chain of survival, which includes early access (to emergency medical services), early CPR, early defibrillation, and early advanced care. It is also performed as part of the choking protocol if all else has failed; revival from apparent or possible death.
**retardation** slowing, delay, lag; slow in development, mental or physical.
**retention** inability to void urine that is present in the bladder.
**reticuloendothelial** pertaining to that group of cells that appear to aid in the making of new blood cells and the disintegration of old ones.
**retina** the innermost layer of the eye that receives the image formed by the lens.
**retinopathy** a degeneration of the retina caused by a decrease in blood supply.
**retraction** a shortening; the act of drawing backward or state of being drawn back.
**retractor** instrument used to hold back tissue, making the operative site easier to visualize.
**retroflexed** refers to the body of the uterus being bent backward.
**retrograde** refers to an x-ray procedure in which a radiopaque material is instilled by catheter into the bladder, ureters, and kidneys.
**retrograde pyelogram** a urologic procedure in which the physician injects contrast into the ureters in order to visualize the ureters and kidney.
**retroperitoneal** behind the peritoneum; posterior to the peritoneal lining of the abdominal cavity.
**retroverted** refers to the entire uterus being tilted backward.
**retrovirus** one with RNA (ribonucleic acid) genetic material.
**revalidation** the renewing or reconfirmation of credentials.
**revocation** temporary of permanent suspension of a license.
**revoke** to cancel, withdraw, take back.
**Rh factor** an antigenic substance in human blood similar to the A and B factors that determine blood groups; apparently present only in red blood cells.
**rhinitis** inflammation of the nasal mucosa.
**rhinoplasty** plastic surgery of the nose.
**rhythm** a measured time or movement; regularity of occurrence.
**ribosome** an organelle within the cytoplasm of the cell.
**rickets** a disease of the bones primarily due to the deficiency of vitamin D.
**Rickettsiae** Any of a family of rod-shaped, coccoid, or diplococcus-shaped, often pleomorphic gram-negative, bacteria that are intracellular parasites of arthropods (such as lice or ticks) and when transmitted to humans cause various diseases (such as typhus).
**risk** chance; hazard; chance of loss or injury; degree of probability of loss.
**R/O** rule out.
**roentgen** refers to x-rays.
**role delineation study** occupational analysis study conducted by AAMA and the National Board of Medical Examination in 1997 that identifies the most up-to-date entry-level areas of competence of the medical assisting profession.
**ROM** see **range of motion.**
**rotate** to move around; to turn on an axis.
**rubella** (German measles) a mild contagious viral disease that may cause severe damage to an unborn child.
**rubeola** (measles) an acute, highly contagious disease marked by a typical cutaneous eruption.

**SA node** see **sinoatrial node.**
**sacrilege** the crime of misappropriating what is consecrated to God or religion.
**sacrum** five fused vertebrae that lie between the coccyx and the lumbar vertebrae of the spinal column.
**safety** freedom from danger or loss.
**sagittal** refers to a plane that is made by dividing the body down the center, creating a right and left side.
**salary** a fixed amount of wages paid to an employee on a regular basis for a prescribed period of time, i.e., weekly or monthly
**saliva** a digestive secretion of the salivary glands that empties into the stomach.
**salivary glands** three pairs of glands that secrete the saliva that begins the digestion of food, primarily the breakdown of starch or complex carbohydrates.
**salpingectomy** surgical removal of the fallopian tube or tubes.
**salpingo-oophorectomy** surgical excision of the ovary and fallopian tube.
**salve** an ointment.
**sanitization** the process of applying antimicrobial agents to nonliving objects to destroy microorganisms.
**sarcoma** malignant tumors of the connective, muscle, or bone tissue.
**sartorius** a long narrow muscle of the thigh; the longest muscle of the body.
**scan** to look over quickly but thoroughly.
**scapula** the shoulder blade.
**schedule** to arrange a timetable; to place in a list of things to be done.
**sciatica** inflammation and pain along the sciatic nerve felt at the back of the thigh running down the inside of the leg.
**scientific** based upon or using the principles and methods of science; systematic; exact.
**sclera** the white or sclerotic outer coat of the eye.
**scoliosis** lateral curvature of the spine.
**screening** a preliminary or indicating procedure.
**Scribe** A person who documents by hand as a profession and helps providers keep track of records.
**script** manuscript; type designed to look like handwriting.
**scrotum** the double pouch containing the testes and part of the spermatic cord.
**scrub** specific and thorough hand washing procedure performed for 6 minutes before taking part in any sterile surgical procedure.
**scrupulously** with great attention to detail; with great care.
**scurvy** a disease caused by lack of fresh fruits, vegetables, and vitamin C in the diet.
**sebaceous** an oily, fatty matter; glands secreting such matter.
**sebum** oily secretion of the sebaceous glands of the skin.
**secondary** one step removed from the first; not primary.
**Secondary insurance** exists when a patient is covered under more than one insurance plan; charges are first submitted to the primary carrier and any charges not covered are then submitted to the secondary carrier.
**secretary** one employed to conduct correspondence; a person responsible for records and correspondence.
**secretion** separation of certain materials from the blood by the activity of a gland.
**sector** a section or division.
**security** freedom from fear or anxiety.
**sedate** to produce a state of calmness; process of allaying nervous excitement; using an agent to produce a tranquilizing effect.
**sedentary** pertaining to sitting; inactivity.
**sedimentation** formation or depositing of sediment; of blood, refers to the speed at which erythrocytes settle when an anticoagulant is added to blood.
**segment** a part or section of an organ or a body.
**seizures** a sudden attack of pain, disease, or certain symptoms.
**self-control** control of ones emotions, desires.
**semen** the mixture of secretions from the various glands and organs of the reproductive system of the male, which is expelled at orgasm.
**semicircular canals** structures located in the inner ear.

**semilunar** the valves of the heart located between the ventricles and the pulmonary artery and aorta.
**senility** feebleness of body or mind caused by old age.
**sensitivity** abnormal susceptibility to a substance.
**sensorineural** refers to a sensory nerve.
**sensorineural deafness** a loss of hearing caused by transmission failure of the nerves within the inner ear or the auditory nerve.
**sensory** refers to the nerves that receive and transmit stimuli from the sense organs.
**septum** a membranous wall dividing two cavities, as within the heart or the nose.
**sequence** order of succession.
**sequentially** arranged in sequence; in an order.
**series** a group; a set of things in the same class coming one after another.
**serrated** notched, toothed.
**serrations** etchings located on the blades of an instrument to keep it from slipping.
**serum** blood plasma in which clotting factors (such as fibrin) have been removed naturally by allowing the blood to clot prior to isolating the liquid component
**service charge** a fee charged for a service, often in addition to a basic fee.
**Seven Rights** Refers to seven elements that must be considered when administering medication, which are: right patient, right medication, right dose (amount), right route (method), right technique, right time (schedule), and right documentation
**sharps** any object that can cut, prick, stab, or scrape the skin.
**sheath** a covering structure of connective tissue, such as the membrane covering a muscle.
**shelf life** that length of time that sterile items are given before they are considered unsuitable as maintaining sterility.
**shiatsu** a massage with the fingers applied to those specific areas of the body used in acupuncture.
**shock** a condition in which the pulse becomes rapid and weak, the blood pressure drops, and the patient is pale and clammy.
**sickle cell anemia** a blood disorder in which the red blood cells are shaped like sickles.
**side effect** unintended or adverse effects of a medication, ranging from mild to intolerable
**sigmoid** an S-shaped section of the large intestine between the descending colon and the rectum.
**sigmoidoscopy** an inspection of the sigmoid with an instrument.
**signature** a signing of one's own name.
**simple** referring to a bone fracture, one without involvement of the skin surface.
**Sims'** an examination position with the patient lying on the left side.
**simultaneous** occurring at the same time.
**Single-booking** a method of scheduling in which only one patient is assigned to one block of time in a visit schedule.
**single-entry bookkeeping system** an accounting method in which each financial transaction is recorded only once in account books.
**singular** the form of a term that indicates the presence of only one.
**sinoatrial (SA) node** the source of the nerve impulse that initiates the heartbeat; the pacemaker.
**sinusitis** inflammation of the sinuses.
**site review** visit, examination, or inspection to the medical office by an outside agency (such as, insurance companies, OSHA, CLIA, etc).
**skeletal** pertaining to the skeleton or bony structure; also to the muscles attached to the skeleton to permit movement.
**skills** a term used to describe procedures that are taught in an educational program or work setting.
**skip** a person who owes money but cannot be located.
**skull x-ray** a radiologic examination of the skull.
**sleep apnea** brief episodes of the cessation of breathing during sleep.
**sling** a hanging support for an injured arm.
**slough** to cast off, as dead tissue.
**smooth** a type of involuntary muscle tissue found in internal organs.
**snap locks** metal locking devices.
**snellen chart** the chart of alphabetic letters used to evaluate distant vision.
**Social Security number (SSN)** unique nine-digit number assigned by the U.S. government.
**software** computer programs necessary for directing the computer hardware to perform specific functions.
**solace** an easing of grief, to comfort.
**sole** only.
**solicit** to ask for.
**Solo Practice** When an individual provider/physician makes all the decisions for the practice.
**somatic** pertaining to the body as distinguished from the mind; physical.
**sonar** a device that transmits high-frequency sound waves in water and registers the vibrations reflected back from an object.
**sonogram** record obtained by ultrasound.
**sophisticated** not simple or natural; very refined; highly complex or developed in form, technique, etc.
**sound** that which is or can be heard; free from damage, safe, secure.
**spasm** an involuntary sudden movement or convulsive muscular contraction.
**spastic colon** spasmodic contractions of the large intestine.
**specific gravity** the ratio of dissolved substances in a solvent as compared with the ratio of dissolved substances in distilled water, most commonly comparing the ratio of dissolved substances in a urine specimen when compared with distilled water.
**specifications** any point or particular specified; mention in detail.
**specificity** something specially suited for a given use or purpose; a remedy regarded as a certain cure for a particular disease.
**specified** named particularly; mentioned in detail.
**specimen** a sample; a representative piece of the whole.
**speculum** an instrument that permits viewing inside a body cavity.
**sperm** the male gamete or sex cell.
**spermatozoan** a sperm cell.
**sphincter** a circular muscle constricting an opening.
**sphygmomanometer** a device that measures blood pressure; also called manometer.
**spina bifida occulta** a disorder characterized by a defect in the spinal vertebrae with or without protrusion of the spinal cord and meninges.
**spinal** pertaining to the spinal column, canal, or cord.
**spinal fusion** the surgical implanting of a bone fragment between the processes of two or more spinal vertebrae to render them immobile.
**spiral** having a circular fashion.
**spirometer** an apparatus that measures the volume of inhaled and exhaled air.
**spleen** an oval, vascular, ductless gland below the diaphragm in the upper left quadrant of the abdomen.
**splinter** a thin sharp piece of wood.
**spontaneous** involuntary; produced by itself; unforced.
**spores** hard capsules formed by certain bacteria that allow them to resist prolonged exposure to heat.
**sports medicine** the branch of medicine dealing with the care of athletes to prevent and treat sports-related injuries.
**sprain** the forcible twisting of a joint with partial rupture or other injury of its attachments.
**sputum** substance ejected from the mouth containing saliva and mucus; usually refers to material coughed up from the bronchi.
**stability** the ability of a reagent to remain constant after being opened.
**stabilize** to make steady; firmly fixed; constant.
**staging** a method for determining the extent of the disease process with cancer.

**standard** conforming to a custom or law.

**Standard of care** the watchfulness, attention, caution and prudence that a reasonable person in the circumstances would exercise.

**Standard of proof** the burden that the plaintiff or prosecution must meet in presenting their case; the measure by which evidence is judged to show a "preponderance of evidence" in a civil action and "beyond a reasonable doubt" in a criminal case.

**standard precautions** guidelines for the prevention of infectious diseases and nosocomial infections established by the centers for disease control and prevention.

**standardization** process of bringing into conformity with a standard; pertaining to ECG, a mark made at the beginning of each lead to establish a standard of reference.

**stapes** one of the three bones of the middle ear.

**stasis ulcer** an open lesion caused by stagnant or inade quate blood supply to an area.

**STAT (statim)** immediately.

**state law** legislation enacted by the state legislature and signed by the governor.

**stationery** writing materials, especially paper and envelopes.

**stature** height.

**Statute / statutory law** a federal or state written law enacted by the Congress or state legislature respectively.

**statutory** legally enacted; deriving authority from law.

**stem cells** Cells with the ability to divide for indefinite periods in culture and to give rise to specialized cells.

**stenosis** narrowing or constriction of a passage or opening.

**sterile** without any organisms.

**sterile gauze square** a piece of dressing for a wound.

**sterilization** the elimination of all transmissible agents (such as bacteria and viruses) from a surface, a piece of equipment, food, or biologic culture medium, including spores.

**sternocleidomastoid** a muscle of the chest arising from the sternum and inner part of the clavicle.

**sternum** the breastbone.

**stethoscope** an instrument used in auscultation to convey to the ear the sounds produced by the body.

**stimulant** a substance that temporarily increases activity.

**stipulations** terms of an agreement.

**stomach** a dilated, saclike, distensible portion of the alimentary canal below the esophagus and before the small intestine.

**stool** bowel movement, feces.

**strabismus** an eye disorder caused by imbalance of the ocular muscles.

**strain** injury to muscles from tension caused by overuse or misuse.

**stratagem** a trick or deception.

**stress** to put pressure on; emphasize; urgency; tension, strained exertion. Topical; causing strain or injury to the skin.

**striated** a type of muscle tissue marked with stripes or striae.

**stricture** the narrowing of an opening, tube, or canal, such as the urethra or esophagus.

**strikethrough** condition in which fluid is able to penetrate through a drape

**stylus** a pen; the ECG writer.

**subarachnoid** the space between the pia mater and the arachnoid containing cerebrospinal fluid.

**subcutaneous** beneath the skin.

**subdural** beneath the dural mater; the space between the arachnoid and the dura mater.

**subjective** relating to the person who is thinking, saying, or doing something; personal; of a disease symptom, felt by the individual but not perceptible to others.

**Subjective Objective Assessment Plan (SOAP)** one of the most widely used methods of charting, to collect patient visit information; appropriate for most types of patient encounters.

**sublimation** to express certain impulses, especially sexual, in constructive, socially acceptable forms.

**sublingual** under the tongue.

**subpoena duces tecum** court process initiated by a party in litigation, compelling production of specific documents and other items, and material in relevance to facts in issue in appending judicial proceedings.

**subsequent** coming after, following.

**substantial** considerable, large.

**subtle** so slight as to be difficult to detect or describe; elusive

**suction** withdrawal by pressure; a sucking action.

**sudden** happening without warning or in a short space of time

**sudden infant death syndrome (SIDS)** the sudden, unexplainable death of an infant.

**suffix** an addition to the end of a term that changes the grammatical function of the term.

**superficial** on the surface.

**superior vena cava** large but short vein that carries deoxygenated blood from the upper half of the body to the heart's right atrium.

**superior** above or higher than.

**supernatant** floating on the surface.

**supervisor** one who oversees; has control; in charge.

**supine** lying horizontally on the back.

**supplement** something added; an additional or extra section.

**support** to hold up; to bear part of the weight of.

**suppository** a medicated conical- or cylindrical-shaped material that is inserted into the rectum or vagina.

**suppression** the shutdown of kidney function; the absence of urine excretion; in psychology, it is the deliberate exclusion of an idea, desire, or feeling from consciousness.

**suppressor** one that holds back or stops an action.

**suprapubic** above the pubic arch.

**Supremacy Clause** article VI, section 2 of the U.S. Constitution, which allows a Supreme Court ruling to be binding on state courts if involving a constitutional issue. The Clause reads: "This Constitution, and the Laws of the United States which shall be made in pursuance thereof; and all treaties made, or which shall be made, under the authority of the United States, shall be the supreme law of the land; and the judges in every state shall be bound thereby, anything in the Constitution or laws of any state to the contrary notwithstanding."

**surfactant** a fatty molecule on the respiratory membranes.

**surgeon** a physician with advanced training in operative procedures.

**surgery** the branch of medicine dealing with manual and operative procedures for correction of deformities and defects and repair of injuries.

**surgical asepsis** techniques used to destroy all pathogenic organisms before they can enter the body.

**surrogate** a substitute; in place of another.

**surveillance** the process of watching or observing.

**susceptible** having little resistance to a disease or foreign protein.

**suspicion** mistrust, not believing statements.

**suture** to unite parts by stitching them together.

**symmetry** the state in which one part exactly corresponds to another in size, shape, and position.

**sympathetic** a portion of the autonomic nervous system.

**symphysis pubis** the junction of the pubic bones on the midline in front.

**symptom** any perceptible change in the body or its functions that indicates disease or the phase of a disease.

**synapse** the minute space between the axon of one neuron and the dendrite of another.

**syncope** fainting; a transient form of unconsciousness.

**syndrome** the combination of symptoms with a disease or disorder.

**synergism** something stimulating the action of another so that the effect of both is greater than the sum of the individual effects.

**synergistic** describes the action of a medication that augments or enhances the actions of another medication.
**synovial** a movable joint; also called diarthroses.
**synthetic** not real or natural.
**syphilis** a communicable venereal disease spread by sexual contact.
**system** a group of organs working together to perform a function of the body.
**systematically** by a system or plan.
**systemic** pertaining to a whole system.
**systole** the contraction phase of the heart; the greatest amount of blood pressure.

**tachycardia** abnormal rapidity of heart action.
**tact** delicate perception of the right things to say and do without offending.
**Tachypenia** Increased rate of respiration.
**tactful** being able to perceive a situation and know the right thing to say or do. Tact is especially difficult and important when dealing with ill people.
**tactile** relating to the sense of touch.
**tar** a sticky, brown or black carcinogenic substance.
**targeted** marked, the object of desire; aimed for.
**tarry** a stool that has the appearance of tar.
**tarsal** pertaining to the seven bones of the instep of the foot.
**taut** tightly drawn; tense.
**technical** relating to some particular art, science, or trade; also, requiring special skill or technique.
**technologist** one skilled in technology; able to apply the technical methods in a particular field of industry or art.
**technology** the practice of any or all of the applied sciences that have practical value and/or industrial use.
**teleconference** a meeting held over phone lines incorporating video equipment.
**teletherapy** radiation therapy administered by a machine that is positioned at some distance from the patient.
**temperature** degree of heat of a living body; degree of hotness or coldness of a substance; usually refers to an elevation of body heat.
**template** an electronic file (or preprinted document) with a pre-designed, customized, format. Examples include fax cover sheets or patient information letters, ready to be filled in.
**temporal** relating to the temporal bone on the skull.
**tendon** fibrous connective tissue serving to attach muscles to bones.
**tendonitis** inflammation of the tendon.
**tentative** experimental, provisional, temporary.
**terminal** final, end; a terminal illness, refers to a condition that cannot be reversed.
**termination** ending.
**testes** the male gonads of the scrotum that produce sperm.
**testosterone** a male hormone secreted by the testes that causes and maintains male secondary sex characteristics.
**tetanus** an acute infectious disease caused by the toxins of the bacillus tetani.
**tetany** intermittent tonic spasms resulting from inadequate parathyroid hormone.
**thalamus** a portion of the brain lying between the cerebrum and the midbrain.
**theories** beliefs not yet tested in practice; the general principles on which a science is based.
**therapeutic** having medicinal or healing properties; pertaining to results obtained from treatment.
**therapist** one who practices the curative and preventive treatment of disease or an abnormal condition.
**thermal** characterized by heat; heat activated.
**thermally** pertaining to heat activation.
**thermography** a technique for sensing and recording on film hot and cold areas of the body by means of an infrared detector that reacts to blood flow.
**thermometer** an instrument used to measure temperature.
**thesaurus** a treasury of words, quotations, knowledge; a collection of words with their synonyms and antonyms.
**thinprep** a method for preparing cytology specimens.
**third-party** someone other than the two principals in a transaction; when referring to checks, a type of check made out to the patient by another unknown person
**third-party** a check made out to someone from an unknown party.
**third-party reimbursement** payment made by a party other than the one providing or receiving the service, such as a physician or patient. Examples of whom you would receive third-party reimbursement from are an insurance company or an attorney.
**thoracic** pertaining to the thorax or chest.
**thorax** the chest; the body cavity enclosed by the ribs and containing the heart and lungs.
**thready** term used to describe a weak pulse that may feel like a thread under the skin surface.
**threshold** a minimum amount of supplies to be maintained; also known as par level
**thrive** vigorous growth.
**thrombophlebitis** inflammation of a vein associated with the formation of a blood clot.
**thrombosis** the formation of a blood clot or thrombus.
**thymus** an unpaired organ located in the mediastinal cavity anterior to and above the heart.
**thyroid** an endocrine gland located anteriorly at the base of the neck.
**thyroidectomy** the surgical removal of the thyroid gland.
**tibia** a long bone in the leg from the knee to the ankle.
**tibialis anterior** a muscle of the leg.
**Time Management** an assortment of skills, tools, and practices used to manage time during daily activities and when accomplishing specific projects.
**tinnitus** a ringing or tinkling sound in the ear that is heard only by the person affected.
**tissue** a collection of similar cells and fibers forming a structure in the body.
**tolerance** the difference between the maximum and minimum; the amount of variation allowed from a standard.
**tongue** the muscular organ of the mouth that assists in the production of speech, contains the taste buds, and provides the ability to swallow.
**tongue depressor** a flat wooden stick used to depress the tongue.
**tonometer** instrument for measuring intraocular tension or pressure.
**tonometry** measuring tension or pressure and especially intraocular pressure.
**topical** pertaining to a specific area; local.
**tort** any wrongful act, damage, or injury done willfully, negligently.
**torticollis** stiff neck caused by spasmotic contraction of neck muscles drawing the head to one side with the chin pointing to the other; can be congenital or acquired.
**total quality management (TQM)** refers to a management style that uses QA and QC to maintain quality of performance throughout the total process, not just to ensure the end result is satisfactory or corrected.
**tourniquet** any constrictor used on an extremity to produce pressure on an artery and control bleeding; also used to distend veins for the withdrawal of blood or the insertion of a needle to instill intravenous injections.
**toxin** poisonous substance or compound of vegetable, animal, or bacterial origin.
**toxoid** a toxin treated so as to destroy its toxicity, but it is still capable of inducing formation of antibodies on injection.
**TQM** see **total quality management.**
**trace** the production of a sketch by means of a stylus passing over the paper, as in electrocardiography.
**trachea** a cartilaginous tube between the larynx and the main bronchus of the respiratory tree.
**tracheotomy** a surgically made opening in the trachea through which a person will breathe.

**traction** the process of pulling; with fractures, traction is applied in a straight line to stretch the contracted muscles and permit realignment of the bone fragments.
**trade name** The name a manufacturer assigns to a given medication compound for marketing purposes or to simplify referencing the medication.
**trait** a feature; a distinguishing feature of character or mind.
**transaction** dealing accomplished.
**transcript** a copy made directly from an original record, especially an official copy of a student's educational record.
**transcription** writing over from one book or medium into another; typing in full in ordinary letters.
**transdermal** through the skin.
**transducer** a device that transforms power from one system to another in the same or different form.
**transfusion** injection of the blood of one person into the blood vessels of another.
**transient ischemic attack (TIA)** temporary interruption of blood flow in the brain caused by small clots closing off blood vessels.
**transillumination** inspection of a cavity or organ by passing a light through its walls.
**transition** passing from one condition, place, or activity to another.
**transmission** the process of sending from one place to another.
**transmitted** sent from one person, thing, or place to another.
**transpose** putting one in place of another, the accidental misplacing of words or letters.
**transurethral** literally means through the urethra; refers to the removal of the prostate by going through the urethral wall.
**transverse** lying across; the segment of large intestine that lies across the abdomen; a line drawn horizontally across the body or a structure.
**trapezius** the large muscle of the back and neck.
**trauma** any injury, physical or mental.
**traumatic** caused by or relating to an injury.
**traumatize** to cause trauma or injury.
**treadmill** an apparatus with a movable platform that permits walking or running in place.
**tremulousness** the process of involuntary shaking or trembling.
**Trendelenburg** a position with the head lower than the feet.
**trephining** cutting out a circular section.
**triage** a system of sorting and identifying the severity of injuries.
**trial balance** bookkeeping strategy to confirm accuracy in debits and credits in ledger.
**triangular** having three angles and three sides.
**triangular bandages** bandages having three angles and three sides.
**triceps** the posterior muscles of the arm that work as a team with the biceps; the triceps straighten the elbow.
**trichomoniasis** infestation with parasitic protozoa; usually refers to vaginal involvement.
**tricuspid** a valve in the right side of the heart, between the chambers; literally means three cusps or leaflets.
**triglycerides** a combination of glycerol and fatty acids in the blood.
**trimester** divided into three sections; the third segment or period.
**tritanopia** the inability to distinguish the color blue.
**trivial** of little value, insignificant.
**truncated** to cut the top or end off; to lop; with insurance.
**Truth in Lending Act (TILA)** federal law designed to protect consumers in credit transactions; it specifies that when there is an agreement between the physician and a patient to accept payment in more than four installments, the physician is required to provide disclosure of finance charges
**tuberculosis** an infectious disease caused by the tubercle bacillus; pulmonary tuberculosis is a specific inflammatory disease of the lungs that destroys lung tissue.
**tumor** a swelling or enlargement; a neoplasm; often used to indicate a malignant growth.
**tuning fork** an instrument used to determine the sensation of hearing.
**turbidity** flaky or granular particles suspended in a clear liquid giving it a cloudy appearance; usually refers to cloudy urine.
**turgor** normal tension; with the skin means the resistance to being deformed and the length of time to return to normal.
**tympanic membrane** the eardrum.
**typhoid** an acute infectious disease acquired by ingesting contaminated food or water.
**tzanck smear** examination of tissue from the lower surface of a lesion in vesicular disease to determine the cell type.

**ulcer** an open lesion on the skin or mucous membrane of the body characterized by loss of tissue and the formation of a secretion.
**ulceration** suppuration of the skin or mucous membrane; an open lesion.
**ulna** a long bone in the forearm from the elbow to the wrist.
**ultimately** in the end, finally.
**ultrasonic scanning** a process of scanning the body with sound waves to produce a picture on a screen of underlying internal structures.
**ultrasound technologist** also known as diagnostic medical sonographers, these individuals are specially trained to use ultrasound equipment to direct high-frequency sound waves into specific areas of a patient's body to produce images of the shape, position, or movement of organs, fluid accumulations, masses, or fetuses.
**umbilical** pertaining to the umbilicus or navel of the abdomen.
**unbundled** reporting multiple codes for a service when there is one code that will report the entire service.
**unemployment** the state of being without work; also, a limited federal program to provide some income for those who are without work.
**unique** one of a kind, unmatched.
**unit clerk** a secretarial position on the health care team of a patient care facility.
**universal** relating to the universe; general or common to all.
**universal emergency medical identification** worn by patients who have conditions that could have emergency episodes, such as heart conditions, diabetes, epilepsy, allergies, or a laryngectomy, to alert health workers of the patients' conditions when they cannot do so on their own.
**universal precautions** steps taken by health care workers to prevent exposure to communicable diseases.
**unobtrusive** not forced upon others; not thrusted forward or pushed out.
**unproductive** not productive; no accomplishment.
**unstructured** without specific arrangement.
**unwittingly** not knowing, unaware; unintentional.
**upcoding** reporting a higher level code than is appropriate for the service that was rendered resulting in higher reimbursement.
**upper respiratory infection (URI)** inflammatory process involving the nose and throat, may include the sinuses; refers to symptoms associated with the common cold.
**uremia** a condition in which products normally found in the urine are found in the blood.
**ureter** a tube carrying urine from the kidney to the urinary bladder.
**urethra** a membranous canal for the external discharge of urine from the bladder.
**urgency** the sudden need to expel urine or stool.
**urgent** requiring immediate attention.
**urgent care center** ambulatory care centers that take care of patients with acute illness or injury and those with minor emergencies. Used quite often when patients can get into to see their own provider.
**URI** see **upper respiratory infection.**

**urinalysis** an analysis of the urine; a test performed on urine to determine its characteristics.
**urinary** pertaining to secreting and containing urine: the kidneys, ureters, bladder and urethra.
**urinary meatus** the opening through which urine passes from the body.
**urinary tract infection (UTI)** infection occurring within the kidneys, ureters, and/ or urinary bladder.
**urination** the act of urinating or voiding of urine.
**urine** fluid secreted from the blood by the kidneys, stored in the bladder, and discharged from the body by voiding.
**urobilinogen** the colorless product of bilirubin reduction formed in the intestines by bacterial action.
**urologist** a doctor who has been specially trained in studies of the urinary system.
**urology** the study of the urine and diseases of the urinogenital organs.
**urticaria** an inflammatory condition characterized by the eruption of wheals that are associated with severe itching; commonly called hives.
**uterus** a muscular, hollow, pear-shaped organ of the female reproductive tract in which a fertilized ovum develops into a baby.
**UTI** see **urinary tract infection.**
**utilization** to put to profitable use.
**utilize** to use or make use of.

**vaccination** inoculation with modified harmless viruses or other microorganisms to produce immunity, a preventive against diseases.
**Vaccination Information Statement (VIS)** information sheets produced by the Centers for Disease Control and Prevention that explain to vaccine recipients by the benefits and risks of a particular vaccine.
**vaccine** any substance for prevention of a disease.
**vagina** a musculomembranous tube that forms the passageway from the uterus to the exterior.
**vaginal** pertaining to the tissues of the vagina.
**vaginitis** inflammation of the vagina.
**vagus** the 10th cranial nerve that has both motor and sensory function, affecting the heart, stomach, and other organs.
**values** beliefs which are important to a person or organization, which influence attitudes or behavior
**valve** any one of various structures for temporarily closing an opening or passageway or for allowing movement of fluid in one direction only.
**varicella** The virus responsible for causing chicken pox
**varices** enlarged, twisted veins.
**varicose** pertaining to varices; distended, swollen veins, most commonly found in the legs.
**vas deferens** the excretory duct of the testes.
**vasectomy** the cutting out of a portion of the vas deferens.
**vector** an organism (such as an insect) that transmits a pathogen.
**vein** a blood vessel carrying blood toward the heart after receiving it from a venule.
**vena cava** one of two large veins that empty into the right atrium of the heart.
**venereal** pertaining to or transmitted by sexual contact.
**venipuncture** the puncture of a vein; the insertion of a needle into a vein for the purpose of obtaining a blood sample or instilling a substance.
**venom** any of a variety of toxins used by several groups of animal species.
**venous** pertaining to a vein.
**ventilation** admission and circulation of fresh air; with the lungs, refers to a diagnostic test to determine air exchange and presence of an embolism.
**ventilatory** that which ventilates, lets in fresh air.
**ventral** pertaining to the anterior or front side of the body.
**ventricle** one of the two lower chambers of the heart; also used in reference to cavities within the brain.
**venule** a minute vein; a blood vessel that connects a capillary with a vein.
**verb** the part of speech that expresses an action.
**verify** to prove to be true; to support by facts.
**veritable** actual, genuine.
**vermiform appendix** the appendix; a small tube attached to the cecum.
**verrucae** warts; small, circumscribed elevations of the skin formed by hypertrophy of the papillae.
**vertebrae** the bones in the spinal column.
**vertex** the top of the head, the crown.
**vesicle** a small sac or bladder containing fluid; a small, blisterlike elevation on the skin containing serous fluid.
**vested** settled; complete; absolute; continuous.
**Viability** capable of normal growth and development
**viable** capable of living.
**vial** a small glass tube or bottle containing medication or a chemical.
**Vicariously liable** attachment of responsibility to a person for harm or damages caused by another person in either a negligence lawsuit or criminal prosecution.
**video display terminal** the computer monitor.
**vigilance** the act of watching for something to happen or watching for danger.
**vigilant** alertly watchful, especially to avoid danger or harm.
**villi** tiny projections from a surface; the villi of the small intestine that absorb nutrients during the process of digestion.
**villous adenoma** a type of polyp that is invasive and malignant.
**viral shedding** that time when a virus is the most active and most contagious.
**Virulence** Disease-evoking power of a pathogen.
**virulent** full of poison; deadly; malignant.
**virus** a very simple, frequently pathogenic, microorganism capable of replicating within living cells.
**viscera** internal organs.
**visceral** pertaining to viscera, the internal organs, especially the abdomen.
**visualization** the formation of mental visual images.
**vital capacity** the total volume of air exchanged from forced inspiration and forced expiration.
**vital** essential; pertaining to the preservation of life (the vital signs).
**vital signs** Signs of life; specifically, the pulse rate, respiratory rate, body temperature, and often blood pressure of a person.
**vitreous humor** the substance that fills the vitreous body of the eye behind the lens.
**void** to pass urine from the urinary bladder; to make ineffective or invalid.
**volatile** easily changed into a gas or tending to change into a vapor; usually considered potentially dangerous.
**voltage** a measure of electromotive force.
**volume** the amount of space occupied by an object as measured in cubic units.
**voluntary** under one's control; done by one's own choice.
**vomit** to expel the contents of the stomach through the mouth.
**voucher** a document that serves as proof that terms of a transaction have been met.
**vulnerable** liable to injury or hurt; capable of being wounded.
**vulva** the female external genitalia, including the clitoris, the labia minora, and the labia majora.

**waived** laboratory testing that is simple in nature and nonthreatening to the patient if performed or interpreted incorrectly.
**waiver** to give up; forgo; waiving of a right or claim.
**walker** a type of mobility device, useful for patients who cannot safely use crutches or a cane.
**warrant** to justify, to give definite assurance as to the value of; to authorize.
**warranted** justification for some act, belief.
**wart** see **verrucae.**
**watermark** a mark imprinted on paper that is visible when it is held to the light, usually a sign of quality.

**WBC differential** a white blood cell count in which each type of white blood cell is classified and counted.
**weight** the amount of heaviness.
**wheals** more or less round and evanescent elevations of the skin, white in center with a pale red edge, accompanied by itching.
**wheelchair** a chair fitted with wheels by which a person can propel oneself.
**whorl** a type of fingerprint in which the central papillary ridges turn through at least one complete circle.
**wick** a small piece of cotton to absorb or provide moisture or medication.
**withdrawal** a removal of something that has been deposited.
**womb** nonmedical name for the uterus.
**word processor** a system or machine that produces typewritten documents.
**word root** a component of a medical term that does not have a combining form vowel attached.
**work-in** to make time or space for.
**wound** an injury to living tissue, especially an injury involving a cut or break in the skin
**write-offs** a reduction in the value of an asset or earnings by the amount of an expense or loss, usually deemed uncollectible by any business.
**writer** the person who writes; the author.
**wrongful death** the death of a human being as the result of a wrongful act of another person. Examples include negligence (such as a misdiagnosis), assault and/or battery, vehicular manslaughter, manslaughter or murder.
**xiphoid** a process that forms the tip of the sternum.
**x-linked** connected to the cell's sex chromosome; a characteristic of the sex chromosome.
**x-ray technician** a person with specialized training in the techniques to prepare x-ray films to visualize the tissues and organs of the body.

**year to date (YTD)** begins with the 1st date of the calendar year to present.
**yoga** a system of exercises for attaining bodily or mental control and well-being.

**Z-track (IM)** a method of injecting medication intramuscularly.
**zygote** a cell produced by the union of an ovum and a sperm.